Medical Oncology and Surgery

Medical Oncology and Surgery

Edited by Jared Barnes

hayle
medical

New York

Hayle Medical,
750 Third Avenue, 9th Floor,
New York, NY 10017, USA

Visit us on the World Wide Web at:
www.haylemedical.com

ISBN: 978-1-63241-696-4

Cataloging-in-Publication Data

Medical oncology and surgery / edited by Jared Barnes.
    p. cm.
Includes bibliographical references and index.
ISBN 978-1-63241-696-4
1. Oncology. 2. Cancer. 3. Cancer--Surgery. I. Barnes, Jared.
RC254 .M43 2019
616.994--dc23

Table of Contents

Preface

In my initial years as a student, I used to run to the library at every possible instance to grab a book and learn something new. Books were my primary source of knowledge and I would not have come such a long way without all that I learnt from them. Thus, when I was approached to edit this book; I became understandably nostalgic. It was an absolute honor to be considered worthy of guiding the current generation as well as those to come. I put all my knowledge and hard work into making this book most beneficial for its readers.

The field of medicine dealing with the prevention, diagnosis and treatment of cancer is known as oncology. The subfield of oncology which deals with the treatment of cancer by chemotherapy, immunotherapy, targeted therapy and hormonal therapy is called medical oncology. The branch of oncology concerned with the surgical treatment of cancerous tumors is known as surgical oncology. Some of the common types of cancer include blood cancer, bone cancer, skin cancer, stomach cancer, brain cancer, breast cancer, lung cancer and oesophageal cancer. Treatment methods of such cancers include chemotherapy, surgery and radiation therapy. Most of the topics introduced in this book cover new techniques and applications of medical oncology and surgery. The various studies that are constantly contributing towards advancing technologies and evolution of these fields are examined in detail. Students, researchers, experts and all associated with medical oncology and oncological surgery will benefit alike from this book.

I wish to thank my publisher for supporting me at every step. I would also like to thank all the authors who have contributed their researches in this book. I hope this book will be a valuable contribution to the progress of the field.

Editor

Surgery Should Complement Endocrine Therapy for Elderly Postmenopausal Women with Hormone Receptor-Positive Early-Stage Breast Cancer

Olivier Nguyen,[1] **Lucas Sideris,**[1] **Pierre Drolet,**[2] **Marie-Claude Gagnon,**[1] **Guy Leblanc,**[1] **Yves E. Leclerc,**[1] **Andrew Mitchell,**[3] **and Pierre Dubé**[1]

[1] Department of Surgery, Maisonneuve-Rosemont Hospital, Université de Montréal, 5415 boulevard de l'Assomption, Montréal, QC, Canada H1T 2M4
[2] Department of Anesthesiology, Maisonneuve-Rosemont Hospital, Université de Montréal, 5415 boulevard de l'Assomption, Montréal, QC, Canada H1T 2M4
[3] Department of Pathology, Maisonneuve-Rosemont Hospital, Université de Montréal, 5415 boulevard de l'Assomption, Montréal, QC, Canada H1T 2M4

Correspondence should be addressed to Pierre Dubé, pierredube@videotron.qc.ca

Academic Editor: C. H. Yip

Introduction. Endocrine therapy (ET) is an integral part of breast cancer (BC) treatment with surgical resection remaining the cornerstone of curative treatment. The objective of this study is to compare the survival of elderly postmenopausal women with hormone receptor-positive early-stage BC treated with ET alone, without radiation or chemotherapy, versus ET plus surgery. *Materials and Methods.* This is a retrospective study based on a prospective database. The medical records of postmenopausal BC patients referred to the surgical oncology service of two hospitals during an 8-year period were reviewed. All patients were to receive ET for a minimum of four months before undergoing any surgery. *Results.* Fifty-one patients were included and divided in two groups, ET alone and ET plus surgery. At last follow-up in exclusive ET patients ($n = 28$), 39% had stable disease or complete response, 22% had progressive disease, of which 18% died of breast cancer, and 39% died of other causes. In surgical patients ($n = 23$), 78% were disease-free, 9% died of recurrent breast cancer, and 13% died of other causes. *Conclusions.* These results suggest that surgical resection is beneficial in this group and should be considered, even for patients previously deemed ineligible for surgery.

1. Introduction

Breast cancer (BC) is the most common cancer in North American women. Elderly postmenopausal women are defined as postmenopausal women over the age of 65, or postmenopausal women with comorbidities that render them ineligible for chemotherapy. Elderly postmenopausal women with early-stage BC represent a particular subset of patients because the majority of their tumors are hormone receptor positive (HR+). Blockage of hormone receptor activation with endocrine therapy (ET) reduces cancer cell division and improves disease control. For this reason, ET is an integral part of standard treatment for postmenopausal women with HR+ BC at any stage. ET is used after mastectomy to prevent recurrence, and is also the only therapeutic option in selected stage IV patients. When locally advanced, ET can be used to reduce unresectable disease to a resectable form. As well, it is now often used prior to surgery in early-stage BC to reduce the extent of surgical resection and thus potentially avoid general anesthesia. For many years, tamoxifen was the only ET agent available but studies in the metastatic setting (ATAC, BIG1-98) confirmed the superiority of aromatase inhibitors over tamoxifen in improving disease-free survival [1, 2]. Furthermore, several studies (PO24, IMPACT, and PROACT) found that aromatase inhibitors (anastrozole, letrozole) given preoperatively were as effective as, if not superior to, tamoxifen in improving surgical outcome in this subset of patients [3–5].

The therapeutic challenge for the surgeon is to determine the likelihood of achieving complete response, disease stability, or palliation with available therapies, and to decide whether surgery is indicated. A decision is made according to the clinical and pathological characteristics of the disease, the patient's preferences, the presence of any comorbid conditions, and estimated survival. For example, postmenopausal patients with comorbid conditions may be considered unsafe for surgery, while others may refuse surgery because of concerns regarding perioperative morbidity and mortality, or the need for hospitalization. In such cases, ET represents the only treatment option.

To our knowledge, no study has yet evaluated ET alone in elderly postmenopausal women with HR+ early BC. ET alone is not widely used in postmenopausal early-stage BC women since it is recognized that a complete clinical response is unlikely. For this reason, most clinicians believe that the cornerstone of curative treatment remains surgical resection followed by adjuvant treatment. However, as discussed above, not all elderly postmenopausal women with HR+ BC will receive surgery. Therefore we devised a study to compare the outcome for elderly postmenopausal women with HR+ early-stage BC treated with ET alone, without radiation therapy or chemotherapy, with that of those treated with ET and breast surgery to determine if surgery could be avoided without affecting survival.

2. Materials and Methods

Medical records collected in a prospective database of elderly postmenopausal BC patients referred to the surgical oncology clinics of one teaching hospital and one community hospital during an 8-year period (January 1, 2000, to December 31, 2007) were reviewed. The diagnosis of BC was confirmed by breast biopsy and the date of diagnosis was taken as the date of biopsy. Elderly postmenopausal women with palpable HR+ (estrogen and/or progesterone receptor expression >10%) tumors, without evidence of metastasis at diagnosis, and who were scheduled to receive at least four months of ET upfront, were included in the study. The reasons to elect for upfront ET were locally advanced disease, the presence of any comorbid condition, and/or the patient's preference. The ET agents used were anastrozole, letrozole, and tamoxifen. Decisions regarding subsequent surgery were taken either at day 0 or after four months of ET using the same criteria. Patients were evaluated every month during the initial four months and every two to three months afterwards. In the case of tumor progression during the initial four months, patients underwent surgery or a change of ET agent. In the case of a partial response, a decision was made based on comorbid conditions and/or patient's preference. When possible, surgery was performed when the maximum best response was attained.

In accordance with the above criteria, two arms were formed. The study arm was composed of elderly postmenopausal early-stage BC women treated with ET alone, without radiation therapy or chemotherapy. The control arm was composed of elderly postmenopausal early-stage BC women treated with ET and surgery, without chemotherapy. All patients underwent breast conserving surgery. Survival was calculated from the date of diagnosis until death. Two patients in the study arm were lost to followup (at 2.6 and 7.1 months) and were included in the intent-to-treat analysis. Response to treatment was evaluated according to RECIST criteria by measuring the tumor with a caliper. Complete response was defined as disappearance of the tumor on physical examination. Partial response was defined as at least a 30% decrease in the diameter of the lesion, progression as at least a 20% increase in the diameter of the lesion, and stable disease as any tumor size in between. Development of metastasis was considered as progressive disease. Initial response was defined as the response observed at four months, or before if surgery was performed because of progressive nonmetastatic disease.

Demographic and oncologic characteristics were compared between patients who had surgery and those who underwent ET alone. Student's t test was used for continuous data while Fisher's exact test was used for all categorical data except the initial tumor's response, which was compared between the two groups with the chi-square test for trend. Log rank test was used to compare survival curves (Kaplan–Meier) between patients who underwent surgery and those who did not. We considered the differences to be significant at $P \leq 0.05$. Statistical analyses were performed using Prism 4.0 (GraphPad software, La Jolla, CA, USA).

3. Results

Fifty-one patients were included in the study. The study group (ET alone) was composed of 28 women (55%; median age, 86 years; range, 65 to 96 years), and the control group (ET plus surgery) of 23 women (45%; median age, 85 years; range, 65 to 92 years). There was no significant age difference between the two groups ($P = 0.3145$). Patient characteristics are summarized in Table 1. Human epidermal growth factor receptor-2 (HER2) was negative or unknown for the majority of patients since it was not routinely assessed for patients older than 70 years old prior to 2007.

ET in the study arm and control groups consisted of tamoxifen (32% and 17%, resp.), and aromatase inhibitors (68% and 83%, resp.). Results of initial response (0 to 4 months) to ET are summarized in Table 2. There was no statistically significant difference in initial response to ET between both groups ($P = 0.8781$). The median interval between diagnosis and best response was 7.4 months (range, 1.6 to 55.3 months) in the study group, and 3.2 months (range, 1.2 to 7.3 months) in the control group.

The median interval between diagnosis and surgery in the control group was 6.2 months (range, 2.4 to 11.2 months).

The median duration of followup was 28.4 months (range, 1.1 to 87.8 months) in the study group, and 63.8 months (range, 37.5 to 109.2 months) in the control group.

Ten patients (36%) refused surgery at the beginning for personal reasons and remained in the study group, half of which (50%) where still alive at the last follow-up visit. Of

TABLE 1: Population characteristics.

	Study group "n" (range) (%)	Control group "n" (range) (%)	P value
Number of patients	28	23	
Mean age (year)	84 [65–96]	82 [65–92]	0.3145
Mean initial tumor diameter (cm)	4 [1–10]	4.6 [0–20]	0.2068
ER status > 10%	28 (100)	23 (100)	
PR status > 10%	23 (82)	16 (70)	
Tumor grade I	4 (14)	8 (35)	
Tumor grade II	19 (68)	9 (39)	
Tumor grade III	5 (18)	6 (26)	
Stage I	6 (21)	5 (22)	
Stage II	19 (68)	13 (56)	
Stage III	3 (11)	5 (22)	

TABLE 2: Choice of endocrine therapy and initial response to endocrine therapy.

	Study group "n" (%)	Control group "n" (%)	P value
Anastrozole	2 (7)	6 (26)	
Letrozole	17 (61)	13 (57)	
Tamoxifen	9 (32)	4 (17)	
Complete response	5 (18)	0 (0)	NS
Partial response	10 (36)	17 (74)	NS
Stable disease	11 (39)	3 (13)	NS
Progressive disease	2 (7)	3 (13)	NS

*NS: nonspecific.

these patients, four (14%) had stable disease, two (7%) had progressive disease, of which one (4%) died from recurrent breast cancer 28 months after diagnosis, and four (14%) died from causes unrelated to their cancer. These causes were uterine bleeding ($n = 1$, 4%), cardiac failure ($n = 1$, 4%), and undetermined or not specified ($n = 2$, 7%).

Two patients (7%) were initially deemed unfit for surgery because of Parkinson's disease ($n = 1$, 4%) and advanced cognitive disorders ($n = 1$, 4%).

Amongst patients who underwent surgery, none attained a complete pathological response.

At last follow-up visit, in the study group (ET alone), 11 patients (39%) had a stable disease or complete clinical response. Six (22%) had a progressive disease, of which five (18%) died of breast cancer (median survival, 15.8 months). Breast cancer causes of death were distant metastatic disease ($n = 4$, 14%) and contralateral breast cancer ($n = 1$, 4%). Finally, 11 (39%) died from a cause unrelated to their cancer (median survival, 29.5 months). These causes were pneumonia ($n = 4$, 14%), mesenteric ischemia ($n = 1$, 4%), cardiac failure ($n = 1$, 4%), Parkinson's disease ($n = 1$, 4%), infectious colitis ($n = 1$, 4%), and undetermined or not specified ($n = 3$, 11%).

At the last follow-up visit, in the control group (ET plus surgery), 18 patients (78%) were disease-free, two (9%) died of recurrent breast cancer (median survival, 68.9 months). Breast cancer causes of death were distant metastatic disease ($n = 1$, 4%), and recurrent breast cancer ($n = 1$, 4%). Finally,

three patients (13%) died from a cause unrelated to their cancer (median survival, 51.2 months). These causes were a fall ($n = 1$, 4%), and undetermined or not specified ($n = 2$, 9%).

At five years, the overall survival for the study group was 18%, and for the control group, 52%. The median survival for the study group was 28 months, and for the control group, 64 months. There was a statistically significant difference in survival between both groups ($P = 0.0003$). Survival curves are shown in Figure 1.

4. Discussion

This study was devised to compare the outcome for elderly postmenopausal women with HR+ early-stage BC treated with ET alone, without radiation therapy or chemotherapy, with that of those treated with ET and breast surgery, without chemotherapy. The objective was to determine if patients treated with ET alone could avoid surgery without affecting their survival.

Overall, patients in the control group (ET plus surgery) had significant longer survival than patients in the study group (ET alone). A larger proportion of patients in the study group died of comorbid conditions rather than of breast cancer. However, in comparison with the control group, there was still a greater proportion of patients in the study group who died of breast cancer (18% versus 9%). For this reason, we think that surgery is clearly indicated in most

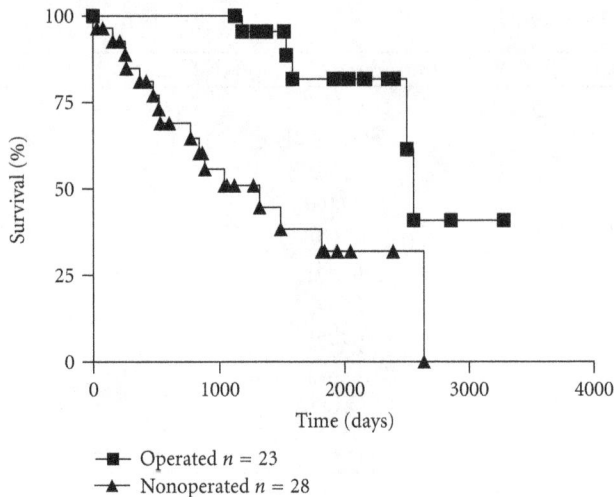

FIGURE 1: Survival in the study group (endocrine therapy (ET) alone) and in the control group (ET plus surgery), log-rank test: $P = 0.003$.

cases, even when comorbid conditions are present. Still, the use of ET prior to surgery until the best maximal response has been reached merits consideration.

The IMPACT trial looked at the effects of neoadjuvant anastrozole, tamoxifen, or a combination of both in postmenopausal HR+ patients with a palpable BC. It concluded that anastrozole is as effective and well tolerated as tamoxifen in these patients [3]. It found no significant differences in the response in patients requiring mastectomy at baseline, but a significant benefit in patients requiring breast-conserving surgery at baseline. The PROACT trial found that neoadjuvant anastrozole is at least as effective as tamoxifen in postmenopausal HR+ BC patients who required breast-conserving surgery at baseline, and more effective in patients who required mastectomy or were deemed inoperable at baseline [4]. Additionally, the PO24 trial showed that neoadjuvant letrozole was more effective than tamoxifen in regards to both tumor response and breast-conserving surgery rates in postmenopausal women who required mastectomy or were deemed inoperable at baseline [5]. In our study, the choice of ET has not been directly studied but letrozole was used most of the time when it became available, initially because of its greater efficacy to reduce estrogen blood levels [6], and then more so after the results of the PO24 study had been revealed [5]. When aromatase inhibitors were contraindicated tamoxifen was used. Anastrozole was used when letrozole was not tolerated; if anastrozole was not tolerated, patients were switched to tamoxifen.

We think that the difference in mortality observed between the study and control groups is due to a selection bias, because patients in the study group had more often severe comorbid conditions and did not receive surgery. On the other hand, patients who had surgery were in better general physical condition. The choice of ET did not appear to play a role.

Randomization of patients could not be performed due to several reasons. First, it is a retrospective study. Second, the decision to operate or not was taken at day 0 or after four months, and was dependent on several factors, including comorbid conditions and patient's preference. For our statistics, use of the multivariable Cox proportional hazards model was considered, but our statistician found it was not feasible.

In this study, the complete response rate was higher in the study group. This can be explained by a longer duration of endocrine treatment, while patients in the control group underwent surgery at some point dictated by a progression of breast cancer or by partial response to the endocrine therapy. A downside to prolonged endocrine treatment is that a proportion of patients may stop responding and eventually progress. On the other hand, continuing treatment beyond the planned four months could have incremental benefits in reducing tumor size and allowing surgery for previously inoperable tumors. This could explain why surgery was performed as late as 337 days after diagnosis.

5. Conclusions

Despite some limitations (sample size, selection bias, no randomization), this study supports the use of upfront ET in most clinical situations in elderly postmenopausal women with HR+ early-stage BC. Appropriate surgery should be performed when the best maximal response has been reached because it reduces BC mortality, even in high-risk patients. At this point, prospective studies should be undertaken.

List of Abbreviations

BC: early breast cancer;
ET: endocrine therapy;
HER2:   human epidermal growth factor receptor-2;
HR+:   hormone receptorpositive.

Acknowledgment

The authors thank Anick Leduc for her contributions in collecting data.

References

[1] B. C. Group, "A comparison of letrozole and tamoxifen in postmenopausal women with early breast cancer," *The New England Journal of Medicine*, vol. 353, pp. 2747–2757, 2005.

[2] J. F. Forbes, J. Cuzick, A. Buzdar, A. Howell, J. S. Tobias, and M. Baum, "Effect of anastrozole and tamoxifen as adjuvant treatment for early-stage breast cancer: 100-month analysis of the ATAC trial," *The Lancet Oncology*, vol. 9, no. 1, pp. 45–53, 2008.

[3] I. E. Smith, M. Dowsett, S. R. Ebbs et al., "Neoadjuvant treatment of postmenopausal breast cancer with anastrozole, tamoxifen, or both in combination: the immediate preoperative anastrozole, tamoxifen, or combined with tamoxifen (IMPACT) multicenter double-blind randomized trial," *Journal of Clinical Oncology*, vol. 23, no. 22, pp. 5108–5116, 2005.

[4] L. Cataliotti, A. U. Buzdar, S. Noguchi et al., "Comparison of anastrozole versus tamoxifen as preoperative therapy in postmenopausal women with hormone receptor-positive breast

cancer: the pre-operative "arimidex" compared to tamoxifen (PROACT) trial," *Cancer*, vol. 106, no. 10, pp. 2095–2103, 2006.

[5] W. Eiermann, S. Paepke, J. Appfelstaedt et al., "Preoperative treatment of postmenopausal breast cancer patients with letrozole: a randomized double-blind multicenter study," *Annals of Oncology*, vol. 12, no. 11, pp. 1527–1532, 2001.

[6] A. S. Bhatnagar, A. M. H. Brodie, B. J. Long, D. B. Evans, and W. R. Miller, "Intracellular aromatase and its relevance to the pharmacological efficacy of aromatase inhibitors," *Journal of Steroid Biochemistry and Molecular Biology*, vol. 76, no. 1–5, pp. 199–202, 2001.

2

The Postoperative Component of MAGIC Chemotherapy Is Associated with Improved Prognosis following Surgical Resection in Gastric and Gastrooesophageal Junction Adenocarcinomas

A. Mirza, S. Pritchard, and I. Welch

Departments of Gastrointestinal Surgery and Histopathology, The University Hospital of South Manchester, Southmoor Road, Wythenshawe, Manchester M23 9LT, UK

Correspondence should be addressed to I. Welch; ian.welch@uhsm.nhs.uk

Academic Editor: Michael Hünerbein

Aims. MAGIC chemotherapy has become the standard of treatment for patients undergoing curative resection for gastric and gastrooesophageal junction (GOJ) cancers. The importance of postoperative component of this regimen is uncertain. The aim of this study was to compare survival and cancer recurrence in patients who have received neoadjuvant and adjuvant chemotherapies according to MAGIC protocol with those patients completing only neoadjuvant chemotherapy. *Methods.* 66 patients with gastric and GOJ adenocarcinomas treated with neoadjuvant and adjuvant chemotherapies according to the MAGIC protocol were studied. All patients underwent potentially curative surgical resection. The histological, demographic, and survival data were collected for all patients. *Results.* The median number of neoadjuvant chemotherapy cycles received was 2 (range 1–3). Thirty-one (47%) patients underwent adjuvant chemotherapy with a median of 2 cycles (range 1–3). Patients who have completed both cycles of chemotherapy had significantly improved survival ($P = 0.04$). Patients with involved lymph nodes and positive longitudinal resection margins had increased incidence of recurrence ($P = 0.02$) and poor five-year survival ($P = 0.03$). *Conclusions.* Patients who received both neoadjuvant and adjuvant chemotherapies for gastric and gastro-oesophageal junction tumours have improved outcomes compared to patients who only received neoadjuvant chemotherapy.

1. Introduction

The annual worldwide incidence of gastric cancer is approximately one million and is ranked the fourth most common cancer worldwide [1]. There are estimated 7,700 new diagnoses and 5,200 deaths from the disease in the UK annually [2]. In the last two decades, more gastric cancer has been diagnosed in the proximal stomach and around the gastrooesophageal junction (GOJ) [3]. Increased levels of gastrooesophageal reflux disease [4] and obesity [5] are identified as probable causative factors.

Both gastric and gastrooesophageal junction (GOJ) cancers are associated with poor five-year survival rates [6–8]. Several treatment strategies have been developed to improve outcome. Potentially curative treatments involve surgical resection and both neoadjuvant and adjuvant chemotherapies, sometimes combined with radiotherapy [9]. The aim

of neoadjuvant treatment is to decrease tumour bulk, improve rates of surgical tumour clearance, and treat occult micrometastatic tumour. Several trials have used a combination of neoadjuvant and adjuvant chemoradiotherapies to improve outcome with varied success.

The use of adjuvant chemoradiation in gastric and GOJ adenocarcinomas (ACC) has achieved mixed results [10, 11]. However, use of neoadjuvant chemoradiotherapy has been shown to improve outcome in GOJ ACC [12]. In gastric cancer, neoadjuvant and adjuvant chemotherapies have been shown to improve overall survival [13, 14].

The landmark MAGIC chemotherapy trial conducted by the MRC (UK) has established guidelines for the administration of perioperative chemotherapy (cisplatin, 5-fluorouracil (5-FU), and epirubicin) in the surgical management of gastric and GOJ ACC [15]. The study recruited patients with gastric, gastrooesophageal junction, and lower third of oesophageal tumours. 45 centres in the UK, Europe, and Asia participated in this randomised control trial (RCT). Between 1994 and 2002, 503 patients were randomised to receive perioperative chemotherapy and surgery (n = 250) or surgery alone (n = 253). 65% (n = 137) of patients started adjuvant chemotherapy but only 42% (n = 104) completed all six cycles of perioperative chemotherapy. The results showed overall improved survival of 36% in the chemotherapy groups versus 23% in surgery-only group on an intention to treat basis. The results also showed improved progression-free survival in perioperative chemotherapy group. The study mentioned a problem of lack of clarity and information regarding chemotherapy, whether it was neoadjuvant or adjuvant chemotherapy or a combination of both responsible for improved overall survival and progression-free survival. The study did not publish the survival comparison for patients receiving both neoadjuvant and adjuvant cycles versus patients who only received neoadjuvant chemotherapy.

Presently, in the UK it is standard practice to offer perioperative chemotherapy for gastric and GOJ ACC for appropriate patients [15]. The aim of this study was to review the outcome for patients who have received MAGIC chemotherapy for gastric and GOJ ACC at our institute. Specifically we aimed to assess survival differences in patients completing perioperative chemotherapy compared with patients who did not complete neoadjuvant chemotherapy.

2. Methods

2.1. Patient Characteristics. A total of 272 patients underwent surgical resection for gastric (n = 115) and GOJ (n = 157) ACC between 1996 and 2010 at the University Hospital of South Manchester. 66 of these patients received neoadjuvant chemotherapy for gastric and GOJ ACC according to MAGIC chemotherapy protocol and subsequently underwent surgical resection. Inclusion criteria were histological diagnosis of ACC, locally advanced disease (T1 to T4, N0 to N2, and M(0)), and fit for both surgical resection and perioperative chemotherapy. All patients underwent a standard staging CT scan (chest, abdomen, and pelvis). The positron emission tomography (PET CT scan) was performed for patients with distal oesophageal and GOJ tumours. Endoscopic ultrasonography has been used for local staging since 2006. Staging laparoscopy was performed in all cases. All patients underwent cardiopulmonary exercise testing as part of preoperative assessment for fitness for general anaesthesia. All cases were discussed in a multidisciplinary team. A consensus decision to offer neoadjuvant chemotherapy was made, and patients were counselled accordingly. All patients were treated according to MAGIC protocol [15]. The chemotherapy was administered in three pre- and three postoperative cycles. Each cycle consisted of epirubicin (50 mg/m^2) by intravenous bolus and cisplatin (60 mg/m^2) intravenously with hydration on day one and 5-FU (200 mg/m^2) daily for 21 days by continuous intravenous infusion. A full blood count, serum electrolyte profile, serum creatinine, coagulation, and liver function test monitoring were performed during each cycle. Patients were closely monitored for development of side effects of chemotherapy. In patients with a history of ischaemic heart disease, echocardiogram was performed to assess the left ventricular function. The dose of chemotherapeutic agents was modified in patients with myelodepression, thrombocytopenia, and compromised renal function. A restaging scan was performed following completion of neoadjuvant chemotherapy. In the absence of further disease progression patients underwent total or subtotal gastrectomy and D2 lymphadenectomy depending upon the tumour site. Patients with GOJ tumours underwent total gastrectomy or Ivor-Lewis oesophagectomy as appropriate. Postoperatively patients were managed by a multi-disciplinary team on the high dependency unit and then on a surgical ward. Following recovery from surgery, patients were reassessed for suitability to receive adjuvant chemotherapy. All patients were reviewed in the outpatient clinic, with progress closely monitored.

The demographic details of patients survival status, disease recurrence, and followup were recorded. The postoperative survival was analysed from the date of surgery to last followup or death. The time to recurrence was calculated from the date of surgery to the radiological and clinically proven evidence of disease recurrence.

2.2. Histological Data. A data set was developed to collect histological information for patients who underwent surgical resection. This included site of tumour, local stage (T), nodal status (N), metastases (M) according to TNM 5 classification, differentiation, and status of longitudinal resection margins.

2.3. Statistical Analysis. SPPS version 16 (SPSS, Chicago, IL, USA) was used for statistical analyses. The histological characteristics including ypTNM, histological grade, and resection margins status were compared against the survival. The survival curves were obtained employing the method of Kaplan-Meier. Both the univariate and multivariate analyses were performed using the log-rank test. A P value of < 0.05 was considered statistically significant.

3. Results

Data was collected for the 66 patients who received neoadjuvant chemotherapy according to MAGIC protocol. Table 1 summarises the characteristics of the study population. The median age was 63 years (range 36 to 76 years). The median number of neoadjuvant and adjuvant cycles completed was 2 (range 1 to 3).

Thirty-one (47%) patients received both neoadjuvant and adjuvant courses of chemotherapy (Table 2). In 11 (17%) patients, who completed full course of chemotherapy (neoadjuvant and adjuvant) the median postoperative survival was 14 months (95% Confidence interval (CI), 12–28) and time to recurrence was 12 months (95% CI, 12–28). In patients who completed only the neoadjuvant chemotherapy the median adjuvant survival was 8 months (95% CI 11–25) and time to recurrence was 7 months (95% CI, 9–19). In our study 35 (53%) patients did not receive adjuvant chemotherapy. This was because of postoperative complications, patient refusal, or time lapse between surgery and initiation of

TABLE 1: Patient characteristics.

Characteristic	No. (%) of patients
Gender	
Male	49 (74%)
Female	17 (26%)
Tumour differentiation	
Well	3 (5%)
Moderate	26 (39%)
Poor	37 (56%)
Tumour site	
Gastric	24 (36%)
GOJ	42 (64%)
T stage	
0	2 (3%)
1	6 (9%)
2	21 (32%)
3	34 (51%)
4	3 (5%)
N stage	
Node negative	19 (29%)
Node positive	47 (71%)
Longitudinal resection margins	
R 0	53 (81%)
R 1	13 (19%)
Tumour recurrence	
Yes	20 (30%)
No	46 (70%)
Neoadjuvant + adjuvant Chemo.	7 (11%)
Neoadjuvant chemo. only	13 (19%)

GOJ: gastro-oesophageal junction; chemo: chemotherapy.

TABLE 2: Number of chemotherapy cycles completed by patients in the perioperative period.

No. of cycles	Neoadjuvant chemotherapy ($n = 66$)	Adjuvant chemotherapy ($n = 31$)
One	12	7
Two	29	13
Three	25	11

adjuvant chemotherapy. There was no significant difference in the rate of recurrence between the two groups. Only three (5%) patients showed complete histological response to neoadjuvant treatment as defined by histological analysis of resected specimens (two patients completed full three cycles and one patient received only two cycles). The univariate and multivariate analyses identified completion of both neoadjuvant and adjuvant chemotherapy courses (HR (hazard ratio) 0.26, $P = 0.008$), nodal status (HR 1.20, $P = 0.014$), and longitudinal resection margin status (HR 1.35, $P = 0.015$) as independent markers of prognosis. Table 3 details the chemotherapy-related side effects and grading of symptoms.

TABLE 3: Grading of chemotherapy-related side effects.

Symptoms	Grade (N)				
	0	1	2	3	4
Nausea		10	12	2	
Vomiting		3	4	1	
Mucositis		7	1		
Myelosuppression		4	3		
Skin infection		3	1		
Diarrhoea		3	1	1	
Phlebitis		3			
Pancreatitis		1			
Tinnitus		1			
Acute renal failure		1			

N: number of patients.

The Kaplan-Meier plot showed significant survival difference between patients completing the neoadjuvant and adjuvant chemotherapies compared with patients receiving only neoadjuvant chemotherapy ($P = 0.02$) (Figure 1). The involvement of the nodes ($P = 0.004$) and longitudinal resection margins ($P = 0.03$) by the tumour were associated with poor outcome.

4. Discussion

This is the first study to investigate the survival outcome difference among patients receiving chemotherapy according to MAGIC protocol (Figure 1). Patients who received both neoadjuvant and adjuvant courses had prolonged survival. There was no statistical difference in the rate of incidence of recurrence between the patients completing both neoadjuvant and adjuvant courses of chemotherapy and patients only receiving neoadjuvant chemotherapy (Table 1). However, recurrence occurred sooner in patients who received only neoadjuvant chemotherapy, although only 11 (17%) patients completed all six courses of perioperative chemotherapy. Also in these two groups of patients no significant difference was observed in terms of neoadjuvant staging and medical fitness before the initiation of chemotherapy.

The difference in postoperative survival may signify the oncological importance of completing the full course of perioperative chemotherapy in the absence of prolonged morbidity following surgery. Though the number of patients included in this study was limited to the experience at a single centre. In the future, a study involving multiple centres with a larger cohort can help to explain if the difference in survival is related to one adjuvant cycle or the completion of all three cycles.

In the management of gastric and GOJ ACC several interventions including neoadjuvant chemotherapy alone, perioperative chemotherapy, and adjuvant chemotherapy alone have been suggested. There is no consensus on the single best treatment option. Specialist centres around the world adopt management strategy which best suits the local practice and guidelines based on the best available evidence.

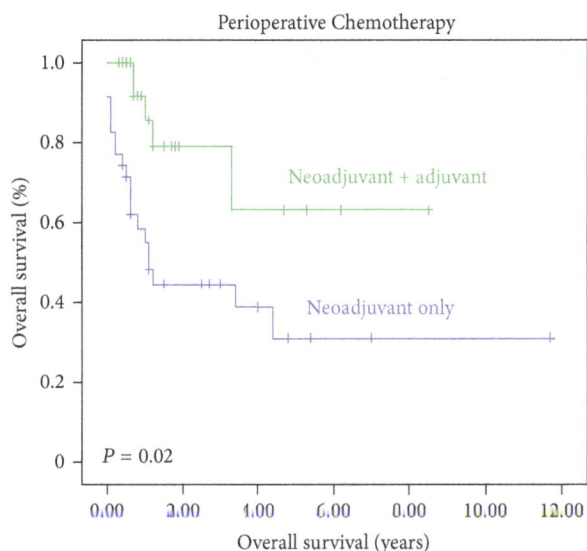

FIGURE 1: The overall survival comparing patients who completed both neoadjuvant and adjuvant chemotherapy courses versus patient who received only neoadjuvant chemotherapy.

In 1970s the first Phase I trial of neoadjuvant infusion of chemotherapeutic agents was carried out in Japan [16, 17]. FAMTX trial (5-FU, doxorubicin, and methotrexate) was the first study to randomise patients into neoadjuvant and surgery alone [18]. This trial did not show any clinical benefit but laid the foundations for further research in neoadjuvant settings for management of gastric cancer. The MAGIC trial has widely been recognised as the first landmark study to report the prognostic benefit of perioperative chemotherapy in a large cohort of patients [15]. A second well-reported trial conducted by Fédération Francophone de la Cancérlogie Digestive (FFCD) group showed significant increase in disease-free survival (34% versus 21%) and overall survival (38% versus 24%) over 5 years following perioperative administration of 5-FU and cisplatin in gastric and distal oesophageal ACC [14]. A meta-analysis of 14 neoadjuvant chemotherapy trials in gastric and GOJ ACC concluded improved overall survival (OR = 1.27, 95% CI: 1.26–2.33) and R0 resection rate (OR = 1.51, 95% CI: 1.19–1.91) in patients treated with perioperative chemotherapy.

In Japan following the publication of ACTS-GS trial adjuvant chemotherapy has become the standard of care. The chemotherapy consists of adjuvant administration of cycles of S-1 (orally active fluoropyrimidine). The study showed overall survival rates of 80.1% in the chemotherapy group and 70.1% in the surgery-only group. Furthermore patients who received chemotherapy had less incidence of recurrence [19]. A recently published meta-analysis by GASTRIC group of 17 trials of adjuvant chemotherapy identified improved overall survival (hazard ration (HR) 0.82, 95% CI 0.76–0.90, $P <$ 0.001) and disease-free survival (HR 0.82, 95% CI 0.75–0.90, $P <$ 0.001) in gastric cancer patients who were administered fluorouracil-based regimen as compared to surgery-only group [20]. On the literature search five randomised control

trails (RCT) were identified which have compared one adjuvant chemotherapy regimen against the other [21–25]. Three trials failed to demonstrate an actual difference in overall and disease-free survival [21, 23, 25]. However one trial showed significant improvement in overall and disease-free survival when administering cisplatin, epirubicin, leucovorin and folinic acid versus etoposide, leucovorin, and folinic acid [22]. Similarly another RCT reported improvement in disease-free survival following administration of 5-FU, folinic acid, irinotecan, docetaxel, and cisplatin versus mitomycin-C [24]. In Japan, an ongoing SAMIT study is evaluating the use of paclitaxel and S-1 versus oral tegafur-uracil (UF) for gastric cancer in the adjuvant settings [26]. The final efficacy results are still awaited [27]. The recently published results of CLASSIC trial in patients with stages II and III gastric cancers have identified improved disease-free survival 74% (95% CI, 69–79) in patients administered adjuvant capecitabine and oxaliplatin versus surgery-only group 59% (95% CI, 53–64) [28].

Adjuvant chemoradiotherapy (CRT) has also been employed in the management of gastric cancer. The INT 0116 trial of gastric and GOJ tumours identified improved three-year survival (50%) and disease-free survival (48%) following administration of adjuvant 5-FU, leucovorin, and radiation (45-Gy for 5 weeks) [10]. The group recently published 10-year follow-up results which showed benefit for the CRT group both in terms of overall survival (HR 0.76, $P =$ 0.004) and disease-free survival (HR 0.66, $P <$ 0.001) [29]. A large RCT CRITICS study is being conducted by a Dutch group. The study aims to evaluate the role of neoadjuvant chemotherapy, surgery and adjuvant CRT versus neoadjuvant chemotherapy, surgery, and adjuvant chemotherapy [30]. A recently concluded RCT of adjuvant chemotherapy versus adjuvant CRT in gastric cancer failed to show any survival difference and clinical benefits between the two groups [31]. Fiorica et al. published a meta-analysis of nine RCT: four trials of neoadjuvant radiotherapy and five of adjuvant CRT [32]. The study reported that reduced mortality in neoadjuvant radiotherapy to surgery alone over 5 years (OR 0.62, 95% CI 0.32–0.64, $P <$ 0.00001) was observed when adjuvant CRT was compared to surgery alone. No trials in the literature were identified which have only compared surgery versus adjuvant radiotherapy.

There is a general consensus that neoadjuvant chemotherapy is well tolerated and tolerance to adjuvant chemotherapy is limited by general morbidity following surgery [33]. Currently STO3 trial conducted by MRC (UK) is employing bevacizumab, a monoclonal antibody targeting vascular endothelial growth factor-A in combination with epirubicin, cisplatin, and capecitabine (ECX) chemotherapy in gastric, GOJ, and lower oesophageal tumours [34].

5. Conclusion

Our study showed considerable prognostic benefit achieved following completion of both neoadjuvant and adjuvant chemotherapy courses. Our study included patients who have received chemotherapy and undergone surgical resection. It does not include patients who received neoadjuvant chemotherapy but did not progress for surgery or patients who received chemotherapy and were found to have unresectable disease. Our study is limited by the total number of patients. Our study is limited by the total number of patients and it will be difficult to draw a firm conclusion. However, this study highlights the importance of completing the perioperative chemotherapy. Long-term follow-up results from MAGIC chemotherapy trial are still awaited. This will further lead to a discussion of whether the neoadjuvant or adjuvant chemotherapy is the best option or a combination of chemotherapy actually improves prognosis.

References

[1] J. Ferlay, H.-R. Shin, F. Bray, D. Forman, C. Mathers, and D. M. Parkin, "Estimates of worldwide burden of cancer in 2008: GLOBOCAN 2008," *International Journal of Cancer*, vol. 127, no. 12, pp. 2893–2917, 2010.

[2] CRC U. Cancer Research UK, *Cancer Stats—Key Facts*, London, UK, 2009.

[3] K. Dolan, R. Sutton, S. J. Walker, A. Morris, F. Campbell, and E. M. Williams, "New classification of oesophageal and gastric carcinomas derived from changinq patterns in epidemiology," *British Journal of Cancer*, vol. 80, no. 5-6, pp. 834–842, 1999.

[4] J. T. Chang and D. A. Katzka, "Gastroesophageal reflux disease, barrett esophagus, and esophageal adenocarcinoma," *Archives of Internal Medicine*, vol. 164, no. 14, pp. 1482–1488, 2004.

[5] A. M. Ryan, M. Duong, L. Healy et al., "Obesity, metabolic syndrome and esophageal adenocarcinoma: epidemiology, etiology and new targets," *Cancer Epidemiology*, vol. 35, no. 4, pp. 309–319, 2011.

[6] E. van Cutsem, M. Dicato, R. Geva et al., "The diagnosis and management of gastric cancer: expert discussion and recommendations from the 12th ESMO/World Congress on Gastrointestinal Cancer, Barcelona, 2010," *Annals of Oncology*, vol. 22, no. 5, pp. 1–9, 2011.

[7] T. D. Reid, L. N. Sanyaolu, D. Chan, G. T. Williams, and W. G. Lewis, "Relative prognostic value of TNM7 vs. TNM6 in staging oesophageal cancer," *British Journal of Cancer*, vol. 105, no. 6, pp. 842–846, 2011.

[8] B. Kayani, E. Zacharakis, K. Ahmed, and G. B. Hanna, "Lymph node metastases and prognosis in oesophageal carcinoma—A systematic review," *European Journal of Surgical Oncology*, vol. 37, no. 9, pp. 747–753, 2011.

[9] T. Sano, "Adjuvant and neoadjuvant therapy of gastric cancer: a comparison of three pivotal studies," *Current Oncology Reports*, vol. 10, no. 3, pp. 191–198, 2008.

[10] J. S. Macdonald, S. R. Smalley, J. Benedetti et al., "Chemoradiotherapy after surgery compared with surgery alone for adenocarcinoma of the stomach or gastroesophageal junction," *New England Journal of Medicine*, vol. 345, no. 10, pp. 725–730, 2001.

[11] C. Fuchs, J. E. Tepper, D. Niedzwiecki, and D. Hollis, "Postoperative adjuvant chemoradiation for gastric or gastroesophageal junction (GEJ) adenocarcinoma using epirubicin, cisplatin, and infusional (CI) 5-FU (ECF) before and after CI 5-FU and radiotherapy (CRT) compared with bolus 5-FU/LV before and after CRT: intergroup trial CALGB 80101," *Journal of Clinical Oncology*, vol. 29, supplement, abstract 4003, 2011.

[12] M. Stahl, M. K. Walz, M. Stuschke et al., "Phase III comparison of preoperative chemotherapy compared with chemoradiotherapy in patients with locally advanced adenocarcinoma of the esophagogastric junction," *Journal of Clinical Oncology*, vol. 27, no. 6, pp. 851–856, 2009.

[13] E. Jansen, "Randomized phase III trial of adjuvant cehmotherapy or chemo-radiotherapy in resectable gastric cancer (CRITICS)," 2008.

[14] V. Boige, J. Pignon, B. Saint-Aubert, P. Lasser, and T. Conroy, "Final results of a randomized trial comparing preoperative 5-fluorouracil (F)/cisplatin (P) to surgery alone in adenocarcinoma of stomach and lower esophagus (ASLE): FNLCC ACCORD07-FFCD 9703 trial," *Journal of Clinical Oncology*, vol. 25, supplement, abstract 4510, no. 18, 2007.

[15] D. Cunningham, W. H. Allum, S. P. Stenning et al., "Perioperative chemotherapy versus surgery alone for resectable gastroesophageal cancer," *New England Journal of Medicine*, vol. 355, no. 1, pp. 11–20, 2006.

[16] S. Fujimoto, Y. Watanabe, K. Enomoto, M. Adachi, and K. Itoh, "Studies on preoperative cancer chemotherapy. Methods of preoperative intra-arterial infusion by the use of methotrexate or vinblastine," *Cancer*, vol. 24, no. 3, pp. 433–441, 1969.

[17] S. Fujimoto, T. Akao, and B. Itoh, "A study of survival in patients with stomach cancer treated by a combination of preoperative intra arterial infusion therapy and surgery," *Cancer*, vol. 37, no. 4, pp. 1648–1653, 1976.

[18] H. H. Hartgrink, C. J. H. van de Velde, H. Putter et al., "Neo-adjuvant chemotherapy for operable gastric cancer: long term results of the Dutch randomised FAMTX trial," *European Journal of Surgical Oncology*, vol. 30, no. 6, pp. 643–649, 2004.

[19] S. Sakuramoto, M. Sasako, T. Yamaguchi et al., "Adjuvant chemotherapy for gastric cancer with S-1, an oral fluoropyrimidine," *New England Journal of Medicine*, vol. 357, no. 18, pp. 1810–1820, 2007.

[20] X. Paoletti, K. Oba, T. Burzykowski et al., "Benefit of adjuvant chemotherapy for resectable gastric cancer: a meta-analysis," *Journal of the American Medical Association*, vol. 303, no. 17, pp. 1729–1737, 2010.

[21] H. M. Chang, K. H. Jung, T.-Y. Kim et al., "A phase III randomized trial of 5-fluorouracil, doxorubicin, and mitomycin C versus 5-fluorouracil and mitomycin C versus 5-fluorouracil alone in curatively resected gastric cancer," *Annals of Oncology*, vol. 13, no. 11, pp. 1779–1785, 2002.

[22] D. Karacetin and O. Incekara, "A randomized trial of 5-fluorouracil, leucovorin, cisplatin and epirubicin (PELF) versus 5-fluorouracil, leucovorin and etoposide (ELF) given as adjuvant chemotherapy to patients with resected advanced gastric adenocarcinomas," *Journal of Balkan Union of Oncology*, vol. 9, no. 3, pp. 263–267, 2004.

[23] S. Cascinu, R. Labianca, C. Barone et al., "Adjuvant treatment of high-risk, radically resected gastric cancer patients with 5-fluorouracil, leucovorin, cisplatin, and epidoxorubicin in a randomized controlled trial," *Journal of the National Cancer Institute*, vol. 99, no. 8, pp. 601–607, 2007.

[24] M. Di Bartolomeo, R. Buzzoni, L. Mariani et al., "Feasibility of sequential therapy with FOLFIRI followed by docetaxel/cisplatin in patients with radically resected gastric adenocarcinoma: a randomized phase III trial," *Oncology*, vol. 71, no. 5-6, pp. 341–346, 2007.

[25] Y. Kang, H. Chang, Y. Min, and D. Zang, "A randomized phase III trial comparing mitomycin-C plus short-term doxifluridine (Mf) versus mitomycin-C plus long-term doxifluridine plus cisplatin (MFP) after curative resection of advanced gastric cancer (AMC 0201)," *Journal of Clinical Oncology*, vol. 26, supplement, abstract 453, 2008.

[26] A. Tsuburaya, J. Sakamoto, S. Morita et al., "A randomized phase III trial of post-operative adjuvant oral fluoropyrimidine versus sequential paclitaxel/oral fluoropyrimidine; and UFT versus S1 for T3/T4 gastric carcinoma: the stomach cancer adjuvant multi-institutional trial group (Samit) trial," *Japanese Journal of Clinical Oncology*, vol. 35, no. 11, pp. 672–675, 2005.

[27] M. Kobayashi, A. Tsuburaya, and K. Yoshida, "Adjuvant paclitaxel followed by oral fluoropyrimidines for gastric cancer: safety data of the factorial phase III SAMIT trial," *Journal of Clinical Oncology*, supplement 4, 2012.

[28] Y.-J. Bang, Y.-W. Kim, H.-K. Yang et al., "Adjuvant capecitabine and oxaliplatin for gastric cancer after D2 gastrectomy (CLASSIC): a phase 3 open-label, randomised controlled trial," *The Lancet*, vol. 379, no. 9813, pp. 315–321, 2012.

[29] J. S. Macdonald, J. Benedetti, and S. Smalley, "Chemoradiation of resected gastric cancer: a 10-year follow-up of the phase III trial INT0116 (SWOG 9008)," *Journal of Clinical Oncology*, vol. 27, supplement, abstract 4515, no. 15, 2009.

[30] J. L. Dikken, J. W. van Sandick, H. Maurits Swellengrebel et al., "Neo-adjuvant chemotherapy followed by surgery and chemotherapy or by surgery and chemoradiotherapy for patients with resectable gastric cancer (CRITICS)," *BMC Cancer*, vol. 11, article 329, 2011.

[31] A. Bamias, M. Karina, P. Papakostas et al., "A randomized phase iii study of adjuvant platinum/docetaxel chemotherapy with or without radiation therapy in patients with gastric cancer," *Cancer Chemotherapy and Pharmacology*, vol. 65, no. 6, pp. 1009–1021, 2010.

[32] F. Fiorica, F. Cartei, M. Enea et al., "The impact of radiotherapy on survival in resectable gastric carcinoma: a meta-analysis of literature data," *Cancer Treatment Reviews*, vol. 33, no. 8, pp. 729–740, 2007.

[33] W. Li, J. Qin, Y.-H. Sun, and T.-S. Liu, "Neoadjuvant chemotherapy for advanced gastric cancer: a meta-analysis," *World Journal of Gastroenterology*, vol. 16, no. 44, pp. 5621–5628, 2010.

[34] E. Smyth, R. Langley, S. Stenning, and L. Stevenson, "ST03: a randomized trial of perioperative epirubicin, cisplatin plus capecitabine (ECX) with or without bevacizumab (B) in patients (pts) with operable gastric, oesophagogastric junction (OGJ) or lower oesophageal adenocarcinoma," *Journal of Clinical Oncology*, vol. 30, 2012.

3

Strategies to Evaluate Synchronous Carcinomas of the Colon and Rectum in Patients That Present for Emergent Surgery

Jennifer L. Agnew, Benjamin Abbadessa, and I. Michael Leitman

Department of Surgery, Albert Einstein College of Medicine, Beth Israel Medical Center, 10 Union Square East, Suite 2M, New York, NY 10003, USA

Correspondence should be addressed to I. Michael Leitman; mleitman@chpnet.org

Academic Editor: S. Curley

It is not always possible to evaluate patients that present acutely with carcinoma of the colon and rectum for synchronous lesions. Patients that require emergent surgery necessitate urgent and efficient operation. Patients with lower gastrointestinal bleeding, perforation, or obstruction represent a challenging subset of patients with colorectal cancer. An organized approach to these patients in the effort not to overlook a synchronous carcinoma is important. The present paper provides an evidenced-based approach to this special situation.

1. Background

Colorectal cancer is the third most common malignancy worldwide and the fourth most common in the United States, with estimated 146,970 new cases diagnosed in 2009. In the United States, approximately 49,920 cancer-related deaths were attributed to a colorectal malignancy in 2009, making it second only to mortality from lung cancer [1]. Despite the high incidence of colorectal carcinoma that is diagnosed yearly, the majority of lesions are resected with curative intent (70%–80%) and colorectal cancer-related deaths account for 20%–30% of those diagnosed and treated surgically, making it a highly curable malignancy if identified in its early-stages. Approximately, 55% of colorectal cancers diagnosed on screening are found to present with Stage I or II disease [2, 3]. Patients with Stage I or Stage II colon cancer have a greater than 60% 5-year survival, and for patients with Stage I or Stage II rectal cancer, there is a greater than 50% 5-year survival [4, 5]. Because of this, colorectal screening exams in asymptomatic patients have become the recommended standard of care for average risk patients at the age of 50 and at the age of 40 or younger for those in the moderate and high risk groups.

Approximately, 70% of colorectal lesions occur distal to the splenic flexure, and looking at colon cancer alone, approximately 25% are found in the sigmoid, 10% at the rectosigmoid junction, and 4%–6% located in the descending colon [6]. Anatomically, the left colon has a smaller diameter than the right, and as a result, left-sided carcinomas can cause varying degrees of intraluminal occlusion and patients more frequently present with obstructive symptoms. Large bowel obstructions present a challenging clinical scenario for the physician in the diagnosis, operative management, and the timing of colonic surveillance. Patients presenting with advanced lesions causing partial or high-grade large bowel obstruction commonly have a distant history or no history of previous colonic surveillance. This fact is of clinical importance because the diagnosis of a primary colorectal malignancy is accompanied by an overall incidence of synchronous colorectal cancers between 2% and 10% and a frequency of synchronous adenomatous polyps ranging from 15% to 50% [7–13]. Interestingly, when compared by stage, no statistically significant difference has been found in the overall and disease-free survival between synchronous and primary cancers [14, 15].

High-grade or completely obstructing lesions may require emergent surgery, and preoperative colonoscopic surveillance by traditional colonoscopy, CT colonography, or barium enema is typically not recommended due to the lack of accuracy. Colonoscopy has a high rate of unsuccessful

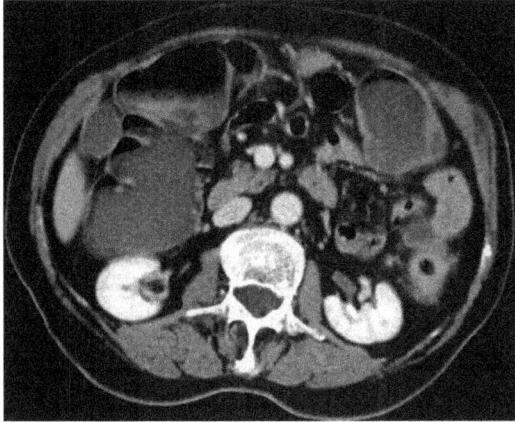

FIGURE 1: CT scan of abdomen in a patient with obstructing carcinoma of the sigmoid colon.

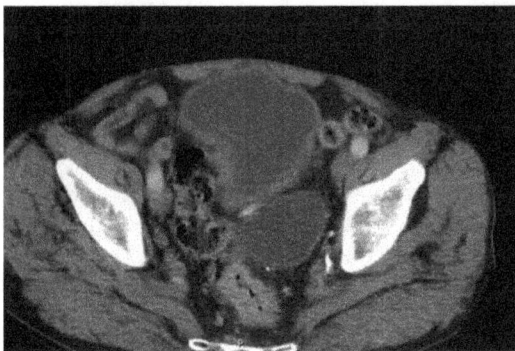

FIGURE 2: CT scan of a patient with obstructing carcinoma of the rectum.

TABLE 1: Alternative strategies for the identification of synchronous colonic lesions for patients that present with acute colonic cancer requiring emergent surgery.

Preoperative
Virtual CT colonoscopy
Magnetic resonance colonoscopy
Colon capsule endoscopy
Intraoperative
Subtotal colectomy
On-table lavage and intraoperative colonoscopy (CO_2 insufflation)

passage of the colonoscope as well as the risk of colonoscopic perforation at the site of obstruction or the more proximal cecum secondary to barotrauma. This particular scenario leaves the patient without adequate visualization and evaluation of the proximal colon prior to their operative resection (Figures 1 and 2). The issue of when and how to best monitor these patients is still debated and evolving, with the recent literature advocating intraoperative, on-table colonic lavage and colonoscopy. The current literature and management options for this unique clinical scenario are presented (Table 1).

2. Preoperative

Colonoscopic screening and surveillance has been proven to be a diagnostic and therapeutic modality that can result in an early diagnosis of colorectal cancer at a curable stage as well as identify and remove premalignant polypoid lesions. Quality control measures require cecal intubation during colonoscopy to classify the study as satisfactory and complete, thus decreasing the likelihood of failure to detect malignant or premalignant lesions. An incomplete colonoscopy is defined as failure of cecal intubation (or ileocolonic anastomosis) with nonvisualization of anatomic features (when present), such as the ileocecal valve, appendiceal orifice, or terminal ileum. Using a population-based cohort, Neerincx and colleagues investigated the rates and reasons for incomplete colonoscopy, as well as the subsequent work-up conducted to evaluate the nonvisualized colon, and the incidence of premalignant and cancerous lesions missed on incomplete colonoscopy. Incomplete colonoscopy was reported in 9.7% of patients. Several factors were cited to explain the occurrence, most commonly looping scope/excessively long colon (dolichocolon) (20.4%), patient discomfort (15.3%), obstructing tumor (13.9%), and insufficient bowel preparation (12.1%), with stenosis (3.7%) and severe inflammation (3.5%) being less common. During an 18-month follow-up period after incomplete index colonoscopy, secondary examinations were performed in 54.4% of these patients. Patients with incomplete colonoscopies due to stenosis (78.9%), severe inflammation (77.8%), and obstructing tumor (74.6%) were most likely to receive a secondary examination during the follow-up period. Barium enema was found to be the most common secondary investigation (47.5%) [16], despite its low diagnostic yield and miss rate for colorectal cancer detection, which has been reported as high as 22% [17]. Other modalities for secondary colon examination included repeat colonoscopy (20.5%), computed tomography colonography (4.3%), abdominal computed tomography (20.9%), and surgical exploration (6.8%). In individuals who underwent follow-up colonic evaluation after incomplete endoscopy, colorectal cancer was diagnosed in 3.5% of patients, with advanced adenoma found in 0.8% of patients, therefore noting overall that advanced neoplasia went undetected in 4.3% of patients due to incomplete colonoscopy [16].

As described by Neerincx et al., obstructing colorectal tumors may lead to incomplete colonoscopy due to inability to pass the colonoscope beyond the lesion. Morrin and colleagues advocated for the use of virtual computed tomographic (CT) colonography to image and detect synchronous lesions in the colon proximal to an obstructing colorectal lesion. Developed in the 1990s, virtual CT colonography uses ionizing radiation to create endoluminal radiologic images in multiple planes of an air-insufflated, cleansed colon, while simultaneously imaging extracolonic regions of the body. Using this modality, lesions greater than 1 cm can be detected with similar accuracy to conventional colonoscopy and with detection rates superior to barium enema. In the Morrin et al. study, virtual CT colonography correctly staged 81% of colorectal cancers. In patients with incomplete colonoscopy, 97%–100% of all colonic segments were adequately visualized on virtual CT colonography, serving as an accurate preoperative imaging option that could be used to investigate for synchronous proximal lesions, thus assisting with operative planning [18–20]. In a study reported by Wong et al., air-inflated magnetic resonance colonoscopy (MRC) was as accurate for identification of colonic lesions as colonoscopy [21]. As described earlier, while colonoscopy, barium enema, and CT colonography are widely accepted as the principle screening tools for the detection of colorectal cancer, they may be contraindicated and therefore not frequently performed during the hospitalization of patients in need of emergent resection for large bowel obstruction due to carcinoma.

In the acute setting of complete or near-total colonic obstruction, where many patients will require an emergent operation, preoperative evaluation of the colon may not be possible. Palpation of the colon and intraoperative colonic lavage and on-table colonoscopy are the only current diagnostic and therapeutic modalities available in the immediate perioperative time period. Although preoperative CT imaging may identify a proximal synchronous lesion(s) along with a high-grade, distal symptomatic obstruction, therapeutic colonoscopic intervention would be delayed until months postoperatively unless intraoperative techniques are used.

3. Intraoperative

Throughout history, intent-to-cure surgical resection has remained the treatment of choice for localized regional colorectal cancer. Surgical resection of obstructing carcinomas of the colon is associated with significant morbidity and mortality [22]. However, surgical management of completely obstructive left-sided colon cancer remains a topic of discussion, particularly as operative techniques and technological advancements have evolved over time. Of major concern is the theory that failure to detect a synchronous lesion proximal to the site of obstruction may lead to inadequate operative procedures at the time of initial surgical intervention, thus leaving unaddressed pathology behind and necessitating subsequent therapeutic interventions, including possible repeat surgical resection.

Historically, early studies favored performing a subtotal colectomy in the setting of left colon obstruction secondary to tumor [23, 24]. At that time, subtotal colectomy allowed removal of synchronous cancers and prevented possible development of metachronous lesions in the colon proximal to an obstructing lesion that had not been properly evaluated endoscopically in the preoperative period. However, depending on the length of remaining colon and rectum, frequent bowel movements and even fecal incontinence have been reported in patients who underwent subtotal colectomy [25].

Over time, the concept of a one-stage resection with intraoperative colonic lavage and primary anastomosis evolved as a potential surgical alternative to subtotal colectomy. On-table colonic irrigation was first described by Muir in 1968. Before that time, when a segmental resection was performed on an unprepared colon, standard practice was to create a colostomy (Hartmann's procedure) at the initial laparotomy. In the uncleansed colon, primary anastomosis was deferred at the time of initial surgery due to the anticipated risk of forceful stress associated with passing a solid load across a newly created surgical anastomosis. Acknowledging the known advantages of operating on a prepped colon, Muir investigated feasible techniques to allow a primary anastomosis to be performed when operating on a colon with a high fecal load preoperatively. Since proper preoperative preparation of the bowel can be difficult or impossible to achieve when an obstructing colorectal lesion is present, Muir proposed washing out the obstructed colon at the time of operation. The standard dissection and mobilization are performed as usual, the bowel is clamped and divided distal to the lesion, and the mobilized intestinal segment containing the lesion was inserted into a sterile polythene bag. Proximal to the lesion, a tube was inserted, and irrigation solution was instilled to lavage the colon. The feculent irrigation waste was subsequently drained out through the same tubing. The irrigation tubing was then removed, the lesion resected, and the operation completed with a primary anastomosis on the clean and empty colon [26].

Modifying Muir's lavage technique, Dudley et al. proposed another method of on-table colonic irrigation in 1980. The region of the lesion was dissected, and the bowel was divided distal to the lesion. The proximal bowel was mobilized and a sterile, rigid plastic tube was inserted through the cut end of this portion of bowel. A small enterotomy in the terminal ileum was made, through which a Foley catheter was inserted and passed across the ileocecal valve. The balloon was inflated, and the catheter was secured into place with a purse-string suture. Irrigation solution was instilled antegrade through the Foley catheter, and feculent waste was drained through the rigid plastic tube distally. After the colon was determined to be clean, the specimen was resected, and primary anastomosis of the bowel was completed. The Foley catheter was either removed and the enterotomy closed after resection of the lesion, or the catheter was brought out through a stab wound in the skin to create a tube cecostomy if clinically indicated. Dudley also noted that by leaving the tube cecostomy in place, a contrast study could be completed in an antegrade fashion if assessment of the anastomosis is necessary in the postoperative period [27].

More recent studies have described implementation of Dudley et al.'s technique for on-table antegrade colonic lavage, with only slight modification of the catheter location (through the appendix, terminal ileum, or cecum) to deliver irrigation and decrease fecal load proximal to the obstructing lesion in preparation for a primary anastomosis. However, colonic lavage via this technique can be cumbersome and time consuming to perform and is associated with possibility of contamination of spilled fecal content into the operative field [28].

Acknowledging these concerns, Park et al. proposed a one-stage resection and primary anastomosis with intraoperative antegrade irrigation in patients with obstructing left-sided colon cancer. The proximal end of the irrigation device was connected with the dilated colon proximal to the obstructing lesion. The distal end of the device contained two ports: one for drainage of colonic contents and one for insertion of the irrigation catheter. After successful colonic irrigation, an on-table colonoscopy was subsequently performed by inserting a colonoscope through the irrigation port. The incidence of synchronous polyps was 47%. Intraoperative endoscopic detection of a synchronous lesion prompted the surgeon to increase the extent of resection in 17% of patients when biopsy-proven malignancy was determined on frozen section. The device employed in this study was one of the first that facilitated a one-stage procedure in patients with obstructing left-sided colon cancer, as well as enabled a simultaneous on-table colonoscopy to be performed both quickly and easily [28].

Determined to decrease incidence of contamination during on-table colonic lavage, Buyukgebiz described a technique utilizing a camera sleeve to control irrigation drainage and spillage from the colon in patients with colonic obstruction due to tumor who underwent one-stage colon resection with primary anastomosis. The colon was divided proximal to the obstructing mass then introduced it into a nylon sleeve traditionally used to sterilely cover intraoperative camera equipment. The sleeve was sutured into place in a telescopic fashion to contain the fecal contents during colonic irrigation and washout via an antegrade catheter inserted through the appendix into the cecum. The in-sleeve method eliminated the need for irrigation drainage catheters, which have diameters smaller than that of the colonic lumen, making them prone to becoming clogged with feculent washout material. Additionally, by washing out the colon, an intraoperative colonoscopy could be effectively performed by introducing the colonoscope through the sleeve and into the transected colon. This technique was found to be a safe and quick means to decrease fecal load in obstructed colons, thus decreasing risk of contamination and allowing proper colon preparation for segmental resection with primary anastomosis. In addition, it provided successful means to perform intraoperative colonoscopy and evaluate the proximal colon on-table for synchronous lesions [19, 29].

Intraoperative colonoscopy can be utilized to evaluate the colon that could not be properly endoscopically assessed during the preoperative period. While the entire colon can be manually examined to assess for synchronous lesions at the time of laparotomy, Heald and Bussey reported that up to 69% of synchronous cancer lesions could not be detected by palpation of the colon [30]. Given the high failure rate and lack of sensitivity of operative palpation, intraoperative colonoscopy may serve as a useful adjunct. However, some concerns have been raised regarding on-table colonoscopy; in order to be properly performed, colonoscopy requires distension of the bowel with intraluminal air insufflation that may subsequently distort visualization and compromise the planned procedure, especially during laparoscopic surgery. If the bowel is over distended during insufflation, the colon may be at risk for mucosal, serosal, or mesenteric tears, regional hypoperfusion of tissue, and potential ischemia. Carbondioxide may be used for colonoscopic insufflation and offers the advantages of rapid absorption and alleviation of bowel distension when compared to atmospheric, nitrogen-rich air.

Nakajima et al. utilized CO_2-insufflated colonoscopy during laparoscopic colonic resections and found this modality to be feasible, safe, and practical, as it minimized bowel distension without negatively affecting operative exposure or the subsequent procedure. Additionally, it allowed the entire colon to be assessed endoscopically, rather than manually palpated, further facilitating the planned resection to be performed in a minimally invasive fashion [31].

Most recently, Sasaki et al. investigated whether intraoperative colonic irrigation and on-table colonoscopy may be useful for more accurate diagnosis of colorectal cancer before colectomy in patients with completely obstructive left-sided cancer. During a one-stage procedure, intraoperative colonic irrigation was completed using a Y-shaped irrigation catheter consisting of a working port and a drainage tube. After irrigation was completed, an intraoperative colonoscope was inserted through this device, and the bowel proximal to the obstructing tumor was endoscopically examined for presence of synchronous neoplastic lesions. In this study, synchronous adenomatous polyps were detected in 26.8% of patients receiving intraoperative colonic irrigation and colonoscopy, 4.0% of which were determined to be carcinoma on pathologic evaluation. In this study, they reported mean operative time to be 28 minutes longer when on-table colonic irrigation and intraoperative colonoscopy were included in the procedure (271 minutes versus 243 minutes). With intraoperative detection of these synchronous lesions, surgical intervention could be performed during the same procedure, thus deferring the need for a second laparotomy. Sasaki et al. found their protocol to be safe with no mortality, low morbidity, and without significant differences in complication rates [32].

Several studies have also shown that operative planning may need to be altered if a synchronous lesion is present. Arenas et al. conducted a prospective study in an effort to evaluate the need to augment the extent of surgical resection due to detection of a synchronous colorectal lesion. In this series, synchronous lesions were present in 45.6% of patients, with 24% of these lesions influencing the degree of surgical resection. Overall, in 11% of cases, the presence of a synchronous lesion influenced operative management and dictated a more extensive operation than would have been performed with only treating the primary lesion [8]. Kim and Park advocated the use of intraoperative colonoscopy to evaluate for synchronous lesions, reporting that 37.2% of on-table endoscopies performed in their study detected synchronous lesions, leading to additional surgical procedures completed at the time of initial operation in 13.7% of cases in order to remove these lesions [33]. In this notion, the overall goal of operative management should therefore be to perform a procedure with intent to cure, assess for synchronous pathology, and address all pathology present at time of the initial surgical intervention to avoid additional operations.

4. Postoperative

While surgical resection is the primary treatment for localized colorectal cancer, development of local, regional, and/or distant recurrence has been reported to occur in 30% to

50% of patients [34]. Greater than 90% of these recurrences have occurred within a 5-year interval following surgery [35]. When detected early, surgical intervention is the treatment of choice for resectable recurrences and for new primary tumors. Recurrence after resection of colorectal cancer is most common in the liver (33%) followed by lung (22%), local recurrence (15% in colon and 35% in rectum), and regional lymph nodes (14%). Less common but still noteworthy is the development of second primary or metachronous lesion in 3% of patients [36]. Though the importance of postoperative surveillance for detection of these lesions is widely acknowledged, no consensus has been established regarding timing and modalities for follow-up protocols in colorectal cancer patients. In 2009, Scheer and Auer performed a literature review exploring current guidelines from various institutions, including the American Society of Clinical Oncology, the National Comprehensive Cancer Network, and the European Society of Medical Oncology, among others. In their meta-analysis, it became apparent that intensive surveillance after curative resection of colorectal cancer improved overall survival, allowing early reoperation to address asymptomatic recurrences [37].

However, different approaches were noted in follow-up protocols, with large variation in frequency of postoperative office visits, serum CEA level monitoring, colonoscopy, and radiologic studies of the chest and abdomen. Office visits are important for surveillance monitoring, allowing the physician to discuss results of investigations, reinforce behavioral modifications, and provide counseling regarding disease process. Advocates of CEA monitoring will trend levels postoperatively, as levels will become elevated in approximately 75% of patients with colorectal recurrence. Depending on the threshold level for abnormal value, sensitivity and specificity for detecting recurrence have been reported between 44% and 80% and 42% and 90%, respectively. Most studies have agreed that CEA monitoring is most sensitive for hepatic and retroperitoneal lesions and least sensitive for local recurrence and pulmonary lesions. Therefore, CEA is used most commonly as a trended value, triggering further work-up if levels are noted to rise [37].

After resection of colorectal cancer, follow-up colonoscopy is recommended to screen recurrence at the anastomosis and to assess metachronous lesions. Mulder et al. reported a significantly higher incidence of metachronous colorectal cancer in patients who had a prior resection for colorectal cancer when compared to an age- and sex-matched population. Of note, these patients had a 1.4 incidence ratio of metachronous lesions within a 3-year interval after initial colorectal cancer diagnosis and resection. The presence of a synchronous lesion at time of initial colorectal cancer resection was noted to be the only significant risk factor for development of metachronous lesion, yielding a relative risk of 13.9 (95% CI 4.7–41.0). Therefore, short-term interval (ideally less than 3 years) surveillance should be recommended for follow-up colonoscopy, possibly sooner for those patients diagnosed with synchronous tumors [38].

Couch and coworkers conducted a retrospective study investigating postoperative colonoscopic surveillance, noting that complete preoperative screening did not translate to a lower incidence of neoplasia detected on first postoperative colonoscopy. Additionally, new neoplastic lesions and recurrences amenable to resection were detected within two years from time of operation. Therefore, Couch et al. advocate a suggested time interval of no more than two years between initial surgery for colorectal cancer and first postoperative surveillance colonoscopy [39]. In their meta-analysis, Scheer and Auer stated that most randomized trials evaluating surveillance for colorectal cancer recurrence after resection of primary lesion reported a median observation period of 5 years or less [37].

Aside from colonoscopy, several imaging modalities are available to assess the colon, as well as extracolonic anatomy. Chest X-ray or thoracic CT can be used if pulmonary lesions are suspected. Abdominal CT and/or ultrasound can be used to image the liver for lesions. American Society of Clinical Oncology current guidelines recommend yearly CT scan of the abdomen for the first 3 years following surgery [37]. A newer imaging modality, CT colonography, may play a role in surveillance after curative resection of colorectal cancer due to its ability to assess for both colonic and extracolonic lesions. Kim and colleagues reported an 81.8% per-patient and 80.8% per-lesion sensitivity for CT colonography when detecting advanced neoplasia, with similar sensitivities of 80% and 78.5%, respectively, for evaluation all adenomatous lesions. CT colonography was noted to have a specificity of 93.1%, with negative predictive values of 100% for adenocarcinoma, 99.1% for advanced neoplasia, and 97% for all adenomatous lesions [40]. More recently, 18FDG-PET has been investigated as a potential diagnostic imaging modality, specifically in patients with an elevated CEA and normal colonoscopy. While this option had a high diagnostic yield for detection of lesions, it is not currently considered a cost-effective method for routine postoperative surveillance [37].

As discussed earlier, the need for postoperative colonoscopic surveillance after resection is paramount due to the elevated incidence of synchronous and metachronous lesions in those patients with a history of colorectal malignancy. Typically, in patients who have undergone preoperative colonoscopic evaluation, colonoscopy is performed within one year after colorectal resection. In the patient without a recent preoperative evaluation (within 5 years), who presents with an acute colonic obstruction that necessitates emergency surgical intervention without intraoperative colonic lavage and colonoscopy, it would be recommended to survey that patient in less than one year after resection, preferably 3–6 months postoperatively. In this specific scenario, if a biopsy-proven malignancy or sessile polyp not amenable to endoscopic resection is found on postoperative colonoscopy, the patient will need to be subjected to two abdominal operations for colorectal resection within a 6-month period. Given the age, functional status, and burden of comorbidity of each patient, this predicament can be a challenging one, but one that is potentially avoidable.

5. Conclusion

At the current state of technology, multiple modalities exist to visualize the colon in the asymptomatic patient, as well as during operative resection and the perioperative period. Despite this fact, a large portion of the population remains unscreened for colorectal lesions, and high-grade obstruction or other emergent conditions from colonic carcinoma can occur without previous detection. On-table colonic lavage and colonoscopy during the time of resection is a technique that has been utilized for many years but recently is becoming more refined. The goal of recent research is to develop a safe, efficient, high-yield procedure that adds little to overall operating room time and postoperative morbidity while give the surgeon the necessary information to make a proper oncologic decision about the extent of resection to provide our patients the best chances for successful outcome. It is a technique and a technology that requires further use and study but with continued evolution and improvement looks to be a viable option in our intraoperative armamentarium.

References

[1] A. Jemal, R. Siegel, E. Ward, Y. Hao, J. Xu, and M. J. Thun, "Cancer statistics, 2009," *CA: A Cancer Journal for Clinicians*, vol. 59, no. 4, pp. 225–249, 2009.

[2] J. M. Jessup, H. R. Menck, A. Fremgen, and D. P. Winchester, "Diagnosing colorectal carcinoma: clinical and molecular approaches," *CA: A Cancer Journal for Clinicians*, vol. 47, no. 2, pp. 70–92, 1997.

[3] M. Peeters, D. G. Haller, S. R. ALberts, R. M. Goldberg, and R. Smith, "Therapy for early-stage colorectal cancer," *Oncology*, vol. 13, no. 3, pp. 307–321, 1999.

[4] AJCC Cancer Staging Manual, 2002.

[5] F. L. Greene, A. K. Stewart, H. J. Norton, and A. M. Cohen, "A new TNM staging strategy for node-positive (stage III) colon cancer: an analysis of 50,042 patients," *Annals of Surgery*, vol. 236, no. 4, pp. 416–421, 2002.

[6] E. T. Hawk, P. J. Limburg, and J. L. Viner, "Epidemiology and prevention of colorectal cancer," *Surgical Clinics of North America*, vol. 82, no. 5, pp. 905–941, 2002.

[7] R. Fante, L. Roncucci, C. Di Gregorio et al., "Frequency and clinical features of multiple tumors of the large bowel in the general population and in patients with hereditary colorectal carcinoma," *Cancer*, vol. 77, no. 10, pp. 2013–2021, 1996.

[8] R. B. Arenas, A. Fichera, D. Mhoon, and F. Michelassi, "Incidence and therapeutic implications of synchronous colonic pathology in colorectal adenocarcinoma," *Surgery*, vol. 122, no. 4, pp. 706–710, 1997.

[9] W. J. Cunliffe, P. S. Hasleton, D. E. F. Tweedle, and P. F. Schofield, "Incidence of synchronous and metachronous colorectal carcinoma," *British Journal of Surgery*, vol. 71, no. 12, pp. 941–943, 1984.

[10] E. Brullet, J. M. Montane, J. Bombardo, X. Bonfill, M. Nogue, and J. M. Bordas, "Intraoperative colonoscopy in patients with colorectal cancer," *British Journal of Surgery*, vol. 79, no. 12, pp. 1376–1378, 1992.

[11] F. J. Burns, "Synchronous and metachronous malignancies of the colon and rectum," *Diseases of the Colon and Rectum*, vol. 23, no. 8, pp. 578–579, 1980.

[12] J. M. Langevin and S. Nivatvongs, "The true incidence of synchronous cancer of the large bowel. A prospective study," *American Journal of Surgery*, vol. 147, no. 3, pp. 330–333, 1984.

[13] A. I. Neugut, E. Lautenbach, B. Abi-Rached, and K. A. Forde, "Incidence of adenomas after curative resection for colorectal cancer," *American Journal of Gastroenterology*, vol. 91, no. 10, pp. 2096–2098, 1996.

[14] M. A. Passman, R. F. Pommier, and J. T. Vetto, "Synchronous colon primaries have the same prognosis as solitary colon cancers," *Diseases of the Colon and Rectum*, vol. 39, no. 3, pp. 329–334, 1996.

[15] H. S. Chen and S. M. Sheen-Chen, "Synchronous and 'Early' metachronous colorectal adenocarcinoma: analysis of prognosis and current trends," *Diseases of the Colon and Rectum*, vol. 43, no. 8, pp. 1093–1099, 2000.

[16] M. Neerincx, J. S. Terhaar Sive Droste, C. J. J. Mulder et al., "Colonic work-up after incomplete colonoscopy: significant new findings during follow-up," *Endoscopy*, vol. 42, no. 9, pp. 730–735, 2010.

[17] J. Toma, L. F. Paszat, N. Gunraj, and L. Rabeneck, "Rates of new or missed colorectal cancer after barium enema and their risk factors: a population-based study," *American Journal of Gastroenterology*, vol. 103, no. 12, pp. 3142–3148, 2008.

[18] M. M. Morrin, R. J. Farrell, V. Raptopoulos, J. B. McGee, R. Bleday, and J. B. Kruskal, "Role of virtual computed tomographic colonography in patients with colorectal cancers and obstructing colorectal lesions," *Diseases of the Colon and Rectum*, vol. 43, no. 3, pp. 303–311, 2000.

[19] D. Giglio, A. Di Muria, A. Marano et al., "Urgent management of obstructing colo-rectal cancer: authors' experience," *Annali Italiani di Chirurgia*, vol. 75, no. 1, pp. 35–39, 2004.

[20] R. Cirocchi, M. Coccetta, D. Giuliani et al., "Virtual colonoscopy in stenosing colorectal cancer," *Chirurgia Italiana*, vol. 60, no. 2, pp. 233–236, 2008.

[21] T. Y. Y. Wong, W. W. M. Lam, N. M. C. So, J. F. Y. Lee, and K. L. Leung, "Air-inflated magnetic resonance colonography in patients with incomplete conventional colonoscopy: comparison with intraoperative findings, pathology specimens, and follow-up conventional colonoscopy," *American Journal of Gastroenterology*, vol. 102, no. 1, pp. 56–63, 2007.

[22] I. M. Leitman, J. D. Sullivan, D. Brams, and J. J. DeCosse, "Multivariate analysis of morbidity and mortality from the initial surgical management of obstructing carcinoma of the colon," *Surgery Gynecology and Obstetrics*, vol. 174, no. 6, pp. 513–518, 1992.

[23] D. K. Brief, B. J. Brener, R. Goldenkranz et al., "Defining the role of subtotal colectomy in the treatment of carcinoma of the colon," *Annals of Surgery*, vol. 213, no. 3, pp. 248–252, 1991.

[24] A. Gainant, "Emergency management of acute colonic cancer obstruction," *Journal of Vascular Surgery*, vol. 149, no. 1, pp. e3–e10, 2012.

[25] The SCOTIA Study Group, "Single-stage treatment for malignant left-sided colonic obstruction: a prospective randomized clinical trial comparing subtotal colectomy with segmental resection following intraoperative irrigation. Subtotal Colectomy versus On-table Irrigation and Anastomosis," *British Journal of Surgery*, vol. 82, no. 12, pp. 1622–1627, 1995.

[26] E. G. Muir, "Safety in colonic resection," *Proceedings of the Royal Society of Medicine*, vol. 61, pp. 401–408, 1968.

[27] H. A. F. Dudley, A. G. Radcliffe, and D. McGeehan, "Intraoperative irrigation of the colon to permit primary anastomosis," *British Journal of Surgery*, vol. 67, no. 2, pp. 80–81, 1980.

[28] U. C. Park, S. S. Chung, K. R. Kim et al., "Single-stage procedure with intraoperative colonoscopy and colonic irrigation in patients with obstructing left-sided colonic cancer," *International Journal of Colorectal Disease*, vol. 19, no. 5, pp. 487–492, 2004.

[29] O. Büyükgebiz, "In-sleeve on-table colonic irrigation in tele-scopic fashion and intraoperative colonoscopy: a novel technique," *Turkish Journal of Trauma & Emergency Surgery*, vol. 16, no. 4, pp. 323–326, 2010.

[30] R. J. Heald and H. J. R. Bussey, "Clinical experiences at St. Mark's Hospital with multiple synchronous cancers of the colon and rectum," *Diseases of the Colon and Rectum*, vol. 18, no. 1, pp. 6–10, 1975.

[31] K. Nakajima, S. W. Lee, T. Sonoda, and J. W. Milsom, "Intraoperative carbon dioxide colonoscopy: a safe insufflation alternative for locating colonic lesions during laparoscopic surgery," *Surgical Endoscopy and Other Interventional Techniques*, vol. 19, no. 3, pp. 321–325, 2005.

[32] K. Sasaki, S. Kazama, E. Sunami et al., "One-stage segmental colectomy and primary anastomosis after intraoperative colonic irrigation and total colonoscopy for patients with obstruction due to left-sided colorectal cancer," *Diseases of the Colon and Rectum*, vol. 55, no. 1, pp. 72–78, 2012.

[33] M. S. Kim and Y. J. Park, "Detection and treatment of synchronous lesions in colorectal cancer: the clinical implication of perioperative colonoscopy," *World Journal of Gastroenterology*, vol. 13, no. 30, pp. 4108–4111, 2007.

[34] K. J. Buechter, C. Boustany, R. Caillouette, and I. Cohn, "Surgical management of the acutely obstructed colon. A review of 127 cases," *American Journal of Surgery*, vol. 156, no. 3, pp. 163–168, 1988.

[35] B. Bohm, W. Schwenk, H. P. Hucke, and W. Stock, "Does methodic long-term follow-up affect survival after curative resection of colorectal carcinoma?" *Diseases of the Colon and Rectum*, vol. 36, no. 3, pp. 280–286, 1993.

[36] S. Galandiuk, H. S. Wieand, C. G. Moertel et al., "Patterns of recurrence after curative resection of carcinoma of the colon and rectum," *Surgery Gynecology and Obstetrics*, vol. 174, no. 1, pp. 27–32, 1992.

[37] A. Scheer and R. A. C. Auer, "Surveillance after curative resection of colorectal cancer," *Clinics in Colon and Rectal Surgery*, vol. 22, no. 4, pp. 242–250, 2009.

[38] S. A. Mulder, R. Kranse, R. A. Damhuis, R. J. Ouwendijk, E. J. Kuipers, and M. E. van Leerdam, "The incidence and risk factors of metachronous colorectal cancer: an indication for follow-up," *Diseases of the Colon and Rectum*, vol. 55, no. 5, pp. 522–531, 2012.

[39] D. Couch, N. Bullen, S. Ward-Booth, and C. Adams, "What interval between colorectal resection and first surveillance colonoscopy? An audit of practice and yield," *Colorectal Disease*, 2012.

[40] H. J. Kim, S. H. Park, P. J. Pickhardt et al., "CT colonography for combined colonic and extracolonic surveillance after curative resection of colorectal cancer," *Radiology*, vol. 257, no. 3, pp. 697–704, 2010.

4

Peritoneal Carcinomatosis: Intraoperative Parameters in Open (Coliseum) versus Closed Abdomen Hipec

E. Halkia,[1,2] A. Tsochrinis,[1] D. T. Vassiliadou,[1] A. Pavlakou,[3] A. Vaxevanidou,[4] A. Datsis,[5] E. Efstathiou,[1] and J. Spiliotis[1]

[1]1st Department of Surgical Oncology, Metaxa Cancer Hospital, 18537 Piraeus, Greece
[2]Peritoneal Surface Malignancy Unit, IASO General Hospital, 15562 Athens, Greece
[3]Department of Anesthesiology, Metaxa Cancer Hospital, 18537 Piraeus, Greece
[4]Department of Anesthesiology, Gennimatas General Hospital, 54635 Thessaloniki, Greece
[5]Department of Surgery, General Hospital of Messolonghi, 30200 Messolonghi, Greece

Correspondence should be addressed to J. Spiliotis; jspil@in.gr

Academic Editor: Edward W. Martin

Background. Peritoneal carcinomatosis (PC) is associated with a poor prognosis. Cytoreductive surgery (CRS) and HIPEC play an important role in well-selected patients with PC. The aim of the study is to present the differences in the intraoperative parameters in patients who received HIPEC in two different manners, open versus closed abdomen. *Patients and Methods.* The population includes 105 patients with peritoneal carcinomatosis from colorectal, gastric, and ovarian cancer, sarcoma, mesothelioma, and pseudomyxoma peritonei. Group A ($n = 60$) received HIPEC using the open technique and Group B ($n = 45$) received HIPEC with the closed technique. The main end points were morbidity, mortality, and overall hospital stay. *Results.* There were two postoperative deaths (3.3%) in the open group versus no deaths in the closed group. Twenty-two patients in the open group (55%) had grade III-IV complications versus 18 patients in the closed group (40%). There are more stable intraoperative conditions in the closed abdomen HIPEC in CVP, pulse rate, and systolic pressure parameters. *Conclusions.* Both methods are equal in the HIPEC procedures. Perhaps the closed method is the method of choice for frail patients due to more stable hemodynamic parameters.

1. Introduction

The presence of peritoneal metastases is often considered a terminal condition, not amenable to standard therapeutic management. However, cytoreductive surgery (CRS) followed by hyperthermic intraperitoneal chemotherapy (HIPEC) offers a promising alternative when implemented on well-selected patients.

HIPEC involves the rinsing of the abdominal cavity with a heated chemotherapy solution. Most regimens suggest the administration of the chemoperfusate for 60 to 120 minutes, at 42°C. The chemotherapeutic agent used depends on the site of the initial neoplasia, the most commonly used being mitomycin-c, oxaliplatin, irinotecan, and cisplatin.

In the open technique (Figure 1(a)), the abdominal wall is elevated to create a funnel in which the chemoperfusate circulates through inflow and outflow lines attached to a pump and heating unit. On the other hand, in the closed technique (Figure 1(b)), the inflow and outflow lines are placed through separate incisions and afterwards the abdominal wall is closed before the delivery of HIPEC.

The open technique has the advantage of a more even distribution of the chemoperfusate in the abdominal cavity and is also preferred by surgeons because the formation of anastomoses is performed after HIPEC, jeopardizing less their integrity. However, its disadvantages include heat dissipation and the risk of personnel exposure to the chemotherapeutic agents, with possible toxic effects.

The closed technique, on the other hand, has been associated with uneven distribution of the perfusate in the peritoneal cavity but eliminates the exposure of the surgical team to the antineoplastic drugs. Moreover, as it has been observed in this study, it ensures more stable intraoperative

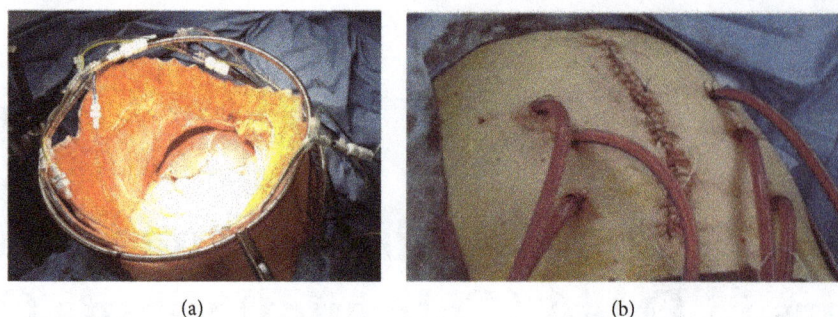

FIGURE 1: (a) The open (coliseum) technique. (b) The closed abdomen technique.

conditions, making it a most appropriate choice for frail patients.

The aim of this study is to assess the differences in the intraoperative parameters during HIPEC administration with the open or the closed technique, as well as to identify perioperative morbidity and mortality.

2. Patients and Methods

Over a period of five years (2009–2013), a population of $n = 105$ patients was included retrospectively in this study. The origins of peritoneal carcinomatosis in those patients were colorectal, ovarian, and gastric cancer, mesothelioma, sarcoma, and pseudomyxoma peritonei. On 60 patients (Group A) the open technique was applied, while on the remaining 45 (Group B) we implemented the closed technique. Patients in both groups shared similar demographic, clinical, and therapeutic features (Table 1). The types of surgery performed are described in Table 2. Intraoperative parameters (abdominal temperature, core temperature, central venous pressure, pulse rate, systolic blood pressure, and urinary output) were recorded at 15-minute intervals from the beginning to the end of HIPEC administration (90 minutes). The outcome measures were perioperative morbidity and mortality as well as duration of hospital stay.

Patient characteristics and outcomes were analyzed by descriptive statistics. Categorical variables were compared using chi-square analysis or Fisher's exact test where appropriate. Normally distributed variables were compared using the t-test as appropriate; nonparametric tests were used when variables were not normally distributed. Survival was measured with the Kaplan-Meier method with $P < 0.05$ considered significant in all analysis. All statistical analyses were conducted using SPSS software (version 17.0) and Microsoft Office Excel.

3. Results

3.1. Morbidity and Mortality. In the immediate postoperative period, in the open HIPEC group, two deaths (3.3%) were recorded, while in the closed HIPEC group no postoperative deaths were recorded (NSS). Grade III and IV complications occurred in 22 patients from the open HIPEC group (55%)

TABLE 1: Patient characteristics, $n = 105$.

	Open HIPEC group (Group A)		Closed HIPEC group (Group B)	
n	60		45	
Mean age	58.3		58.1	
	n	%	n	%
Origin of peritoneal carcinomatosis				
Colorectal cancer	17	28.3	13	28.9
Ovarian cancer	14	23.3	9	20
Gastric cancer	6	10	4	8.8
Mesothelioma	8	13.3	8	17.8
Sarcoma	3	5	5	11.1
Pseudomyxoma	12	20	6	13.3
Ascites				
Yes	18	30	16	35.6
No	42	70	29	64.4
Peritoneal carcinomatosis index				
PCI < 5	7	11.7	8	17.8
5 ≤ PCI < 10	24	40	12	26.7
PCI ≥ 10	29	48.3	25	55.6
Completeness of cytoreduction				
CC-0	39	65	32	71.1
CC-1	12	20	7	15.6
CC-2	9	15	6	13.3

and in 18 patients from the closed HIPEC group (40%) (NSS). The complications are reported in Table 3.

3.2. Hospital Stay. Mean duration of hospital stay was 8.7 days in the open HIPEC group versus 9.1 days in the closed HIPEC group (NSS).

3.3. Intraoperative Parameters. Haemodynamic parameters recorded during the administration of HIPEC are presented in Table 4. No statistically significant differences were observed in any of the parameters studied, that is, abdominal temperature, core temperature, central venous pressure, heart

TABLE 2: Operations performed.

	Open		Closed	
	n	%	n	%
Splenectomy	8	13.3	7	15.6
Cholecystectomy	60	100	45	100
Omentectomy	60	100	45	100
Hysterectomy	26	43.3	11	24.4
Gastrectomy	9	15	7	15.6
Complete colectomy	19	31.7	8	17.8
Douglas resection	29	48.3	14	31.1
Small bowel resection	43	71.7	32	71.1
Partial colectomy	15	25	8	17.8
Total	**60**	**100**	**45**	**100**

rate, systolic blood pressure, and urinary output (Figures 2(a)–2(f)).

4. Discussion

Delivery of hyperthermic intraperitoneal chemotherapy can be safely performed using either the open or the closed technique, without significant difference in operative time or efficacy [1].

This study has shown that there are no significant differences in the postoperative morbidity and mortality with the implementation of either technique. While the analysis of the haemodynamic parameters evaluated did not yield any statistical significance either, it appears that the closed technique is associated with more stable intraoperative conditions, exposing the patient to a lesser stress. This proves to be helpful especially in frail patients, with suboptimal preoperative status (older age, comorbidities, and cachexia), suggesting the application of the closed technique in those patients.

4.1. Haemodynamic Parameters and Morbidity. Regarding the haemodynamic monitoring, the present study has shown that parameters such as the abdominal and core temperatures, central venous pressure, heart rate, systolic blood pressure, and urine output do not differ significantly with the two techniques.

These findings are in accordance with those of Pascual-Ramírez et al. who did not detect any difference in haemodynamic parameters during CRS and HIPEC when describing the closed technique in ovarian cancer patients, as it was also known from the study of Desgranges et al. [2, 3]. Similarly, in the Pascual-Ramírez series there was not a rise in body temperature or a disturbance in renal function, as in our study and the one conducted by Schmidt et al. [3, 4].

In our series, no difference was observed in heart rate between the open and the closed techniques. In the Pascual-Ramírez study, an increase in heart rate was reported, attributed to increased vasodilatation and relative volume deficit due to heat increase [3]. However, this finding is not present in our study, possibly due to the decreased fluid turnover that occurs in the closed method as opposed to

the open one and the positive fluid balance perioperatively. Indeed, we observed more stable perioperative conditions with the closed technique, not statistically significant to those of the open one, however with narrowest ranges. This observation cannot be evaluated with statistic methods, perhaps owing to a small statistic sample being a limitation of our study.

A retrospective analysis of 78 patients undergoing cytoreductive surgery and HIPEC demonstrated a large intraoperative fluid turnover, increased airway pressure, and central venous pressure (due to the increased intra-abdominal pressure with the closed technique), while increased body temperature resulted in a mild metabolic acidosis [4].

According to the findings of another prospective study of 60 patients, haemodynamic disturbances occurred during HIPEC administration, characterized by an increase in heart rate and cardiac output and a decreased systemic vascular resistance on account of increased body temperature and decreased effective circulating volume. Urinary output showed a decreasing tendency over time [5].

A recent study by Facy et al., conducted on a swine model, reported that increased intra-abdominal pressure when applying the closed HIPEC technique resulted in tachycardia, a decrease in blood pressure despite more aggressive fluid resuscitation, and an increase in ventilation pressure [6].

Intraoperative parameters may be associated with postoperative outcome, in terms of morbidity and mortality, as demonstrated by a previous study conducted by our team [7]. However, these parameters do not correspond with long-term survival outcomes.

Postoperative ICU admission is often considered protocol after cytoreductive surgery and HIPEC, mainly due to the need for haemodynamic surveillance and stabilization after this major operation. However, it was recently reported that there was no difference in the rate and degree of complications observed in patients who were admitted to the ICU, noting that ICU admission should not be standardized but should be based on individual patient characteristics [8].

Most frequent complications of the open technique, as identified by a previous study by our team, were pulmonary complications, gastrointestinal fistulae, haematologic toxicity, and postoperative haemorrhage [9].

4.2. Efficacy. A comparative study between the two techniques by Ortega-Deballon et al., conducted on an animal model, identified that good thermal homogeneity was reached with both techniques; however better chemotherapeutic absorption and tissue uptake were achieved with the open technique [10].

Even with the application of high pressure with the closed technique, hypothesized to increase drug tissue penetration, the open technique still seems to attain better intraperitoneal distribution and enhanced tissue uptake [6].

The same team had previously reported a combined technique of closed HIPEC with open abdomen, utilizing a latex wall expander and a hand-access port (similar to those used in laparoscopic surgery), in an attempt to minimize personnel exposure to the chemoperfusate [11].

TABLE 3: Complications.

			Open		Closed		
			n	%	n	%	
Grade I	No intervention required for resolution	Nausea, vomiting, metabolic acidosis, neutropenia, and ileus	9	15	10	22.2	NSS
Grade II	Medical treatment sufficient for resolution	Reintubation, blood product transfusion, and pneumonia	29	48.3	17	37.8	NSS
Grade III	An invasive intervention, for example, radiological intervention, required for resolution	Intra-abdominal collection	18	30	16	35.5	NSS
Grade IV	Urgent definitive intervention, for example, returning to the OR or to surgical ICU, required for resolution	Reoperation, readmission to ICU	4	6.7	2	4.4	NSS
	Total		60	100	45	100	

TABLE 4: Haemodynamic parameters during HIPEC.

Time		0 min	15 min	30 min	45 min	60 min	75 min	90 min	End of operation
Abdominal temperature	Open	34.7 ± 1.6	39.8 ± 1.9	41.2 ± 2.4	42.2 ± 2.1	41.8 ± 2.1	42.4 ± 2.4	42.8 ± 2.1	38.1 ± 1.8
	Closed	35.9 ± 1.8	41.2 ± 1.9	42.5 ± 2.1	43.0 ± 2.3	42.8 ± 2.0	42.8 ± 5.0	43.1 ± 2.0	40.1 ± 2.0
Core temperature	Open	35.7 ± 1.2	36.5 ± 1.0	37.0 ± 1.6	37.2 ± 1.4	37.5 ± 1.6	37.8 ± 1.8	37.9 ± 1.6	37.2 ± 1.8
	Closed	35.9 ± 1.1	36.2 ± 1.2	37.4 ± 1.4	37.8 ± 2.0	37.9 ± 1.4	38.0 ± 2.0	37.9 ± 1.4	37.5 ± 1.6
CVP	Open	7.4 ± 2.1	10.2 ± 2.3	11 ± 2.8	11.8 ± 3	13.4 ± 2.9	12.1 ± 3.0	11.8 ± 2.0	10 ± 1.5
	Closed	8.1 ± 1.7	8.3 ± 1.7	8.9 ± 2.1	9.5 ± 2.4	9.8 ± 1.9	10 ± 1.9	10.1 ± 1.9	8 ± 1.1
Pulse rate	Open	58 ± 10	85 ± 11	92 ± 12	100 ± 15	118 ± 12	120 ± 11	100 ± 13	90 ± 9
	Closed	55 ± 10	60 ± 14	65 ± 12	63 ± 18	75 ± 16	80 ± 10	68 ± 18	65 ± 13
Systolic blood pressure	Open	115 ± 17	114 ± 12	110 ± 10	90 ± 10	81 ± 18	65 ± 20	110 ± 12	118 ± 20
	Closed	122 ± 10	128 ± 8	115 ± 17	110 ± 14	102 ± 20	100 ± 15	125 ± 10	122 ± 18
Urinary output (mL)	Open		220	310	380	400	500	180	
	Closed		160	180	210	280	310	140	

4.3. Personnel Safety. The issue of personnel safety arises with the administration of HIPEC, especially when implementing the open technique, as exposure to chemotherapeutics may result in toxic and possibly mutagenic effects on the surgical team.

Recently, it has been reported that no platinum was detected in the internal aspect of surgical gloves with neither the closed nor the open method of intraperitoneal delivery of oxaliplatin [6].

A previous study evaluated the risk of exposure to platinum in members of the surgical team and demonstrated minimal concentration in the blood and urine of the personnel, below safety threshold [12].

This suggests that, with either method, HIPEC is safe for the operating theatre personnel, given that standard protective measures are taken.

4.4. Laparoscopic HIPEC. A most novel method of administrating intraperitoneal chemotherapy is the laparoscopic

approach [13]. In terms of efficacy, an animal study demonstrated increased drug perfusion with the laparoscopic technique [14]. Two recent cohorts of patients treated with laparoscopic cytoreductive surgery and HIPEC versus laparotomy presented no significant differences in postoperative morbidity and mortality between the two approaches, identifying laparoscopic HIPEC as a safe and efficient alternative [15, 16].

The consensus statement issued by the Peritoneal Surface Oncology Group International after the meeting in Milan in 2006 reached the conclusion that the best technique to deliver HIPEC is the open one, without sufficient evidence in the literature to prove the superiority of one technique over the other regarding outcome, morbidity, and personnel safety [17, 18].

5. Conclusion

Both the open and the closed abdomen technique are safe and efficient methods of HIPEC delivery in the treatment of

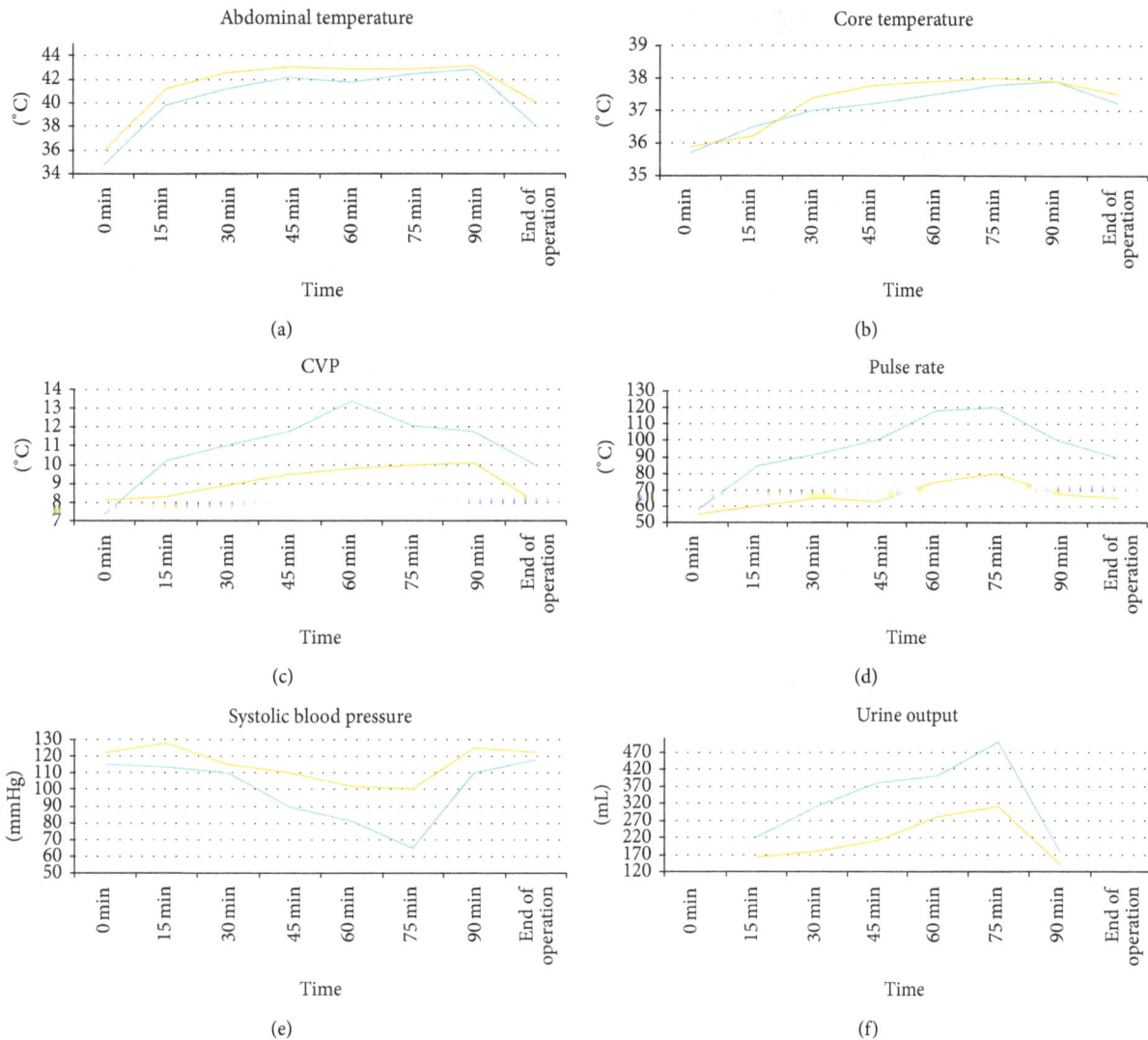

FIGURE 2: (a) Abdominal temperature. Blue = open, yellow = closed. (b) Core temperature. Blue = open, yellow = closed. (c) Central venous pressure. Blue = open, yellow = closed. (d) Heart rate. Blue = open, yellow = closed. (e) Systolic blood pressure. Blue = open, yellow = closed. (f) Urine output. Blue = open, yellow = closed.

peritoneal carcinomatosis, causing no significant haemodynamic disturbances, and are of equal morbidity and mortality. However, the more stable conditions ensured by the closed technique make it more appropriate for frail patients.

References

[1] S. González-Moreno, L. A. González-Bayón, and G. Ortega-Pérez, "Hyperthermic intraperitoneal chemotherapy: rationale and technique," *World Journal of Gastrointestinal Oncology*, vol. 2, no. 2, pp. 68–75, 2010.

[2] F.-P. Desgranges, A. Steghens, H. Rosay et al., "Epidural analgesia for surgical treatment of peritoneal carcinomatosis: a risky technique?" *Annales Francaises d'Anesthesie et de Reanimation*, vol. 31, no. 1, pp. 53–59, 2012.

[3] J. Pascual-Ramírez, S. Sánchez García, F. González Ruiz de la Herrán et al., "Security and efficiency of a closed-system, turbulent-flow circuit for hyperthermic intraperitoneal chemotherapy after cytoreductive ovarian surgery: perioperative outputs," *Archives of Gynecology and Obstetrics*, vol. 290, no. 1, pp. 121–129, 2014.

[4] C. Schmidt, M. Creutzenberg, P. Piso, J. Hobbhahn, and M. Bucher, "Peri-operative anaesthetic management of cytoreductive surgery with hyperthermic intraperitoneal chemotherapy," *Anaesthesia*, vol. 63, no. 4, pp. 389–395, 2008.

[5] V. I. Rankovic, V. P. Masirevic, M. J. Pavlov et al., "Hemodynamic and cardiovascular problems during modified hyperthermic intraperitoneal perioperative chemotherapy," *Hepato-Gastroenterology*, vol. 54, no. 74, pp. 364–366, 2007.

[6] O. Facy, C. Combier, M. Poussier et al., "High pressure does not counterbalance the advantages of open techniques over closed techniques during heated intraperitoneal chemotherapy with oxaliplatin," *Surgery*, vol. 157, no. 1, pp. 72–78, 2015.

[7] J. Spiliotis, A. Vaxevanidou, A. Datsis, A. Rogdakis, and S. Kekelos, "Peritoneal carcinomatosis: intra-operative and post-operative assessment of patients undergoing cytoreduction and HIPEC," *Hepato-Gastroenterology*, vol. 57, no. 102-103, pp. 1052–1059, 2010.

[8] H. N. López-Basave, F. Morales-Vasquez, C. Mendez-Herrera et al., "Intensive care unit admission after cytoreductive surgery and hyperthermic intraperitoneal chemotherapy. Is it necessary?" *Journal of Oncology*, vol. 2014, Article ID 307317, 6 pages, 2014.

[9] J. D. Spiliotis, A. Rogdakis, A. Vaxevanidou, A. Datsis, G. Zacharis, and A. Christopoulou, "Morbidity and mortality of cytoreductive surgery and hyperthermic intraperitoneal chemotherapy in the management of peritoneal carcinomatosis," *Journal of B.U.ON.*, vol. 14, no. 2, pp. 259–264, 2009.

[10] P. Ortega-Deballon, O. Facy, S. Jambet et al., "Which method to deliver hyperthermic intraperitoneal chemotherapy with oxaliplatin? An experimental comparison of open and closed techniques," *Annals of Surgical Oncology*, vol. 17, no. 7, pp. 1957–1963, 2010.

[11] L. Benoit, N. Cheynel, P. Ortega-Deballon, G. D. Giacomo, B. Chauffert, and P. Rat, "Closed hyperthermic intraperitoneal chemotherapy with open abdomen: a novel technique to reduce exposure of the surgical team to chemotherapy drugs," *Annals of Surgical Oncology*, vol. 15, no. 2, pp. 542–546, 2008.

[12] H. Mahteme, S. N. Andréasson, H. Anundi, S.-B. Thorén, and H. Ehrsson, "Is platinum present in blood and urine from treatment givers during hyperthermic intraperitoneal chemotherapy?" *Journal of Oncology*, vol. 2010, Article ID 649719, 4 pages, 2010.

[13] E. A. Halkia, J. Kyriazanos, E. Efstathiou, and J. D. Spiliotis, "Laparoscopic hyperthermic intraperitoneal chemotherapy for the management of advanced peritoneal carcinomatosis," *Hepato-Gastroenterology*, vol. 58, no. 112, pp. 1915–1917, 2011.

[14] A. Gesson-Paute, G. Ferron, F. Thomas, E. C. de Lara, E. Chatelut, and D. Querleu, "Pharmacokinetics of oxaliplatin during open versus laparoscopically assisted heated intraoperative intraperitoneal chemotherapy (HIPEC): an experimental study," *Annals of Surgical Oncology*, vol. 15, no. 1, pp. 339–344, 2008.

[15] R. Fish, C. Selvasekar, P. Crichton et al., "Risk-reducing laparoscopic cytoreductive surgery and hyperthermic intraperitoneal chemotherapy for low-grade appendiceal mucinous neoplasm: early outcomes and technique," *Surgical Endoscopy and Other Interventional Techniques*, vol. 28, no. 1, pp. 341–345, 2014.

[16] G. Passot, N. Bakrin, S. Isaac et al., "Postoperative outcomes of laparoscopic vs open cytoreductive surgery plus hyperthermic intraperitoneal chemotherapy for treatment of peritoneal surface malignancies," *European Journal of Surgical Oncology*, vol. 40, no. 8, pp. 957–962, 2014.

[17] J. Esquivel, "Technology of hyperthermic intraperitoneal chemotherapy in the United States, Europe, China, Japan, and Korea," *Cancer Journal (Sudbury, Mass)*, vol. 15, no. 3, pp. 249–254, 2009.

[18] O. Glehen, E. Cotte, S. Kusamura et al., "Hyperthermic intraperitoneal chemotherapy: nomenclature and modalities of perfusion," *Journal of Surgical Oncology*, vol. 98, no. 4, pp. 242–246, 2008.

5

Minimising Unnecessary Mastectomies in a Predominantly Chinese Community

Mona P. Tan,[1] Nadya Y. Sitoh,[2] and Yih Y. Sitoh[3]

[1]Breast Surgical Oncology, MammoCare, 38 Irrawaddy No. 06-21, Singapore 329563
[2]MammoCare, 38 Irrawaddy No. 06-21, Singapore 329563
[3]Medical Education, Mount Elizabeth Hospital, 3 Mount Elizabeth No. 17-16, Singapore 228510

Correspondence should be addressed to Mona P. Tan; jabezhopems@gmail.com

Academic Editor: C. H. Yip

Background. Recent data shows that the use of breast conservation treatment (BCT) for breast cancer may result in superior outcomes when compared with mastectomy. However, reported rates of BCT in predominantly Chinese populations are significantly lower than those reported in Western countries. Low BCT rates may now be a concern as they may translate into suboptimal outcomes. A study was undertaken to evaluate BCT rates in a cohort of predominantly Chinese women. *Methods.* All patients who underwent surgery on the breast at the authors' healthcare facility between October 2008 and December 2011 were included in the study and outcomes of treatment were evaluated. *Results.* A total of 171 patients were analysed. Two-thirds of the patients were of Chinese ethnicity. One hundred and fifty-six (85.9%) underwent BCT. Ninety-eight of 114 Chinese women (86%) underwent BCT. There was no difference in the proportion of women undergoing BCT based on ethnicity. After a median of 49 months of follow-up, three patients (1.8%) had local recurrence and 5 patients (2.9%) suffered distant metastasis. Four patients (2.3%) have died from their disease. *Conclusion.* BCT rates exceeding 80% in a predominantly Chinese population are possible with acceptable local and distant control rates, thereby minimising unnecessary mastectomies.

1. Introduction

As a result of prospective randomised controlled trials (RCTs) beginning in the 1970s, breast conservation therapy (BCT) was adopted as an appropriate alternative for the treatment of breast cancer and has been an accepted option for more than three decades [1–5]. A consensus statement in 1991 endorsed BCT as the surgical therapy of choice, for it offered similar survival rates while preserving the form of the breast 4]. Recent data suggests that in the presence of modern adjuvant therapies, instead of equivalent survival outcomes, BCT could be superior to mastectomy for the treatment of breast cancer [6–10]. A large retrospective analysis evaluating women with early breast cancer similar to those in one RCT demonstrated a higher 10-year breast-cancer-specific survival for women who had undergone BCT when compared with mastectomy with or without radiation [2, 6]. For patients who had characteristics unlike those in the RCTs, higher mastectomy rates were found to be associated with poorer survival outcomes [7–9], and, in a prospective series studying hormone-positive tumours, BCT resulted in lower local recurrence rates and improved survival [10].

Despite the longstanding acceptance of BCT, its utilisation in predominantly Chinese communities has been reported to be lower than in Western populations [6, 11–18]. Approximately 75–85% of women with early stage breast cancer are expected to be candidates for BCT [19], yet BCT rates in predominantly Chinese populations are reported to average 30%, even for T1-T2 tumours [11–15] (Table 1). An absolute improvement of 4% in breast-cancer-specific survival rates was reported with BCT rates of 70% [6]. It was also estimated that, for each 1-percentage-point rise in the mastectomy rate, there would be a concomitant fall in 7-year survival by 0.1% [7]. It can be inferred from these calculations that, on a population basis, no survival benefit is expected with a mastectomy rate of 70%. There is therefore a pressing need to relook at surgical treatment in predominantly Chinese communities as a persistently

TABLE 1: Comparison of published data for BCT rates.

Author	Centre/country/study period	n	Characteristics	% BCT
	Predominantly Chinese populations			
Sim et al. [11]	National Cancer Centre, Singapore (2001–2010)	5130	Stages 0–IV	29.2%
Wang et al. [12]	Changi General Hospital, Singapore (2002–2008)	761	Stages 0–IV	23.3%
Chang et al. [13]	National University Hospital, Singapore (1990–2007)	2449	Stages 0–IV	29.2%
Yip et al. [14]	University of Malaya Medical Centre (2001–2005)	953	T1, T2	29.7%
Yau et al. [15]	Pamela Y. Nethersole Eastern Hospital, Hong Kong (1994–2007)	2375	T1, T2	30%
	International/Western			
Agarwal et al. [6]	SEER database (1998–2008)	132149	Tumour ≤4 cm, ≤3 lymph node +	70%
McGuire et al. [16]	Moffitt Cancer Centre, FL, USA (1994–2007)	5865	Stages 0–IV	63.7%
Lee et al. [17]	University of Michigan Medical Centre, Michigan, USA (2003–2005)	993	Tis–T4	63%
Garcia-Etienne et al. [18]	EUSOMA (2003–2010)	15 369	Stages 0, I, and II (stage III, T3/T4 excluded)	73.3%
Current study	MammoCare, Singapore (2008–2011)	125	Symptomatic	82.4%
		46	Screen detected	95.6%
		171	Tis–T4	85.9%

BCT: breast conservation treatment.
SEER: surveillance, epidemiology, and end-result.
FL: Florida, USA: United States of America.
EUSOMA: European Society of Breast Cancer Specialists.

low BCT rate could translate to suboptimal outcomes. The reasons cited for low BCT rates include cultural preferences, surgeon bias, and factors relating to physical attributes [11–15]. Chinese women have been shown to have smaller breast tissue volume [20], which poses challenges for good cosmetic outcomes in BCT [21]. This study was therefore performed to review the authors' experience in treating women with BCT in a predominantly Chinese community, evaluate BCT rates in this cohort, and compare it with prior reports.

2. Materials and Methods

A retrospective analysis of all patients with breast malignancies who underwent operative treatment by clinicians at this medical facility between October 2008 and December 2011 was performed. Preoperative diagnostic workup consisted of clinical examination and standard imaging with mammography and sonography, and percutaneous needle biopsies were done for diagnosis where possible. In certain clinical settings where percutaneous biopsy was not possible or inconclusive, like where there was insufficient compression thickness or discordant imaging and biopsy results, a surgical diagnostic procedure was performed. Routine magnetic resonance imaging (MRI) was not done.

Following diagnosis, patients deemed eligible for BCT were given the option of an attempt at breast conservation or to proceed directly to mastectomy, with or without reconstruction. Eligibility for BCT was made based on the surgeon's assessment of the ability to achieve a reasonable cosmetic result after tumour resection with clear margins. Multifocal and multicentric breast cancers (MFMCBC) were not considered to be ineligible if preoperative evaluation indicated the possibility of en bloc excision of all foci through a single incision. If the tumour(s) was assessed to be too large, the patient was offered neoadjuvant medical therapy and had placement of radioopaque clip(s) prior to its commencement. These were localised before wide excision, which was guided by the position(s) of the marker clip(s).

Patients who were assessed to be eligible for BCT and who agreed to undergo a trial of BCT had wide excision of their lesion(s) performed through a single incision. Incisions were planned such that they coursed over the lesions where possible. In the instances where there were more than one tumour foci, the incision was sited above at least one of the lesions. If the other lesion(s) were more than 2 cm away from the incision, radioopaque clips were positioned in the tumour bed for ease of radiotherapy administration. Following tumour extirpation with negative margins, partial mastectomy defects were repaired using local tissue rearrangement techniques only. This was performed by mobilising full thickness parenchymal flaps off the pectoralis fascia, advancing the pillars and directly apposing them with sutures. None of the patients had volume replacement using autologous flaps or implants.

All patients who were intended for BCT had intraoperative frozen section analysis (IFSA) for margins status. If margins were positive at the time of surgery, further margins were excised until proven to be negative. These were reassessed at paraffin sections. Successful BCT of MFMCBC was defined as operative attainment of clear margins (no ink on tumour) [22] and a reasonable cosmetic outcome. In clinical scenarios where this was thought to be unattainable, mastectomy was recommended. Mastectomy was also performed for patients according to preference for breast removal rather than BCT.

The patients were referred both to a medical oncologist and to radiation oncologists for discussions relating to the need for further adjuvant treatment. Patients were considered to have completed therapy if they adhered to recommended treatment regimens. Systemic therapy was given based on the discretion of the treating medical oncologist. Whole breast irradiation was given for women who underwent BCT with a boost to the tumour bed according to the preference of the radiation oncologist. Patients who underwent mastectomy with large tumours, more than 3 positive axillary lymph nodes, and lymphovascular invasion were treated with post-mastectomy radiotherapy.

Statistical analyses of the respective associations were performed using SPSS (Chicago, IL) version 11 advanced statistical software module. Comparisons of categorical variables were performed using the chi-squared test. Continuous variables with median or mean values were compared using the Student's t-test or Mann-Whitney U test where appropriate.

3. Results

A total of 177 female patients were treated during the study period. However, 6 were lost to follow-up before any cancer-related events were noted, leaving 171 for analysis. Clinico-pathological characteristics of the cohort are summarised in Table 2. Of note, 147 patients (86%) underwent BCT. Twenty-four patients had a mastectomy. Fifteen of these (62.5%) had contraindications to BCT based on size and improbability of attaining negative margins without compromising cosmesis, while nine elected to have a mastectomy despite being eligible for BCT. The mean age of these patients who chose a mastectomy was 58 years, which was significantly higher than that of those who underwent BCT, whose mean age was 47.9 years ($P = 0.003$). There was no significant difference between the mean ages of patients who had BCT and those who underwent mastectomy out of necessity (mean age: 50.1 years) based on therapeutic principles ($P = 0.40$). The majority of the cohort was Chinese (66.7%) and was generally expected to have smaller volume breast tissue than women of other ethnicities [15, 20]. There were a fair proportion of Caucasian women and women of other ethnic origins as well, and no difference in the proportion of women undergoing BCT based on ethnicity was demonstrated ($P = 0.88$).

One hundred and fifty-six of the total of 171 (91.2%) were assessed to be suitable candidates for BCT. However, nine patients of 156 (5.8%) decided against BCT. The main reasons given by these few patients were a perceived superiority of survival with mastectomy and reduction of anxiety relating to follow-up. The mean tumour size for patients who underwent BCT was 19.2 mm, while that for women who elected for mastectomy despite being suitable candidates for BCT was 18.3 mm. There was no significant difference between the two groups ($P = 0.83$). In contrast, there was a significant

Table 2: Summary of demographic, clinicopathologic, and outcome data for study population.

Clinicopathologic characteristic	All patients (n = 171)	(%)	BCT (n = 147)	(%)	Mastectomy (n = 24) By need (15)	(%)	By choice (9)	(%)	P value
Age in years									
Median (range)	48 (28–78)								
Mean (SD)	48.6 (10)		47.9 (10)		50.1 (8.8)				0.40
Mean (SD)			47.9 (10)				58.0 (6.9)		*0.003*
Ethnicity									0.88
Chinese	114	(66.7)	98/114	(86.0)	8/114	(7.0)	8/114	(7.0)	
Malay/Indonesian	12	(7.0)	10/12	(83.3)	2/12	(16.7)	0/12		
Indian	11	(6.4)	10/11	(91.0)	1/11	(9.0)	0/12		
Other Asian	14	(8.2)	13/14	(92.9)	1/14	(7.1)	0/14		
Caucasian	20	(11.7)	16/20	(80.0)	3/20	(15.0)	1/20	(5.0)	
Mode of presentation									0.07
Symptomatic tumours	125	(73.1)	103/125	(82.4)	13/125	(10.4)	9/125	(7.2)	
Screen detected lesions	46	(26.9)	44/46	(95.6)	2/46	(4.3)	0		
All patients	171		147/171	(85.9)	15/171	(8.8)	9/171	(5.3)	
Tumour size in mm (range)									
Median (range)	19.0 (3–97)		18.0 (3–72)		35.0 (4–97)		15.9 (3–35)		
Mean (SD)	21.1 (15.4)		19.2 (12.1)		40.5 (28.0)				*0.000*
(DCIS included)			19.2 (12.1)				18.3 (12.9)		0.83
≤20 mm	108	(63.2)	100/108	(92.6)	4/108	(3.7)	4/108	(3.7)	
21–50 mm	51	(29.8)	39/51	(76.5)	7/51	(13.7)	4/51	(7.8)	
>50 mm	9	(5.3)	6/9	(66.7)	3/9	(33.3)	0		
T4	3	(1.8)	2/3	(66.7)	1/3	(33.3)			
Pathologic stage									*<0.001*
0	22	(12.9)	20/22	(90.1)	1/22	(4.5)	1/22	(4.5)	
I	70	(41.0)	69/70	(98.6)	1	(1.4)	0		
II	55	(32.2)	46/55	(83.6)	4/55	(7.3)	5/55	(9.1)	
III	21	(12.3)	11/221	(52.4)	8/21	(38.1)	2/21	(9.5)	
IV	1	(0.6)	0		1				
Unknown	2	(1.2)	1/2				1/2		
Histological type									0.34
DCIS	22	(12.9)	20/22	(91.0)	1/22	(4.5)	1/22	(4.5)	
Invasive ductal	132	(77.2)	114/132	(86.4)	11/132	(8.3)	7/125	(5.6)	
Invasive lobular	7	(4.1)	5/7	(71.4)	1/7	(1.4)	1/7	(1.4)	
Other invasive	10	(5.8)	8/10	(80.0)	2/10	(20)			
Grade									0.48
DCIS	22	(12.9)	20/22	(91.0)	1/22	(4.5)	1/22	(4.5)	
1	29	(17.0)	28/29	(96.5)	1/29	(3.6)	0		
2	61	(35.6)	50/61	(81.7)	6/61	(9.8)	5/61	(8.2)	
3	54	(31.6)	44/54	(81.5)	7/54	(13.0)	3/54	(5.6)	
Unknown	5	(2.9)	4/4	(100)					
Neoadjuvant medical therapy									*<0.001*
Yes	25	(14.6)	16/25	(64.0)	8/25	(32.0)	1/25	(4.0)	
No	146	(85.4)	131/146	(89.7)	7/146	(4.8)	8/146	(4.8)	
Disease extent									0.97
Unifocal	128	(74.6)	110/128	(85.9)	11/128	(8.6)	7/128	(5.5)	
Multiple foci at diagnosis	43	(25.1)	34/40	(85)	4/40	(10)	2/40	(5)	

BCT: breast conservation surgery; SD: standard deviation; DCIS: ductal carcinoma in situ.

difference in the mean tumour sizes of women who had BCT and those who were advised to undergo a mastectomy, the latter group of which had a mean tumour size of 40.5 mm ($P < 0.001$).

Four patients in the cohort (2.3%) required a second therapeutic surgical procedure, three for undetected multicentric tumours seen on postoperative imaging and a fourth for a falsely negative sentinel lymph node (SLN) at IFSA. The last patient had multifocal disease with two separate foci of invasive ductal carcinoma, grade III, 35 mm and 8 mm, and 2 of 22 lymph nodes involved. All four patients who needed reoperation had multifocal or multicentric breast cancers (MFMCBC) and are currently disease-free. The mean pathologic tumour size for those requiring reoperation was 32.3 mm, while those who had a single operation had a mean tumour size of 20.8 mm ($P = 0.14$). There were no patients who required a reexcision on the basis of false negative margins at IFSA.

The median follow-up period was 49 months (range 21–68 months). None of the 22 patients who presented with ductal carcinoma in situ only developed locoregional recurrence or distant metastasis. Of the other 149 patients with invasive carcinoma, two patients who underwent BCT developed local failure (1.4%). A total of four patients with invasive disease, two who had undergone BCT and two mastectomy, developed distant disease and have succumbed to their disease (2.3%). A summary of locoregional and distant events is given in Table 3.

4. Discussion

The last two decades of the twentieth century witnessed a paradigm shift of treatment concepts for breast cancer, with definitive evidence from prospective randomised trials demonstrating that performing less surgery resulted in equivalent survival outcomes. This led to the establishment of BCT and a steady increase in its utilisation. Unexpectedly, in the last decade, a rising trend of mastectomy rates has been observed in some Western communities [16, 23]. Despite this rise, mastectomy rates for early breast cancer in these countries are still lower than the high rates reported in predominantly Chinese populations. Mastectomy rates need to be reexamined in the presence of contemporary reports indicating possible higher cancer-specific survival, lower surgical complication rates, cost-effectiveness of treatment, and improved quality of life outcomes with BCT [6–10, 21, 24–28]. This is juxtaposed against the possible psychological benefit that mastectomy and contralateral prophylactic mastectomy (CPM) offer [24, 29], but the diminution of anxiety might not completely compensate for poorer quality of life outcomes with longer breast cancer survivorship [26, 30].

Specifically for predominantly Chinese populations, reasons cited for low BCT rates include cultural preferences, surgeon bias, and factors relating to physical attributes [11–15]. Addressing the issue of physical attributes first, Chinese women tend to have smaller volume breast (SVB) tissue which may pose a barrier to BCT [15, 20]. In this series, overall BCT rate was 85.9%. Among Chinese women, who formed two-thirds of the cohort, BCT rate was 86%. There

was no significant difference of the proportion of Chinese women undergoing BCT compared with women of other ethnic groups. In particular, 80% of Caucasian women had BCT. This rate is similar to other reported series in a Western context (Table 1). This data appears to suggest that the physical attributes of Chinese women may not have a significant impact on BCT rates. In a study by Collins et al., of 125 women who were eligible for either BCT or mastectomy, 35% elected to have a mastectomy [31]. In the present study, of 156 patients who were considered eligible for BCT or mastectomy, only 5.8% decided against breast conservation. This data suggests that the local Chinese culture may be a factor in favour of BCT, rather than a condition in support of high mastectomy rates.

Another factor influencing patient decision for mastectomy is surgeon's advice [32]. In this study, 156 of 171 patients (91.2%) were assessed preoperatively to be suitable candidates for BCT. Nine patients decided in favour of mastectomy, making utilisation of BCT in this cohort 94.2%. Eligible patients who decided for mastectomy had a mean tumour size not significantly different from those who underwent successful BCT. Hence, it is reasonable to conclude that successful BCT would have been possible for this group of women, suggesting that, on the whole, eligibility of Chinese women for BCT is not significantly different from women of other ethnic origins. The difference perhaps is surgeon philosophy, which may account for varying reported mastectomy rates in different geographical locations [23, 33]. Surgeons with a strong bias toward mastectomy will require clinical circumstances extremely favourable for BCT before contemplating it, while surgeons whose default position is conservative surgery would be more inclined to explore innovative methods of achieving BCT even in challenging clinical situations. The development of oncoplastic breast surgery was likely the result of this creative pressure. There are several categories of techniques that fall into this broad description. The authors prefer the use of only volume displacement or local tissue rearrangement techniques with direct apposition of adequately mobilised residual uninvolved parenchymal pillars with sutures. This approach results in better patient satisfaction than mastopexy and avoids the issues with surgical clip migration with the use of mammoplasty techniques which require extensive tissue mobilization [21, 34, 35]. Moreover, local tissue rearrangement techniques result in lower complication rates and superior cosmetic outcomes compared to complex reconstructive techniques [21].

Although the presence of multicentric disease, or MFMCBC, is a conventional contraindication for BCT [36], a recent expert consensus considers this scenario a relative rather than an absolute contraindication [37]. MFMCBC pose technical challenges for BCT but may be surmounted with careful attention to surgical planning and technique. Patients initially considered ineligible for BCT by some surgeons might in fact be suitable candidates once appropriate measures are applied, avoiding "unnecessary mastectomies." Examples of these situations are depicted in Figures 1 and 2. Based on imaging findings and percutaneous biopsy results, these two patients were recommended to have a mastectomy at another tertiary referral cancer centre. A second

TABLE 3: List of patients with posttreatment events.

Presentation	Treatment	Time to local recurrence	Time to distant recurrence	Treatment for recurrence	Comments/outcome
T3N1	Neoadjuvant chemotherapy, BCT, RT	Four months	Nil	Mastectomy	Disease-free at 57 months
T3N2	Neoadjuvant chemotherapy, mastectomy, RT	Nil	35 months, visceral, bony	Chemotherapy	Succumbed at 42 months
T2N2	BCT, adjuvant chemotherapy, RT	33 months	33 months, visceral	Declined treatment	Lost to follow-up
T3N3	Disease progression during neoadjuvant chemotherapy, mastectomy, RT	8 months	15 months, CNS	Declined further chemotherapy, VP shunt	Succumbed at 20 months
T3N1	Neoadjuvant chemotherapy, BCT, RT	Nil	9 months, CNS	Declined further chemotherapy	Died 13 months after surgery
T3N0	Neoadjuvant chemotherapy, BCT, RT	Nil	12 months, CNS	Chemotherapy	Died 19 months after surgery

BCT: breast conservation treatment.

RT: radiotherapy.

CNS: recurrence in the central nervous system.

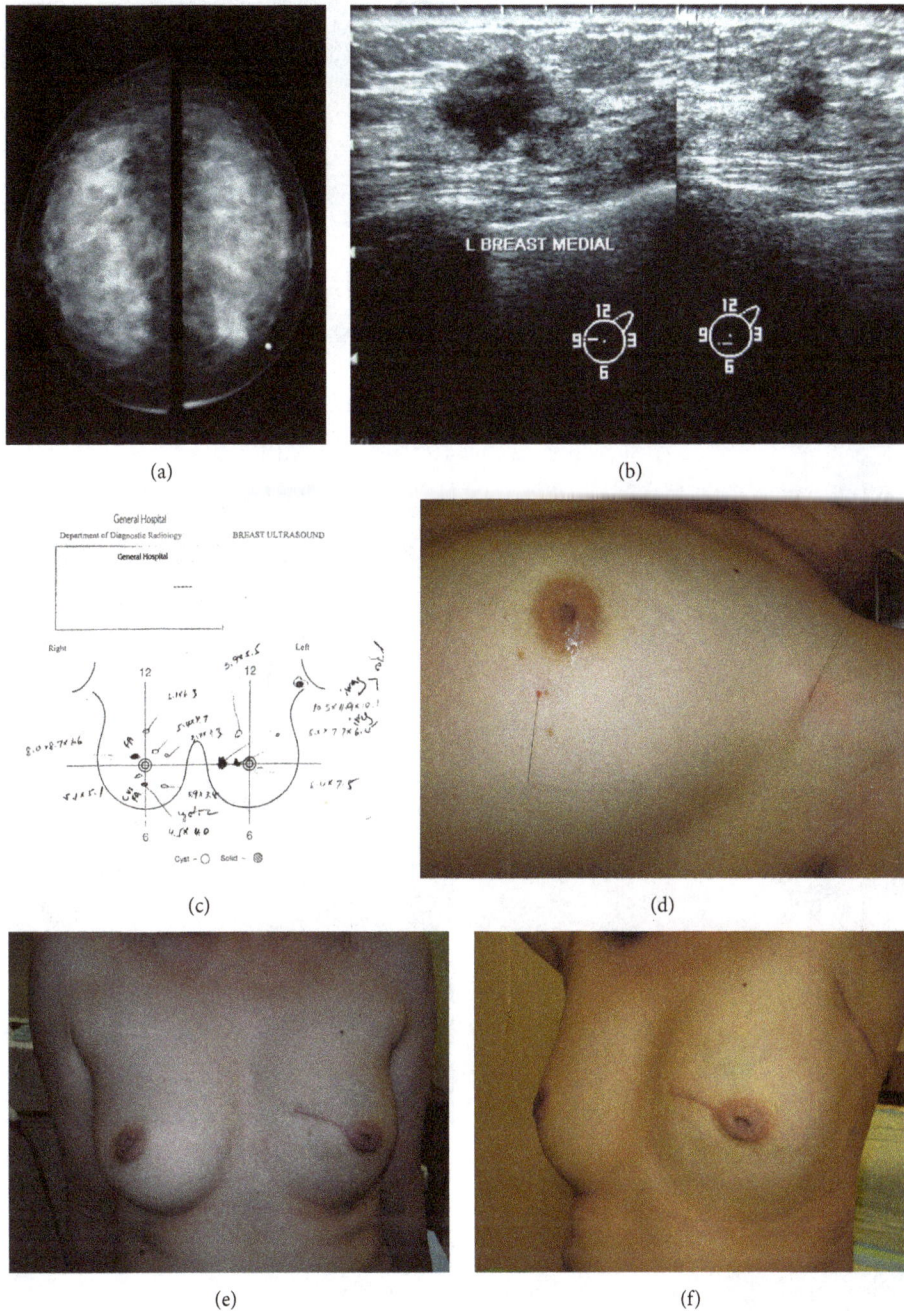

FIGURE 1: ((a)–(f)) Avoiding mastectomy in a patient with "multifocal tumour" on imaging. This 45-year-old patient was diagnosed with what was thought to be multifocal invasive ductal carcinoma at another facility following core biopsy. Mastectomy was originally recommended at the first centre due to the presence of multiple synchronous ipsilateral tumours and proximity of one lesion to the nipple. She sought a second opinion at the authors' facility and was agreeable to a "trial of breast conservation treatment." Localisation of the impalpable periareolar lesion and of the suspicious axillary lymph node was performed. She underwent an en bloc wide excision of the two left breast lesions through a boomerang incision and axillary staging through a separate axillary incision. The sentinel node coincided with the localised node and was found to be positive for metastasis on frozen section analysis. She underwent axillary dissection at the same operation. Histology was reported as a 4 cm invasive ductal carcinoma, with no intervening normal tissue between the clinical lesions. Three of sixteen axillary lymph nodes were involved. She is currently disease-free after more than 5 years.

opinion was sought with the authors and they were willing to undergo a "trial of BCT." Both underwent successful BCT and are now disease-free more than five years after surgical treatment. Sometimes, approaches which contravene conventional guideline recommendations are necessary. For example, unlike guidelines which recommend skin crease incisions [36], radial incisions may be necessary to incorporate larger lesions, multiple tumours, and allow adequate

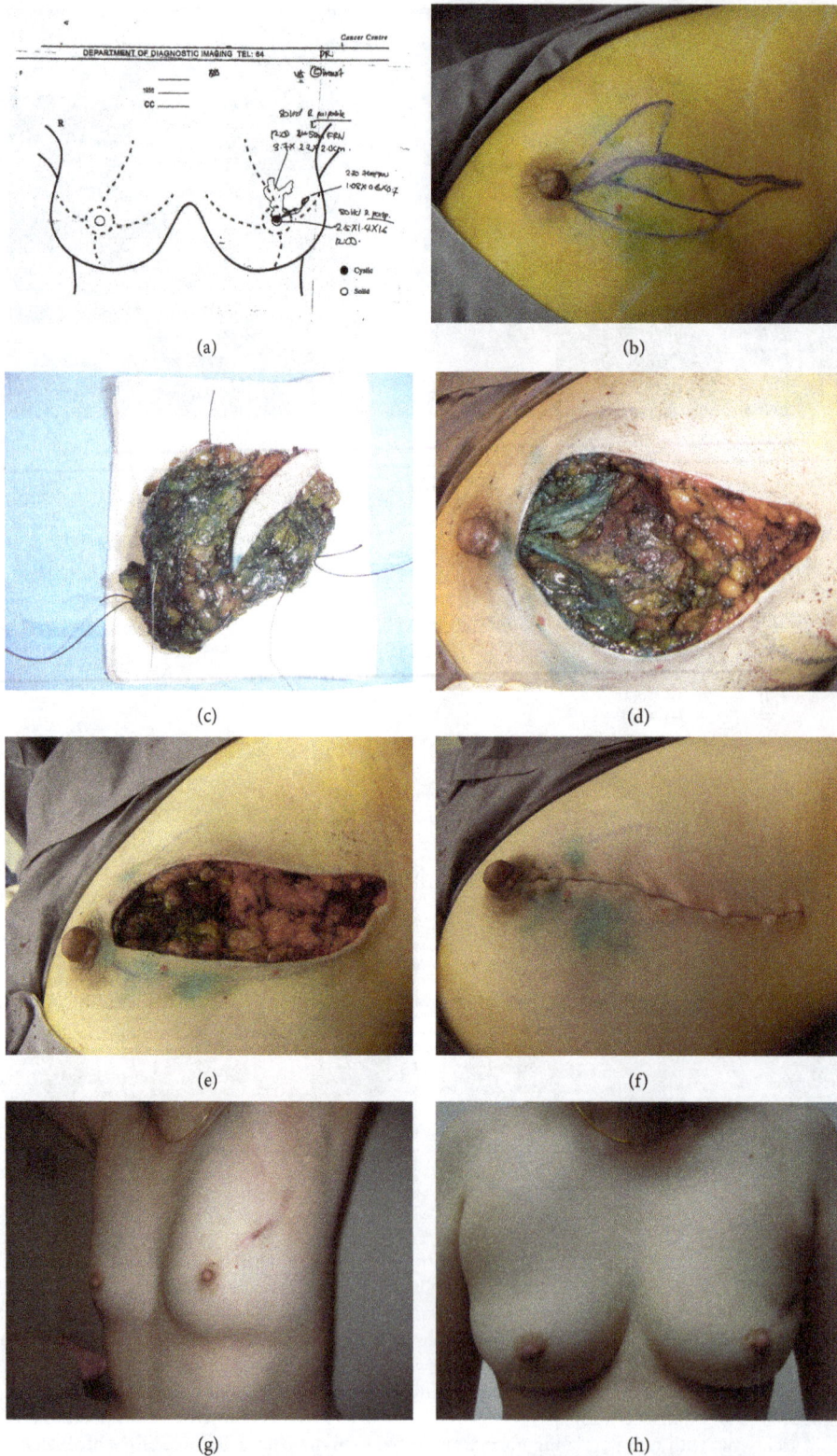

FIGURE 2: ((a)–(h)) Avoiding mastectomy in a patient with "multicentric tumour" on imaging. This patient was diagnosed to have high grade ductal carcinoma in situ (DCIS) at an oncology centre and was offered mastectomy on the assumption that this was a multicentric lesion. She sought a second opinion with the authors and was agreeable to a "trial of breast conservation treatment." Just prior to surgery, the lateral and medial extents of her dual-segment disease were localised under ultrasound guidance. Tissue resection was planned as indicated to balance the need for negative margins and retention of sufficient uninvolved parenchyma for defect repair. Through a radial incision and eccentric ellipse, an en bloc resection of the lesion using a multisegment resection pattern was performed. Sentinel node biopsy was performed through the same incision for this palpable high grade DCIS. Histology was reported as a unifocal 25 mm high grade DCIS. No multicentric component could be identified. She completed all adjuvant treatment and is now disease-free more than 5 years after surgery.

exposure for remodelling to avoid deformity [38, 39] (Figures 1 and 2).

Advances in imaging resulted in an improved ability to identify multiple tumour foci. However, recent data suggest that this increase in identification of MFMCBC with MRI results in higher mastectomy rates without definitive improvement in survival outcomes [40, 41]. Hence, a selective approach should be taken with the use of preoperative MRI. In this study, because preoperative MRI was not used, four patients, all of whom had multiple ipsilateral cancers, required a reoperation. MRI may be applied when multiple cancers or extensive microcalcifications are detected on conventional imaging to avoid reoperations. However, further work may be necessary in this area to assess specific selection criteria for its use to balance this need against a potential for increasing mastectomy use in this group of patients.

The reported rise in mastectomy rates is observed with a concomitant increase in the use of contralateral prophylactic mastectomy (CPM) [24, 25]. Factors contributing to this phenomenon include the use of preoperative MRI, the presence of multicentric disease, the availability of reconstructive surgery, fear of cancer recurrence, concerns over the risk of contralateral breast cancer (CBC), and a perceived survival benefit with mastectomy [24, 29]. The first three factors, which may also influence high mastectomy rates in Chinese populations, are clinician related and have been discussed earlier. The latter three involve patient psychology and information dissemination for decision-making. Data on how communication methods and decision aids affect patient's surgical decisions is varied [31–33, 42]. It is interesting to note that BCT tends to be preferred in women without breast cancer [43], but once diagnosed, higher mastectomy rates as the definitive operation were reported with greater patient involvement in decision-making [44]. In the light of recent data that higher mastectomy rates could lead to poorer survival outcomes, a reexamination of patient decision-making processes is needed. One factor which may influence patient choice in favour of mastectomy despite eligibility for BCT is the availability of reconstruction [24]. While reconstruction does lead to improved body image [26], its availability prior to a "trial of BCT" may have an adverse effect on BCT rates, possibly encouraging not only mastectomy but CPM as well. Some authors have concluded that, based on current evidence, the use of CPM for the purposes of risk reduction in sporadic breast cancer is unjustified [25, 44]. Other investigators share a different opinion [24]. Arriving at the delicate balance between a paternalistic approach recommending treatment associated with evidence-based superior outcomes and allowing patient autonomy in decision-making is complex and elusive. This difficulty can make a "simple can be harder than complex" situation in the pursuit of improvements in BCT [19]. Further work on this subject is warranted.

In a surgical era where there is increasing public acceptance towards less invasive procedures for equivalent outcomes in breast cancer, as has been seen in the paradigm shifts with percutaneous breast biopsies and the management of the axilla, it is perplexing that BCT rates are persistently low in predominantly Chinese communities, and mastectomy and CPM rates are rising in other populations. Recent data showing the potential for improved survival, lower complication rates, cost-effectiveness, and better body image during survivorship with BCT [6–10, 21, 25, 26] behoves clinicians to consider means of increasing its utilisation. The surgeon factor has been shown to affect BCT rates [32, 45, 46]. The data in this study appears to support this conclusion. It may be reasonable to surmise that surgeons recommending BCT apply operative techniques to surmount patient's physical attributes of SVB. Careful attention to clinical approaches and surgical technique may raise BCT rates in a predominantly Chinese community from approximately 30% to 86%, minimising unnecessary mastectomies in this population. Further work is needed to investigate if the concepts for improving utilisation of BCT in a population with prevailing low BCT rates may be applied in other settings to reverse a trend of rising mastectomy rates.

The retrospective nature of this study and small cohort are limitations to this study. In addition, the authors' practice in a private healthcare facility may serve as a selection bias where women who actively sought BCT were treated at the authors' facility. Notwithstanding, the distribution of tumour sizes is not dissimilar from other reports where oncoplastic reduction mammoplasty was performed [34, 35], indicating that the concepts discussed herein may be applicable to other healthcare settings to raise BCT rates.

5. Conclusion

Higher BCT rates demonstrated in this study than previously reported for predominantly Chinese communities suggest that it is possible to minimise unnecessary mastectomies in this select population. Further work is needed to define modifying factors.

References

[1] U. Veronesi, N. Cascinelli, L. Mariani et al., "Twenty-year follow-up of a randomized study comparing breast-conserving surgery with radical mastectomy for early breast cancer," *New England Journal of Medicine*, vol. 347, no. 16, pp. 1227–1232, 2002.

[2] B. Fisher, S. Anderson, J. Bryant et al., "Twenty-year follow-up of a randomized trial comparing total mastectomy, lumpectomy, and lumpectomy plus irradiation for the treatment of invasive breast cancer," *The New England Journal of Medicine*, vol. 347, no. 16, pp. 1233–1241, 2002.

[3] M. M. Poggi, D. N. Danforth, L. C. Sciuto et al., "Eighteen-year results in the treatment of early breast carcinoma with mastectomy versus breast conservation therapy," *Cancer*, vol. 98, no. 4, pp. 697–702, 2003.

[4] "NIH consensus conference. Treatment of early-stage breast cancer," *The Journal of the American Medical Association*, vol. 265, no. 3, pp. 391–395, 1991.

[5] S. A. McLaughlin, "Surgical management of the breast: breast conservation therapy and mastectomy," *Surgical Clinics of North America*, vol. 93, no. 2, pp. 411–428, 2013.

[6] S. Agarwal, L. Pappas, L. Neumayer, K. Kokeny, and J. Agarwal, "Effect of breast conservation therapy vs mastectomy on disease-specific survival for early-stage breast cancer," *JAMA Surgery*, vol. 149, no. 3, pp. 267–274, 2014.

[7] J. M. Brooks, E. A. Chrischilles, M. B. Landrum et al., "Survival implications associated with variation in mastectomy rates for early-staged breast cancer," *International Journal of Surgical Oncology*, vol. 2012, Article ID 127854, 9 pages, 2012.

[8] N. L. Keating, M. B. Landrum, J. M. Brooks et al., "Outcomes following local therapy for early-stage breast cancer in non-trial populations," *Breast Cancer Research and Treatment*, vol. 125, no. 3, pp. 803–813, 2011.

[9] M. A. Schonberg, E. R. Marcantonio, D. Li, R. A. Silliman, L. Ngo, and E. P. McCarthy, "Breast cancer among the oldest old: tumor characteristics, treatment choices, and survival," *Journal of Clinical Oncology*, vol. 28, no. 12, pp. 2038–2045, 2010.

[10] M. van Hezewijk, E. Bastiaannet, H. Putter et al., "Effect of local therapy on locoregional recurrence in postmenopausal women with breast cancer in the Tamoxifen Exemestane Adjuvant Multinational (TEAM) trial," *Radiotherapy & Oncology*, vol. 108, no. 2, pp. 190–196, 2013.

[11] Y. Sim, V. K. M. Tan, G. H. Ho et al., "Contralateral prophylactic mastectomy in an Asian population: a single institution review," *Breast*, vol. 23, no. 1, pp. 56–62, 2013.

[12] W. V. Wang, S. M. Tan, and W. L. Chow, "The impact of mammographic breast cancer screening in Singapore: a comparison between screen-detected and symptomatic women," *Asian Pacific Journal of Cancer Prevention*, vol. 12, no. 10, pp. 2735–2740, 2011.

[13] G. Chang, C. W. Chan, and M. Hartman, "A commentary on delayed presentation of breast cancer in Singapore," *Asian Pacific Journal of Cancer Prevention*, vol. 12, no. 6, pp. 1635–1639, 2011.

[14] C. H. Yip, N. A. Taib, G. H. Tan, K. L. Ng, B. K. Yoong, and W. Y. Choo, "Predictors of axillary lymph node metastases in breast cancer: is there a role for minimal axillary surgery?" *World Journal of Surgery*, vol. 33, no. 1, pp. 54–57, 2009.

[15] T.-K. Yau, I. S. Soong, H. Sze et al., "Trends and patterns of breast conservation treatment in Hong Kong: 1994–2007," *International Journal of Radiation Oncology, Biology, Physics*, vol. 74, no. 1, pp. 98–103, 2009.

[16] K. P. McGuire, A. A. Santillan, P. Kaur et al., "Are mastectomies on the rise? A 13-year trend analysis of the selection of mastectomy versus breast conservation therapy in 5865 patients," *Annals of Surgical Oncology*, vol. 16, no. 10, pp. 2682–2690, 2009.

[17] M. C. Lee, K. Rogers, K. Griffith et al., "Determinants of breast conservation rates: reasons for mastectomy at a Comprehensive Cancer Center," *Breast Journal*, vol. 15, no. 1, pp. 34–40, 2009.

[18] C. A. Garcia-Etienne, M. Tomatis, J. Heil et al., "Mastectomy trends for early-stage breast cancer: a report from the EUSOMA multi-institutional European database," *European Journal of Cancer*, vol. 48, no. 13, pp. 1947–1956, 2012.

[19] I. T. Rubio, "Breast conservative surgery in breast cancer: simple can be harder than complex," *Journal of Surgical Oncology*, vol. 110, no. 1, p. 1, 2014.

[20] Q. Qiao, G. Zhou, and Y.-C. Ling, "Breast volume measurement in young Chinese women and clinical applications," *Aesthetic Plastic Surgery*, vol. 21, no. 5, pp. 362–368, 1997.

[21] S. J. Kronowitz, J. A. Feledy, K. K. Hunt et al., "Determining the optimal approach to breast reconstruction after partial mastectomy," *Plastic and Reconstructive Surgery*, vol. 117, no. 1, pp. 1–11, 2006.

[22] M. S. Moran, S. J. Schnitt, A. E. Giuliano et al., "Society of surgical oncology-American Society for Radiation Oncology consensus guideline on margins for breast-conserving surgery with whole-breast irradiation in stages I and II invasive breast cancer," *Annals of Surgical Oncology*, vol. 21, no. 3, pp. 704–716, 2014.

[23] A. E. Dragun, B. Huang, T. C. Tucker, and W. J. Spanos, "Increasing mastectomy rates among all age groups for early stage breast cancer: a 10-year study of surgical choice," *Breast Journal*, vol. 18, no. 4, pp. 318–325, 2012.

[24] A. Soran, A. K. Polat, R. Johnson, and K. P. McGuire, "Increasing trend of contralateral prophylactic mastectomy: what are the factors behind this phenomenon?" *Surgeon*, vol. 12, no. 6, pp. 316–322, 2014.

[25] A. Roberts, M. Habibi, and K. D. Frick, "Cost-effectiveness of contralateral prophylactic mastectomy for prevention of contralateral breast cancer," *Annals of Surgical Oncology*, vol. 21, no. 7, pp. 2209–2217, 2014.

[26] S.-Y. Fang, B.-C. Shu, and Y.-J. Chang, "The effect of breast reconstruction surgery on body image among women after mastectomy: a meta-analysis," *Breast Cancer Research and Treatment*, vol. 137, no. 1, pp. 13–21, 2013.

[27] J. Engel, J. Kerr, A. Schlesinger-Raab, H. Sauer, and D. Hölzel, "Quality of life following breast-conserving therapy or mastectomy: results of a 5-year prospective study," *Breast Journal*, vol. 10, no. 3, pp. 223–231, 2004.

[28] M. C. Lee, R. S. Bhati, E. E. von Rottenthaler et al., "Therapy choices and quality of life in young breast cancer survivors: a short-term follow-up," *The American Journal of Surgery*, vol. 206, no. 5, pp. 625–631, 2013.

[29] C. S. Fisher, T. Martin-Dunlap, M. B. Ruppel, F. Gao, J. Atkins, and J. A. Margenthaler, "Fear of recurrence and perceived survival benefit are primary motivators for choosing mastectomy over breast-conservation therapy regardless of age," *Annals of Surgical Oncology*, vol. 19, no. 10, pp. 3246–3250, 2012.

[30] N. L. Stout, J. M. Binkley, K. H. Schmitz et al., "A prospective surveillance model for rehabilitation for women with breast cancer," *Cancer*, vol. 118, no. 8, pp. 2191–2200, 2012.

[31] E. D. Collins, C. P. Moore, K. F. Clay et al., "Can women with early-stage breast cancer make an informed decision for mastectomy?" *Journal of Clinical Oncology*, vol. 27, no. 4, pp. 519–525, 2009.

[32] T. T. Fancher, J. A. Palesty, R. Thomas et al., "A woman's influence to choose mastectomy as treatment for breast cancer," *Journal of Surgical Research*, vol. 153, no. 1, pp. 128–131, 2009.

[33] R. S. Ballinger, K. F. Mayer, G. Lawrence, and L. Fallowfield, "Patients' decision-making in a UK specialist centre with high mastectomy rates," *Breast*, vol. 17, no. 6, pp. 574–579, 2008.

[34] B. R. Eaton, A. Losken, D. Okwan-Duodu et al., "Local recurrence patterns in breast cancer patients treated with oncoplastic reduction mammaplasty and radiotherapy," *Annals of Surgical Oncology*, vol. 21, no. 1, pp. 93–99, 2014.

[35] C. Eichler, M. Kolsch, A. Sauerwald, A. Bach, O. Gluz, and M. Warm, "Lumpectomy versus mastopexy—a post-surgery patient survey," *Anticancer Research*, vol. 33, no. 2, pp. 731–736, 2013.

[36] M. Morrow, E. A. Strom, L. W. Bassett et al., "Standard for breast conservation therapy in the management of invasive breast

carcinoma," *CA Cancer Journal for Clinicians*, vol. 52, no. 5, pp. 277–300, 2002.

[37] A. Goldhirsch, E. P. Winer, A. S. Coates et al., "Personalizing the treatment of women with early breast cancer: highlights of the st gallen international expert consensus on the primary therapy of early breast Cancer 2013," *Annals of Oncology*, vol. 24, no. 9, pp. 2206–2223, 2013.

[38] M. P. Tan, "The boomerang incision for periareolar breast malignancies," *The American Journal of Surgery*, vol. 194, no. 5, pp. 690–693, 2007.

[39] M. Tan and O. Ung, "Alternative approaches for oncoplastic breast surgery," *Annals of Surgical Oncology*, vol. 18, no. 1, pp. 297–299, 2011.

[40] N. Houssami, R. Turner, and M. Morrow, "Preoperative magnetic resonance imaging in breast cancer," *Annals of Surgery*, vol. 257, no. 2, pp. 249–255, 2013.

[41] A. Fancellu, D. Soro, P. Castiglia et al., "Usefulness of magnetic resonance in patients with invasive cancer eligible for breast conservation: a comparative study," *Clinical Breast Cancer*, vol. 14, no. 2, pp. 114–121, 2014.

[42] S. Molenaar, M. A. G. Sprangers, E. J. Rutgers et al., "Decision support for patients with early-stage breast cancer: effects of an interactive breast cancer CDROM on treatment decision, satisfaction, and quality of life," *Journal of Clinical Oncology*, vol. 19, no. 6, pp. 1676–1687, 2001.

[43] D. Lazovich, K. K. Raab, J. G. Gurney, and H. Chen, "Knowledge and preference for breast conservation therapy among women without breast cancer," *Women's Health Issues*, vol. 10, no. 4, pp. 210–216, 2000.

[44] S. J. Katz, P. M. Lantz, N. K. Janz et al., "Patient involvement in surgery treatment decisions for breast cancer," *Journal of Clinical Oncology*, vol. 23, no. 24, pp. 5526–5533, 2005.

[45] H. S. Fiegelson, T. A. James, R. M. Single et al., "Factors associated with the frequency of initial total mastectomy: results of a multi-institutional study," *Journal of the American College of Surgeons*, vol. 216, pp. 966–975, 2013.

[46] Y. Y. Woon and M. Y. P. Chan, "Breast conservation surgery—the surgeon's factor," *The Breast*, vol. 14, no. 2, pp. 131–135, 2005.

6

Regional Failures after Selective Neck Dissection in Previously Untreated Squamous Cell Carcinoma of Oral Cavity

Hassan Iqbal,[1] Abu Bakar Hafeez Bhatti,[1] Raza Hussain,[1] and Arif Jamshed[2]

[1] Department of Surgical Oncology, Shaukat Khanum Memorial Cancer Hospital and Research Centre, 7A Block R-3, M.A. Johar Town, Lahore, Pakistan
[2] Department of Radiation Oncology, Shaukat Khanum Memorial Cancer Hospital and Research Centre, 7A Block R-3, M.A. Johar Town, Lahore, Pakistan

Correspondence should be addressed to Abu Bakar Hafeez Bhatti; abubakar.hafeez@yahoo.com

Academic Editor: S. Curley

Aim. To share experience with regional failures after selective neck dissection in both node negative and positive previously untreated patients diagnosed with squamous cell carcinoma of the oral cavity. *Patients and Methods.* Data of 219 patients who underwent SND at Shaukat Khanum Cancer Hospital from 2003 to 2010 were retrospectively reviewed. Patient characteristics, treatment modalities, and regional failures were assessed. Expected 5-year regional control was calculated and prognostic factors were determined. *Results.* Median follow-up was 29 (9–109) months. Common sites were anterior tongue in 159 and buccal mucosa in 22 patients. Pathological nodal stage was N0 in 114, N1 in 32, N2b in 67, and N2c in 5 patients. Fourteen (6%) patients failed in clinically node negative neck while 8 (4%) failed in clinically node positive patients. Out of 22 total regional failures, primary tumor origin was from tongue in 16 (73%) patients. Expected 5-year regional control was 95% and 81% for N0 and N+ disease, respectively ($P < 0.0001$). Only 13% patients with well differentiated, T1 tumors in cN0 neck were pathologically node positive. *Conclusions.* Selective neck dissection yields acceptable results for regional management of oral squamous cell carcinoma. Wait and see policy may be effective in a selected subgroup of patients.

1. Introduction

Since description of neck dissection in late 19th century, modifications have been proposed, practiced, and argued. Tracing back the heritage of neck dissection, sequential evolution from a morbid to a cosmetically tailored and oncologically acceptable procedure becomes evident. Although several different classifications have been adapted in the past, debate on a balanced and widely acceptable nomenclature continues. Lately selective neck dissection (SND) has been the buzz word for regional management in head and neck cancer. Shah [1] demonstrated frequency and patterns of regional lymph node metastases from oral squamous cell carcinoma in patients who underwent radical neck dissection. By definition SND refers to preservation of 1 or more lymph node levels. Although SND is an accepted procedure for pathological staging of clinically node negative (cN0) neck, the house remains divided between elective neck dissection versus a more conservative wait and see policy [2]. The therapeutic role of SND in clinically node positive (cN+) disease is still unclear but is gaining popularity in carefully selected patients [3, 4]. The exact protocol for regional management of squamous cell carcinoma of oral cavity is yet to be established. The objective of present study was to report regional control with selective neck dissection in both N0 and N+ previously untreated patients diagnosed with squamous cell carcinoma of the oral cavity.

2. Methods

A review of patients who underwent SND between 2003 and 2010 at Shaukat Khanum Memorial Cancer Hospital and Research Center was performed. A total of 219 patients who underwent SND for histology proven squamous cell carcinoma (SCCa) of oral cavity during the study period were included. Patients who received any treatment elsewhere were excluded from the study. All patients underwent a comprehensive clinical examination of head and neck followed by MRI of the face and neck and chest X-ray. Patients were staged according to the AJCC (American Joint Commission on Cancer) guidelines. The management protocol of these patients was tailored in the weekly multidisciplinary team clinic. SND was the mainstay surgical protocol for regional control alongside wide local excision of tumor. For patients diagnosed with SCCa of upper alveolus, maxillectomy was performed and SND was reserved for patients with clinically or radiologically node positive disease. Inclusion criteria for performing SND included tumor >1.5 cm and tumor thickness of more than 4 mm. Adjuvant treatment options such as postoperative radiotherapy (PORT) or concurrent chemoradiotherapy (CRT) were planned for the patients after pathological staging.

3. Induction Chemotherapy

Main indication for induction chemotherapy (IC) was bulky local and inoperable disease. Other indications included patients with tumors crossing midline, involvement of tip of tongue, and extension into the base of tongue or floor of the mouth. A total of 45 patients received IC prior to surgery. Induction chemotherapy was administered on outpatient basis. The regimen comprised of a combination of 2 drugs: intravenous gemcitabine $1000 \, mg/m^2$ on day 1 and day 8 and cisplatin $75 \, mg/m^2$ on day 1 of each cycle, respectively. A 3-week interval was observed between the 2 cycles. After 2 weeks from the second cycle, a response assessment was clinically devised and patients were planned for wide local excision of the tumor along with SND.

4. Surgical Management

Wide local excision was performed in tongue, lips, retromolar trigone, and buccal mucosa with 1 cm clear margin. Patients with squamous cell carcinoma of lower alveolar mucosa underwent marginal or segmental mandibulectomy depending on extent of involvement of lower alveolus. Maxillectomy was performed for patients with SCCa of upper alveolus. Frozen section was reserved for patients with clinically suspicious mucosal tissue. Majority of patients with T1 and early T2 tumors (<3 cm) and cN0 underwent SND I–III. Patients with advanced T2 (>3 cm), T3, and T4 tumors or clinically N+ disease underwent SND I–IV. After extraction of neck specimen, sublevels were separated and placed individually in formalin filled containers and sent for histopathological analysis. A template was prepared by pathologist to interpret the report including the number of nodes harvested, size of the fibro fatty tissue, and number of positive nodes. The presence of perineural invasion, lymphovascular invasion, and extra capsular spread was also documented for each level of neck specimen. Bilateral neck dissection was performed in patients with radiological evidence of contralateral neck disease.

5. Adjuvant Treatment

Postoperative radiotherapy (PORT) was used in patients with pathologically node positive disease, >1 cm tumor size, >5 mm tumor thickness, and poorly differentiated tumors. In pathologically node negative patients, 60 Gy in 30 fractions was given to the primary site and ipsilateral neck. In pathologically node positive patients, 60 Gy in 30 fractions was given to the primary site and bilateral neck. Concurrent chemoradiotherapy (CRT) was reserved for patients with extra capsular spread, perineural invasion, lymphovascular invasion, and more than 2 positive lymph nodes.

6. Statistical Analysis

Patient characteristics and treatment modalities were observed. Patients who did not have contralateral neck dissection were not included as regional failures. Regional control was calculated by subtracting date of failure from date of surgery. Expected 5-year regional control was calculated using Kaplan-Meier curves and significance between variables was determined with log rank test. Statistical Package for Social Sciences (SPSS), version 17, was used for statistical analysis.

7. Results

7.1. Patient Characteristics. A total of 219 patients underwent SND of which 158 were clinically node negative and 61 were node positive. Median age at presentation for node negative patients was 51 (13–76) years and median follow-up was 2.9 (0.07–9) years. Median age at presentation for node positive patients was 50 (28–79) years and median follow-up was 1.8 (0.2–7) years. Anterior tongue was the most common subsite with nearly 72% patients. Majority of patients received postoperative radiotherapy. Forty-five patients received induction chemotherapy. Table 1 summarizes patient characteristics and treatment modalities with respect to clinically node negative and positive patients. There was a significant difference between two groups with respect to site of primary tumor ($P = 0.009$), treatment received ($P = 0.0001$), and sublevels dissected ($P = 0.002$). Anterior tongue was the site of primary in 75% patients with N0 neck disease versus 66% with N+ neck disease. Surgery alone was the treatment modality in 16% patients with clinically N0 disease and 2% patients with N+ disease. Sublevels I–III were dissected in 21% patients with N0 versus 3% patients with N+ disease. Out of a total of 52 patients with unknown extracapsular status, 65% patients received postoperative radiation, and 25% received concurrent chemoradiotherapy based on presence of other poor prognostic factors. Postoperative radiotherapy was used in 193 (88%) patients. Out of these, 51 (26%) had concurrent chemoradiotherapy.

7.1.1. Clinical and Pathological Stage. Table 2 represents the clinical and pathological distribution of the study cohort. Locally advanced (T3/T4) tumors were found in 26% patients. One hundred and fifty-eight (72%) patients were

TABLE 1: Patient characteristics and treatment modalities in clinically node negative and positive patients.

	Node negative patients		Node positive patients		
	Number (N)	Percent (%)	Number (N)	Percent (%)	
Gender					Not significant
Male	104	66	38	62	
Female	54	34	23	38	
Subsite					0.009
Anterior tongue	119	75	40	66	
Upper alveolus	1	1	0	0	
Lower alveolus	22	14	10	16	
Buccal mucosa	16	10	6	10	
Retromolar trigone	0	0	2	3	
Lips	0	0	3	5	
Grade					Not significant
Well	79	50	31	51	
Moderate	64	40	21	34	
Poor	13	10	9	15	
Treatment modality					0.0001
S	25	16	1	2	
S + RT	91	58	30	49	
S + CRT	16	10	11	18	
C + S + RT	15	10	6	10	
C + S + CRT	11	7	13	21	
Level					0.002
I–III	33	21	2	3	
I–IV	125	79	59	97	

S: surgery, RT: radiation therapy, and C: chemotherapy.

cN0 at the time of presentation. One hundred and twenty-one (55%) patients had advanced disease (stage III/IV) on histopathology. Mean number of extracted nodes was 50 nodes and a total of 11936 nodes (level 1, 1836; level 2a, 2500; level 2b, 1600; level 3, 3000; level 4; 3000) were extracted in 219 patients. Occult nodal disease was present in 58 (37%) patients. Level II A was the most commonly involved sublevel in tumors of anterior tongue while level I was most frequently involved in tumors of buccal mucosa and lower alveolus.

7.2. New Classification. In Table 3, the newly proposed classification of neck dissection was compared with older version. None of the patients who underwent level I–III neck dissection had removal of any nonlymphatic tissues. Thirty-three patients out of 184 who underwent level I–IV SND had one or more nonlymphatic structures removed and were clearly demonstrable in new classification. Out of these 33 patients, 4 (12%) patients had extra capsular spread on histopathology (IJV = 3, IJV+SAN = 1). Rest had nonlymphatic structures removed due to perinodal fibrous adhesions.

7.3. Induction Chemotherapy. A total of 45 patients received induction chemotherapy. Male to female ratio was 2 : 1. Table 4 represents their characteristics. On clinical exam, 65% patients had locally advanced (T3/T4) tumors. There was 1 patient with a T1 tumor on clinical exam who received induction. This patient had squamous cell carcinoma of tongue crossing midline. Histopathology of resected specimen after induction chemotherapy demonstrated that only 7% patients had T3/T4 tumors. Complete pathological response was seen in 6 patients. This difference was not observed for nodal involvement after induction chemotherapy. The expected 5-year overall survival for patients who received induction chemotherapy versus those who did not was 69 and 74%, respectively, and was not significantly different (P = 0.4).

7.4. Regional Failures in Clinically Node Negative and Node Positive Patients. Table 5 demonstrates failures in clinically node negative and positive patients. Total number of regional failures was 22. Fourteen (8.8%) patients failed in clinically node negative neck while 8 (13%) failed in clinically node positive patients. The most common tumor size stage was T2 in 45% patients. Tongue was the most common site of primary in 16 (72%) patients. Out of total 7 patients with extracapsular extension, 3 (42%) patients developed regional failure. Median recurrence-free survival in pN+ patients with and without extracapsular spread was 1.6 (0.08–9) and 1.7 (0.02–7) years and was not significantly different. A total of 14 patients had ipsilateral failures, including 3 patients that failed both locally and regionally. All patients that failed ipsilaterally underwent SND I–IV. Almost all patients

TABLE 2: Clinical and pathological staging of patients according to AJCC guidelines.

Stage	Clinical number (N)	Percent (%)	Pathological number (N)	Percent (%)
T stage				
T0	—	—	8	4
T1	65	29	97	44
T2	98	45	81	37
T3	28	13	13	6
T4	28	13	20	9
N Stage				
N0	158	72	114	52
N1	34	16	32	14
N2a	6	3	0	0
N2b	16	7	67	31
N2c	5	2	5	2
N3	0	—	1	1
Overall stage				
0	—		6	3
I	53	24	55	25
II	70	32	38	17
III	46	21	32	15
IV	50	23	88	40

TABLE 3: Comparison of old and proposed classification.

Selective neck dissection			Proposed classification		
	Number (%)	Percent (%)		Number	Percent (%)
Level I–III	35 (16)	16	ND (I–III)	35	16
Level I–IV	184 (84)	84	ND (I–IV)	151	69
			ND (I–IV, IJV, CN XI)	2	1
			ND (I–IV, IJV)	29	13
			ND (I–IV, CN XI)	2	1

ND: neck dissection, IJV: internal jugular vein, and CN XI: accessory nerve.

that failed ipsilaterally in the neck were either treated with palliative chemotherapy or symptomatically. A total of 4 patients failed contralaterally in the neck.

There were 38 local, 19 regional, 3 locoregional, and 6 distant failures (not shown). None of the patients who underwent SND I–III failed ipsilaterally. Eight patients had occult metastatic disease after SND I–III, that is, 3 patients in level III, 5 in level II, and 3 in level I. Two patients underwent bilateral SND I–III as they were staged radiologically N2c; on histopathology they had N1 and N2b disease, respectively. Both these patients had SCCa of the anterior tongue. One patient had skip metastasis with pathologically positive node in level III, escaping levels I and II. Level II B dissection was performed in all patients. A total of 184 patients underwent SND I–IV of which thirteen patients had bilateral neck dissection. Ten patients showed skip metastasis of which nine patients had SCCa oral tongue and one had SCCa buccal mucosa. Level II B was removed in all patients. A total of 14 (7.6%) patients had positive lymph nodes in level IV but no

isolated level IV involvement was seen. Also, 12/14 patients with level IV involvement had more than two positive nodes. Five of the fourteen patients had cN0 disease at presentation and on staging MRI ten patients had radiologically significant nodal disease.

7.5. *Prognostic Factors.* Grade, lymphovascular invasion, and pathological N stage were statistically significant for 5-year regional control (Table 6). A highly significant difference in regional control was present between N0 and N+ patients with expected 5-year control of 95% and 81%, respectively ($P = 0.005$). The 5-year overall survival and disease-free survival for the whole group were 73% and 61%, respectively (not shown).

Table 7 represents the rates of pathological nodal positivity after SND in patients with well differentiated tumors and clinically node negative neck. Almost 90% patients with T1 tumors in this subgroup had pN0 disease.

TABLE 4: Characteristics of patient who received induction chemotherapy.

	Number ($N = 45$)	Percent (%)
Gender		
Male	30	66
Female	15	34
Clinical T stage		
T1	1	2
T2	15	33
T3	23	51
T4	6	14
Clinical N stage		
N0	26	58
N+	19	42
Grade		
Well	21	47
Moderate	17	38
Poor	7	15
Pathological T stage		
pT0	6	14
pT1	25	55
pT2	10	22
pT3	3	7
pT4	1	2
Pathological N stage		
N0	19	42
N+	26	58

8. Discussion

Regional spread of oral cancer continues to be the most significant prognostic factor and decreases survival by 50% [5, 6]. A better understanding of lymphatic spread has shown that lymph drains within aponeurotic compartments [7]. Studies have shown that lymphatic spread with respect to anatomical subsite can be predicted [8, 9]. Shah [1] mapped the lymphatic spread for squamous cell carcinoma of upper aerodigestive tract in 501 patients with oral cancer. Studies have shown 0–3% rate of metastatic spread in level V supporting the notion of sparing posterior triangle while performing neck dissection [10, 11]. It was also concluded that level V dissection can be avoided even if suspicious lymph nodes are encountered at level IV [3]. In the current study, a marked difference in regional control was observed between node negative and node positive patients who underwent neck dissection. Level I–IV SND was performed more frequently (82% versus 18%). Overall, 8% of total patients who underwent level I–IV SND had level IV involvement. Tongue was the most common site of primary and level II A or subdigastric level was the most common involved sublevel. Overall 22 patients failed regionally with a high preponderance of ipsilateral failures (18 versus 4). Regional failure was more common in the first year after surgery and highlights importance of meticulous surveillance in this time period. Limitations of the current study include its retrospective design and missing data. Sublevels of regional failures in neck could not be determined as majority of patients had huge fixed neck recurrences involving more than one sublevels of neck. In addition the prognostic role of extracapsular extension could not be determined due to small number of patients who had extracapsular involvement.

There are no set guidelines for management of clinically node negative neck in early oral cancer. Studies have been reported both in favor of elective neck dissection and wait and see policy [12–14]. Current guidelines recommend elective neck dissection when probability of occult metastasis is 20% [2]. Recently a meta-analysis showed elective neck dissection to be a better option [15]. A high occult metastatic rate of 37%, low socioeconomic status, and distant geographic location of our patients made elective neck dissection a more suitable option in our setting. In critical assessment of supraomohyoid neck dissection, removal of level I–III was found appropriate for staging of cN0 patients. Occult metastasis was present in 31% out of a total of one hundred and fifteen patients included in the study [16]. In the current study, a high proportion of cN0 patients underwent level I–IV neck dissection but only 14 patients were found to have pathological evidence of disease in level IV. Since the results on the findings of the current study, practice has already been modified and level IV dissection is only performed in patients with clinical nodal disease in level III/IV in neck in our institute now.

Radiotherapy either in pre- or postoperative setting has shown its benefit with reduction in the incidence of neck failures by 50% irrespective of the N stage [17–19]. The choice of pre- or postoperative radiation remains largely institutional with surgeons preferring PORT as it reduces the operative complications and makes performance of neck dissection relatively easy [20]. Adjuvant radiotherapy has also been recommended in clinically node negative contralateral neck to reduce the rate of contralateral neck failure [21]. Two trials conducted in Europe (European Organization Research and Treatment of Cancer (EORTC)) and the United States (Radiation Therapy Oncology Group (RTOG)) have shown better locoregional control in patients with extracapsular spread and/or positive surgical margins who received postoperative chemoradiation [22, 23]. Chemoradiation has been advocated in presence of poor prognostic factors like stage III–IV disease, perineural infiltration, vascular embolisms, and/or clinically enlarged level IV–V lymph nodes [14]. In the current study, 88% patients received radiation of which 23% were in the setting of concurrent chemoradiotherapy. Tumor grade, extracapsular spread, lymphovascular invasion, and pathological N stage were significant variables for regional control in present study. However the number of patients with these variables was very small.

Radical neck dissection (RND) remained the procedure of choice in node positive patients for greater part of the 20th century. Strong [24] in their study showed a regional recurrence rate of 54.3% in node positive patients and 71.3% in patients with positive nodes at multiple levels. This leads to several questions regarding the oncological benefit and morbidity associated RND. In the past two decades the use of SND has gained popularity in the management of node positive patients partly because of the comparable regional

TABLE 5: Regional failures in clinically node negative and node positive neck.

	Node negative N = 14		Node positive N = 8		Total
	Number	Percent	Number	Percent	
Tumor size					
T1	5	36	2	33	7
T2	6	43	4	43	10
T3	3	21	0	8	3
T4	0	0	2	16	2
Site					
Ipsilateral	11	80	7	86	18
Contralateral	3	20	1	14	4
Primary					
Tongue	10	72	6	75	16
Lower alveolus	1	7	1	12.5	2
Buccal mucosa	2	14	1	12.5	3
Upper alveolus	1	7	0	0	1
Extracapsular					
Present	2	50	1	33	3

TABLE 6: Prognostic variables for 5-year regional control.

Prognostic factor	Number (n)	5-year regional control (%)	P value
Tumor grade			
Well	110	84	
Mod	84	87	0.006
Poorly	25	62	
Lymphovascular invasion			
Positive	12	68	
Negative	153	85	0.044
Unknown	54	85	
Perineural invasion			
Positive	28	75	
Negative	140	84	Not significant
Unknown	51	84	
Pathological N stage			
N0	114	95	<0.0001
N+	105	81	
Pathological T stage			
T1-T2	186	82	Not significant
T3-T4	33	91	
Number of positive nodes			
1, 2	57	70	
3, 4, 5	26	71	Not significant
>5	22	61	

control rate in patients with occult disease undergoing elective neck dissection and also due to an increasing use of PORT for better disease control. Andersen et al. [3] in their study of 106 patients with 129 therapeutic SND had 9 regional failures. The study included all sites of head and neck region and >50% patients had N1 disease. In another study on effectiveness of SND in clinically node positive neck including all primary sites of head and neck region, 54 patients underwent SND including 33 patients with pN2/3 disease. There were 2 ipsilateral recurrences and SND showed

TABLE 7: Frequency of node positivity on histopathology in patients with well-differentiated tumors and clinically node negative neck.

	pN0	%	pN1	%	pN2a	%	pN2b	%	Total
cT1	27	87	2	6.5	0	—	2	6.5	31
cT2	17	53	7	22	0		8	25	32
cT3	5	71	0	—	1	14.5	1	14.5	7
cT4	6	67	1	11	0	—	2	22	9
	55	70	10	13	1	1	13	16	79

p: pathological.
c: clinical.

better disease control but did not reach statistical significance [25].

With an increasing trend of performing limited and site specific lymphadenectomy procedures, a comprehensive classification of neck dissection has been proposed that is logical, simple, and easy to remember [26]. In the current study, the authors have compared the old nomenclature with the proposed classification and found the new classification better at defining precisely the lymphatic and non-lymphatic structures excised.

The role of induction chemotherapy in head and neck squamous cell carcinoma before a definitive surgical intervention is not well defined [27]. In the current study, 45 patients received induction chemotherapy. On histopathology, only 1 patient had T4 tumor out of 6 patients with cT4 tumors who received induction chemotherapy. Out of 23 patients with cT3 disease who received induction chemotherapy, only 3 had pT3 disease. This favors the role of induction chemotherapy in downstaging of head and neck tumors before surgical resection; however conclusions cannot be drawn due to heterogeneous nature of our cohort.

We also made an effort to identify a subgroup of patients in which pathological nodal positivity was absent. This could potentially represent a group in which SND could be avoided. Almost 90% patients with well-differentiated, T1 tumors and cN0 neck did not have pathological nodal disease after SND. This group could potentially represent a subgroup that might benefit from wait and see policy under close surveillance. Further studies are needed to address this issue taking into consideration several other prognostic variables.

The current study reports regional failures after SND in previously untreated squamous cell carcinoma of oral cavity in both node negative and positive patients. It highlights several important issues. Induction chemotherapy may have a beneficial role in locally advanced head and neck squamous cell carcinomas but this needs to be confirmed in future trials. There might be a subgroup of patients with well-differentiated, clinically node negative T1 tumors that can be safely managed with observation alone. As the role of neck dissection becomes more conservative with ever-expanding application of PORT and CRT providing improved regional control, application of level I–IV SND should be limited. Superselective neck dissection might become the standard for regional management of neck in oral squamous cell carcinoma.

References

[1] J. P. Shah, "Patterns of cervical lymph node metastasis from squamous carcinomas of the upper aerodigestive tract," *The American Journal of Surgery*, vol. 160, no. 4, pp. 405–409, 1990.

[2] A. K. D'Cruz and M. R. Dandekar, "Elective versus therapeutic neck dissection in the clinically node negative neck in early oral cavity cancers: do we have the answer yet?" *Oral Oncology*, vol. 47, no. 9, pp. 780–782, 2011.

[3] P. E. Andersen, F. Warren, J. Spiro et al., "Results of selective neck dissection in management of the node-positive neck," *Archives of Otolaryngology*, vol. 128, no. 10, pp. 1180–1184, 2002.

[4] R. S. Patel, J. R. Clark, K. Gao, and C. J. O'Brien, "Effectiveness of selective neck dissection in the treatment of the clinically positive neck," *Head & Neck*, vol. 30, no. 9, pp. 1231–1236, 2008.

[5] J. P. Shah and P. E. Andersen, "Evolving role of modifications in neck dissection for oral squamous carcinoma," *British Journal of Oral and Maxillofacial Surgery*, vol. 33, no. 1, pp. 3–8, 1995.

[6] J. P. Shah, "Cancer of the upper aerodigestive tract," in *The Practice of Cancer Surgery*, A. E. Alfonso and B. Gardener, Eds., Appleton-Century-Crofts, New York, NY, USA, 1982.

[7] E. Bocca and O. Pignataro, "A conservation technique in radical neck dissection," *The Annals of Otology, Rhinology and Laryngology*, vol. 76, no. 5, pp. 975–987, 1967.

[8] U. P. Fisch and M. E. Siegel, "Cervical lymphatic system as viewed by lymphography," *The Annals of Otology, Rhinology and Laryngology*, vol. 73, pp. 869–882, 1964.

[9] R. Lindberg, "Distribution of cervical lymph node metastases from squamous cell carcinoma of the upper respiratory and digestive tracts," *Cancer*, vol. 29, no. 6, pp. 1446–1449, 1972.

[10] B. J. Davidson, V. Kulkarny, M. D. Delacure, and J. P. Shah, "Posterior triangle metastases of squamous cell carcinoma of the upper aerodigestive tract," *The American Journal of Surgery*, vol. 166, no. 4, pp. 395–398, 1993.

[11] E. M. Skolnik, K. F. Yee, M. Friedman, and T. A. Golden, "The posterior triangle in radical neck surgery," *Archives of Otolaryngology*, vol. 102, no. 1, pp. 1–4, 1976.

[12] A. R. Fakih, R. S. Rao, A. M. Borges, and A. R. Patel, "Elective versus therapeutic neck dissection in early carcinoma of the oral tongue," *The American Journal of Surgery*, vol. 158, no. 4, pp. 309–313, 1989.

[13] A. P. Yuen, C. M. Ho, T. L. Chow et al., "Prospective randomized study of selective neck dissection versus observation for N0

neck of early tongue carcinoma," *Head & Neck*, vol. 31, no. 6, pp. 765–772, 2009.

[14] R. M. Byers, A. K. El-Naggar, Y. Y. Lee et al., "Can we detect or predict the presence of occult nodal metastases in patients with squamous cell carcinoma of the oral tongue?" *Head & Neck*, vol. 20, no. 2, pp. 138–144, 1998.

[15] A. J. Fasunla, B. H. Greene, N. Timmesfeld, S. Wiegand, J. A. Werner, and A. M. Sesterhenn, "A meta-analysis of the randomized controlled trials on elective neck dissection versus therapeutic neck dissection in oral cavity cancers with clinically node-negative neck," *Oral Oncology*, vol. 47, no. 5, pp. 320–324, 2011.

[16] J. D. Spiro, R. H. Spiro, J. P. Shah, R. B. Sessions, and E. W. Strong, "Critical assessment of supraomohyoid neck dissection," *The American Journal of Surgery*, vol. 156, no. 4, pp. 286–289, 1988.

[17] R. M. Byers, "Modified neck dissection. A study of 967 cases from 1970 to 1980," *The American Journal of Surgery*, vol. 150, no. 4, pp. 414–421, 1985.

[18] D. R. Goffinet, W. E. Fee Jr., and R. L. Goode, "Combined surgery and postoperative irradiation in the treatment of cervical lymph nodes," *Archives of Otolaryngology*, vol. 110, no. 11, pp. 736–738, 1984.

[19] B. Vikram, E. W. Strong, J. P. Shah, and R. Spiro, "Failure in the neck following multimodality treatment for advanced head and neck cancer," *Head & Neck Surgery*, vol. 6, no. 3, pp. 724–729, 1984.

[20] L. Tupchong, C. B. Scott, P. H. Blitzer et al., "Randomized study of preoperative versus postoperative radiation therapy in advanced head and neck carcinoma: long-term follow-up of RTOG study 73-03," *International Journal of Radiation Oncology, Biology, Physics*, vol. 20, no. 1, pp. 21–28, 1991.

[21] H. T. Barkley Jr., G. H. Fletcher, R. H. Jesse, and R. D. Lindberg, "Management of cervical lymph node metastases in squamous cell carcinoma of the tonsillar fossa, base of tongue, supraglottic larynx, and hypopharynx," *The American Journal of Surgery*, vol. 124, no. 4, pp. 462–467, 1972.

[22] J. Bernier, C. Domenge, M. Ozsahin et al., "Postoperative irradiation with or without concomitant chemotherapy for locally advanced head and neck cancer," *The New England Journal of Medicine*, vol. 350, no. 19, pp. 1945–1952, 2004.

[23] J. S. Cooper, T. F. Pajak, A. A. Forastiere et al., "Postoperative concurrent radiotherapy and chemotherapy for high-risk squamous-cell carcinoma of the head and neck," *The New England Journal of Medicine*, vol. 350, no. 19, pp. 1937–1944, 2004.

[24] E. W. Strong, "Preoperative radiation and radical neck dissection," *Surgical Clinics of North America*, vol. 49, no. 2, pp. 271–276, 1969.

[25] R. S. Patel, J. R. Clark, K. Gao, and C. J. O'Brien, "Effectiveness of selective neck dissection in the treatment of the clinically positive neck," *Head & Neck*, vol. 30, no. 9, pp. 1231–1236, 2008.

[26] A. Ferlito, K. T. Robbins, J. P. Shah et al., "Proposal for a rational classification of neck dissections," *Head & Neck*, vol. 33, no. 3, pp. 445–450, 2011.

[27] M. Benasso, "Induction chemotherapy for squamous cell head and neck cancer: a neverending story?" *Oral Oncology*, vol. 49, no. 8, pp. 747–752, 2013.

7

Evaluating the Feasibility of Performing Window of Opportunity Trials in Breast Cancer

Angel Arnaout,[1,2] Susan Robertson,[3] Iryna Kuchuk,[4] Demetrios Simos,[4] Gregory R. Pond,[5] Christina L. Addison,[2] Mehrzad Namazi,[1] and Mark Clemons[2,4]

[1]Division of Surgical Oncology, Department of Surgery, Ottawa Hospital, Ottawa, ON, Canada
[2]Cancer Therapeutics Program, Ottawa Hospital Research Institute, Ottawa, ON, Canada
[3]Division of Anatomical Pathology, Ottawa Hospital, Ottawa, ON, Canada
[4]Division of Medical Oncology, Department of Medicine, Ottawa Hospital and Ottawa Hospital Cancer Center, Ottawa, ON, Canada
[5]Department of Oncology, McMaster University, Hamilton, ON, Canada

Correspondence should be addressed to Angel Arnaout; anarnaout@toh.on.ca

Academic Editor: Kefah Mokbel

Background. The waiting period to surgery represents a valuable "window of opportunity" to evaluate novel therapeutic strategies. Interventional studies performed during this period require significant multidisciplinary collaboration to overcome logistical hurdles. We undertook a one-year prospective window of opportunity study to assess feasibility. *Methods.* Eligible newly diagnosed postmenopausal, estrogen receptor positive breast cancer patients awaiting primary surgery received anastrozole daily until surgery. Feasibility was assessed by (a) the proportion of patients who consented and (b) completed the study. Comparison of pre- and poststudy Ki67 labelling index and cleaved caspase 3 scores (CC3) was performed. *Results.* 22/131 (16.8%) patients were confirmed eligible and 20/22 (91%) patients completed the study. 19/20 (95%) patients agreed to undergo optional additional tissue biopsies. The mean duration of anastrozole use was 24.7 (15–44) days. There were a statistically significant decline in mean Ki67 indices of 48.8% ($p < 0.001$) and a trend towards significance in the decline of CC3 ($p = 0.17$) when comparing pre- with posttreatment values. *Conclusion.* window of opportunity trials in breast cancer are a feasible way of assessing the biologic efficacy of different therapies in the presurgical setting. The majority of eligible women were willing to participate including undergoing additional tissue biopsies.

1. Introduction

Window of opportunity (also called phase 0) trials can provide insight into biological effects and potential therapeutic efficacy of novel therapeutic strategies [1–4]. One example of window of opportunity trial is for women with newly diagnosed breast cancer to receive a study drug between the diagnostic breast biopsy and planned surgical resection. The advantage of window of opportunity trials is that they allow short-term testing of novel agents in patients who already have surgery planned as their primary therapy; and therefore agents may be tested in patients who are not pretreated. Window of opportunity trials differ from the more traditional neoadjuvant trials in that no therapeutic benefit is envisaged,

whereas in neoadjuvant trials an investigational agent is given preoperatively along with chemotherapy or endocrine therapy for a longer duration (usually months) and surgery is delayed to allow for a therapeutic response in the tumor. Ultimately, window studies have the potential to expedite drug development process by improving the understanding of an agent's biologic effect early in its development through monitoring tissue samples obtained before and after drug exposure. These trials may assess target or pharmacodynamic effects of an intervention, allowing for greater potential to select for subsets of patients who might benefit from a therapy in clinical trials that are powered to detect changes in clinical outcome [2–4].

Despite the short duration of window studies, they are challenging to perform as they require close collaboration between multiple disciplines, including surgeons, oncologists, pathologists, radiologists, and laboratory scientists [2, 4–11]. In addition, one common concern of the preoperative window of opportunity model for patients and investigators is that it can lead to treatment delays if these evaluations cannot be completed within the standard normal surgical wait times [4–12]. As a result, window of opportunity studies are still relatively rare in the medical literature.

We undertook a one-year, pilot, window of opportunity trial using anastrozole to assess the feasibility of performing such trials at our institution. Feasibility was assessed through several endpoints, including the proportion of eligible patients, patient compliance, patient acceptability of additional research biopsies, and the ability to assess change in tumor Ki67 (marker of proliferation) and cleaved caspase 3 (CC3, marker of apoptosis).

2. Methods

2.1. Study Participants and Eligibility. This study was a single center, single arm, prospective study to assess the feasibility of performing a window of opportunity study at our center. The design was deliberately pragmatic and was designed to investigate the use of anastrozole in newly diagnosed postmenopausal, hormone receptor positive breast cancer patients awaiting primary surgery in the time from diagnostic tissue biopsy to surgery.

Eligibility criteria for the study included (1) postmenopausal status; (2) histologically confirmed estrogen receptor positive invasive carcinoma on diagnostic core biopsy; (3) the invasive cancer which was clinically and/or radiologically ≥ 2 cm in size; (4) patients who did not have any contraindications to take anastrozole; and (5) surgery date which was planned for 2–8 weeks after initial consultation. All patients had to be stage II or operable stage III as the practice in our institution is such that only inoperable stage III as well as stage IV patients went on to primary chemotherapy treatment. Patients could not have received hormone replacement therapy, tamoxifen, or an aromatase inhibitor within the previous 6 months or have known metastatic or recurrent breast cancer. Institutional Research Ethics Board and Health Canada approval was obtained prior to study commencement.

2.2. Study Procedures. All potential study patients with a core biopsy confirmed invasive breast cancer were evaluated at initial consultation by one surgeon (AA). The surgeon decided whether the patient was potentially eligible based on tumor size and postmenopausal status. If the patient was interested in the study she was then approached for study screening by a research nurse for study eligibility (see Figure 1 study schema). Those patients who were screened and deemed potentially eligible had a formal request made to a pathologist (SR) for assessment of estrogen receptor (ER), progesterone receptor (PR), and human epidermal growth factor receptor 2 (HER2) on the diagnostic specimen. At the time of the study,

routine biomarker analysis on initial diagnostic core biopsies was not performed at our institution and therefore could only be requested once the patient had consented to participate in the study. If ER and/or PR staining was greater than or equal to 1% they were considered positive and the patient was then eligible of the study.

All qualifying patients were referred to a medical oncologist (MC, IK, and DS) for assessment prior to starting anastrozole (1 mg po od). The time between starting anastrozole and surgery had to be a minimum of 2 weeks, and the last dose was to be taken the night before surgery. Patient compliance was assessed by pill count. Toxicity assessments (Common Terminology Criteria for Adverse Events (CTCAE) version 3.0 [7]) were performed prior to starting anastrozole, just before surgery, and 3-4 weeks after surgery.

2.3. Additional Optional Tissue, Blood, and Urine Collection. Patients with insufficient tissue in the initial diagnostic core biopsy for study analyses underwent an additional tumor biopsy. Even if there was sufficient initial core biopsy material for study analyses, at the time of the initial consent process, patients were also given the choice to undergo additional optional tissue biopsies and collection of blood and urine samples for use in the future as yet unplanned research. All tumor biopsies were immediately fixed in 10% neutral buffered formalin and excisional specimens were sliced and exposed to formalin within 1 hour with the majority having 24–72 hours of fixation time and less than 1/2 hour ischemic time. After standard tissue processing and embedding in paraffin wax sections were cut and were stained with hematoxylin and eosin or left unstained for immunohistochemistry.

2.4. Ki67 and CC3 Immunohistochemistry. Ki67 and CC3 were assessed on tissue sections cut from the FFPE diagnostic core biopsy (i.e., before anastrozole) and compared with expression in sections of surgical specimens as determined on selected representative tissue blocks (i.e., after anastrozole). The core biopsy specimens were generally 5-6 samples obtained with a 14 g needle. A minority of patients who were planned for surgery, and thus eligible for the study, were found to have medical comorbidities delaying their primary surgical treatment. For these patients, they continued on anastrozole while waiting for their surgery and a mandatory further core biopsy at 6 weeks was performed and used for the "postanastrozole" specimen.

Immunohistochemistry for Ki67 was performed using Leica PA0118 clone MM1 using the Refine Detection Kit from Leica. The "Ki67 index" (percentage of nuclei showing nuclear immunoreactivity of any intensity) was determined by computer image assisted count by a single pathologist (SR). In each case, after a low-power scan of the entire tissue section, hot spot regions of highest activity were selected and from these 1,000 tumor nuclei were counted at 400–600x magnification.

For CC3 immunohistochemical analysis, serial sections were reacted with cleaved caspase 3 (Asp175) specific antibody, New England Technology, using the Refine Detection

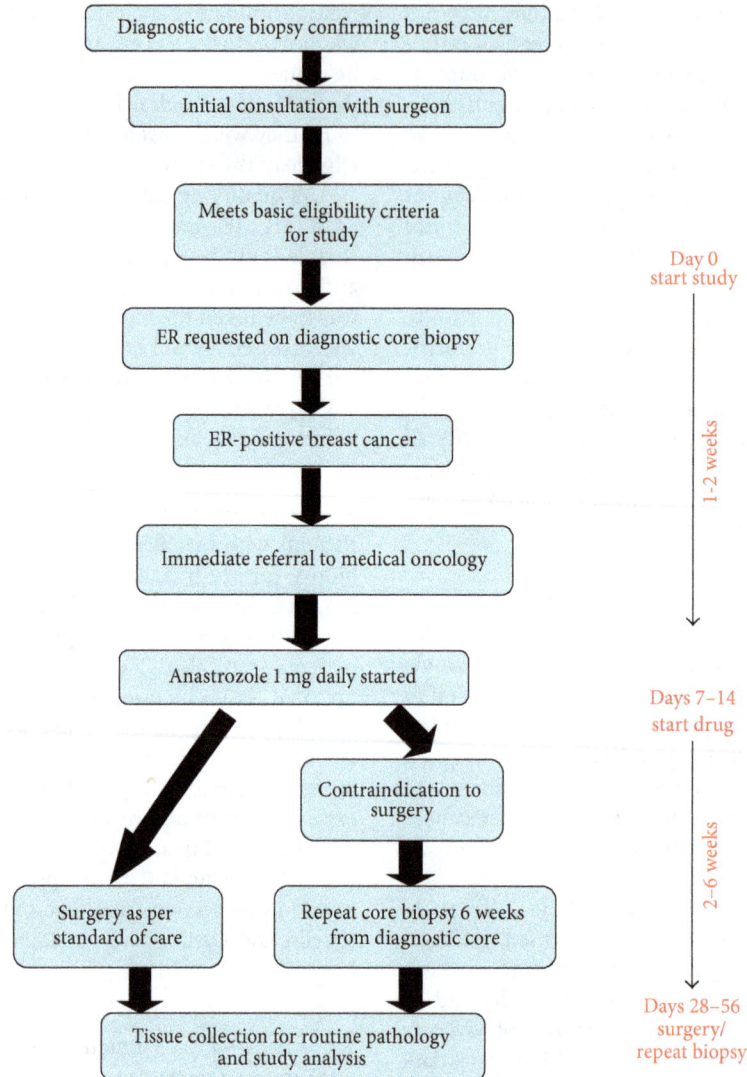

FIGURE 1: Study schema.

Kit from Leica. Five hundred cells from each specimen under ×400 magnification in the best-stained tumor area of each section were counted by a single pathologist (SR) for each specimen. CC3 immunoreactivity score was defined as the percentage of stained cells.

2.5. Statistical Analyses. The following criteria were established by the trial investigators as being required in order to demonstrate a meaningful success of feasibility for the group: (1) accrual of >50% of patients who were approached and (2) successful completion of >50% of patients who initially received anastrozole. Descriptive statistics were used to summarize the Ki67 values at baseline, at time of surgery, and the relative change from baseline to surgery. The percentage Ki67 change is defined as [surgical Ki67 − baseline Ki67]/[baseline Ki67 ∗ 100%] for each patient and the absolute change is defined as surgical Ki67 − baseline Ki67. Hence, a negative value indicates a decrease in Ki67 from baseline to surgery. Similar analyses were performed for CC3. Spearman ρ was

calculated to evaluate the association between caspase and Ki67, the change between these measures, and the association between the duration of drug and the change in these measures. All tests were two-sided, and $p < 0.05$ was considered statistically significant in all cases.

3. Results

3.1. Study Population and Characteristics. Between September 2012 and September 2013, a total of 131 newly diagnosed breast cancer patients underwent initial surgical consultation (consort diagram, Figure 2). A total of 32 (24.4% of all patients) patients were deemed as being potentially eligible based on tumor size and menopausal status and thus were screened for the study. Of the 32 patients that were approached, all (100%) consented to participate in the study. There were 10 screen failures, seven were due to estrogen receptor negative status on the diagnostic core biopsy, one patient was found to have distant metastatic disease, and two

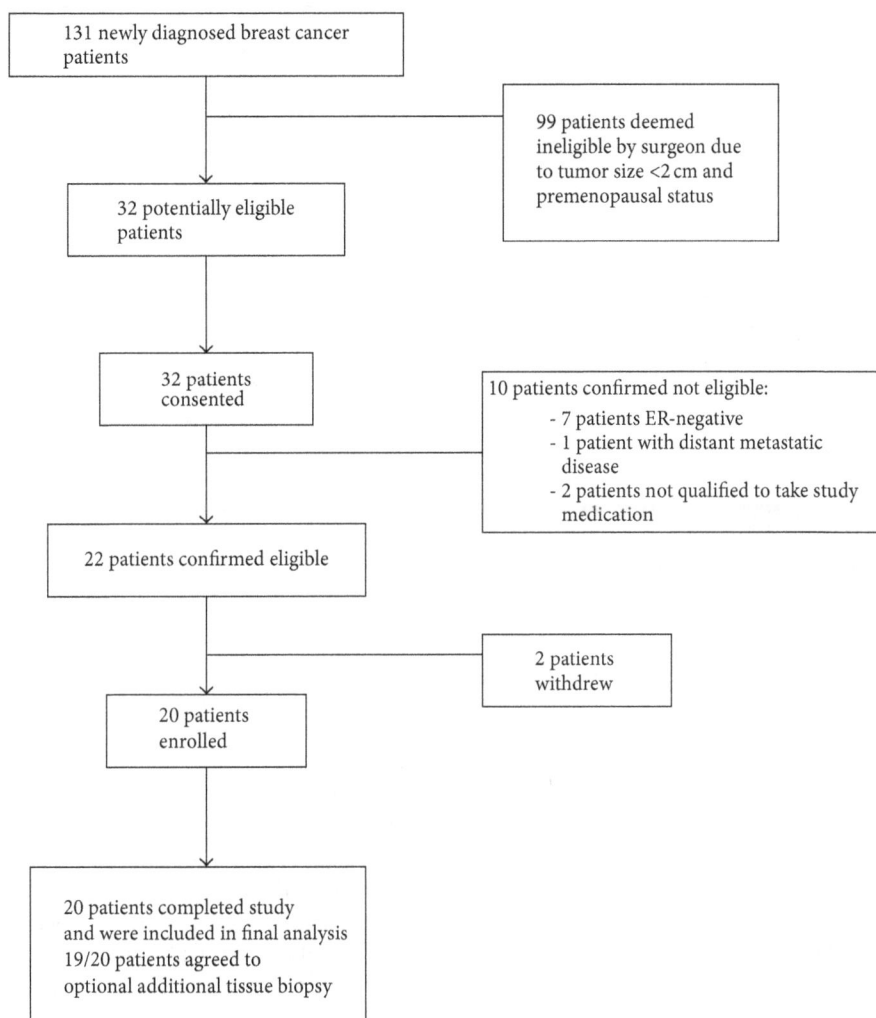

```
┌─────────────────────────┐
│ 131 newly diagnosed     │
│ breast cancer patients  │
└─────────────────────────┘
            │              ┌──────────────────────────┐
            ├─────────────▶│ 99 patients deemed        │
            │              │ ineligible by surgeon due │
            ▼              │ to tumor size <2 cm and   │
┌─────────────────────────┐│ premenopausal status     │
│ 32 potentially eligible │└──────────────────────────┘
│ patients                │
└─────────────────────────┘
            │
            ▼              ┌──────────────────────────┐
┌─────────────────────────┐│ 10 patients confirmed    │
│ 32 patients             ││ not eligible:            │
│ consented               │└──────────────────────────┘
```

FIGURE 2: Patient flowchart.

patients did not qualify to take anastrozole due to medical comorbidities. 20/22 (91%) patients were therefore confirmed to be eligible for the study. Two patients withdrew from the study prior to taking anastrozole. Of the 20 remaining patients who received anastrozole, 100% completed the study.

Patient characteristics of the 20 patients that started anastrozole and completed the study are shown in Table 1. Mean patient age was 66.3 (range 52–89), and 80% of the patients had invasive ductal carcinoma. The mean tumor size was 3.8 cm (range 1.4–6.5 cm). The majority of patients had pathological stage II (T2N0) invasive ductal carcinoma and breast conserving surgery.

3.2. Duration of Treatment, Side Effects, and Compliance.
The mean duration of drug intake was 24.7 days (SD 6.4 days; range 14–35 days), while the mean wait time from surgical decision to actual surgery date was 32.3 days (SD 8 days; range 15–44 days). The duration from the consent date to the patients' medical oncology appointment was a mean of 8.1 days (SD 4.6 days; range 1–19 days). All surgeries proceeded according to plan and scheduled date

which was decided at the initial surgical consultation. Of the 20 patients that completed the study, 18/20 experienced mild to moderate adverse effects (grades 1-2) including hot flashes, joint pains, fatigue, and nausea. There were no grades 3 or 4 toxicities.

3.3. Changes in Tumor Ki67 and CC3.
One patient had insufficient diagnostic tissue for baseline Ki67 and CC3 assessment and an additional tumor biopsy was performed prior to starting anastrozole. Another patient had sufficient core biopsy for pretreatment Ki67 but not CC3 analysis and also required an additional biopsy. The remaining 18 patients had sufficient paired pre- and posttreatment tissue samples for analysis. One patient did not proceed to surgery as planned within the 8-week time frame as she had ongoing cardiac comorbidities and more time was needed to better optimize her perioperative morbidity. She had a repeat biopsy 4 weeks after anastrozole treatment used for repeat Ki67 and CC3 analyses. After the additional biopsies, Ki67 and CC3 were assessable in all 20 patients from pre- and postanastrozole tumor tissue.

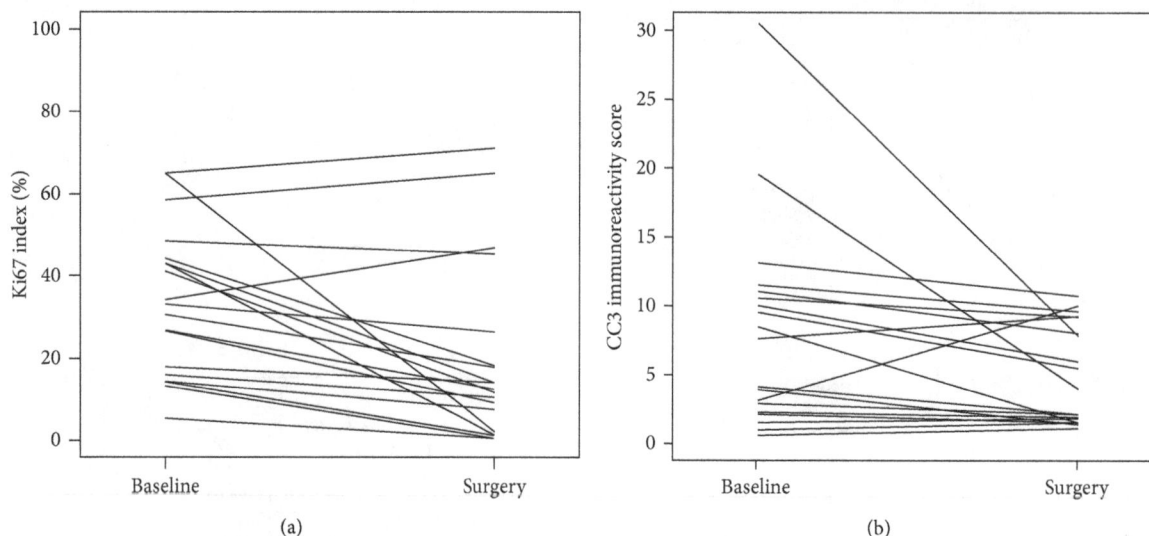

FIGURE 3: Ki67 labelling index (a) and cleaved caspase 3 (CC3) (b) at baseline and after anastrozole treatment at surgery.

TABLE 1: Clinical and pathological characteristics of patients who enrolled in the study.

Patient and surgical specimen tumor characteristics	
Age (years), mean (SD)	66.3 (10)
Age range (years)	52–89
Invasive disease, *n* (%)	
Invasive, ductal	16/20 (80%)
Invasive, lobular	2/20 (10%)
Mixed invasive, ductal, and lobular	2/20 (10%)
Surgical tumor stage, *n* (%)	
T1	5/20 (25%)
T2	10/20 (50%)
T3	5/20 (25%)
Surgical nodal stage, *n* (%)	
N0	10/20 (50%)
N1	3/20 (15%)
N2	5/20 (25%)
N3	2/20 (10%)
ER, *n* (%)	
Positive	20/20 (100%)
Negative	0/20 (0%)
PR, *n* (%)	
Positive	17/20 (85%)
Negative	3/20 (15%)
HER2, *n* (%)	
Positive	4/20 (20%)
Negative	18/20 (80%)
Type of breast surgery	
Lumpectomy	11/20 (55%)
Mastectomy	9/20 (45%)

Table 2 and Figure 3 summarize the Ki67 values before and after anastrozole treatment. One patient was excluded for analysis involving Ki67, as their postanastrozole Ki67 value increased by >1200%, which was an extreme outlier result and suggested technical inaccuracy; this patient was included for CC3 analyses.

Baseline pretreatment Ki67 mean was 33.2% (standard deviation 17.6%), compared to posttreatment Ki67 mean of 19.1% (standard deviation 21.2%) resulting in an absolute decline of 14.1% ($p < 0.001$) and relative decline of 48.8% ($p = 0.001$). 17/19 (89%) patients experienced a decline in the Ki67 value after treatment. Table 2 summarize the CC3 values before and after anastrozole treatment. Baseline pretreatment CC3 mean value was 7.7 (standard deviation 7.4) compared to posttreatment CC3 mean of 4.8 (standard deviation 3.6). This results in a statistically significant absolute decline of 2.9 points ($p = 0.007$) and a 10.5% relative decline that did not reach statistical significance ($p = 0.17$). Table 3 shows the association between Ki67 and CC3 values at baseline and posttreatment. There was a weak-to-none association ($r < |0.30|$ and p value > 0.05 for all) between Ki67 and CC3, at baseline, posttreatment, and for the change scores. Similarly, no association between Ki67 and drug duration was observed. However, for CC3, longer drug duration was moderately associated with a greater reduction in value, with a statistically significant association ($r = -0.50$, p value = 0.026) for relative percent change, and a trend towards significance for ($r = -0.43$, p value = 0.060) absolute change.

Results of any changes to Ki67 or CC3 as a result of the anastrozole treatment were blinded to the oncologist such that decisions regarding adjuvant chemotherapy or hormonal therapy decisions would not be affected.

3.4. Patient Acceptability for Additional Optional Tissue Collection. All 20 patients were approached to have additional optional breast tumor biopsies, additional blood sample retrieval, and urine collection for future research studies and

TABLE 2: Ki67 labeling index (%) and cleaved caspase 3 (CC3) at baseline (before anastrozole) and surgery (after anastrozole) on the 20 patients who completed the study.

	Statistic	Patients	p value
Ki67 labeling index (%)			
Baseline	Mean (std)	33.2 (17.6)	
	Median (10p, 90p)	31.7 (13.2, 61.8)	
End of study	Mean (std)	19.1 (21.2)	
	Median (10p, 90p)	12.1 (0.7, 55.8)	
% change	Mean (std)	−48.8 (40.1)	
	Median (10p, 90p)	−55.8 (−97.5, 10.1)	p = 0.001
Absolute change	Mean (std)	−14.1 (17.5)	
	Median (10p, 90p)	−12.2 (−35.6, 6.2)	p < 0.001
Cleaved caspase 3 (CC3)			
Baseline	Mean (std)	7.7 (7.4)	
	Median (10p, 90p)	5.9 (1.3, 16.3)	
End of study	Mean (std)	4.8 (3.6)	
	Median (10p, 90p)	3.1 (1.2, 9.8)	
% change	Mean (std)	−10.5 (67.7)	
	Median (10p, 90p)	−25.5 (−76.9, 66.7)	p = 0.17
Absolute change	Mean (std)	−2.9 (6.3)	
	Median (10p, 90p)	−1.6 (−11.2, 1.1)	p = 0.007

10p = 10th percentile; 90p = 90th percentile; p value = Wilcoxon rank sum; std = standard deviation.

TABLE 3: Association between Ki67 labelling index and cleaved caspase 3 (CC3) values at baseline (before anastrozole) and surgery (after anastrozole) using the Spearman r (p value) for associations.

	Baseline Ki67	Surgical Ki67	% change Ki67	Absolute change Ki67	Drug duration
Baseline CC3	−0.25 (0.14)				
Surgical CC3		0.06 (0.74)			
% change CC3			−0.02 (0.90)		−0.50 (0.026)
Absolute change CC3				−0.17 (0.33)	−0.43 (0.060)
Drug duration			0.23 (0.32)	0.07 (0.76)	

19/20 (95%) agreed to all three types of additional sample acquisition.

4. Discussion

While exciting for drug development strategies, performing window of opportunity trials faces multiple logistical and system barriers [4–13]. This albeit small pilot study demonstrated that performing such studies was possible at our cancer center. Our study did meet our established criteria for feasibility: we exceeded our target accrual of 50% of patients approached (32/32 patients approached consented to the study) and exceeded our 50% target completion rate in patients who received anastrozole (20/20 patients who received anastrozole complete the study). The results of our study demonstrated that women are willing to participate in such trials and undergo additional biopsies and give

additional blood and urine samples for future research. Combined and closely coordinated efforts among the different disciplines involved in the patient's care (surgery, pathology, and radiology) meant that it was possible to conduct such trials without delaying surgery.

As feasibility to accrue patients involves a range of issues including eligibility criteria, patient compliance, and study mandated procedures we decided to use a number of feasibility measures. At our center ER, PR, and Her2 are not routinely performed on diagnostic core specimens. Therefore, in order to test for these potential patients had to sign consent *before* they were screened by a study research associate for eligibility. Clearly, depending on the eligibility criteria, the number of patients which must be approached to identify those likely meeting eligibility criteria for any given study will vary considerably. Even with our pragmatic design (newly diagnosed breast cancer, postmenopausal,

>2 cm clinical or radiological confirmed, subsequently identified hormone receptor positive disease) 197 patients had to be approached or screened in order to identify the 32 potentially eligible patients who consented to the study. Subsequently, 69% (22/32) of the consented were eligible for the study, and 91% (20/22) ultimately completed the study. These numbers are similar to overall accrual rates in other window of opportunity studies [12–16]. We recognize that most of centers now routinely perform biomarkers on the diagnostic core biopsy specimens already, a process that was not in effect at our institution at the time of the study. The additional few days it took to obtain these results certainly may have helped allow for more time to enroll these patients without delay of their set surgical date, without which our accrual rate may have potentially been further reduced.

Our study also demonstrated that patient willingness to participate in such studies does not appear to be a barrier to accrual, as we were able to realize a high accrual rate. The fact that 19/20 (95%) patients enrolled agreed to undergo additional biopsies and blood and urine storage for future research studies reflected high patient enthusiasm for this type of research. This high rate of accrual likely reflects the fact that anastrozole, in addition to being a relatively safe and well tolerated drug, is already an established treatment for breast cancer, therefore making it a simple and easy drug to use for a pilot feasibility study [17, 18]. Its side effects did not preclude the patient from surgery which made it an acceptable agent for surgeons to consider. In the current study, the recognized therapeutic benefit of anastrozole likely helped patient compliance as all 20 patients who commenced anastrozole completed the study. Time will tell whether the use of agents that could interfere with surgical intervention (e.g., through effects on cardiac, neurological, marrow, coagulopathic, or thromboembolic events) would receive the same enthusiasm [1, 12]. Clearly, we do not know if a window of opportunity trial with an agent with no implied therapeutic advantage and unknown side effects will become more of an issue for patient compliance [4].

Changes in tumor Ki67 expression is a well-recognized surrogate endpoint for treatment response [18–21] and predictor of clinical outcome [22, 23]. Variability in Ki67 staining can occur as a result of a number of factors, including the duration of tissue ischemia, formalin quality, duration of fixation, immunohistochemical technique used, and assessor differences. Further, when comparing pretreatment biopsy to posttreatment excision or posttreatment biopsy, there may be effects of tumor heterogeneity on biomarker scores and at least a theoretical risk of alteration induced by the first biopsy procedure. We were able to have one pathologist (SR) perform all the analyses with the hope that variability in the assessor was reduced.

Many anticancer drugs induce apoptosis by molecular mechanisms mediated through mitochondrial dysfunction [24–26]. Release of cytochrome c from the internal part of the mitochondrial membrane into the cytosol results in the activation of caspase cascades, in particular caspase 9, caspase 3, caspase 6, and caspase 7. Because caspase 3 is the main executioner of apoptosis, immunohistochemical analysis to the active form of caspase 3, known as cleaved caspase 3 (CC3), has been used as an indicator of apoptosis in paraffin sections from various tissue sites [27–30]. Compared to the traditional TUNEL assay, whose interpretation and specificity have been reported as being difficult and controversial, CC3 immunohistochemistry is an easy, sensitive, and reliable method for detecting and quantifying apoptosis in tissues, with good correlation reported ($r = 0.75$) between it and the TUNEL assay [29]. Few studies have used it as a marker of response to treatment in breast cancer.

While the results may be counterintuitive in that CC3 (and therefore apoptosis) declined with anastrozole treatment, and a greater reduction was seen with longer duration of treatment, these results mirror what has been demonstrated with the TUNEL assay in anastrozole treated patients [20, 31, 32]. Unlike what is observed with cytotoxic chemotherapy, patients in the IMPACT study and others have demonstrated a decrease in apoptosis with endocrine therapy [20, 32]. It is possible that the capacity of breast cancer cells to pass into apoptosis is retarded by the profound antiproliferative effects of antiestrogenic therapy. It has been observed that *c-Myc* is a determinant of both proliferation and apoptosis [20], and its expression is enhanced by estrogen and suppressed by antiestrogens. This data suggests that estrogen may not be important for cell survival in breast cancers.

There remain a number of limitations to the current study. It was single center and single arm with a small sample size. Additional logistical and practical issues would be present in a multicenter or multiarm trial. Further difficulties may additionally be encountered if a novel agent with no known therapeutic benefit was used instead of anastrozole or if the biomarker was experimental and pathologists had little prior experience with measuring it. Additionally, the authors of this paper acknowledge that the involvement of a single dedicated surgeon and few medical oncologists would have potentially allowed for greater accrual. The success of the accrual may be less generalizable to larger group practices where it may be more difficult to overcome logistical hurdles. Finally, the authors recognize that the effect of presurgical hormonal therapy on Ki67 has already been demonstrated previously in studies such as IMPACT and POETIC [18, 20, 33]. The main objective of our study was to assess feasibility of such window trials at our institution.

In summary, this study demonstrates that accrual to nontherapeutic protocols is feasible in a single large academic cancer center and is acceptable to patients. The success achieved with this trial has been used as a strategy to convince other surgeons and patients to be involved in future research (NCT01948128).

Acknowledgments

This trial was supported by the University of Ottawa Department of Surgery research grant. Special thanks are due to Nancy Page for her assistance with REB and Health Canada approval and for overseeing the administrative aspects of the study. The authors are grateful to Luisa Ianni for her assistance in recruiting participants and for data collection. They would also like to thank Emily Desormeaux and Joelle Levac who assisted with all the immunohistochemistry performed. Finally, they would like to acknowledge all their participating patients and Women's Breast Health Center nurses including Pat Gorman, Antonella Iaderosa, Kelly Legallais, Lee-Anne Wolfesberger, Sandra Lowry, and Jennifer Smylie for helping out with the study.

References

[1] I. C. Henderson, "Window of opportunity," *Journal of the National Cancer Institute*, vol. 83, no. 13, pp. 894–896, 1991.

[2] K. Kalinsky and D. L. Hershman, "Cracking open window of opportunity trials," *Journal of Clinical Oncology*, vol. 30, no. 21, pp. 2573–2575, 2012.

[3] K. B. Wisinski, A. Faerber, S. Wagner et al., "Predictors of willingness to participate in window of opportunity breast trials," *Clinical Medicine and Research*, vol. 11, no. 3, pp. 107–112, 2013.

[4] B. Glimelius and M. Lahn, "Window of opportunity trials to evaluate clinical activity of new molecular entities in oncology," *Annals of Oncology*, vol. 22, no. 8, pp. 1717–1725, 2011.

[5] J. Hilton, A. Arnaout, and M. Clemons, "Primary endocrine therapy as an approach for patients with localized breast cancer deemed not to be surgical candidates," *Current Opinion in Supportive and Palliative Care*, vol. 8, no. 1, pp. 53–58, 2014.

[6] A. Arnaout, J. F. Boileau, and M. Brackstone, "Surgical considerations in locally advanced breast cancer patients receiving neoadjuvant chemotherapy," *Current Opinion in Supportive and Palliative Care*, vol. 8, no. 1, pp. 39–45, 2014.

[7] F. C. Wright, J. Zubovits, S. Gardner et al., "Optimal assessment of residual disease after neo-adjuvant therapy for locally advanced and inflammatory breast cancer—clinical examination, mammography, or magnetic resonance imaging?" *Journal of Surgical Oncology*, vol. 101, no. 7, pp. 604–610, 2010.

[8] J. Lemieux, M. Clemons, L. Provencher et al., "The role of neoadjuvant HER2-targeted therapies in HER2-overexpressing breast cancers," *Current Oncology*, vol. 16, no. 5, pp. 48–57, 2009.

[9] H. Al-Husaini, E. Amir, B. Fitzgerald et al., "Prevalence of overt metastases in locally advanced breast cancer," *Clinical Oncology*, vol. 20, no. 5, pp. 340–344, 2008.

[10] P. J. Goodwin, V. Stambolic, J. Lemieux et al., "Evaluation of metformin in early breast cancer: a modification of the traditional paradigm for clinical testing of anti-cancer agents," *Breast Cancer Research and Treatment*, vol. 126, no. 1, pp. 215–220, 2011.

[11] O. C. Freedman, S. Verma, and M. J. Clemons, "Using aromatase inhibitors in the neoadjuvant setting: evolution or revolution?" *Cancer Treatment Reviews*, vol. 31, no. 1, pp. 1–17, 2005.

[12] E. Singletary, R. Lieberman, N. Atkinson et al., "Novel translational model for breast cancer chemoprevention study: accrual to a presurgical intervention with tamoxifen and N-[4-hydroxyphenyl] retinamide," *Cancer Epidemiology Biomarkers and Prevention*, vol. 9, no. 10, pp. 1087–1090, 2000.

[13] S. E. Singletary, E. N. Atkinson, A. Hoque et al., "Phase II clinical trial of N-(4-hydroxyphenyl)retinamide and tamoxifen administration before definitive surgery for breast neoplasia," *Clinical Cancer Research*, vol. 8, no. 9, pp. 2835–2842, 2002.

[14] S. Niraula, R. J. O. Dowling, M. Ennis et al., "Metformin in early breast cancer: a prospective window of opportunity neoadjuvant study," *Breast Cancer Research and Treatment*, vol. 135, no. 3, pp. 821–830, 2012.

[15] S. Hadad, T. Iwamoto, L. Jordan et al., "Evidence for biological effects of metformin in operable breast cancer: a preoperative, window of opportunity, randomized trial," *Breast Cancer Research and Treatment*, vol. 128, no. 3, pp. 783–794, 2011.

[16] W. Demark-Wahnefried, S. L. George, B. R. Switzer et al., "Overcoming challenges in designing and implementing a phase II randomized controlled trial using a presurgical model to test a dietary intervention in prostate cancer," *Clinical Trials*, vol. 5, no. 3, pp. 262–272, 2008.

[17] M. Dowsett, I. Smith, J. Robertson et al., "Endocrine therapy, new biologicals, and new study designs for presurgical studies in breast cancer," *Journal of the National Cancer Institute—Monographs*, no. 43, pp. 120–123, 2011.

[18] M. Dowsett, I. E. Smith, S. R. Ebbs et al., "Prognostic value of Ki67 expression after short-term presurgical endocrine therapy for primary breast cancer," *Journal of the National Cancer Institute*, vol. 99, no. 2, pp. 167–170, 2007.

[19] R. B. Clarke, I. J. Laidlaw, L. J. Jones, A. Howell, and E. Anderson, "Effect of tamoxifen on Ki67 labelling index in human breast tumours and its relationship to oestrogen and progesterone receptor status," *British Journal of Cancer*, vol. 67, no. 3, pp. 606–611, 1993.

[20] I. E. Smith, M. Dowsett, S. R. Ebbs et al., "Neoadjuvant treatment of postmenopausal breast cancer with anastrozole, tamoxifen, or both in combination: the Immediate Preoperative Anastrozole, Tamoxifen, or Combined With Tamoxifen (IMPACT) multicenter double-blind randomized trial," *Journal of Clinical Oncology*, vol. 23, no. 22, pp. 5108–5116, 2005.

[21] M. J. Ellis, A. Coop, B. Singh et al., "Letrozole inhibits tumor proliferation more effectively than tamoxifen independent of HER1/2 expression status," *Cancer Research*, vol. 63, no. 19, pp. 6523–6531, 2003.

[22] M. J. Ellis, Y. Tao, J. Luo et al., "Outcome prediction for estrogen receptor-positive breast cancer based on postneoadjuvant endocrine therapy tumor characteristics," *Journal of the National Cancer Institute*, vol. 100, no. 19, pp. 1380–1388, 2008.

[23] O. C. Freedman, E. Amir, W. Hanna et al., "A randomized trial exploring the biomarker effects of neoadjuvant sequential treatment with exemestane and anastrozole in post-menopausal women with hormone receptor-positive breast cancer," *Breast Cancer Research and Treatment*, vol. 119, no. 1, pp. 155–161, 2010.

[24] D. R. Green and G. Kroemer, "The pathophysiology of mitochondrial cell death," *Science*, vol. 305, no. 5684, pp. 626–629, 2004.

[25] A. Bressenot, S. Marchal, L. Bezdetnaya, J. Garrier, F. Guillemin, and F. Plénat, "Assessment of apoptosis by immunohistochemistry to active caspase-3, active caspase-7, or cleaved PARP in monolayer cells and spheroid and subcutaneous xenografts of human carcinoma," *Journal of Histochemistry and Cytochemistry*, vol. 57, no. 4, pp. 289–300, 2009.

[26] Z. Jin and W. S. El-Deiry, "Overview of cell death signaling pathways," *Cancer Biology and Therapy*, vol. 4, no. 2, pp. 139–163, 2005.

[27] W. R. Duan, D. S. Gamer, S. D. Williams, C. L. Funckes-Shippy, I. S. Spath, and E. A. G. Blomme, "Comparison of immunohistochemistry for activated caspase-3 and cleaved cytokeratin 18 with the TUNEL method for quantification of apoptosis in

histological sections of PC-3 subcutaneous xenografts," *Journal of Pathology*, vol. 199, no. 2, pp. 221–228, 2003.

[28] A. M. Gown and M. C. Willingham, "Improved detection of apoptotic cells in archival paraffin sections: immunohisto-chemistry using antibodies to cleaved caspase 3," *Journal of Histochemistry and Cytochemistry*, vol. 50, no. 4, pp. 449–454, 2002.

[29] A. R. Resendes, N. Majó, J. Segalés et al., "Apoptosis in normal lymphoid organs from healthy normal, conventional pigs at different ages detected by TUNEL and cleaved caspase-3 immunohistochemistry in paraffin-embedded tissues," *Veterinary Immunology and Immunopathology*, vol. 99, no. 3-4, pp. 203–213, 2004.

[30] S. Jakob, N. Corazza, E. Diamantis, A. Kappeler, and T. Brunner, "Detection of apoptosis in vivo using antibodies against caspase-induced neo-epitopes," *Methods*, vol. 44, no. 3, pp. 255–261, 2008.

[31] J. Geisler, S. Detre, H. Berntsen et al., "Influence of neoadjuvant anastrozole (Arimidex) on intratumoral estrogen levels and proliferation markers in patients with locally advanced breast cancer," *Clinical Cancer Research*, vol. 7, no. 5, pp. 1230–1236, 2001.

[32] C. L. Harper-Wynne, N. P. M. Sacks, K. Shenton et al., "Comparison of the systemic and intratumoral effects of tamoxifen and the aromatase inhibitor vorozole in postmenopausal patients with primary breast cancer," *Journal of Clinical Oncology*, vol. 20, no. 4, pp. 1026–1035, 2002.

[33] L.-A. Martin, G. L. S. Davies, M. T. Weigel et al., "Pre-surgical study of the biological effects of the selective cyclo-oxygenase-2 inhibitor celecoxib in patients with primary breast cancer," *Breast Cancer Research and Treatment*, vol. 123, no. 3, pp. 829–836, 2010.

8

The Aetiology of Delay to Commencement of Adjuvant Chemotherapy following Colorectal Resection

G. S. Simpson,[1] R. Smith,[1] P. Sutton,[1,2] A. Shekouh,[1] C. McFaul,[1] M. Johnson,[1] and D. Vimalachandran[1]

[1] *Countess of Chester Hospital NHS Foundation Trust, Countess of Chester Health Park, Liverpool Road, Chester CH2 1UL, UK*
[2] *University of Liverpool, Liverpool, Merseyside L69 3BX, UK*

Correspondence should be addressed to G. S. Simpson; gregorysimpson@doctors.org.uk

Academic Editor: S. Curley

Purpose. Timely administration of adjuvant chemotherapy following colorectal resection is associated with improved outcome. We aim to assess the factors which are associated with delay to adjuvant chemotherapy in patients who underwent colorectal resection as part of an enhanced recovery protocol. *Method.* A univariate and multivariate analysis of patient data collected as part of a prospectively maintained database of colorectal cancer patients between 2007 and 2012. *Results.* 166 patients underwent colorectal resection followed by adjuvant chemotherapy. Median postoperative hospital stay was 6 days, and time to commencement of adjuvant chemotherapy was 50 days. Longer inpatient stay correlated with increased time to adjuvant chemotherapy ($P = 0.05$). Factors found to be independently associated with duration of hospital stay and time to commencement of adjuvant chemotherapy included stoma formation ($P = 0.032$), anastaomotic leak ($P = 0.027$), and preoperative albumin ($P = 0.027$). The use of laparoscopic surgery was associated with shorter time to adjuvant chemotherapy but did not reach significance ($P = 0.143$). *Conclusion.* A number of independent variables associated with delay to adjuvant therapy previously not described have been identified. Further work may be required to elucidate the effect that these variables have on long-term outcome.

1. Introduction

Colon and rectal cancer is a common malignancy worldwide, having the third highest incidence of all cancers with around 1 million diagnoses worldwide each year [1]. Multimodality treatment strategies are employed in the management of colorectal malignancy; with neoadjuvant and adjuvant treatments complimenting the mainstay of treatment-surgical resection.

The use of adjuvant chemotherapy (AC) following surgical resection of colorectal cancer has been shown to improve outcome [2–5]. Adjuvant chemotherapy has been advocated in patients with stage II disease associated with adverse disease features including T4 disease, perforation or obstruction [6], and in all patients with stage III disease [7].

The timing of administration of adjuvant chemotherapy following surgical resection has been proposed as a factor that potentially affects overall outcome, although this has not been proven conclusively. Some studies have demonstrated that initiation of chemotherapy occurring more promptly following surgical resection is being associated with improved outcome [8–10]. A meta-analysis found poorer outcomes if chemotherapy is administered 8 weeks or more after surgery [11], whilst another meta-analysis has reported a decrease in overall survival of 14% for each 4-week delay in administration of adjuvant chemotherapy [12].

Multiple factors dictating postoperative course and outcome in colorectal cancer have been identified including markers of the extent of systemic inflammatory response such as the Glasgow Prognostic Score (GPS), C-reactive protein, and albumin [13–15]. In addition, physiological parameters [16], patient comorbidity [17], and operative strategy [18, 19] have been shown to influence postoperative course and outcome. In contrast, limited information regarding the factors associated with increased delay to commencement of adjuvant therapy is available; however, age and race have been

TABLE 1: Patient demographics and operative details.

Number of patients identified	**166**
Gender: men	112 (67%)
Age: median (IQR)	66 (61 to 73) years
Comorbidity	91 (55%)
BMI: median (IQR)	27.3 (24.2 to 30.3)
Neoadjuvant chemoradiotherapy	
None	124 (75%)
Long course	36 (22%)
Short course	6 (3%)
Operation details	
Anterior resection	63 (38%)
Right hemicolectomy	50 (30%)
Left/sigmoid colectomy	30 (18%)
Abdominoperineal resection	13 (8%)
Hartmann's procedure	6 (4%)
Subtotal colectomy	3 (2%)
Panproctocolectomy	1 (<1%)
Mode of surgery	
Open	124 (75%)
Laparoscopic	42 (19%)
Converted	10 (6%)
Elective : emergency	153 (92%) : 13 (8%)
Stoma required	72 (43%)
Preoperative bloods: median (IQR)	
Haemoglobin (g/dL)	13.0 (11.9 to 14.3)
Platelets ($\times 10^6$/mL)	249 (218 to 333)
Neutrophils ($\times 10^6$/mL)	4.6 (3.6 to 5.7)
Lymphocytes ($\times 10^6$/mL)	1.5 (1.0 to 2.0)
Albumin (mg/L)	38 (35 to 41)
C-reactive protein (mg/L)	3 (2 to 11)

IQR: interquartile range.

TABLE 2: Histological tumour characteristics.

Histology	
Tumour size: median (IQR)	35 (27–50) mm
Differentiation	
Well/moderate	146 (88%)
Poor	13 (8%)
Complete response	7 (4%)
Node status	
N0	57 (34%)
N1	72 (43%)
N2	37 (22%)
Median nodal yield	14 (10 to 20)
Median number of involved nodes	3 (1 to 5)
Median lymph node ratio	0.18 (0.10 to 0.33)
T stage	
T0/T1	12 (7%)
T2	14 (8%)
T3	92 (55%)
T4	48 (29%)
Resection margin status	
R0	160 (94.4%)
R1	6 (3.6%)
Vascular invasion	
Positive	46 (28%)
Negative	120 (72%)

linked to delay in administration of adjuvant chemotherapy [20], whilst the occurrence of surgical complications has been associated with complete omission of adjuvant chemotherapy rather than delay of commencement [21].

Our aim is to identify factors which are associated with increased delay in administration of adjuvant chemotherapy in a cohort of patients undergoing curative resection for colorectal cancer.

2. Patients and Methods

An analysis of a prospectively maintained database containing details of all patients undergoing colorectal cancer resections from 2007 to 2012 was performed. All those with stages II-III colorectal cancer who received adjuvant chemotherapy following surgical resection were identified and included in the study. Relevant data pertaining to patient characteristics, operative strategy, complications, histology, biochemical parameters, and adjuvant therapy were extracted and analysed.

2.1. Outcome Measures. The time period (days) between surgical resection and commencement of adjuvant chemotherapy was calculated. Pre- and postoperative variables, histology, and biochemical parameters were analysed as to know their influence on the time to administration of adjuvant chemotherapy.

2.2. Statistical Analysis. All continuous data were analysed with median, interquartile range, and 95% confidence intervals. Nonparametric tests were employed for comparative purposes (Mann-Whitney U test). The interval between surgery and commencement of adjuvant chemotherapy was analysed as time to event data using Cox regression to analyse continuous and categorical variables for univariate and multivariate analysis. Software used included StatView V5 (SAS Institute, Cary, NC).

3. Results

166 patients who underwent intended curative resection for colorectal adenocarcinoma followed by adjuvant chemotherapy were identified. Table 1 outlines the patient demographics and operative details for this patient cohort. Table 2 outlines the histological characteristics of the resected cancers. Preoperative blood was typically recorded within 24 hours of surgery—median time interval = 1 day (IQR = 1 to 6).

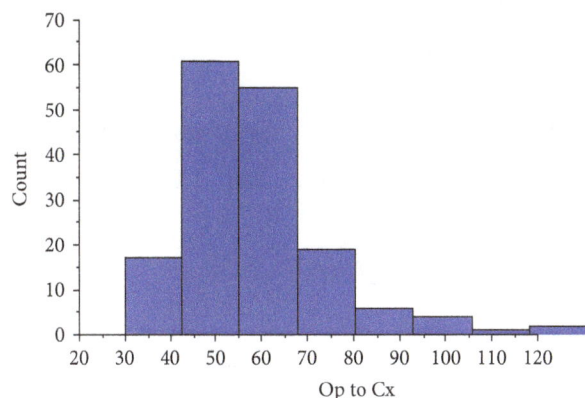

FIGURE 1: Distribution of time intervals from operation to commencement of chemotherapy (for inclusion in online publication only).

3.1. Postoperative Data. The median duration of hospital stay was 6 (IQR = 5 to 8) days. Five patients (3%) had a postoperative anastomotic leak; four of whom required further surgery. Two patients (1%) had significant postoperative bleeding; one of whom required reoperation and one required readmission. The median time interval from hospital discharge to commencing chemotherapy was 50 (IQR = 41 to 58) days. Patients with a longer postoperative inpatient stay exhibited a significant trend towards having a longer time interval from discharge to chemotherapy (linear regression; $t = 1.94$; $P = 0.050$)

3.2. Interval from Operation to Chemotherapy. Overall, the median time interval from the date of surgery to date of commencing adjuvant chemotherapy was 58 days (IQR = 39 to 77). Figure 1 illustrates this distribution. No patients received chemotherapy within 30 days of surgery. 107 (64%) patients received chemotherapy between 30 and 60 days of surgery and 59 (36%) patients received chemotherapy after 60 days.

Table 3 demonstrates the relationship between the clinicopathological factors investigated and time from surgery to commencement of adjuvant chemotherapy (Cox regression). From this analysis preoperative hypoalbuminaemia, anastomotic leak, requirement for stoma, and increasing lymph node ratio were all identified as having a potential association with a longer wait to commencement of adjuvant chemotherapy ($P < 0.100$). Patients undergoing laparoscopic surgery exhibited a trend towards shorter time intervals to starting adjuvant chemotherapy but this failed to reach significance ($P = 0.143$). On multivariate Cox regression, all four factors were independently significant. Figure 2 illustrates the associations between these four variables and time to chemotherapy. Due to incomplete preoperative biochemical data in 7 cases, the final multivariate analysis included 159 patients.

3.3. Duration of Hospital Admission. All four variables identified from the above analysis were also found to demonstrate a significant association with increased duration of postoperative stay (Table 4). Alongside this, patients undergoing laparoscopic resections were found to have a shorter postoperative hospital stay than those undergoing open surgery (Mann-Whitney; $P < 0.001$)—Figures 3 and 4.

4. Discussion and Conclusion

Adjuvant chemotherapy is a key component in the treatment of colorectal cancer and is shown to improve survival [3–5]. Data assessing the effect of timing of adjuvant chemotherapy have shown an increased mortality in patients where administration of chemotherapy has been delayed beyond 60 days [10, 22]. Only a small number of reports have demonstrated little effect of the timing of adjuvant chemotherapy following colorectal cancer resection on outcome [23, 24]. Recent meta-analyses have shown the benefit of early administration of chemotherapy, demonstrating a decrease in survival of 14% with every 4-week increase in delay to chemotherapy following resection [11, 12]. The finding of improved outcome with timely administration of adjuvant chemotherapy has also been documented in patients with cancer at other sites, most notably the breast [25–27] and pancreas [28].

Our data has identified multiple independently significant factors which are associated with increased delay to provision of adjuvant chemotherapy. Preoperative serum albumin has been shown to be inversely correlated with delay to commencement of adjuvant therapy. Similarly, our data has demonstrated that low preoperative serum albumin is associated with increased postoperative hospital stay. Albumin has previously been identified as a valuable preoperative marker linked to outcome following colorectal resection; however, no accounts are available in the literature showing it to be linked to timely receipt of adjuvant chemotherapy [13–15]. Preoperative albumin represents a potential marker of disease severity which could represent the degree of disease progression relating to operative difficulty and extension of recovery time, detrimentally affecting timely administration of chemotherapy. Additionally, albumin acts as an indicator of poor preoperative nutritional repleteness and overall systemic upset, factors which will dictate postoperative recovery and readiness for adjuvant chemotherapy.

Anastomotic leak following colorectal resection has a profound impact upon postoperative course and has a known detrimental effect on recurrence and overall survival [29, 30], in addition to being associated with significant morbidity and often permanent stoma formation [31]. From our data, it can be seen that this impacts the duration of inpatient stay and its effect extends to timely administration of chemotherapy, with those patients experiencing an anastomotic leak further jeopardized by a delay in the commencement of their systemic therapy.

The use of a defunctioning stoma following colorectal resection has been associated with extended inpatient hospital stay and delay to chemotherapy in this patient population. Available literature shows the formation of a defunctioning stoma to carry morbidity in the early postoperative period [32, 33] and to extend postoperative hospital stay

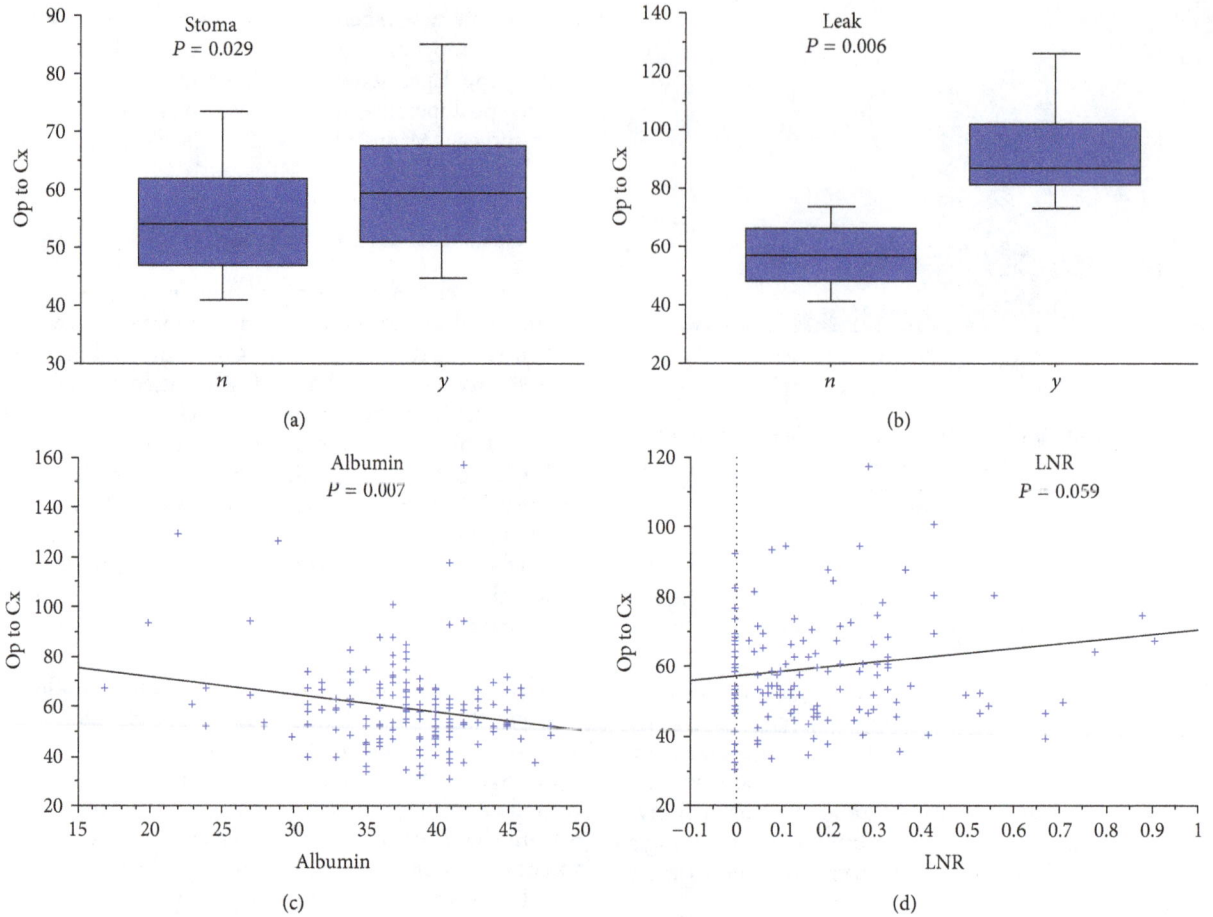

(a)

(b)

(c)

(d)

FIGURE 2: Relationship between requirement of stoma (a), anastomotic leak (b), preoperative serum albumin (c), and lymph node ratio (d) with time to adjuvant chemotherapy (categorical variables = Mann-Whitney; continuous variable = linear regression).

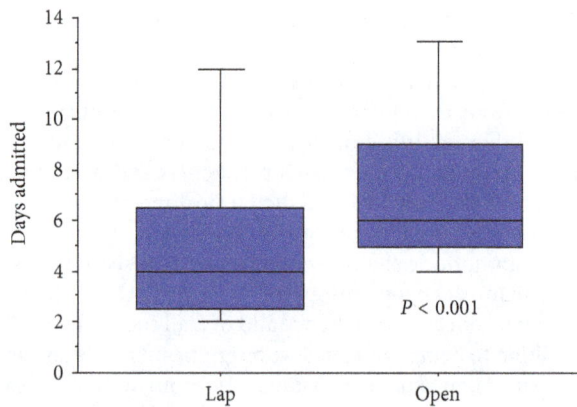

FIGURE 3: Association between laparoscopic surgery and shorter postoperative stay.

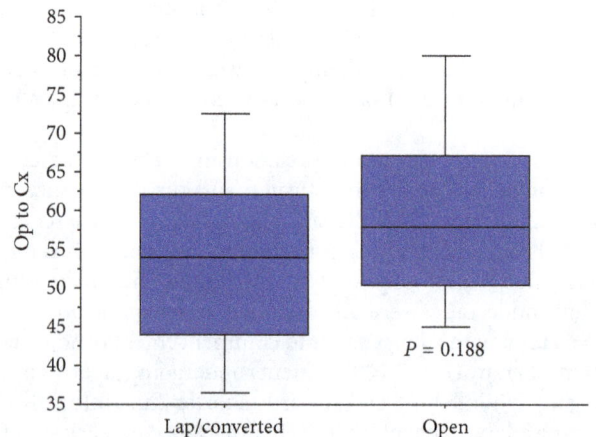

FIGURE 4: Association between approach to resection and time to adjuvant chemotherapy, laparoscopic/converted versus open (for inclusion in online publication only).

[34], mirroring our findings; however, the presence of a defunctioning stoma being associated with delay to adjuvant therapy has not been previously documented. The use of a defunctioning stoma is commonly associated with patients who have undergone preoperative chemoradiotherapy, rectal resections, and major or difficult resections, factors which may represent the cause of delay as opposed to the presence of a stoma.

TABLE 3: Cox regression analysis of factors associated with time from surgery to commencement of adjuvant chemotherapy.

	Univariate analysis			Multivariate analysis ($n = 159$)		
	Hazard ratio (95% CI)	χ^2	P	Hazard ratio (95% CI)	χ^2	P
Age	0.993 (0.978 to 1.007)	0.973	0.324			
Gender (F)	1.310 (0.937 to 1.832)	2.500	0.114			
BMI	0.991 (0.961 to 1.023)	0.292	0.589			
Comorbidity (Y)	1.083 (0.789 to 1.488)	0.247	0.619			
Neoadjuvant therapy (Y)	0.889 (0.625 to 1.265)	0.425	0.514			
Laparoscopic procedure (Y)	1.337 (0.906 to 1.973)	2.141	0.143			
Stoma (Y)	0.757 (0.555 to 1.031)	3.115	**0.078**	0.704 (0.512 to 0.970)	4.613	**0.032**
Tumour size	1.002 (0.994 to 1.010)	0.180	0.672			
Differentiation (poor versus well/moderate)	1.201 (0.679 to 2.122)	0.396	0.529			
T stage	1.009 (0.863 to 1.179)	0.013	0.911			
N stage	0.940 (0.680 to 1.299)	0.141	0.707			
Lymph node ratio	0.494 (0.215 to 1.131)	2.785	0.095	0.408 (0.168 to 0.992)	3.915	**0.048**
Resection margin status (+)	0.917 (0.546 to 1.541)	0.107	0.744			
Vascular invasion (+)	1.151 (0.816 to 1.623)	0.645	0.422			
Anastomotic leak (Y)	0.304 (0.123 to 0.749)	6.701	**0.010**	0.352 (0.140 to 0.887)	4.907	**0.027**
Preoperative haemoglobin	1.006 (0.915 to 1.105)	0.013	0.908			
Preoperative platelets	1.000 (0.999 to 1.002)	0.613	0.434			
Preoperative neutrophils	0.977 (0.915 to 1.042)	0.518	0.472			
Preoperative lymphocytes	0.966 (0.824 to 1.131)	0.187	0.666			
Preoperative C-reactive protein	0.998 (0.994 to 1.001)	1.751	0.186			
Preoperative albumin	1.036 (1.007 to 1.067)	5.933	**0.015**	1.034 (1.004 to 1.065)	4.916	**0.027**
Tumour site (colon versus rectum)	1.092 (0.802 to 1.487)	0.311	0.577			
Emergency (Y)	0.755 (0.426 to 1.339)	0.925	0.336			

TABLE 4: Multivariate Cox regression analysis of hypoalbuminaemia, anastomotic leak, requirement for stoma, lymph node ratio, and association with duration of postoperative admission (for inclusion in online publication only).

	Hazard ratio (95% CI)	χ^2	P
Albumin	1.044 (1.012 to 1.076)	7.573	**0.006**
Anastomotic leak (Y)	0.127 (0.042 to 0.388)	13.150	**<0.001**
Stoma (Y)	0.609 (0.437 to 0.848)	8.613	**0.003**
Lymph node ratio	0.264 (0.102 to 0.686)	7.479	**0.006**

Lymph node ratio defined as the number of involved lymph nodes divided by the total nodal yield has been proposed as a valuable prognostic indicator in colorectal cancer with studies showing that poorer long-term outcome is associated with an increasing lymph node ratio [35, 36] potentially as a result of more aggressive tumour biology in those tumours with higher lymph node ratios. Lymph node ratio in this study may represent those patients who have required a more extensive surgical dissection or are more systemically unwell as a consequence of their more aggressive malignancy and thus are more likely to experience a greater time to commencement of adjuvant chemotherapy.

Whilst the effect of delayed chemotherapy has been investigated, research into the aetiology of such a delay has been minimal. In the available evidence, factors which have previously been cited as having an association with increased delay to commencement of chemotherapy include advanced age, patient comorbidity, tumour grade, marital status, postoperative stay, and race [20, 22]. Our findings are not consistent with these previously documented associations. Administration of neoadjuvant therapies, tumour characteristics, patient comorbidity, age, and sex do not have a significant effect on the timely provision of adjuvant therapy in our data.

This study has identified a number of independently significant variables which are associated with delay to administration of adjuvant chemotherapy. The variables identified have not previously been described in the literature. Interestingly, the use of a laparoscopic approach to colorectal resection has been seen to yield a shorter wait to commencement of chemotherapy, although this did not achieve significance. This represents a potential further advantage of laparoscopic surgery in addition to shorter inpatient stay, postoperative pain, cost-effectiveness, and recovery time previously described [37–39]. This study is potentially limited by the retrospective nature of the data analysis.

The importance of timely administration of adjuvant chemotherapy following surgical resection has been identified as of importance in a number of specialties and its benefit has been made evident in colorectal cancer. Vigilance regarding prompt administration of adjuvant chemotherapy to colorectal cancer patients following surgical resection should be promoted, with colorectal teams providing this aspect of treatment as promptly as possible following surgical resection. Our study demonstrates a number of factors associated with delay in receiving adjuvant chemotherapy and may be used to identify patients who are at risk of delayed adjuvant chemotherapy so that this may be addressed in preoperative and intraoperative treatment decisions.

What Does This Paper Add to the Literature?

We present a number of previously undescribed variables associated with delay to adjuvant chemotherapy. We show that extended postoperative stay is related to delay to commencement of adjuvant chemotherapy.

Authors' Contribution

Gregory S. Simpson contributed in conception and design, data collection and interpretation, and drafting of paper. Richard Smith contributed in design, data collection and interpretation, and drafting of paper. Paul Sutton contributed in data interpretation and drafting of paper. Ali R. Shekouh contributed in drafting of paper. Christopher D. McFaul contributed in drafting of paper; final approval of paper is to be submitted. Michael A. Johnson contributed in drafting of paper; final approval of paper is to be submitted. Dale Vimalachandran (senior author) contributed in design and drafting of paper; final approval of paper is to be submitted.

References

[1] D. M. Parkin, F. Bray, J. Ferlay, and P. Pisani, "Global cancer statistics, 2002," *Ca-A Cancer Journal for Clinicians*, vol. 55, no. 2, pp. 74–108, 2005.

[2] QUASAR Collaborative Group, "Adjuvant chemotherapy versus observation in patients with colorectal cancer: a randomised study," *The Lancet*, vol. 370, no. 9604, pp. 2020–2029, 2007.

[3] J. Sakamoto, "Efficacy of oral adjuvant therapy after resection of colorectal cancer: 5-Year results from three randomized trials," *Journal of Clinical Oncology*, vol. 22, no. 3, pp. 484–492, 2004.

[4] S. Dubé, F. Heyen, and M. Jenicek, "Adjuvant chemotherapy in colorectal carcinoma: results of a meta- analysis," *Diseases of the Colon and Rectum*, vol. 40, no. 1, pp. 35–41, 1997.

[5] S. Gill, C. L. Loprinzi, D. J. Sargent et al., "Pooled analysis of fluorouracil-based adjuvant therapy for stage II and III colon cancer: who benefits and by how much?" *Journal of Clinical Oncology*, vol. 22, no. 10, pp. 1797–1806, 2004.

[6] A. Figueredo, M. E. Coombes, and S. Mukherjee, "Adjuvant therapy for completely resected stage II colon cancer," *Cochrane Database of Systematic Reviews*, vol. 16, no. 3, Article ID CD005390, 2008.

[7] A. B. Benson III, D. Schrag, M. R. Somerfield et al., "American society of clnical oncology recommendations on adjuvant chemotherapy for stage II colon cancer," *Journal of Clinical Oncology*, vol. 22, no. 16, pp. 3408–3419, 2004.

[8] D. Hershman, M. J. Hall, X. Wang et al., "Timing of adjuvant chemotherapy initiation after surgery for stage III colon cancer," *Cancer*, vol. 107, no. 11, pp. 2581–2588, 2006.

[9] I. S. Lima, Y. Yasui, A. Scarfe, and M. Winget, "Association between receipt and timing of adjuvant chemotherapy and survival for patients with stage III colon cancer in Alberta, Canada," *Cancer*, vol. 117, no. 16, pp. 3833–3840, 2011.

[10] U. D. Bayraktar, E. Chen, S. Bayraktar et al., "Does delay of adjuvant chemotherapy impact survival in patients with resected stage ii and iii colon adenocarcinoma?" *Cancer*, vol. 117, no. 11, pp. 2364–2370, 2011.

[11] G. Des Guetz, P. Nicolas, G. Perret, J. Morere, and B. Uzzan, "Does delaying adjuvant chemotherapy after curative surgery for colorectal cancer impair survival? A meta-analysis," *European Journal of Cancer*, vol. 46, no. 6, pp. 1049–1055, 2010.

[12] J. J. Biagi, M. J. Raphael, W. J. Mackillop, W. Kong, W. D. King, and C. M. Booth, "Association between time to initiation of adjuvant chemotherapy and survival in colorectal cancer a systematic review and meta-analysis," *Journal of the American Medical Association*, vol. 305, no. 22, pp. 2335–2342, 2011.

[13] M. J. Proctor, D. S. Morrison, D. Talwar et al., "A comparison of inflammation-based prognostic scores in patients with cancer. A Glasgow Inflammation Outcome Study," *European Journal of Cancer*, vol. 47, no. 17, pp. 2633–2641, 2011.

[14] R. Carruthers, L. M. Tho, J. Brown, S. Kakumanu, E. McCartney, and A. C. McDonald, "Systemic inflammatory response is a predictor of outcome in patients undergoing preoperative chemoradiation for locally advanced rectal cancer," *Colorectal Disease*, vol. 14, no. 10, pp. e701–e707, 2012.

[15] L. H. Moyes, E. F. Leitch, R. F. McKee, J. H. Anderson, P. G. Horgan, and D. C. McMillan, "Preoperative systemic inflammation predicts postoperative infectious complications in patients undergoing curative resection for colorectal cancer," *British Journal of Cancer*, vol. 100, no. 8, pp. 1236–1239, 2009.

[16] C. H. Richards, E. F. Leitch, P. G. Horgan, J. H. Anderson, R. F. McKee, and D. C. McMillan, "The relationship between patient physiology, the systemic inflammatory response and survival in patients undergoing curative resection of colorectal cancer," *British Journal of Cancer*, vol. 103, no. 9, pp. 1356–1361, 2010.

[17] P. O. Hendry, J. Hausel, J. Nygren et al., "Determinants of outcome after colorectal resection within an enhanced recovery programme," *British Journal of Surgery*, vol. 96, no. 2, pp. 197–205, 2009.

[18] S. Trastulli, R. Cirocchi, C. Listorti et al., "Laparoscopic vs open resection for rectal cancer: a meta-analysis of randomized clinical trials," *Colorectal Disease*, vol. 14, no. 6, pp. e277–e296, 2012.

[19] H. Ohtani, Y. Tamamori, T. Azuma et al., "A meta-analysis of the short- and long-term results of randomized controlled trials that compared laparoscopy-assisted and conventional open surgery for rectal cancer," *Journal of Gastrointestinal Surgery*, vol. 15, no. 8, pp. 1375–1385, 2011.

[20] W. Y. Cheung, B. A. Neville, and C. C. Earle, "Etiology of delays in the initiation of adjuvant chemotherapy and their impact on

outcomes for stage II and III rectal cancer," *Diseases of the Colon and Rectum*, vol. 52, no. 6, pp. 1054–1063, 2009.

[21] S. Hendren, J. D. Birkmeyer, H. Yin, M. Banerjee, C. Sonnenday, and A. M. Morris, "Surgical complications are associated with omission of chemotherapy for stage III colorectal cancer," *Diseases of the Colon and Rectum*, vol. 53, no. 12, pp. 1587–1593, 2010.

[22] D. Hershman, M. J. Hall, X. Wang et al., "Timing of adjuvant chemotherapy initiation after surgery for stage III colon cancer," *Cancer*, vol. 107, no. 11, pp. 2581–2588, 2006.

[23] R. Zeig-Owens, S. T. Gershman, R. Knowlton, and J. S. Jacobson, "Survival and time interval from surgery to start of chemotherapy among colon cancer patients," *Journal of Registry Management*, vol. 36, no. 2, pp. 30–62, 2009.

[24] S. Ahmed, I. Ahmad, T. Zhu et al., "Early discontinuation but not the timing of adjuvant therapy affects survival of patients with high-risk colorectal cancer: a population-based study," *Diseases of the Colon and Rectum*, vol. 53, no. 10, pp. 1432–1438, 2010.

[25] N. Alkis, A. G. Durnali, U. Y. Arslan et al., "Optimal timing of adjuvant treatment in patients with early breast cancer," *Medical Oncology*, vol. 28, no. 4, pp. 1255–1259, 2011.

[26] C. Lohrisch, C. Paltiel, K. Gelmon et al., "Impact on survival of time from definitive surgery to initiation of adjuvant chemotherapy for early-stage breast cancer," *Journal of Clinical Oncology*, vol. 24, no. 30, pp. 4888–4894, 2006.

[27] D. L. Hershman, X. Wang, R. McBride, J. S. Jacobson, V. R. Grann, and A. I. Neugut, "Delay of adjuvant chemotherapy initiation following breast cancer surgery among elderly women," *Breast Cancer Research and Treatment*, vol. 99, no. 3, pp. 313–321, 2006.

[28] Y. Murakami, K. Uemura, T. Sudo et al., "Early initiation of adjuvant chemotherapy improves survival of patients with pancreatic carcinoma after surgical resection," *Cancer Chemotherapy and Pharmacology*, vol. 71, no. 2, pp. 419–429, 2013.

[29] M. A. Boccola, P. G. Buettner, W. M. Rozen et al., "Risk factors and outcomes for anastomotic leakage in colorectal surgery: a single-institution analysis of 1576 patients," *World Journal of Surgery*, vol. 35, no. 1, pp. 186–195, 2011.

[30] W. L. Law, H. K. Choi, Y. M. Lee, J. W. C. Ho, and C. L. Seto, "Anastomotic leakage is associated with poor long-term outcome in patients after curative colorectal resection for malignancy," *Journal of Gastrointestinal Surgery*, vol. 11, no. 1, pp. 8–15, 2007.

[31] A. A. Khan, J. M. D. Wheeler, C. Cunningham, B. George, M. Kettlewell, and N. J. M. Mortensen, "The management and outcome of anastomotic leaks in colorectal surgery," *Colorectal Disease*, vol. 10, no. 6, pp. 587–592, 2008.

[32] O. Akesson, I. Syk, G. Lindmark, and P. Buchwald, "Morbidity related to defunctioning loop ileostomy in low anterior resection," *International Journal of Colorectal Disease*, vol. 27, no. 12, pp. 1619–1623, 2012.

[33] V. L. Tsikitis, D. W. Larson, V. P. Poola et al., "Postoperative morbidity with diversion after low anterior resection in the era of neoadjuvant therapy: a single institution experience," *Journal of the American College of Surgeons*, vol. 209, no. 1, pp. 114–118, 2009.

[34] M. T. Cartmell, O. M. Jones, B. J. Moran, and T. D. Cecil, "A defunctioning stoma significantly prolongs the length of stay in laparoscopic colorectal resection," *Surgical Endoscopy and Other Interventional Techniques*, vol. 22, no. 12, pp. 2643–2647, 2008.

[35] K. P. Wong, J. T. C. Poon, J. K. M. Fan, and W. L. Law, "Prognostic value of lymph node ratio in stage III colorectal cancer," *Colorectal Disease*, vol. 13, no. 10, pp. 1116–1122, 2011.

[36] R. Rosenberg, J. Engel, C. Bruns et al., "The prognostic value of lymph node ratio in a population-based collective of colorectal cancer patients," *Annals of Surgery*, vol. 251, no. 6, pp. 1070–1078, 2010.

[37] M. Z. Li, L. B. Xiao, W. H. Wu, S. B. Yang, and S. Z. Li, "Meta-analysis of laparoscopic versus open colorectal surgery within fast-track perioperative care," *Diseases of the Colon & Rectum*, vol. 55, no. 7, pp. 821–827, 2012.

[38] C. C. Jensen, L. M. Prasad, and H. Abcarian, "Cost-effectiveness of laparoscopic vs open resection for colon and rectal cancer," *Diseases of the Colon & Rectum*, vol. 55, no. 10, pp. 1017–1023, 2012.

[39] M. M. Reza, J. A. Blasco, E. Andradas, R. Cantero, and J. Mayol, "Systematic review of laparoscopic versus open surgery for colorectal cancer," *British Journal of Surgery*, vol. 93, no. 8, pp. 921–928, 2006.

9

Clear Cell Adenocarcinoma of the Urethra

Anthony Kodzo-Grey Venyo

North Manchester General Hospital, Department of Urology, Manchester, UK

Correspondence should be addressed to Anthony Kodzo-Grey Venyo; akodzogrey@yahoo.co.uk

Academic Editor: Rajendra A. Badwe

Background. Clear cell adenocarcinoma of the urethra (CCAU) is extremely rare and a number of clinicians may be unfamiliar with its diagnosis and biological behaviour. *Aims.* To review the literature on CCAU. *Methods.* Various internet databases were used. *Results/Literature Review.* (i) CCAU occurs in adults and in women in the great majority of cases. (ii) It has a particular association with urethral diverticulum, which has been present in 56% of the patients; is indistinguishable from clear cell adenocarcinoma of the female genital tract but is not associated with endometriosis; and probably does not arise by malignant transformation of nephrogenic adenoma. (iii) It is usually, readily distinguished from nephrogenic adenoma because of greater cytological a-typicality and mitotic activity and does not stain for prostate-specific antigen or prostatic acid phosphatase. (iv) It has been treated by anterior exenteration in women and cystoprostatectomy in men and at times by radiotherapy; chemotherapy has rarely been given. (v) CCAU is aggressive with low 5-year survival rates. (vi) There is no consensus opinion of treatment options that would improve the prognosis. *Conclusions.* Few cases of CCAU have been reported. Urologists, gynaecologists, pathologists, and oncologists should report cases of CCAU they encounter and enter them into a multicentric trial to determine the best treatment options that would improve the prognosis.

1. Introduction

Clear cell adenocarcinoma of the urethra (CCAU) is rare in both sexes but has been more commonly described in the female urethra. Even in the female CCAU is very rare. Information regarding CCAU has been obtained from single case reports and small case series [1, 2]. The ensuing paper contains a review of the literature which has been divided into (A) Overview which has broadly summarized CCAU and (B) Discussion and narrations from reported cases and case series of CCAU.

2. Methods

Various internet search databases were used to obtain literature on CCAU using the following key words: clear cell adenocarcinoma of urethra; renal cell carcinoma of urethra; primary; metastatic; secondary. Twenty-six references were identified which were suitable for the review of the literature.

3. Literature Review

3.1. Overview

3.1.1. General

Epidemiology. Clear cell adenocarcinoma of the urethra most commonly occurs in women with a mean age of 58 years (range 35 to 80 years) [3].

Aetiology. CCACU is conjectured to arise from surface urothelial metaplasia or Müllerian rests or Müllerianosis [4].

3.1.2. Presentation. CCACU tends to have similar clinical manifestation to the other urethral carcinomas [1, 3], haematuria [2].

3.1.3. Investigations

Urine Cytology. Patients tend to present with haematuria and when they are first seen their urine specimens are sent for cytological examination in addition to the urine specimens being sent for microscopy and culture.

Cytological Features. The cytological features of CCAU include: (i) enlarged tumour cells which contain abundant clear cytoplasm with conspicuous vacuoles; (ii) hobnail patterned cells; (iii) and hyaline globules.

Urethrocystoscopy

(i) Urethrocystoscopy enables the surgeon to visualise the urethral tumour and provides a means by which biopsies are taken for histological examination to establish the diagnosis of CCACU.

(ii) Examination under anaesthesia at urethrocystoscopy enables the surgeon to bimanually examine and assess the urethral tumour for fixity of the tumour and to determine how easy or difficult it might be to completely excise the lesion at operation.

3.1.4. Radiological Imaging.

The following radiological investigations can be used to localize a mass in the urethra as well as show whether there is any urinary bladder wall thickness, pelvic lymph node involvement, or distant metastases.

Ultrasound scan may reveal urethral mass [5].

MRI scan may reveal urethral diverticulum containing a nodular enhancing malignancy [6] or a heterogeneous mass in the urethra [5].

CT scan may reveal urethral diverticulum containing a heterogeneous mass [5, 6]. It could be imagined that if there is no urethral diverticulum the CT scan may demonstrate urethral mass only.

Isotope bone scan can also reveal whether or not there is bony metastasis [5, 6].

3.1.5. Macroscopic Features.

Most commonly (56%) CCACUs are found as tumours arising in urethral diverticulum [3].

For microscopic features, see Figures 1, 2, 3, 4, 5, 6, 7, 8, 9, 10, 11, 12, and 13 which show various microscopic and immunohistochemical staining characteristics of the tumour.

(i) The microscopic characteristics of CCAU are similar to clear cell adenocarcinoma of female genital tract.

(ii) CCAUs tend to exhibit the classic triad of (a) tubulocystic, (b) papillary, and (c) diffuse patterns [2, 3] which characterize the tumour.

(iii) Microscopic examination of CCAUs shows hobnail and flattened cells with abundant clear cytoplasm, moderate to marked nuclear pleomorphism, and frequent mitotic figures are seen [2, 3].

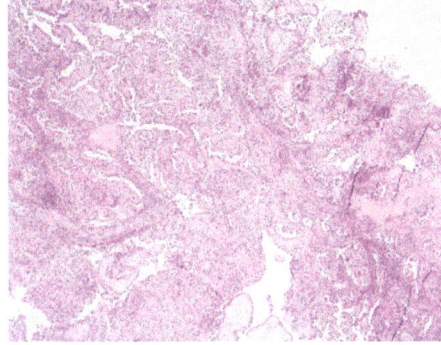

FIGURE 1: Haematoxylin and eosin staining, original magnification ×4, showing complex papillary architecture with abundant fibrovascular stroma; minimal tubular structures and focal solid areas are also seen. The figure was reproduced from [4, 7] with permission granted by Dr. Eddie Fridman. This permission is exclusive to this request specifically for this paper. Additional usage of any printed or electronic material for which Dr. Eddie Fridman holds would require copyright permission from Dr. Eddie Fridman.

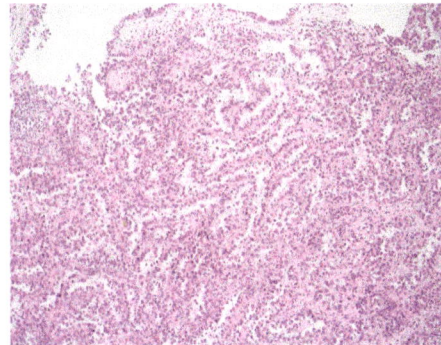

FIGURE 2: Haematoxylin and eosin staining, original magnification ×10, showing papillary and tubular structures, with cytologically atypical epithelial lining with clear cells and focal hob-nail appearance. The figure was reproduced from [4, 7] with permission granted by Dr. Eddie Fridman. This permission is exclusive to this request specifically for this paper. Additional usage of any printed or electronic material for which Dr. Eddie Fridman holds would require Dr. Eddie Fridman.

For immunohistochemical staining characteristics, see Figures 1 to 13 which show various microscopic and immunohistochemical staining characteristics of the tumour.

3.1.6. Positive Staining.

CCAUs exhibit positive immunohistochemical staining for

(i) PAX2 [3],

(ii) PAX8 [3],

(iii) cytokeratin 7 [5, 9],

(iv) p16 [5],

(v) p53 [5],

(vi) CA125 [5],

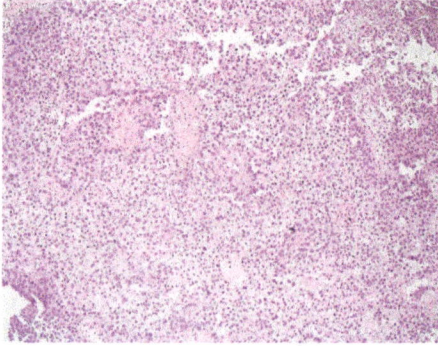

FIGURE 3: Haematoxylin and eosin staining, original magnification ×10, showing areas of solid growth pattern composed of atypical clear cells. The figure was reproduced from [4, 7] with permission granted by Dr. Eddie Fridman. Copyright to Dr. Eddie Fridman. This permission is exclusive to this request specifically for this paper. Additional usage of any printed or electronic material for which Dr. Eddie Fridman holds would require copyright permission from Dr. Eddie Fridman.

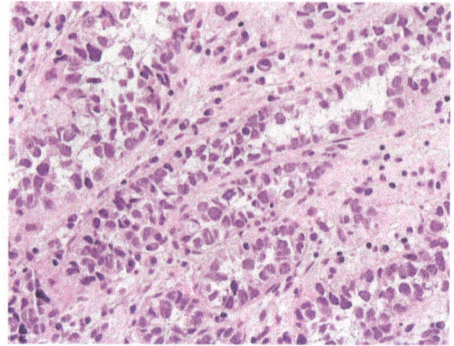

FIGURE 5: Haematoxylin and eosin staining, original magnification ×40, showing prominent cytological pleomorphism in clear cells and atypical mitotic figures. The figure was reproduced from [4, 7] with permission granted by Dr. Eddie Fridman. Copyright to Dr. Eddie Fridman. This permission is exclusive to this request specifically for this paper. Additional usage of any printed or electronic material for which Dr. Eddie Fridman holds would require copyright permission from Dr. Eddie Fridman.

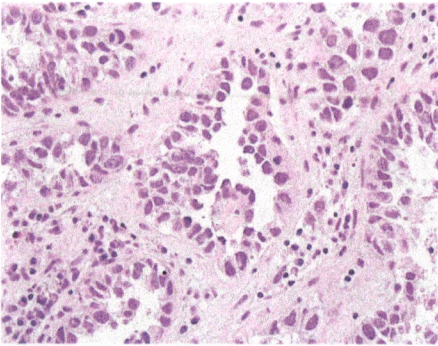

FIGURE 4: Haematoxylin and eosin staining, original magnification ×40, high magnification, showing prominent cytological nuclear atypia and few eosinophilic globules. The figure was reproduced from [4, 7] with permission granted by Dr. Eddie Fridman. Copyright to Dr. Eddie Fridman. This permission is exclusive to this request specifically for this paper. Additional usage of any printed or electronic material for which Dr. Eddie Fridman holds would require copyright permission from Dr. Eddie Fridman.

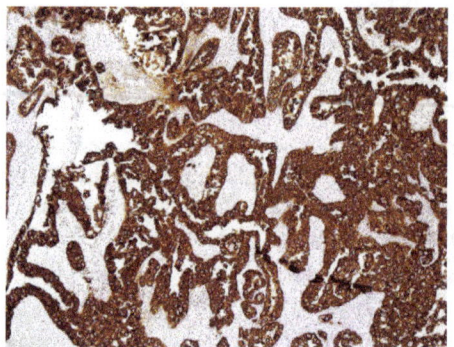

FIGURE 6: Immunohistochemical staining of clear cell adenocarcinoma showing strongly positive staining for CK7. The figure was reproduced from [4, 7] with permission granted by Dr. Eddie Fridman. Copyright to Dr. Eddie Fridman. This permission is exclusive to this request specifically for this paper. Additional usage of any printed or electronic material for which Dr. Eddie Fridman holds would require copyright permission from Dr. Eddie Fridman.

    (vii) CAM5.2 [5],

   (viii) AE1/AE3 [5].

3.1.7. Negative Staining. CCAUs exhibit negative immunohistochemical staining for

     (i) PSA [2, 3],

    (ii) PAP [3],

   (iii) thrombomodulin [5],

   (iv) oestrogen [5],

    (v) progesterone [5],

   (vi) cytokeratin 20 [5],

   (vii) p63 [5],

  (viii) CD10 [5],

   (ix) CEAP [5],

    (x) WTI [5],

   (xi) AFP [5],

  (xii) s100 [5].

3.1.8. Differential Diagnoses

    (i) Metastatic involvement from the female genital tract should be excluded [4].

   (ii) Nephrogenic adenoma in which no marked nuclear pleomorphism can be seen on microscopy, in which no mitotic figures can be seen, and in which there exists no infiltrative or solid growth pattern.

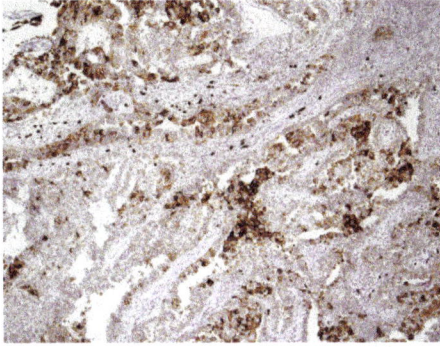

FIGURE 7: Immunohistochemical staining for clear cell adenocarcinoma showing positive staining for CD15. The figure was reproduced from [4, 7] with permission granted by Dr. Eddie Fridman. Copyright to Dr. Eddie Fridman. This permission is exclusive to this request specifically for this paper. Additional usage of any printed or electronic material for which Dr. Eddie Fridman holds would require copyright permission from Dr. Eddie Fridman.

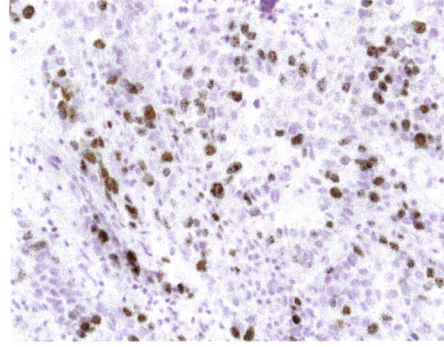

FIGURE 9: Immunohistochemical staining of clear cell adenocarcinoma showing positive staining for Ki-67 (original magnification ×40). The figure was reproduced from [4, 7] with permission granted by Dr. Eddie Fridman. Copyright to Dr. Eddie Fridman. This permission is exclusive to this request specifically for this paper. Additional usage of any printed or electronic material for which Dr. Eddie Fridman holds would require copyright permission from Dr. Eddie Fridman.

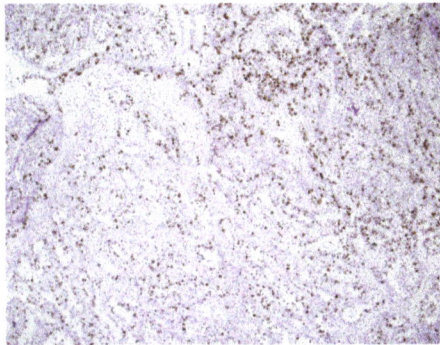

FIGURE 8: Immunohistochemical staining of clear cell adenocarcinoma showing positive staining for Ki-67 (original magnification ×10). The figure was reproduced from [4, 7] with permission granted by Dr. Eddie Fridman. Copyright to Dr. Eddie Fridman. This permission is exclusive to this request specifically for this paper. Additional usage of any printed or electronic material for which Dr. Eddie Fridman holds would require copyright permission from Dr. Eddie Fridman.

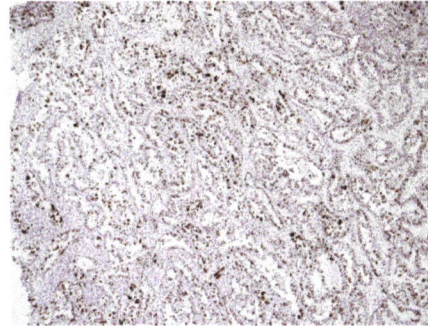

FIGURE 10: Immunohistochemical staining of clear cell adenocarcinoma showing positive staining for p53 (original magnification ×10). The figure was reproduced from [4, 7] with permission granted by Dr. Eddie Fridman. Copyright to Dr. Eddie Fridman. This permission is exclusive to this request specifically for this paper. Additional usage of any printed or electronic material for which Dr. Eddie Fridman holds would require copyright permission from Dr. Eddie Fridman.

3.1.9. Treatment

(i) A small urethral tumour of CCAU may be effectively treated by urethrectomy alone.

(ii) Urethrectomy in conjunction with cystoprostatectomy or urethrectomy in combination with anterior exenteration would be considered good options of treatment for CCAU.

(iii) Anterior exenteration and pelvic lymph node dissection were the treatment used in most reported cases of CCAU (as in [5, 6, 9]).

(iv) Consolidation radiotherapy to the pelvis had been given in a case of pelvic lymph node involvement.

(v) There is lack of knowledge of the effectiveness of chemotherapy in the treatment of CCAU and there has not been any documentation to suggest that chemotherapy is effective in the treatment of CCAU (see [10] in which chemotherapy was given).

3.1.10. Prognosis.

Few cases of CCAU have been reported and it would appear so far that CCAU is an aggressive tumour with low 5-year survival rates. There is therefore the need to explore for treatment options that would improve the prognosis.

3.2. Discussion and Miscellaneous Narrations from Some Reported Cases and Case Series.

Oliva and Young [3] reported 19 clear cell adenocarcinomas of the urethra in 1996. They reported that out of the 19 patients with CCAU 18 were from women and 1 from a man. The ages of the patients ranged from 35 years to 80 years and the average age was 58 years. They stated that the clinical manifestation and macroscopic findings were similar to those of urethral

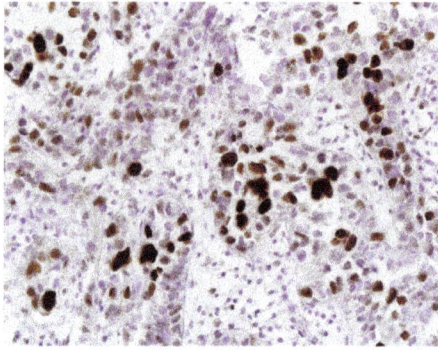

FIGURE 11: Immunohistochemical staining of clear cell adenocarcinoma showing positive staining for p53 (original magnification ×40). The figure was reproduced from [4, 7] with permission granted by Dr. Eddie Fridman. Copyright to Dr. Eddie Fridman. This permission is exclusive to this request specifically for this paper. Additional usage of any printed or electronic material for which Dr. Eddie Fridman holds would require copyright permission from Dr. Eddie Fridman.

carcinomas, except for the fact that 12 tumours which were all found in women arose within urethral diverticulum. They also reported that microscopic examination revealed that the neoplasms exhibited the classic triad of (a) tubulocystic, (b) papillary, and (c) diffuse patterns which characterized the tumour. Furthermore, they reported the following.

(i) The tumours exhibited the typical cytological characteristics of clear cell adenocarcinoma which included hobnail cells, flattened cells, and cells with abundant clear cytoplasm.

(ii) Nuclear pleomorphism was typically at least moderate and was marked in almost half of the specimens.

(iii) They easily found mitotic figures in almost all the specimens.

(iv) The aforementioned cytological characteristics should be helpful in the distinction of CCAU from benign nephrogenic adenoma, even though one of their patients was initially misdiagnosed as having nephrogenic adenoma.

(v) They had performed immunohistochemical staining of the tumours for prostate-specific antigen (PSA) and prostatic acid phosphatase (PAP) on 13 tumours and all were negative.

(vi) Follow-up was available for 13 patients. Six of the patients did not have any evidence of recurrence up to 10 years postoperatively. Four patients had died of disease from between 5 months and 42 months postoperatively. Three more patients developed recurrence but they were alive up to 6.5 years following their presentation.

Scantling et al. [6] reported a 47-year-old woman with a history of chronic recurrent urinary tract infection who was diagnosed with urethral carcinoma during investigation for visible haematuria, hesitancy, straining, and urge incontinence. She had cystoscopy which revealed a papillary urethral

mass emanating from urethral diverticulum, and histological examination of the biopsy specimen revealed clear cell adenocarcinoma. She had a contrast enhanced magnetic resonance imaging (MRI) scan and computed tomography (CT) scan of the pelvis which confirmed the urethral diverticulum containing a nodular enhancing malignancy and enlarged pelvic side wall bilaterally. She also had CT scan of thorax and bone scan which were normal. She underwent robotic assisted radical anterior exenteration with Indiana pouch creation (radical cystectomy, hysterectomy, urethrectomy, and neobladder construction). The pathology of specimens revealed a 3 cm × 1.6 cm × 1.2 cm grade 2 (moderately differentiated) clear cell urethral adenocarcinoma within urethral diverticulum invading the anterior vagina with negative margins, distal bilateral ureters with negative margins, distal bilateral ureters with negative margins, 21 negative lymph nodes, and a negative hysterectomy specimen. The pathological staging was pT3N0M0. She did not have adjuvant therapy. She was well at her one-year follow-up without any recurrent disease.

Sheahan and Vega Vega [5] reported a 54-year-old woman who presented with haematuria and urethral mass on ultrasound scan. She later on had MRI scan which showed a heterogeneous mass in urethral diverticulum. She had biopsies of the mass and histological examination of the specimens revealed clear cell adenocarcinoma with clearing of the cytoplasm, moderate nuclear pleomorphism. Immunohistochemical staining revealed that the tumour cells were positive for cytokeratin 7 and p16, p53, CA125, CAM5.2, and AE1/AE3. Immunohistochemical staining also showed that the tumour cells were negative for thrombomodulin, oestrogen, progesterone, cytokeratin 20, p63, CD10, CEAP, WTI, AFP, and s100. She underwent anterior exenteration with pelvic lymphadenectomy and ileal conduit construction. Histological examination of the specimen revealed surgically clear margins but 3 out of 6 positive lymph nodes. She underwent 50.4 Gy consolidate radiotherapy due to lack of known benefit of chemotherapy in CCAU. She subsequently had PET scans which showed progression of lymphatic disease but she was alive, one year after her diagnosis.

Nakatsuka et al. [9] reported a 42-year-old woman who presented with bloody discharge from her urethra and lower back pain. Cytological examination of her urine sediment was reported to be highly indicative of adenocarcinoma. Papanicolau-stained specimens of her urine showed a small number of papillary or spherical clusters of atypical cells with many benign urothelial cells and squamous cells in the background. A few neutrophils and lymphocytes were observed; however, no necrotic debris was seen. The nuclei of the atypical cells showed an increase in the chromatin content with fine granular pattern and irregular contours; the nucleoli were prominent. Most of the atypical cells had a moderate amount of cytoplasm that was lightly stained green; however, some atypical cells showed clear, abundant cytoplasm that formed spherical clusters resembling "mirror balls." The cytological findings were reported to be suggestive of a malignant tumour of the urinary tract system and favoured adenocarcinoma. She had computed tomography (CT) and magnetic resonance imaging scans

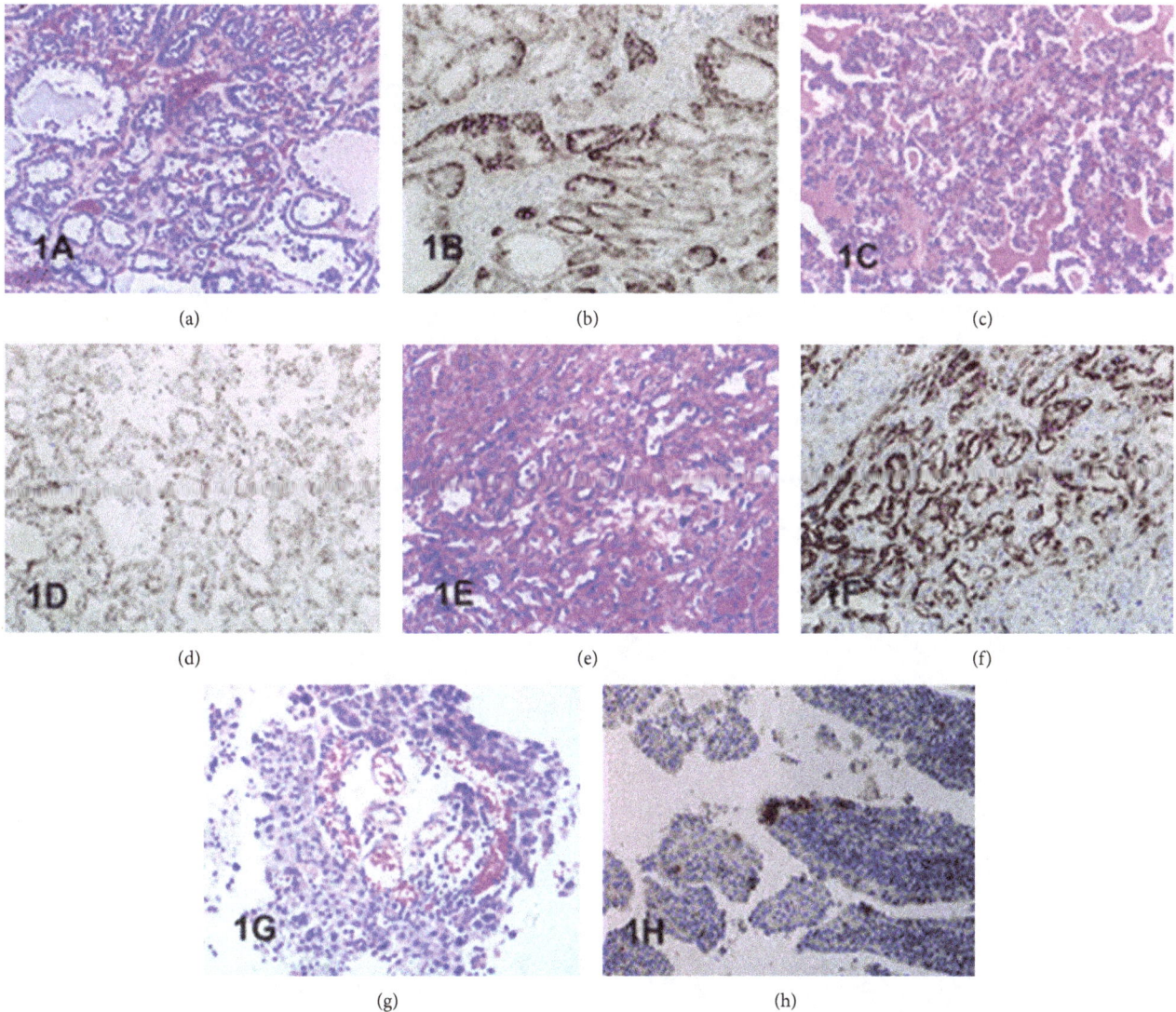

FIGURE 12: This figure shows architectural patterns of clear cell adenocarcinomas and granular cytoplasmic reactivity with P504S. (a) Tubulocystic pattern with tubules lined by cells with clear cytoplasm component (bladder case 1). (b) Positive staining with P504S bladder case 1). (c) Diffuse growth of clear cells (bladder, case 2). (d) Positive staining with P504S (bladder, case 2). (e) Tubulocystic pattern with tubules lined by hobnail cells showing moderate to severe nuclear atypia (urethra, case 3). (f) Positive staining with P504S (urethra, case 3). (g) Papillary growth pattern with papillae lined by hobnail cells with severe nuclear atypia and mitoses (urethral diverticulum, case 4). (h) Positive staining with P504S (urethral diverticulum, case 4). Haematoxylin-eosin and immunoperoxidase original magnification ×200. Reprinted from [8] Sun et al. Clear cell adenocarcinoma of the urinary bladder and urethra: another urinary tract lesion immunoreactive for P504S. Arch Pathol Lab Med 2008 Sep; 132(9): 1417–1422 reprinted with permission from Archives of Pathology and Laboratory Medicine Copyright 2008 College of American Pathologists. This permission is exclusive to this request specifically for this paper. Additional usage of any printed or electronic material for which the Archives of Pathology and Laboratory Medicine owns copyright would require permission from the editorial office.

which showed a tumour in the entire urethra. The rest of the intra-abdominal and pelvic organs and lymph nodes were normal. She had cystourethroscopy which showed two diverticula in the urethral wall in which whitish papillary and villous lesions were found. The tumours were biopsied and resected transurethrally and histological examination of the specimens was suggestive of clear cell adenocarcinoma (CCA) but was indeterminate for malignancy. She underwent total cystourethrectomy and partial resection of the vaginal wall. The final pathological diagnosis of the resected tumour was clear cell adenocarcinoma (CCA) stage III pT3N0M0.

Histological examination of the biopsy and transurethral resected specimen showed that the tumour was comprised of papillotubular lesions.

The epithelial cells which covered the tumour were cuboidal and single layered, and some of these showed a "hobnail pattern." Most of the cells had eosinophilic cytoplasm, with the exception of a few which had clear cytoplasm. The cells that had a clear cytoplasm were positive for periodic

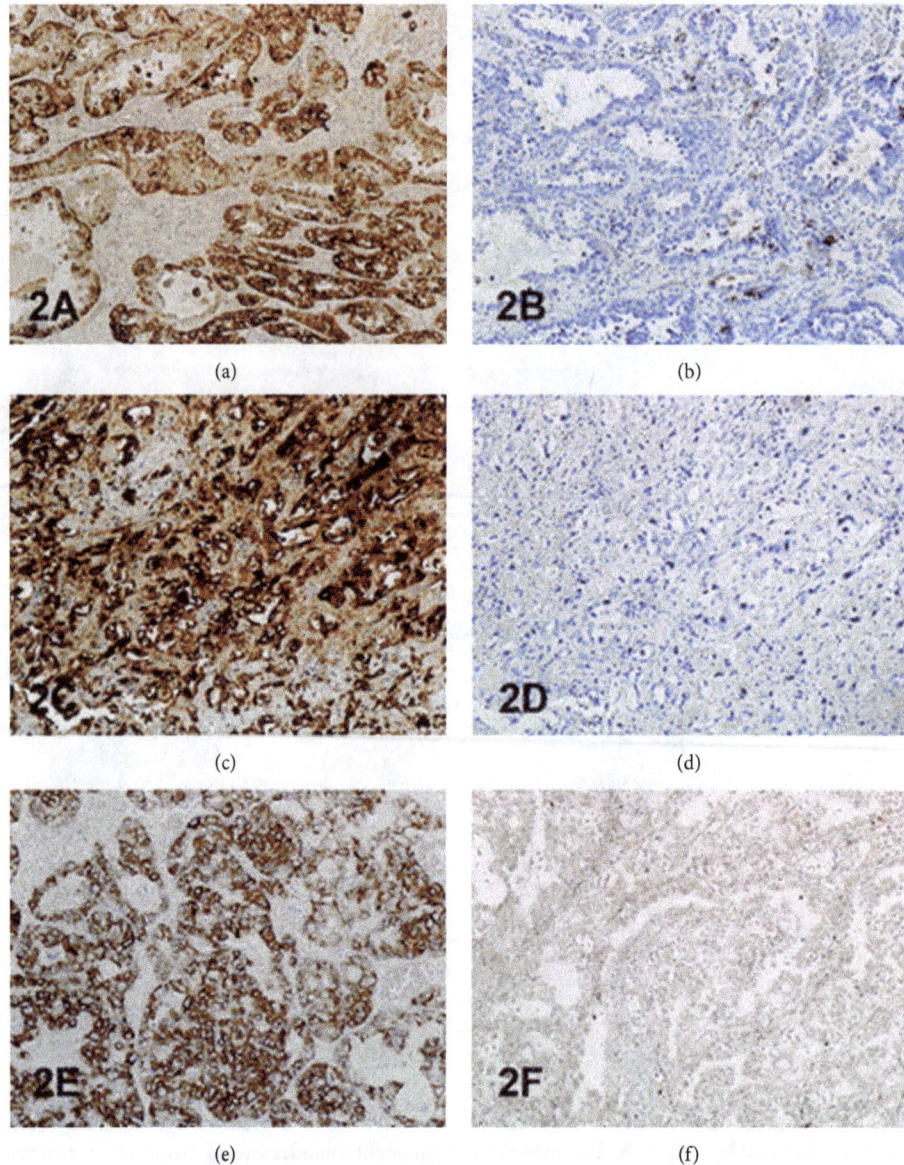

FIGURE 13: This figure shows immunoreactivity of cytokeratin (CK) 7, CK 20, K903, and p63 in clear cell adenocarcinoma. (a) Positive staining with CK7 (bladder, case 1). (b) Focally positive staining with CK20 (bladder, case 1). (c) Positive staining with CK 7 (urethra, case 3). (d) Negative staining with CK 20 (urethra, case 3). (e) Positive staining with K 903 (bladder, case 2). (f) Negative staining with p63 (bladder, case 2). Immunoperoxidase, original magnification ×200 ((a) to (e)) and ×100 (f). Reprinted from [8] Sun et al. Clear cell adenocarcinoma of the urinary bladder and urethra: another urinary tract lesion immunoreactive for P504S. Arch Pathol Lab Med 2008 Sep; 132(9): 1417–1422 reprinted with permission from Archives of Pathology and Laboratory Medicine Copyright 2008 College of American Pathologists. This permission is exclusive to this request specifically for this paper. Additional usage of any printed or electronic material for which the Archives of Pathology and Laboratory Medicine owns copyright would require permission from the editorial office.

acid-Schiff reaction. The epithelial cells exhibited relatively mild cytological atypia and they did not invade the stroma. Mitotic figures were seen at a frequency of 10/10 high-power fields. Necrotic debris was regularly seen in the lumen of the tubular structures.

Immunohistochemical staining showed that the tumour cells were positive for

(i) cytokeratin (CK7),

(ii) EMA,

(iii) carbohydrate antigen (CA) 125.

Immunohistochemical staining also showed that the tumour cells were focally positive for CD15 (see Figure 5(b)).

Immunohistochemical staining showed that the tumour cells were negative for

(i) CK5/6,

(ii) CK20,

(iii) carcinoembryonic antigen,

(iv) thrombomodulin,

(v) uroplakin,

(vi) prostate-specific antigen,

(vii) calretinin,

(viii) oestrogen receptor,

(ix) progesterone receptor.

The aforementioned histological findings were reported to have suggested a diagnosis of CCAU, even though definitive diagnosis of malignancy could not be elicited in view of the absence of stromal invasion in both the biopsy and the transurethrally resected specimens. Nevertheless, in the surgically resected specimens, clear atypical cells with papillotubular structure were seen to have invaded all the layers of the urethra and vaginal muscular layer. Based upon these findings the final diagnosis was CCA. The authors further reported that the Ki-67 labeling index of the tumour cells was about 20% (see Figure 5(c)) and about 5% of the tumour cells exhibited strong p53 positivity in the nucleus.

Göğuş et al. [10] stated that CCAU is extremely rare. Most of the data on CCAU have been obtained from case reports and case series [1, 3, 10]. CCAU mostly affects females and up to half of the cases develop in urethral diverticulum [3, 11, 12].

Göğuş et al. [10] reported a 44-year-old man with a history of two previous urinary retentions who presented with obstructive urinary symptoms. He had a rectal examination which revealed an indurated prostate. His serum prostatic-specific antigen (PSA) was 0.15 ng/mL (normal). He had cystourethroscopy which revealed a friable solid tumour in the entire urethra and bladder neck. The tumour was resected transurethrally and histological examination revealed a tumour which was composed of tubular structures lined with cells comprising hyperchromatic nuclei and clear cytoplasm. Papillary pattern was observed adjacent to these areas. Tubular and papillary structures were lined with hobnail cells in some areas of the tumour. Immunohistochemical staining of the tumour was negative for PSA. He had a CT scan of abdomen and pelvis which showed multiple bilateral internal iliac lymph nodes. He had bone scan and chest X-ray which was normal. He underwent radical cystoprostatectomy, bilateral pelvic and inguinal lymph node dissection, urethrectomy, and construction of ileal conduit. Histological examination of the cystoprostatectomy specimen confirmed features of clear cell adenocarcinoma of the bladder neck and the tumour in the entire urethra which was similar to the findings of the transurethrally resected specimens. The perivesical fat, the prostate gland, and seminal vesicles were infiltrated by the tumour. He received three cycles of methotrexate-vinblastine-epirubicin-cisplatin (MVEC) chemotherapy but he died of progressive disease 10 months after his cystoprostatectomy.

Konnak [13] in 1973 reported the first case of CCAU; since then sporadic cases of CCAU have been reported. Konnak [13] used the terminology "mesonephric carcinoma" for CCAU and postulated that the tumour perhaps emanates from the mesonephric duct or intermediate mesodermal vestiges. On the contrary, Kawano and associates [14] are of the opinion that CCAU is of origin.

Some authors [15, 16] suggested that there is a clear association between clear cell adenocarcinoma and diverticula of the urethra and that CCAU is the most common malignancy arising from diverticula of the urethra. It has been stated whilst only 10% of carcinoma of the urethra is clear cell adenocarcinoma, one-third of such carcinomas originate in a diverticulum [15].

Pollen and Dreilinger [17] in 1984 iterated their support for the homogeneity between the female paraurethral duct and the prostate gland in men based upon the finding of positive immunohistochemical staining for prostate-specific antigen (PSA) and prostatic specific acid phosphatase (PAP).

Trabelsi et al. [2] reported a 56-year-old woman who presented with visible haematuria. On examination bleeding was observed from her urethral meatus. She underwent cystoscopy which revealed a tumour protruding from the posterior urethral wall at the neck of the urinary bladder. She underwent transurethral biopsy of the tumour and histological examination of the specimen showed an invasive poorly differentiated carcinoma of the urethra. She underwent total urethrocystectomy including her anterior vaginal wall and pelvic lymph node dissection and ileal conduit construction. The bladder mucosa was normal but the tumour involved all the urethral layers. Microscopic examination of the specimen showed a tumour which was composed of nests and papillary structures which were lined with cells that had clear cytoplasm with hobnail cells in some areas of the tumour; the cells exhibited cytological atypia and high mitotic rate; the tumour cells invaded all the urethral layers but did not involve the urinary bladder. The lymph nodes were not involved. Immunohistochemical staining for prostate-specific antigen (PSA) was negative. She did not receive any adjuvant therapy and she was free of disease 3 months after her operation.

Trabelsi et al. [2] stated the following.

(i) Pollen and Dreilinger [17] were of the opinion that CAUs arose from the female paraurethral duct and, in their case, the tumour cells were negative for PSA.

(ii) Zaviačič and associates [18] had reported a neoplasm with similar histological appearance and immunohistochemical features as adenocarcinoma of Skene's paraurethral gland and ducts.

(iii) Their aforementioned findings would support the postulate of Abascal Junquera and associates [11] that the female clear cell adenocarcinoma arises from the paraurethral duct. Nevertheless, it would seem that female urethral adenocarcinoma has more than one tissue of origin with minority arising from the Skene's glands as suggested by Dodson and associates [19]. Morphologically, CCAU of the urethra must be differentiated from nephrogenic adenoma of the urethra especially on biopsy. The predominance of clear cells, severe cytological atypia, high mitotic rate, and necrosis favored the diagnosis of CCAU.

(iv) Some authors [10, 20] stated that, in view of the rarity CCAU, the optimal treatment is not known. It would appear to be based upon the localization of the primary tumour and the presence of metastasis. Ebisuno and associates [20] stated that radical cystourethrectomy with or without irradiation was performed in most cases. Some authors [20, 21] also stated that the response to chemotherapy is also not clear.

Han et al. [22] reported a 54-year-old woman who presented with painless visible haematuria. She had vaginal ultrasound scan which revealed a sausage-like elongated mass in the urethra. Cytological examination of her voided urine revealed small clusters of rounded or papillary cells. The necrotic debris and inflammatory cells were present within some clusters of tumour cells. The tumour cells were enlarged and had abundant clear or granular cytoplasm with cytoplasmic vacuoles. The nucleus was granular and contained vesicular chromatin with prominent nucleoli. Hobnail cells and hyaline globules were also as in a histological section. They stated the following.

(i) The histological findings were compatible with clear cell adenocarcinoma.

(ii) Nevertheless, cytologically, it would be necessary to make a differential diagnosis from the other adenocarcinoma or high-grade urothelial carcinoma.

(iii) Oliva and Young [3] indicated that CCAU accounts for about 1% of male urethral carcinomas and about 15% of female urethral carcinomas.

Fridman [7] in 2011 reported an 82-year-old woman who underwent transurethral resection of a space occupying lesion which was diagnosed in her urethra and bladder neck (see Figures 1 to 11 for various microscopic and immunohistochemical characteristics of the tumour). Fridman stated that CCAUs are high-grade tumours which are common in women and macroscopically, they are papillary. Fridman summarized the features of CCAU as follows.

(i) CCAUs have various architectural patterns including tubules, cysts, papillae, and diffuse tumour.

(ii) Most tumours have prominent clear cytoplasm due to glycogen and hobnailing.

(iii) The tumour cells have prominent pleomorphism and marked cytotic activity.

(iv) There is often muscular invasion and necrosis [23].

(v) The tumour cells are immunoreactive for CK7, CK903, Ki-67, and p53 and usually negative for CK20. In contrast to majority of urothelial carcinomas, they are also immunoreactive for P504S and negative for p63 [8].

Fridman [7] stated that the differential diagnosis of CCAU includes nephrogenic adenoma, a metaplastic process which often occurs in young adults with a history of genitourinary trauma, surgery, or stones. Fridman [7] further stated that, in nephrogenic adenoma, reactive changes may exist in the tumour cells as well as mitotic activity, but in such cases there is no marked pleomorphism or invasion. There are usually no clear cells in nephrogenic adenoma, and if present they are focal, and Ki-67 and p53 are usually negative or have minimal staining [24].

Fridman [7] additionally stated the following.

(i) Herawi et al. [25] in 2010 described a clear cell adenocarcinoma which mimicked nephrogenic adenoma due to less prominent nuclear pleomorphism, less prominent nucleoli, and fewer clear cells. Nevertheless, this variant of adenocarcinoma did exhibit extensive muscular invasion and focal hyperchromatic and pleomorphic tumour cells that would not be in nephrogenic adenoma.

(ii) Miller and Karnes [26] in 2008 stated that clear cell adenocarcinoma is an aggressive tumour with low rates of 5-year survival. In their case, the patient had received an incomplete course of chemotherapy after she had undergone surgery. She was well during the subsequent three and half years until 5 months prior to the presentation of the case, when she underwent excision of pelvic lymph node histology of which confirmed clear cell carcinoma similar to the primary tumour. At the time of presentation of the case the patient was alive without any further recurrence.

Young and Scully [23] described the clinical and pathological characteristics of three previously unreported and 16 previously reported examples of clear cell adenocarcinoma of the urinary bladder and urethra. They stated that six of the tumours arose in the urinary bladder and 13 in the urethra. Sixteen of the patients were female, and the ages ranged between 35 years and 78 years. Most of the tumours were papillary tumours but some of the tumours were sessile. Young and Scully [23] reported that microscopic examination of the tumours showed various patterns which included tubular glands, cysts, papillae, and diffuse areas. They had identified cells with abundant glycogen-rich clear cytoplasm and hobnail cells in majority of the tumours. Young and Scully [23] advised that these tumours should be differentiated from nephrogenic adenomas. They stated the following.

(i) A young age or a history of genitourinary trauma, operation, or calculus may constitute a clue to the latter diagnosis; microscopic characteristics such as sheets of clear cells, significant pleomorphism, or mitotic activity would be in favour of the diagnosis of clear cell adenocarcinoma.

(ii) The follow-up of majority of the patients, most of who underwent a radical operation, was short, but five tumours were known to have metastasized.

Sun et al. [8] stated that adequate characterization had been hampered by its rarity; alpha-methyl-acyl-CoA-racemase (AMACR)/P504S had been reported to be positive in prostatic adenocarcinoma, papillary renal cell carcinoma, and gastrointestinal neoplasms; nevertheless, it had never been previously studied in clear cell carcinomas of lower urinary tract. They investigated the immunohistochemical staining profile in 4 primary clear cell carcinomas of the urinary tract including P504S. They retrieved four cases of clear cell adenocarcinoma from their archives: 2 cases from the urinary bladder (one each from a man and a woman)

TABLE 1: This table shows immunohistochemical staining characteristics of clear cell carcinoma. Reproduced from Sun et al. [8]. Clear cell adenocarcinoma of the urinary bladder and urethra: another urinary tract lesion immunoreactive for P504S. Arch Pathol Lab Med 2008 Sep; 132(9): 1417–1422 reprinted with permission from Archives of Pathology and Laboratory Medicine Copyright 2008 College of American Pathologists. This permission is exclusive to this request specifically for this paper. Additional usage of any printed or electronic material for which the Archives of Pathology and Laboratory Medicine owns copyright would require permission from the editorial office.

Case number	P504S	CK7	CK20	CA 125	K903	p63
1	+++	+++	++	++	+++	0
2	+++	+++	++	+	+++	0
3	+++	+++	0	0	+++	0
4	+	+++	0	++	+++	0

*CK indicates cytokeratin; 0, less than 5% of tumor cells staining positive; +, 5% to 25%; ++, 26% to 50%; and +++, greater than 50%.

and 2 cases from the urethra (both from women, 1 in a diverticulum). They performed immunohistochemistry for P504S, K903, cytokeratin (CK) 7, CK20, CA 125, and p63. Sun et al. [8] reported that clear cell carcinomas had distinct immunoreactive profile: strongly positive for P504S, K903, and CK 7 and negative reactivity for p63. Two of the cases were also positive for CA 125 and CK 20 (see Figures 12 and 13 as well as Table 1 for various microscopic features and immunohistochemical characteristics of some of the tumours). Sun et al. [8] concluded the following.

(i) The immunohistochemical profile of clear cell carcinoma shares some similarity to conventional urothelial carcinoma; nevertheless, it deviates from urothelial carcinomas in being positive for P504S and negative for p63.

(ii) This staining profile may indicate a nonurothelial origin for these tumours and may serve as a useful tool in the differential diagnosis of clear cell adenocarcinoma and may reflect its aetiology.

(iii) In view of the fact that similar expression of P504S is also seen in nephrogenic adenoma, this marker should not be used to differentiate nephrogenic adenomas from clear cell adenocarcinomas.

4. Conclusions

Few cases of CCAU have been reported and the tumours have been reported to be aggressive with low 5-year survival rates.

CCAUs have been treated by anterior exenteration in women and cystoprostatectomy in men and at times by radiotherapy; chemotherapy has rarely been given.

Acknowledgments

The author would like to acknowledge Dr. Nat Pernick, President of http://PathologyOutlines.com/, and http://Pathology-Outlines.com/, for directing the author to Dr. Eddie Fridman the copyright owner to a number of figures used in the paper which enabled the author to obtain copyright permission to reproduce Figures 1 to 11 from their website. The author would like to thank Dr. Eddie Fridman, Head of Uro-Pathology Service, Department of Pathology, The chaim Sheba Medical Center, and Associated Professor at The Sacker Medical School, Tel-Aviv University, Israel, for granting permission for figures from his reported case to be reproduced in the paper and for kindly providing legends for all the figures relating to his case. The Archives of Pathology and Laboratory Medicine and the American College of Pathologists, for granting the author permission to reproduce figures from their journal (Archives of Pathology and Laboratory Medicine).

References

[1] P. A. Drew, W. M. Murphy, F. Civantos, and V. O. Speights, "The histogenesis of clear cell adenocarcinoma of the lower urinary tract: case series and review of the literature," Human Pathology, vol. 27, no. 3, pp. 248–252, 1996.

[2] A. Trabelsi, S. Abdelkrim, S. Rammeh et al., "Clear cell adenocarcinoma of a female urethra: a case report and review of the literature," North American Journal of Medical Science, vol. 1, no. 6, pp. 321–323, 2009.

[3] E. Oliva and R. H. Young, "Clear cell adenocarcinoma of the urethra: a clinicopathologic analysis of 19 cases," Modern Pathology, vol. 9, no. 5, pp. 513–520, 1996.

[4] T. Al-Hussain, "Urethra Clear cell adenocarcinoma," Pathology outlines.com, 2012, http://www.pathologyoutlines.com/topic/urethraclearcell.html.

[5] G. Sheahan and A. Vega Vega, "Primary clear cell adenocarcinoma in a female urethral diverticulum: a case report and review," World Journal of Nephrology & Urology, vol. 2, no. 1, pp. 29–32, 2013.

[6] D. Scantling, C. Ross, and J. Jaffe, "Primary cleat cell adenocarcinoma of a urethral diverticulum treated with multidisciplinary robotic anterior pelvic exenteration," Case Reports in Medicine, vol. 2013, Article ID 387591, 4 pages, 2013.

[7] E. Fridman, Case of the Week #194, January 2011, narrated by N. Pernick, L. Parker, January 2011, In: Al- Hussain T Urethra Clear cell adenocarcinoma Pathology outlines.com, June 2012, http://www.pathologyoutlines.com/topic/urethra-clearcell.html.

[8] K. Sun, Y. Huan, and P. D. Unger, "Clear cell adenocarcinoma of urinary bladder and urethra: another urinary tract lesion immunoreactive for P504S," Archives of Pathology and Laboratory Medicine, vol. 132, no. 9, pp. 1417–1422, 2008.

[9] S.-I. Nakatsuka, I. Taguchi, T. Nagatomo et al., "A case of clear cell adenocarcinoma arising from the urethral diverticulum: utility of urinary cytology and immunohistochemistry," CytoJournal, vol. 9, article 11, 2012.

[10] Ç. Göğuş, S. Baltaci, D. Orhan, and Ö. Yaman, "Clear cell adenocarcinoma of the male urethra," International Journal of Urology, vol. 10, no. 6, pp. 348–349, 2003.

[11] J. M. Abascal Junquera, L. Cecchini Rosell, R. Martos Calvo et al., "Presentation of a new case of primary clear cell adeno-carcinoma of the urethra and its surgical management," *Actas Urológicas Españolas*, vol. 31, no. 4, pp. 411–416, 2007.

[12] R. M. Seballos and R. R. Rich, "Clear cell adenocarcinoma arising from a urethral diverticulum," *The Journal of Urology*, vol. 153, no. 6, pp. 1914–1915, 1995.

[13] J. W. Konnak, "Mesonephric carcinoma involving the urethra," *The Journal of Urology*, vol. 110, no. 1, pp. 76–78, 1973.

[14] K. Kawano, M. Yano, S. Kitahara, and K. Yasuda, "Clear cell adenocarcinoma of the female urethra showing strong immunostaining for prostate-specific antigen," *BJU International*, vol. 87, no. 4, pp. 412–413, 2001.

[15] J. Manning, "Case report: transitional cell carcinoma in situ within a urethral diverticulum," *International Urogynecology Journal*, vol. 23, no. 12, pp. 1801–1803, 2012.

[16] C. Flynn, J. Oxley, P. McCullagh, and W. G. McCluggage, "Primary high-grade serous carcinoma arising in the urethra or urethral diverticulum: a report of 2 cases of an extremely rare phenomenon," *International Journal of Gynecological Pathology*, vol. 32, no. 1, pp. 141–145, 2013.

[17] J. J. Pollen and A. Dreilinger, "Immunohistochemical identification of prostatic acid phosphatase and prostate specific antigen in female periurethral glands," *Urology*, vol. 23, no. 3, pp. 303–304, 1984.

[18] M. Zaviačič, J. Šidlo, and M. Borovský, "Prostate specific antigen and prostate specific acid phosphatase in adenocarcinoma of Skene's paraurethral glands and ducts," *Virchows Archiv A Pathological Anatomy and Histopathology*, vol. 423, no. 6, pp. 503–505, 1993.

[19] M. K. Dodson, W. A. Cliby, P. P. Pettavel, G. L. Keeney, and K. C. Podratz, "Female urethral adenocarcinoma: evidence for more than one tissue of origin?" *Gynecologic Oncology*, vol. 59, no. 3, pp. 352–357, 1995.

[20] S. Ebisuno, M. Miyai, and T. Nagareda, "Clear cell adeno-carcinoma of the female urethra showing positive staining with antibodies to prostate-specific antigen and prostatic acid phosphatase," *Urology*, vol. 45, no. 4, pp. 682–685, 1995.

[21] U. Maier, K. Dorfinger, and M. Susani, "Clear cell adenocarcinoma of the female urethra," *The Journal of Urology*, vol. 160, no. 2, pp. 492–493, 1998.

[22] J.-Y. Han, K.-H. Kim, L. Kim et al., "Cytologic findings of clear cell adenocarcinoma of the urethra: a case report," *Korean Journal of Pathology*, vol. 46, no. 2, pp. 210–214, 2012.

[23] R. H. Young and R. E. Scully, "Clear cell adenocarcinoma of the bladder and urethra: a report of three cases and review of the literature," *The American Journal of Surgical Pathology*, vol. 9, no. 11, pp. 816–826, 1985.

[24] M. Z. Gilcrease, R. Delgado, F. Vuitch, and J. Albores-Saavedra, "Clear cell adenocarcinoma and nephrogenic adenoma of the urethra and urinary bladder: a histopathologic and immuno-histochemical comparison," *Human Pathology*, vol. 29, no. 12, pp. 1451–1456, 1998.

[25] M. Herawi, P. A. Drew, C.-C. Pan, and J. I. Epstein, "Clear cell adenocarcinoma of the bladder and urethra: cases diffusely mimicking nephrogenic adenoma," *Human Pathology*, vol. 41, no. 4, pp. 594–601, 2010.

[26] J. Miller and R. J. Karnes, "Primary clear-cell adenocarcinoma of the proximal female urethra: case report and review of the literature," *Clinical Genitourinary Cancer*, vol. 6, no. 2, pp. 131–133, 2008.

10

Gastrointestinal Stromal Tumors Associated with Neurofibromatosis 1: A Single Centre Experience and Systematic Review of the Literature Including 252 Cases

Pier Federico Salvi, Laura Lorenzon, Salvatore Caterino, Laura Antolino, Maria Serena Antonelli, and Genoveffa Balducci

Surgical and Medical Department of Translational Medicine, Sant'Andrea Hospital, Faculty of Medicine and Psychology, University of Rome La Sapienza, St. Andrea Hospital, Via di Grottarossa 1035-39, 00189 Rome, Italy

Correspondence should be addressed to Laura Lorenzon; laura.lorenzon@uniroma1.it

Academic Editor: Steven N. Hochwald

Aims. The objectives of this study were (a) to report our experience regarding the association between neurofibromatosis type 1 (NF1) and gastrointestinal stromal tumors (GISTs); (b) to provide a systematic review of the literature in this field; and (c) to compare the features of NF1-associated GISTs with those reported in sporadic GISTs. *Methods*. We reported two cases of NF1-associated GISTs. Moreover we reviewed 23 case reports/series including 252 GISTs detected in 126 NF1 patients; the data obtained from different studies were analyzed and compared to those of the sporadic GISTs undergone surgical treatment at our centre. *Results*. NF1 patients presenting with GISTs had a homogeneous M/F ratio with a mean age of 52.8 years. NF1-associated GISTs were often reported as multiple tumors, mainly incidental, localized at the jejunum, with a mean diameter of 3.8 cm, a mean mitotic count of 3.0/50 HPF, and KIT/PDGFRα wild type. We reported a statistical difference comparing the age and the symptoms at presentation, the tumors' diameters and localizations, and the risk criteria of the NF1-associated GISTs comparing to those documented in sporadic GISTs. *Conclusions*. NF1-associated GISTs seem to have a distinct phenotype, specifically younger age, distal localization, small diameter, and absence of KIT/PDGRFα mutations.

1. Introduction

Neurofibromatosis type 1 (NF1, von Recklinghausen's disease) is an autosomal-dominant disorder occurring in 1 out of 3,000 births that is caused by the inactivation of the NF1 gene. NF1 is a tumor suppressor that encodes for the neurofibromin protein, a member of the Ras family. The inactivation might be a familial condition with an autosomal-dominant inheritance pattern; otherwise it might be sporadic [1, 2].

The disease is characterized by cutaneous neurofibromas, café au lait macules, axillary and inguinal freckling, and Lisch nodules.

NF1 is also associated with several tumors, including tumors of the nervous system (central and peripheral) and of the gastrointestinal (GI) tract, with the gastrointestinal stromal tumors (GISTs) indicated as the most common GI NF1-associated tumors [3].

GISTs are mesenchymal and usually kit positive tumors, originating from the interstitial cell of Cajal or their related stem cells [4, 5]. The incidence of the GISTs has been reported in 10–20 new cases per million/year [6]. GISTs represent 80% of mesenchymal GI tumors and 0.1–3% of all GI malignancies [7–10]. GIST's pathogenesis is related to kit and platelet-derived growth factor receptor alpha (PDGFRa) mutation. Kit and PDGFRa encode for similar type III receptor tyrosine kinase proteins: these mutations are somatic and occur only in the neoplastic tissue of sporadic GISTs, whereas constitutional mutations in familial GISTs occur in every cell of the body and are inheritable [11–14].

Over the last few years several case reports documented the association between GISTs and NF1 syndrome; however to date there is a lack of reviews in this field with the objective of describing the clinical and pathological features of GISTs presenting in NF1 patients.

Aims of this study were (a) to report our experience regarding this association; (b) to provide a systematic review of the literature in this field including 252 GISTs described in 126 NF1 patients with the objective of analyzing the clinical, pathological, and molecular features of these tumors in patients affected by this condition; and (c) to compare the clinical/pathological features of GISTs presenting associated with NF1 with those reported in sporadic GISTs.

2. Materials and Methods

2.1. Systematic Review: Data Source and Search Strategies. This investigation has been conducted adhering at the PRISMA statements for review and meta-analysis (Figure 1). We conducted a systematic review of the literature by searching PubMed database for all published series and case reports investigating the association of NF1 and GIST (Keywords: "GIST and NF1", language: English; filter "human" studies); the Medline search was conducted at the beginning of September 2013 and retrieved 24 papers. We also included references from the retrieved publications (n 3 manuscripts).

Published series with the aim to investigate exclusively the molecular profile (n 1 study), the NF1 radiological features (n 1 study), or its association with other gastrointestinal tumors, for example, gastrointestinal schwannomas (n 1 article), were excluded.

Moreover we also excluded those reviews in this field that did not include patients' presentation (n 2 studies), one paper that reported GISTs without signs of NF1 syndrome and another study investigating the intestinal neurofibromatosis.

The same search strategies have been applied to the Ovid database and provided the addition of 3 more papers (after the manual removal of duplicate references).

Overall the systematic review has been conducted on 23 articles published from 2004 to date [15–37], plus the two patients we herein presented.

Authors conducting this review of the literature were blinded to authors' and journals' names and did not consider any journal's score (e.g., journal's Impact Factors) of the published case/series as an exclusion criteria for this study.

We collected data regarding study populations, number of investigated patients and GISTs, familiar or sporadic history of NF1, age at presentation of the GISTs, symptoms, sex of the patients, tumors' location, tumors' diameter, and number of mitoses. The morphologic appearance and cellular descriptions (generally referred to as epithelioid, spindle, and mixed cells) were also recorded along with the immuno-histochemistry for CD117 (c-kit), S-100 protein, CD-34, and SMA-alpha. Whenever available, we included data regarding GIST risk classification and the studies investigating c-kit and PDGFRa mutations.

2.2. Statistical Analysis. With respect to the systematic review, we pooled together the data obtained from different studies in order to analyze a large series of patients and of clinical and pathological variables. Patients' clinical features and tumors' pathological records were thus analysed using

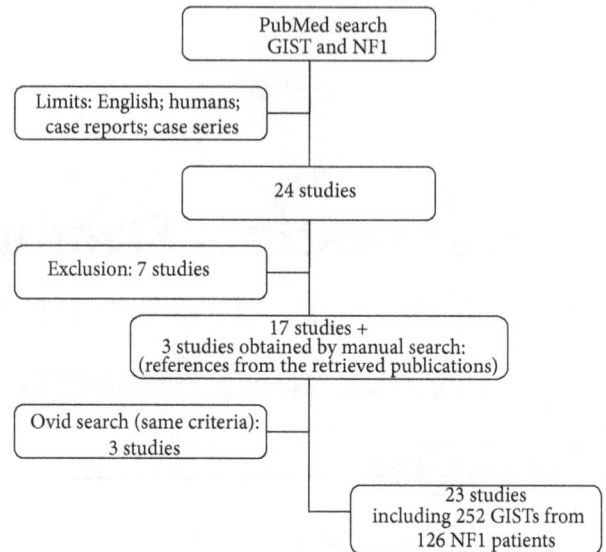

FIGURE 1: Systematic review: study design according to the PRISMA statement.

means and standard deviations for quantitative variables and using frequencies and percents for categorical variables.

Moreover, the clinical and pathological features of the GISTs presenting associated with the NF1 syndrome (including age at presentation, M/F ratio, symptoms, tumors' diameter and localization, and risk criteria) retrieved from the international literature have been compared for statistical purpose to those obtained in a personal case series of sporadic GISTs undergone surgical resection at our department. Variables were compared using the t-test for continuous variable and the Chi-square test for categorical variables; all test were two-tailed and a $P < 0.05$ was considered of statistical significance value. All statistical evaluations were conducted with the statistical software MedCalc version 11.4.4.0.

3. Results

3.1. Personal Cases Series Presentation

Case 1. A 71-year-old male patient with a history of NF1 presented with an abdominal mass incidentally detected in the work-up of an abdominal aortic aneurism.

The patient's past medical history was consistent with hypertension and cholecystectomy for lithiasis. The abdominal CT scan documented a gastric mass of 3.6 cm (Figure 2); the patient underwent a gastroscopy that documented an atrophic gastritis. The patient was scheduled for a surgical procedure and a laparoscopic wedge resection of the posterior gastric wall was performed. The postoperative course was uneventful and the patient was discharged on 6th postoperative day.

The pathological examination documented a gastric GIST (c-KIT+, DOG1+) with spindle cell morphology, with a mitotic count of 2/50 HPF thus classified as a "low grade risk," according to Miettinen's classification. The patient is currently disease-free, 8 months after the surgical resection.

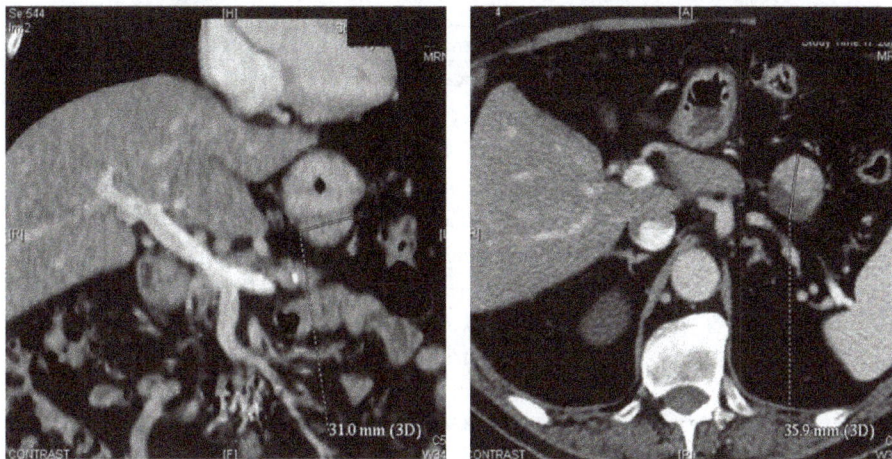

FIGURE 2: Abdominal CT scan documenting a 3.6 cm GIST of the stomach.

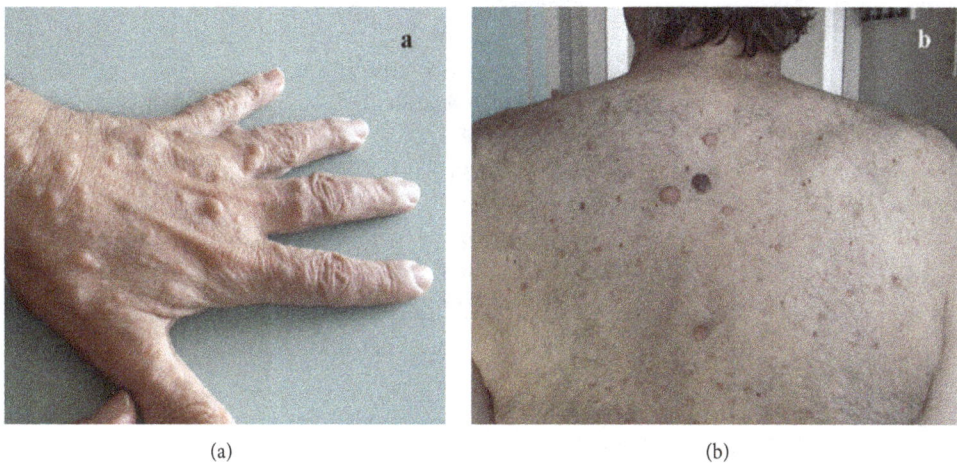

(a)   (b)

FIGURE 3: Cutaneous neurofibromas in patient affected by NF1 and duodenal GIST of the hand (a) and back (b).

Case 2. A 56-year-old man was admitted to our department with a familial history of NF1 (Figure 3) and a past medical history consistent with a pheochromocytoma in 1994. The patient underwent a surgical resection elsewhere for a duodenal GIST (third portion) and presented to our attention with a relapse of the disease 7 months after the primary surgical resection. The patient was scheduled for a surgical procedure of duodenotomy and excision of the recurrence. The pathological description was consistent with a 4 cm c-KIT and CD34 positive GIST with 9 mitosis/50 HPF thus classified as at "intermediate risk" according to Miettinen's classification. The postoperative course was uneventful and the patient was discharged in 9th postoperative day. The patient is disease-free, 8 years after the surgical treatment.

3.2. Systematic Review. Table 1 summarizes the studies included in the present review of the literature. For the purpose of this investigation we pooled patients from different studies (23 articles, plus the present single centre experience),

obtaining the clinical and pathological records of 252 GISTs detected in 126 NF1 patients [15–37].

As documented in Table 1, the vast majority of the studies reported single cases or small case series, excluding the article by Miettinen reporting 45 patients followed by the experience of Liegl and Andersson (resp., 16 and 15 NF1 patients) [18, 19, 27].

Table 2 shows the results of the data analysis. Patients were documented homogeneous regarding the M/F ratio (M/F 1), with a mean age at presentation of 52.8 years. Data regarding the NF1 syndrome (as a sporadic or familial disorder) has been detected exclusively in 17 out of the 126 NF1 included patients (13.5% of the series) and notably it has been documented as familial syndrome in the vast majority of the cases (70.6%). GISTs were reported as multiple tumors in the 35.3% of the patients and the prevalent localization was documented at the jejunum site 39.2%, followed by ileus in 30.6% of the cases. GISTs appeared to be incidental in the majority of the cases (52.5%) and were reported with a mean diameter of 3.8 cm. The mean mitotic count

TABLE 1: Systematic review of the literature from 2004 to date.

Reference	Author	Journal	Year	No. of patients	No. of GISTs
[15]	Cheng et al.	Digestive Diseases and Sciences	2004	3	5
[16]	Kinoshita et al.	The Journal of pathology	2004	7	29
[17]	Takazawa et al.	The American Journal of Surgical pathology	2005	9	36
[18]	Andersson et al.	The American Journal of Surgical pathology	2005	15	27
[19]	Miettinen et al.	The American Journal of Surgical pathology	2006	45	45
[20]	Maertens et al.	Human Molecular Genetics	2006	3	7
[21]	Nemoto et al.	Journal of Gastroenterology	2006	1	1
[22]	Bümming et al.	Scandinavian Journal of Gastroenterology	2006	1	4
[23]	Teramoto et al.	International Journal of Urology	2007	2	2
[24]	Stewart et al.	Journal of Medical Genetics	2007	2	3
[25]	Kramer et al.	World Journal of Gastroenterology	2007	1	1
[26]	Invernizzi et al.	Tumori	2008	1	1
[27]	Liegl et al.	The American Journal of Surgical pathology	2009	16	16
[28]	Yamamoto et al.	Journal of Cancer Research and Clinical Oncology	2009	5	31
[29]	Dell'Avanzato et al.	Surgery Today	2009	1	2
[30]	Hirashima et al.	Surgery Today	2009	1	17
[31]	Cavallaro et al.	The American Journal of Surgery	2010	2	2
[32]	Relles et al.	Journal of Gastrointestinal Surgery	2010	2	5
[33]	Izquierdo and Bonastre	Anticancer Drugs	2012	1	4
[34]	Agaimy et al.	International Journal of Clinical and Experimental pathology	2012	2	3
[35]	Ozcinar et al.	International Journal of Surgery Case Reports	2013	1	4
[36]	Vlenterie et al.	American Journal of medicine	2013	2	4
[37]	Sawalhi et al.	World Journal of Clinical Oncology	2013	1	1
		Present experience	2013	2	2
Total				126	252

was documented to be 3.0/50 HPF and the pathological morphology was consistent with spindle-shaped cell tumors in almost the totality of the GISTs (93.0%). Indeed 97.4% were c-kit positive and 81.6% CD34 positive; moreover, even though data regarding the DOG-1 expression were available exclusively in 17 patients, 88.2% were reported as DOG-1 positive. Opposite anti-SMA antibodies were positive in 24.1% of the cases and S-100 protein was expressed in 30.3% of the tumors. Notably desmin expression has been documented negative in all the 109 tumors analyzed. Wild-type c-kit and PDGRF alpha genes were reported in 95.2% of the tumors analyzed for any mutations.

Of note, the 64.9% of the GISTs were reported as low risk tumors, otherwise the 17.5% were considered at intermediate risk and the 17.5% as high risk GISTs.

3.3. Comparison with Sporadic GISTs. Clinical and pathological features of GISTs associated with NF1 syndrome (including mean age at presentation, M/F ratio, tumors' localizations, symptoms at presentation, mean diameters, and risk classification) were compared for statistical purpose with those documented in sporadic GISTs in a subset of patients undergone surgical resection at our centre from 1999 to 2009 (n 47 patients) [38]. Table 3 summarizes results of the statistical analysis. We documented a difference of

statistical value analyzing the mean age at presentation: indeed according to our results patients affected by NF1 were younger compared to sporadic GISTs patients (t-test P 0.0001). Moreover, in this subset of patients, tumors were significantly smaller (t-test P 0.0003). Tumors were located mainly in the jejunum/ileus in the NF1 subgroup whereas the main localization in the sporadic group was the stomach (Chi-square test $P < 0.0001$); moreover in the former group the vast majority of the GISTs were incidentally detected (Chi-square test P 0.002). Moreover, even though we did not document a significant difference analyzing the M/F ratios (Chi-square test P ns), we reported a prevalence of low-risk criteria in the NF1 subgroup compared with the sporadic GISTs (Chi-square test P 0.03).

4. Discussion

In this review we highlighted the clinical, pathological, and molecular features of GISTs detected in NF1 patients and, to the best of our knowledge, this is the first and most numerically relevant systematic analysis of the literature in this field. Moreover we reported our single centre experience regarding 2 GISTs detected in NF1 patients. Of note, from 1999 to date we treated 91 GISTs; thus the cases herein reported represent 2.2% of our series.

TABLE 2: Clinical and pathological features from 252 GISTs in 126 NF1 patients.

Sex	n	%
M	59.0	50.0
F	59.0	50.0
Total available	**118.0**	**100.0**
Age (years)		
Mean; SD		52.8; 13
Range		19.0–82.0
Familial history	n	%
Sporadic	5.0	29.4
Familial	12.0	70.6
Total available	**17.0**	**100.0**
Number of GISTs	n	%
1	77.0	64.7
>1	42.0	35.3
Total available	**119.0**	**100.0**
Localization	n	%
Stomach	12.0	5.4
Duodenum	44.0	19.8
Jejunum	87.0	39.2
Ileus	68.0	30.6
Colon	4.0	1.8
Other	6.0	2.7
Not specified	1.0	0.5
Total available	**222.0**	**100.0**
Symptoms	n	%
Incidental	21.0	52.5
Bleeding	11.1	27.5
Pain	4.0	10.0
Palpable mass	4.0	10.0
Total available	**40.0**	**100.0**
GIST's diameter (cm)		
Mean		3.8; 4.3
Range		0.1–29.0
Mitotic index (n/50 HPF)		
Mean		3.0; 8.2
Range		0.0–57.0
Morphology	n	%
Spindle-shaped	159.0	93.0
Epithelioid	9.0	5.3
Mix	3.0	1.7
Total available	**171.0**	**100.0**
c-kit	n	%
Positive	151.0	97.4
Negative	4.0	2.6
Total available	**155.0**	**100.0**
CD34	n	%
Positive	84.0	81.6
Negative	19.0	18.4
Total available	**103.0**	**100.0**

TABLE 2: Continued.

Anti-SMA	n	%
Positive	19.0	24.1
Negative	60.0	75.9
Total available	**79.0**	**100.0**
S-100	n	%
Positive	33.0	30.3
Negative	76.0	69.7
Total available	**109.0**	**100.0**
Desmin	n	%
Positive	0.0	0,0
Negative	109.0	100.0
Total available	**109.0**	**100.0**
DOG-1	n	%
Positive	15.0	88.2
Negative	2.0	11.8
Total available	**17.0**	**100.0**
c-kit/PDGRFa Mutations	n	%
Presence	8.0	4.8
Absence—wild type	157.0	95.2
Total available	**165.0**	**100.0**
Risk classification	n	%
Low risk	37.0	64.9
Intermediate risk	10.0	17.5
High risk	10.0	17.5
Total available	**57.0**	**100.0**

GISTs are commonly associated with NF1 syndrome, since a past study conducted on an autopsy series documented a GIST in one third of the NF1 patients [39].

GISTs associated with NF1 syndrome seem to have however a distinct phenotype: Miettinen reported that they occur in younger patients compared with sporadic GISTs that are often multiple and occur in the duodenum or small intestine [40].

Consistently with these findings, in our systematic review we highlighted that the mean age at presentation was 52.8 years and they are detected as multiple lesions in 35.3% of the cases, occurring in distal sites as the jejunum and small intestine.

Indeed in our previous research conducted on 47 primary GISTs patients, we reported a mean age at presentation of 61.4 years (median 62 years), none of the patients presented multiple lesions, and the most reported localization was the stomach, representing 59.6% of the tumors' sites [38].

Moreover, GISTs associated with NF1 patients have been described as clinically indolent and often asymptomatic, with low mitotic rates [40]. Indeed, we reported that 52.5% of the cases were described as incidental findings, whereas in our previous case series on GISTs, the patients were reported asymptomatic in 19.2% of the cases. Mean mitotic rate has been herein documented as 3/50 HPF; however also in our previous research 74.5% of the tumors had a mitotic count <5/50 HPF [38].

TABLE 3: Comparison between GISTs presenting in NF1 patients and sporadic GISTs.

	GISTs in NF1 patients	GIST personal case series	P value
Age			
Mean (years)	52.8	61.4	0.0001*
Sex			
M/F ratio	1	1.61	0.2§
Localization (%)			
Stomach	5.4	56.9	
Jejunum/ileus	69.8	23.4	<0.0001§
Other	24.8	19.7	
Symptoms (%)			
Incidental	52.5	19.1	0.002§
Other	47.5	80.9	
Diameter			
Mean (cm)	3.8	7.4	0.0003*
Risk classification (%)			
Low risk	64.9	41.3	
Intermediate risk	17.5	21.7	0.03§
High risk	17.5	37.0	

*t-test; §Chi-square test.

Notably a mutation in kit or PDGFR alpha genes has been reported exclusively in 4.8% of the cases.

Recently those GISTs associated with Carney Triad, Carney-Stratakis syndrome, along with young and pediatric GISTs have been documented to have a loss of succinate dehydrogenase subunit B (SDHB) expression, a mitochondrial protein [41–43]. On the basis of the SDHB expression, it has been recently proposed that GISTs could be differentiated into 2 characteristic subgroups: type 1 SDHB-positive and type 2 SDHB-negative [41]. Type 1 GISTs usually occur in adults with no predilection of tumor's locations, show homogeneous M/F, present KIT or PDGFRA mutations, and, generally, may benefit from the imatinib treatment. Type 2 GISTs occur usually in paediatric/young female patients almost exclusively in the stomach and present an epithelioid morphology. These tumors are usually c-kit and PDGFRa wild type and do not respond to the molecular treatment with imatinib [44].

Even though NF1 associated GISTs have been documented to be type 1 SDHB-positive tumors [43], they could be differentiated by several features including the predilection of localization to jejunum/small intestines, common tumor multiplicity, and the lack of GIST-specific mutations (kit and PDGFRa); moreover and alike the SDHB type 2 tumors, they do not respond well to imatinib treatment [43, 45, 46].

In conclusion, a wide review of the literature in this field documented that GISTs detected in NF1 patients seem to have a peculiar and distinct phenotype, different than the one commonly reported GISTs including younger age at presentation, distal localization, small diameter, low mitotic rate, and absence of kit and/or PDGRFa mutations. Moreover the vast majority of these tumors were documented to be kit positive consistent with spindle-shaped cells and were considered as low-risk neoplasms.

Authors' Contribution

Pier Federico Salvi and Laura Lorenzon contributed equally to the study.

References

[1] Neurofibromatosis Conference statement, "National institutes of health consensus development conference," *Archives of Neurology*, vol. 45, pp. 575–578, 1988.

[2] Y. Takazawa, S. Sakurai, Y. Sakuma et al., "Gastrointestinal stromal tumors of neurofibromatosis type I (von Recklinghausen's disease)," *American Journal of Surgical Pathology*, vol. 29, no. 6, pp. 755–763, 2005.

[3] C. E. Fuller and G. T. Williams, "Gastrointestinal manifestations of type 1 neurofibromatosis (von Recklinghausen's disease)," *Histopathology*, vol. 19, no. 1, pp. 1–11, 1991.

[4] M. Miettinen and J. Lasota, "Gastrointestinal stromal tumors: review on morphology, molecular pathology, prognosis, and differential diagnosis," *Archives of Pathology and Laboratory Medicine*, vol. 130, no. 10, pp. 1466–1478, 2006.

[5] M. Miettinen and J. Lasota, "Gastrointestinal stromal tumors—definition, clinical, histological, immunohistochemical, and molecular genetic features and differential diagnosis," *Virchows Archiv*, vol. 438, no. 1, pp. 1–12, 2001.

[6] B. Nilsson, P. Bümming, J. M. Meis-Kindblom et al., "Gastrointestinal stromal tumors: the incidence, prevalence, clinical course, and prognostication in the preimatinib mesylate era—a population-based study in western Sweden," *Cancer*, vol. 103, no. 4, pp. 821–829, 2005.

[7] G. J. C. Burkill, M. Badran, O. Al-Muderis et al., "Malignant gastrointestinal stromal tumor: distribution, imaging features, and pattern of metastatic spread," *Radiology*, vol. 226, no. 2, pp. 527–532, 2003.

[8] F. Duffaud and J.-Y. Blay, "Gastrointestinal stromal tumors: biology and treatment," *Oncology*, vol. 65, no. 3, pp. 187–197, 2003.

[9] R. P. DeMatteo, J. J. Lewis, D. Leung, S. S. Mudan, J. M. Woodruff, and M. F. Brennan, "Two hundred gastrointestinal stromal tumors: recurrence patterns and prognostic factors for survival," *Annals of Surgery*, vol. 231, no. 1, pp. 51–58, 2000.

[10] J. J. Lewis and M. F. Brennan, "Soft tissue sarcomas," *Current Problems in Surgery*, vol. 33, pp. 817–872, 1996.

[11] S. Hirota, K. Isozaki, Y. Moriyama et al., "Gain-of-function mutations of c-kit in human gastrointestinal stromal tumors," *Science*, vol. 279, no. 5350, pp. 577–580, 1998.

[12] Y. Kitamura and S. Hirota, "Kit as a human oncogenic tyrosine kinase," *Cellular and Molecular Life Sciences*, vol. 61, no. 23, pp. 2924–2931, 2004.

[13] T. Pawson, "Regulation and targets of receptor tyrosine kinases," *European Journal of Cancer*, vol. 38, supplement 5, pp. S3–S10, 2002.

[14] B. P. Rubin, S. Singer, C. Tsao et al., "KIT activation is a ubiquitous feature of gastrointestinal stromal tumors," *Cancer Research*, vol. 61, no. 22, pp. 8118–8121, 2001.

[15] S.-P. Cheng, M.-J. Huang, T.-L. Yang et al., "Neurofibromatosis with gastrointestinal stromal tumors: insights into the association," *Digestive Diseases and Sciences*, vol. 49, no. 7-8, pp. 1165–1169, 2004.

[16] K. Kinoshita, S. Hirota, K. Isozaki et al., "Absence of c-kit gene mutations in gastrointestinal stromal tumours from neurofibromatosis type I patients," *Journal of Pathology*, vol. 202, no. 1, pp. 80–85, 2004.

[17] Y. Takazawa, S. Sakurai, Y. Sakuma et al., "Gastrointestinal stromal tumors of neurofibromatosis type I (von Recklinghausen's disease)," *American Journal of Surgical Pathology*, vol. 29, no. 6, pp. 755–763, 2005.

[18] J. Andersson, H. Sihto, J. M. Meis-Kindblom, H. Joensuu, N. Nupponen, and L.-G. Kindblom, "NF1-associated gastrointestinal stromal tumors have unique clinical, phenotypic, and genotypic characteristics," *American Journal of Surgical Pathology*, vol. 29, no. 9, pp. 1170–1176, 2005.

[19] M. Miettinen, J. F. Fetsch, L. H. Sobin, and J. Lasota, "Gastrointestinal stromal tumors in patients with neurofibromatosis 1: a clinicopathologic and molecular genetic study of 45 cases," *American Journal of Surgical Pathology*, vol. 30, no. 1, pp. 90–96, 2006.

[20] O. Maertens, H. Prenen, M. Debiec-Rychter et al., "Molecular pathogenesis of multiple gastrointestinal stromal tumors in NF1 patients," *Human Molecular Genetics*, vol. 15, no. 6, pp. 1015–1023, 2006.

[21] H. Nemoto, G. Tate, A. Schirinzi et al., "Novel NF1 gene mutation in a Japanese patient with neurofibromatosis type 1 and a gastrointestinal stromal tumor," *Journal of Gastroenterology*, vol. 41, no. 4, pp. 378–382, 2006.

[22] P. Bümming, B. Nilsson, J. Sörensen, O. Nilsson, and H. Ahlman, "Use of 2-tracer PET to diagnose gastrointestinal stromal tumour and pheochromocytoma in patients with Carney triad and neurofibromatosis type 1," *Scandinavian Journal of Gastroenterology*, vol. 41, no. 5, pp. 626–630, 2006.

[23] S. Teramoto, T. Ota, A. Maniwa et al., "Two von Recklinghausen's disease cases with pheochromocytomas and gastrointestinal stromal tumors (GIST) in combination," *International Journal of Urology*, vol. 14, no. 1, pp. 73–74, 2007.

[24] D. R. Stewart, C. L. Corless, B. P. Rubin et al., "Mitotic recombination as evidence of alternative pathogenesis of gastrointestinal stromal tumours in neurofibromatosis type 1," *Journal of medical genetics*, vol. 44, no. 1, article e61, 2007.

[25] K. Kramer, C. Hasel, A. J. Aschoff, D. Henne-Bruns, and P. Wuerl, "Multiple gastrointestinal stromal tumors and bilateral pheochromocytoma in neurofibromatosis," *World Journal of Gastroenterology*, vol. 13, no. 24, pp. 3384–3387, 2007.

[26] R. Invernizzi, B. Martinelli, and G. Pinotti, "Association of GIST, breast cancer and schwannoma in a 60-year-old woman affected by type-1 von Recklinghausen's neurofibromatosis," *Tumori*, vol. 94, no. 1, pp. 126–128, 2008.

[27] B. Liegl, J. L. Hornick, C. L. Corless, and C. D. M. Fletcher, "Monoclonal antibody DOG1.1 Shows higher sensitivity than KIT in the diagnosis of gastrointestinal stromal tumors, including unusual subtypes," *American Journal of Surgical Pathology*, vol. 33, no. 3, pp. 437–446, 2009.

[28] H. Yamamoto, T. Tobo, M. Nakamori et al., "Neurofibromatosis type 1-related gastrointestinal stromal tumors: a special reference to loss of heterozygosity at 14q and 22q," *Journal of Cancer Research and Clinical Oncology*, vol. 135, no. 6, pp. 791–798, 2009.

[29] R. Dell'Avanzato, F. Carboni, M. B. Palmieri et al., "Laparoscopic resection of sporadic synchronous gastric and jejunal gastrointestinal stromal tumors: report of a case," *Surgery Today*, vol. 39, no. 4, pp. 335–339, 2009.

[30] K. Hirashima, H. Takamori, M. Hirota et al., "Multiple gastrointestinal stromal tumors in neurofibromatosis type 1: report of a case," *Surgery Today*, vol. 39, no. 11, pp. 979–983, 2009.

[31] G. Cavallaro, U. Basile, A. Polistena et al., "Surgical management of abdominal manifestations of type 1 neurofibromatosis: experience of a single center," *American Surgeon*, vol. 76, no. 4, pp. 389–396, 2010.

[32] D. Relles, J. Baek, A. Witkiewicz, and C. J. Yeo, "Periampullary and duodenal neoplasms in neurofibromatosis type 1: two cases and an updated 20-year review of the literature yielding 76 cases," *Journal of Gastrointestinal Surgery*, vol. 14, no. 6, pp. 1052–1061, 2010.

[33] M. E. Izquierdo and M. T. Bonastre, "Patient with high-risk GIST not associated with c-KIT mutations: same benefit from adjuvant therapy?" *Anticancer Drugs*, vol. 23, supplement, pp. S7–S9, 2012.

[34] A. Agaimy, N. Vassos, and R. S. Croner, "Gastrointestinal manifestations of neurofibromatosis type 1 (Recklinghausen's disease): clinicopathological spectrum with pathogenetic considerations," *International Journal of Clinical and Experimental Pathology*, vol. 5, no. 9, pp. 852–862, 2012.

[35] B. Ozcinar, N. Aksakal, O. Agcaoglu et al., "Multiple gastrointestinal stromal tumors and pheochromocytoma in a patient with von Recklinghausen's disease," *International Journal of Surgery Case Reports*, vol. 4, no. 2, pp. 216–218, 2013.

[36] M. Vlenterie, U. Flucke, L. C. Hofbauer et al., "Pheochromocytoma and gastrointestinal stromal tumors in patients with neurofibromatosis type I.," *American Journal of Medicine*, vol. 126, no. 2, pp. 174–180, 2013.

[37] S. Sawalhi, K. Al-Harbi, Z. Raghib, A. I. Abdelrahman, and A. Al-Hujaily, "Behavior of advanced gastrointestinal stromal tumor in a patient with von-Recklinghausen disease: case report," *World Journal of Clinical Oncology*, vol. 4, pp. 70–74, 2013.

[38] S. Caterino, L. Lorenzon, N. Petrucciani et al., "Gastrointestinal stromal tumors: correlation between symptoms at presentation, tumor location and prognostic factors in 47 consecutive patients," *World Journal of Surgical Oncology*, vol. 9, article 13, 2011.

[39] M. E. Zoller, B. Rembeck, A. Oden, M. Samuelsson, and L. Angervall, "Malignant and benign tumors in patients with neurofibromatosis type 1 in a defined Swedish population," *Cancer*, vol. 79, pp. 2125–2131, 1997.

[40] M. Miettinen and J. Lasota, "Histopathology of gastrointestinal stromal tumor," *Journal of Surgical Oncology*, vol. 104, no. 8, pp. 865–873, 2011.

[41] A. J. Gill, A. Chou, R. Vilain et al., "Immunohistochemistry for SDHB divides gastrointestinal stromal tumors (GISTs) into 2 distinct types," *American Journal of Surgical Pathology*, vol. 34, no. 5, pp. 636–644, 2010.

[42] J. Gaal, C. A. Stratakis, J. A. Carney et al., "SDHB immunohistochemistry: a useful tool in the diagnosis of Carney-Stratakis and Carney triad gastrointestinal stromal tumors," *Modern Pathology*, vol. 24, no. 1, pp. 147–151, 2011.

[43] J. H. Wang, J. Lasota, and M. Miettinen, "Succinate dehydrogenase subunit B (SDHB) is expressed in neurofibro-matosis 1-associated gastrointestinal stromal tumors (Gists): implications for the SDHB expression based classification of gists," *Journal of Cancer*, vol. 2, pp. 90–93, 2011.

[44] B. Pasini, S. R. McWhinney, T. Bei et al., "Clinical and molecular genetics of patients with the Carney-Stratakis syndrome and germline mutations of the genes coding for the succinate dehydrogenase subunits SDHB, SDHC, and SDHD," *European Journal of Human Genetics*, vol. 16, no. 1, pp. 79–88, 2008.

[45] C. Mussi, H.-U. Schildhaus, A. Gronchi, E. Wardelmann, and P. Hohenberger, "Therapeutic consequences from molecular biology for gastrointestinal stromal tumor patients affected by neurofibromatosis type 1," *Clinical Cancer Research*, vol. 14, no. 14, pp. 4550–4555, 2008.

[46] J.-L. Lee, J. Y. Kim, M.-H. Ryu et al., "Response to imatinib in KIT- and PDGFRA-wild type gastrointestinal stromal associated with neurofibromatosis type 1," *Digestive Diseases and Sciences*, vol. 51, no. 6, pp. 1043–1046, 2006.

11

Trail Overexpression Inversely Correlates with Histological Differentiation in Intestinal-Type Sinonasal Adenocarcinoma

M. Re,[1] A. Santarelli,[2] M. Mascitti,[2] F. Rambini,[2] L. Lo Muzio,[3] A. Zizzi,[4] and C. Rubini[4]

[1] Department of Otorhinolaryngology, Marche Polytechnic University, 60121 Ancona, Italy
[2] Department of Clinical Specialistic and Dental Sciences, Marche Polytechnic University, 60121 Ancona, Italy
[3] Department of Sperimental and Clinical Medicine, University of Foggia, 71121 Foggia, Italy
[4] Department of Neurosciences, Marche Polytechnic University, 60121 Ancona, Italy

Correspondence should be addressed to M. Mascitti; marcomascitti86@hotmail.it

Academic Editor: Timothy M. Pawlik

Introduction. Despite their histological resemblance to colorectal adenocarcinoma, there is some information about the molecular events involved in the pathogenesis of intestinal-type sinonasal adenocarcinomas (ITACs). To evaluate the possible role of TNF-related apoptosis-inducing ligand (TRAIL) gene defects in ITAC, by investigating the immunohistochemical expression of TRAIL gene product in a group of ethmoidal ITACs associated with occupational exposure. *Material and Methods.* Retrospective study on 23 patients with pathological diagnosis of primary ethmoidal ITAC. Representative formalin-fixed, paraffin-embedded block from each case was selected for immunohistochemical studies using the antibody against TRAIL. Clinicopathological data were also correlated with the staining results. *Results.* The immunohistochemical examination demonstrated that poorly differentiated cases showed a higher percentage of TRAIL expressing cells compared to well-differentiated cases. No correlation was found with other clinicopathological parameters, including T, stage and relapses. *Conclusion.* The relationship between upregulation of TRAIL and poorly differentiated ethmoidal adenocarcinomas suggests that the mutation of this gene, in combination with additional genetic events, could play a role in the pathogenesis of ITAC.

1. Introduction

Malignant tumors of the nasal cavity and paranasal sinuses account for 0.2% of all human primary malignant neoplasms, with an incidence of 0.1–1.4 new cases/year/100,000 inhabitants [1–3].

Adenocarcinomas account for 10–20% of all primary malignant neoplasms of the sinonasal tract [4, 5]. Many of these have salivary gland origin, while others have histologic patterns resembling those of colon adenocarcinoma. This second type of sinonasal adenocarcinoma has been named intestinal-type adenocarcinoma (ITAC) and is responsible for less than 4% of the total malignancies of this region [6].

ITACs of the nasal cavity and paranasal sinuses can occur sporadically or are associated with occupational exposure to hardwood and leather dusts [7]. Exposure to wood and leather dusts increases the risk of adenocarcinoma by 500-fold [8, 9]. Findings from several studies have suggested

clinical differences between ITAC arising in individuals with occupational dust exposure and ITAC arising sporadically. In fact tumors related to occupational exposure affect men in 85–90% of cases, showing a strong tendency to arise in the ethmoid sinuses [10–12].

ITACs are aggressive tumors characterized by frequent local recurrences, low incidence of distant metastases, and an overall mortality of approximately 53% [12]. Histopathological grading appears to be a significant prognostic indicator [11–13]. Surgery is considered the standard treatment.

ITAC seems to be preceded by intestinal metaplasia of the respiratory mucosa, induced by hardwood dust, leather dust, and other unknown agents, which is accompanied by a switch to an intestinal phenotype. The molecular mechanisms involved in metaplastic transformation of terminally differentiated epithelium to a phenotypically different epithelium are largely unknown.

The morphological appearance of these tumors is variable, and they may resemble conventional colorectal adenocarcinoma. The similarities between ITAC and intestinal adenocarcinoma involve their ultrastructural and immunohistochemical aspects [14–17].

Numerous studies have shown that mutations of the K-ras and TP53 genes are common in colorectal adenocarcinomas [18, 19]. In comparison, there is very little information about the molecular events involved in the pathogenesis of ITAC [16, 19–26], in contrast to even more increasing information about the molecular mechanisms involved in the pathogenesis of head and neck squamous cell carcinomas (HNSCC) [27–32].

Tumor necrosis factor (TNF)-related apoptosis-inducing ligand (TRAIL) is a TNF-family member, found in a variety of tissues [33] and with a conditional expression in several immune effector cells [34, 35]. To date, five different receptors have been identified to interact with TRAIL: TRAILR1 (DR4), TRAIL-R2 (DR5), TRAIL-R3 (DcR1), TRAIL-R4 (DcR2), and osteoprotegerin. DR4 and DR5 are two different death domain-containing membrane receptors, whereas DcR1 and DcR2 are two decoy receptors that compete for TRAIL binding with DR4 and DR5 [36–39]. The final effect of the TRAIL signaling is the induction of apoptosis by the intrinsic death pathway, recruiting the inactive form of caspase-8 [40]. Expression of TRAIL and its receptors has been detected in various human tumors, suggesting that TRAIL signaling pathway is involved in endogenous tumor surveillance [40], but the mechanism of how TRAIL and its receptors contribute to carcinogenesis remains unknown.

To gain further insight into the phenotype and possible mechanisms of ethmoidal ITAC, we investigated the expression of TRAIL, correlating with clinicopathological data.

2. Materials and Methods

2.1. Patients Selection. The samples of 23 primary ethmoidal intestinal-type adenocarcinomas were retrospectively retrieved from the archives of the Institute of Pathology, Marche Polytechnic University, Ancona, Italy. All the tumors in which the diagnosis of ITAC was confirmed were subsequently subtyped, as papillary, colonic, solid, mixed, or mucinous types, as described by Barnes [12].

The medical records of these patients were reviewed. Inclusion criteria were complete clinical data, uniformity of histological differentiation throughout the tumor sample, and the availability of sufficient material from the primary tumor for investigations. Patients with previous or synchronous second malignancies or with previous radiation therapy or chemotherapy were excluded from the study. The follow-up time ranged from 2 to 10 years (mean 4.8 years).

2.2. Immunohistochemistry. Four-micrometer serial sections from formalin-fixed, paraffin-embedded blocks of tumour representative areas were cut for each case. Immunohistochemical staining for TRAIL was performed using the following antigen retrieval system. Sections were deparaffinized in two changes of xylene for 10 minutes each, then, were

rehydrated through graded alcohols, and immersed in 0,3% hydrogen peroxide in methanol for 30 minutes to block endogenous peroxidase activity. Sections were then washed in PBS. The tissue sections were placed in a microwave oven (Philips, Cooktyronic M720, 700 W) in a plastic Coplin jar filled with 10 mM sodium citrate buffer (pH 6,0) at 5-minute interval, the fluid level in the Coplin jar was removed from the microwave oven and allowed to cool. Slides were incubated overnight with a 1 : 50 dilution of the primary mouse antihuman TRAIL monoclonal antibody (Dako DO-7, Glostrup, Denmark). A biotin-streptavidin detection system was used with diaminobenzidine as the chromogen. Slides were washed twice with PBS and incubated with the linking reagent (biotinylated anti-immunoglobulins) for 15 minutes, at room temperature. After rinsing in PBS, the slides were incubated with the peroxidase-conjugated streptavidin label for 15 minutes at room temperature. The sections were again rinsed in PBS and incubated with diaminobenzidine for 10 minutes, in the dark. After chromogen development, slides were washed in two changes of water and counterstained with a 1 : 10 dilution of hematoxylin. The sections were then dehydrated, cleared in xylene, and mounted.

TRAIL expression and location were evaluated on histological section using a Leitz Orthoplan microscope equipped with a X 400 objective. The percentage of TRAIL positive cells was evaluated from a minimum of 1,000 cells in each case. Only nuclear staining of epithelial cells was observed, and the nuclei with a clear brown color, regardless of staining intensity, were regarded as TRAIL positive.

A negative control for TRAIL immunostaining was performed in all cases by omitting the primary antibody, which, in all instances, resulted in negative immunoreactivity. The positive control consisted of staining a human normal mammary gland epithelium.

2.3. Scoring of Preparations. Both the histological diagnoses and evaluation of the positivity for TRAIL were carried out indipendently by two of the authors (C.R. and A.Z.). Immunohistochemical labeling for TRAIL was classified as positive, when more than 5% of nuclei or cells were stained.

2.4. Statistical Analysis. The following pathological and clinical parameters were analyzed: tumour grade of differentiation (G1,G2,G3), tumour extension (T1,T2,T3,T4), tumor stage (I, II, III, IV), and TRAIL immunoreactivity. Differences in TRAIL immunoreactivity between the different groups were compared by the nonparametric Kruskal-Wallis test. Statistical significance was set at $P < 0.05$. All statistical analyses were performed using the SPSS statistical package (SPPS Inc., Chicago, IL).

3. Results

3.1. Clinical Findings. There were 21 males and 2 females, with a mean age of 66.3 years (range 54–77). There were 8 grade I, 8 grade II, and 7 grade III adenocarcinomas. 3 patients were in I stage, 7 patients were in II stage, 11 patients were in III stage,

TABLE 1: Clinicopathological data of patients and TRAIL oncoprotein expression percentage.

Patient	Age	Sex	T	Grade	CH	CHT	RT	Relapse	Trail%
1	70	M	T2	3	No	No	Yes	Yes	70
2	55	M	T3	1	Yes	Yes	Yes	No	10
3	67	M	T3	2	No	Yes	Yes	No	60
4	60	F	T1	1	Yes	No	No	No	5
5	62	M	T3	3	Yes	Yes	Yes	Yes	80
6	54	M	T3	2	Yes	No	Yes	No	35
7	54	M	T3	2	Yes	No	Yes	No	50
8	74	M	T3	1	Yes	No	Yes	No	20
9	74	M	T2	2	Yes	No	Yes	Yes	55
10	58	M	T1	1	Yes	No	Yes	No	2
11	74	M	T2	3	Yes	No	Yes	Yes	80
12	70	M	T2	2	Yes	No	Yes	No	50
13	72	M	T3	1	Yes	No	Yes	No	3
14	68	M	T3	3	Yes	No	Yes	No	70
15	77	M	T3	2	Yes	No	Yes	No	75
16	67	M	T3	1	Yes	No	Yes	No	45
17	77	M	T2	2	Yes	No	No	Yes	60
18	65	M	T3	3	Yes	No	Yes	Yes	75
19	63	M	T2	1	Yes	No	Yes	No	55
20	61	F	T1	1	Yes	No	Yes	No	5
21	65	M	T2	2	Yes	No	No	No	25
22	61	M	T4a	3	Yes	No	Yes	Yes	90
23	76	M	T4b	3	Yes	No	No	Yes	80

T: tumor extension, CH: surgery, CHT: chemotherapy, RT: radiotherapy.

and 2 patients were in IV stage. Clinicopathological staging was determined by the TNM classification (UICC 2009).

All the patients had a known history of occupational exposure to hardwood dust, and intestinal-type adenocarcinoma was localized in all cases in the ethmoid region as confirmed by endoscopic and imaging (TC and/or MR) evaluation.

The main clinicopathologic features of the patients and the oncoprotein expression are summarized in Table 1.

3.2. Immunohistochemistry. The cases classified as ITAC showed a variable cellular appearance and were composed of a mixture of tall columnar absorptive cells, atypical stratified cylindrical cells similar to the cells seen in conventional colorectal adenocarcinoma, goblet cells, and large round to polygonal nondescriptive epithelial cells.

3.3. TRAIL Expression. The percentage of neoplastic cells immunoreactive for TRAIL ranged from 2% to 90%. In all cases, TRAIL expression was nuclear. There was a relationship between TRAIL overexpression and the histological grading. Indeed, poorly differentiated cases (G2 and G3) showed a higher percentage of TRAIL expressing cells in comparison to well differentiated (G1) cases. No correlation between TRAIL expression and other clinicopathological parameters, including T, stage and relapses was found (Figures 1 and 2).

4. Discussion

Despite their histological similarity to colorectal carcinomas, there is very little information about the molecular events involved in the pathogenesis of ITAC. Several crucial pathways of tumorigenesis have been identified in colorectal adenocarcinomas [18, 19]. These pathways involve the mutation and inactivation of multiple oncogenes, tumor suppressor genes, and DNA mismatch repair genes including K-ras, APC, p53, MLH1, and MSH2 [18–20].

Working on the hypothesis that morphological similarities to colorectal adenocarcinomas might reflect equivalent genetic alterations, several authors have investigated the presence of activating mutations of Ras oncogenes and TP53 mutations in ITAC [21–25]. TP53 mutations were found in 18–44% of mostly occupational ITACs, whereas, K-Ras mutations were found in 10–15% of ITACs [21–25]. The results of these studies suggest that mutations of K-Ras and other Ras genes are relatively uncommon in ITAC, and similarly, TP53 mutations in ITACs have not been widely demonstrated.

Other studies have shown that K-Ras mutation and C-erb-2 expression could be associated with more aggressive ITACs [16, 26].

Licitra et al. found the existence of two genetic ITACs subgroups, defined by differences in TP53 mutational status or protein functionality, that strongly influence pathologic response to primary chemotherapy and, ultimately, prognosis [41].

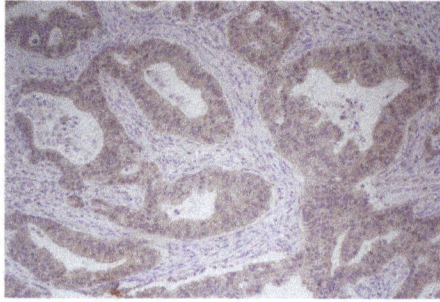

FIGURE 1: Poorly differentiated ethmoidal intestinal-type adenocarcinoma (G3) showing high percentage of TRAIL expressing cells (magnification 20x).

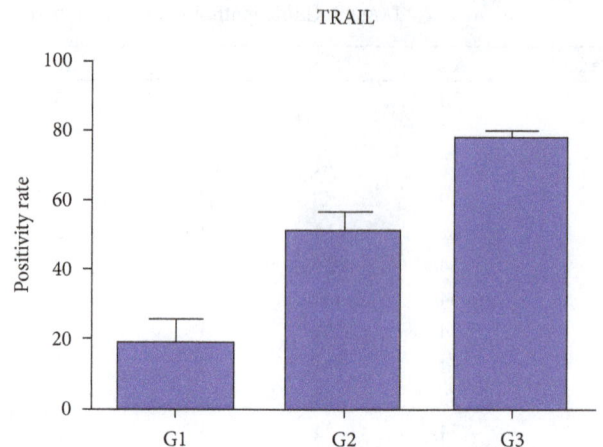

FIGURE 2: Poorly differentiated cases showed a higher percentage of TRAIL expressing cells in comparison to well-differentiated ethmoidal ITAC.

Perez-Ordonez et al. evaluated the possible role of DNA mismatch repair (MMR) gene defects or disruptions of E-cadherin/β-catenin complex in ITAC by investigating the immunohistochemical expression of the MMR gene products, E-cadherin, and β-catenin in a group of sporadic ITACs. The preserved nuclear expression of MLH1, MSH2, MSH3, and MSH6 suggested that mutations or promoter methylation of MMR genes do not play a role in the pathogenesis of ITAC [42].

Kennedy et al. found that sinonasal ITACs have a distinctive phenotype, with all cases expressing CK20, CDX-2, and villin and most ITACs also expressing CK7, so that the expression pattern of CK7, CK20, CDX-2, and villin positive may be useful in separating these tumors from other non-ITAC adenocarcinomas of the sinonasal tract [43].

Given these findings, to explore other pathways involved in the molecular pathogenesis of ITACs, we immunohistochemically investigated the expression of the apoptosis-regulating protein TRAIL in a group of 23 ethmoidal ITAC associated with occupational exposure. This immunohistochemical expression was also retrospectively correlated with the patient outcome to evaluate their independent prognostic relevance. To the best of our knowledge, there are no previous reports on the expression of TRAIL protein in ITACs.

TRAIL is an apoptosis-inducing protein and a molecule important in inhibiting cellular immunity [44–46]. Similarly, cancer cells may use TRAIL to evade the antitumor immune response [47]. In literature, there are many works that have detected the expression of TRAIL and its receptors in several tumors, correlating this expression with clinicopathological analysis.

Trail-R1 was identified as an independent prognostic factor for disease-free survival in 128 patients with colon cancer [48]. McCarthy et al. showed that high TRAIL-R2 expression was significantly associated with decreased survival and lymph node involvement in patients with primary breast cancer [49]. Yoldas et al. revealed that TRAIL and DR4 expression were correlated with the pathological grading in patients with laryngeal squamous cell carcinoma, while the alteration in DR5 expression was correlated with the clinical staging [50]. Despite the several works, the specific mechanism of how TRAIL and its receptors contribute to carcinogenesis remains unknown.

The results of our immunohistochemical examination showed a relationship between TRAIL upregulation and the increase of the histological tumor grading. No correlation was found with other clinicopathological parameters, including T, stage and relapses.

5. Conclusion

Our results suggest that mutations of TRAIL expression, in combination with additional genetic events, could play a role in the pathogenesis of ITAC. However, this study showed that TRAIL expression cannot be considered as an independent prognostic factor in patients with ITACs, because there was not sufficient statistical power to detect significant associations between immunohistochemical expression of this protein and the clinicopathologic parameters of the tumors, therefore, further investigations with a larger sample are needed.

References

[1] P. E. Robin, D. J. Powell, and J. M. Stansbie, "Carcinoma of the nasal cavity and paranasal sinuses: incidence and presentation of different histological types," *Clinical Otolaryngology and Allied Sciences*, vol. 4, no. 6, pp. 431–456, 1979.

[2] J. G. Batsakis, D. H. Rice, and A. R. Solomon, "The pathology of head and neck tumors: squamous and mucous-gland carcinomas of the nasal cavity, paranasal sinuses, and larynx, part VI," *Head and Neck Surgery*, vol. 2, no. 6, pp. 497–508, 1980.

[3] M. Re and E. Pasquini, "Nasopharyngeal mucoepidermoid carcinoma in children," *International Journal of Pediatric Otorhinolaryngology*, vol. 77, no. 4, pp. 565–569, 2013.

[4] A. L. Weber and A. C. Stanton, "Malignant tumors of the paranasal sinuses: radiological, clinical, and histopathologic evaluation of 200 cases," *Head and Neck Surgery*, vol. 6, no. 3, pp. 761–776, 1984.

[5] M. Iacoangeli, A. Di Rienzo, M. Re et al., "Endoscopic endonasal approach for the treatment of a large clival giant cell tumor complicated by an intraoperative internal carotid artery rupture," *Cancer Management and Research*, vol. 5, pp. 21–24, 2013.

[6] J. I. Lopez, M. Nevado, B. Eizaguirre, and A. Perez, "Intestinal-type adenocarcinoma of the nasal cavity and paranasal sinuses. A clinicopathologic study of 6 cases," *Tumori*, vol. 76, no. 3, pp. 250–254, 1990.

[7] O. Kleinsasser and H.-G. Schroeder, "Adenocarcinomas of the inner nose after exposure to wood dust: morphological findings and relationships between histopathology and clinical behavior in 79 cases," *Archives of Oto-Rhino-Laryngology*, vol. 245, no. 1, pp. 1–15, 1988.

[8] A. Leclerc, M. M. Cortes, M. Gerin, D. Luce, and J. Brugere, "Sinonasal cancer and wood dust exposure: results from a case-control study," *American Journal of Epidemiology*, vol. 140, no. 4, pp. 340–349, 1994.

[9] S. D. Stellman, P. A. Demers, D. Colin, and P. Boffetta, "Cancer mortality and wood dust exposure among participants in the American Cancer Society Cancer Prevention Study-II (CPS-II)," *American Journal of Industrial Medicine*, vol. 34, no. 3, pp. 229–237, 1990.

[10] E. H. Hadfield, "A study of adenocarcinoma of the paranasal sinuses in woodworkers in the furniture industry," *Annals of the Royal College of Surgeons of England*, vol. 46, no. 6, pp. 301–319, 1970.

[11] C. Klintenberg, J. Olofsson, and H. Hellquist, "Adenocarcinoma of the ethmoid sinuses. A review of 28 cases with special reference to wood dust exposure," *Cancer*, vol. 54, no. 3, pp. 482–488, 1984.

[12] L. Barnes, "Intestinal-type adenocarcinoma of the nasal cavity and paranasal sinuses," *American Journal of Surgical Pathology*, vol. 10, no. 3, pp. 192–202, 1986.

[13] A. Franchi, O. Gallo, and M. Santucci, "Clinical relevance of the histological classification of sinonasal intestinal-type adenocarcinomas," *Human Pathology*, vol. 30, no. 10, pp. 1140–1145, 1999.

[14] S. E. Mills, R. E. Fechner, and R. W. Cantrell, "Aggressive sinonasal lesion resembling normal intestinal mucosa," *American Journal of Surgical Pathology*, vol. 6, no. 8, pp. 803–809, 1982.

[15] J. G. Batsakis, B. Mackay, and N. G. Ordonez, "Enteric-type adenocarcinoma of the nasal cavity: an electron microscopic and immunocytochemical study," *Cancer*, vol. 54, no. 5, pp. 855–860, 1984.

[16] C. D. McKinney, S. E. Mills, and D. W. Franquemont, "Sinonasal intestinal-type adenocarcinoma: immunohistochemical profile and comparison with colonic adenocarcinoma," *Modern Pathology*, vol. 8, no. 4, pp. 421–426, 1995.

[17] A. Franchi, D. Massi, G. Baroni, and M. Santucci, "CDX-2 homeobox gene expression," *American Journal of Surgical Pathology*, vol. 27, no. 10, pp. 1390–1391, 2003.

[18] E. R. Fearon and B. Vogelstein, "A genetic model for colorectal tumorigenesis," *Cell*, vol. 61, no. 5, pp. 759–767, 1990.

[19] D. C. Chung, "The genetic basis of colorectal cancer: insights into critical pathways of tumorigenesis," *Gastroenterology*, vol. 119, no. 3, pp. 854–865, 2000.

[20] P. M. Calvert and H. Frucht, "The genetics of colorectal cancer," *Annals of Internal Medicine*, vol. 137, no. 7, pp. 603–612, 2002.

[21] A. T. Saber, L. R. Nielsen, M. Dictor, L. Hagmar, Z. Mikoczy, and H. Wallin, "K-ras mutations in sinonasal adenocarcinomas in patients occupationally exposed to wood or leather dust," *Cancer Letters*, vol. 126, no. 1, pp. 59–65, 1998.

[22] P. Pérez, O. Dominguez, S. González, A. Triviño, and C. Suárez, "ras gene mutations in ethmoid sinus adenocarcinoma: prognostic implications," *Cancer*, vol. 86, no. 2, pp. 255–264, 1999.

[23] T.-T. Wu, L. Barnes, A. Bakker, P. A. Swalsky, and S. D. Finkelstein, "K-ras-2 and p53 genotyping of intestinal-type adenocarcinoma of the nasal cavity and paranasal sinuses," *Modern Pathology*, vol. 9, no. 3, pp. 199–204, 1996.

[24] F. Perrone, M. Oggionni, S. Birindelli et al., "TP53, P14ARF, P16INK4a and H-ras gene molecular analysis in intestinal-type adenocarcinoma of the nasal cavity and paranasal sinuses," *International Journal of Cancer*, vol. 105, no. 2, pp. 196–203, 2003.

[25] M. Re, G. Magliulo, P. Tarchini et al., "p53 and Bcl-2 over-expression inversely correlates with histological differentiation in occupational ethmoidal intestinal-type sinonasal adenocarcinoma," *International Journal of Immunopathology and Pharmacology*, vol. 24, no. 3, pp. 603–609, 2011.

[26] O. Gallo, A. Franchi, I. Fini-Storchi et al., "Prognostic significance of c-erbB-2 oncoprotein expression in intestinal-type adenocarcinoma of the sinonasal tract," *Head & Neck*, vol. 20, no. 3, pp. 224–231, 1998.

[27] D. L. Crowe, J. G. Hacia, C.-L. Hsieh, U. K. Sinha, and D. H. Rice, "Molecular pathology of head and neck cancer," *Histology and Histopathology*, vol. 17, no. 3, pp. 909–914, 2002.

[28] L. Lo Muzio, A. Santarelli, R. Caltabiano et al., "p63 overexpression associates with poor prognosis in head and neck squamous cell carcinoma," *Human Pathology*, vol. 36, no. 2, pp. 187–194, 2005.

[29] M. Re, G. Magliulo, L. Ferrante et al., "p63 expression in laryngeal squamous cell carcinoma is related to tumor extension, histologic grade, lymph node involvement and clinical stage," *Journal of Biological Regulators & Homeostatic Agents*, vol. 27, no. 1, pp. 121–129, 2013.

[30] M. Artico, E. Bianchi, G. Magliulo et al., "Neurotrophins, their receptors and KI-67 in human GH-secreting pituitary adenomas: an immunohistochemical analysis," *International Journal of Immunopathology and Pharmacology*, vol. 25, no. 1, pp. 117–125, 2012.

[31] M. Re, R. Romeo, and V. Mallardi, "Paralateral-nasal malignant schwannoma with rhabdomyoblastic differentiation (Triton tumor). Report of a case," *Acta Otorhinolaryngologica Italica*, vol. 22, no. 4, pp. 245–247, 2002.

[32] R. Verdolini, P. Amerio, G. Goteri et al., "Cutaneous carcinomas and preinvasive neoplastic lesions. Role of MMP-2 and MMP-9 metalloproteinases in neoplastic invasion and their relationship with proliferative activity and p53 expression," *Journal of Cutaneous Pathology*, vol. 28, no. 3, pp. 120–126, 2001.

[33] S. R. Wiley, K. Schooley, P. J. Smolak et al., "Identification and characterization of a new member of the TNF family that induces apoptosis," *Immunity*, vol. 3, no. 6, pp. 673–682, 1995.

[34] L. Zamai, M. Ahmad, I. M. Bennett, L. Azzoni, E. S. Alnemri, and B. Perussia, "Natural killer (NK) cell-mediated cytotoxicity: differential use of TRAIL and Fas ligand by immature and mature primary human NK cells," *Journal of Experimental Medicine*, vol. 188, no. 12, pp. 2375–2380, 1998.

[35] T. S. Griffith, S. R. Wiley, M. Z. Kubin, L. M. Sedger, C. R. Maliszewski, and N. A. Fanger, "Monocyte-mediated tumoricidal activity via the tumor necrosis factor-related cytokine, TRAIL," *Journal of Experimental Medicine*, vol. 189, no. 8, pp. 1343–1353, 1999.

[36] G. S. Wu, "TRAIL as a target in anti-cancer therapy," *Cancer Letters*, vol. 285, no. 1, pp. 1–5, 2009.

[37] D. Mahalingam, E. Szegezdi, M. Keane, S. D. Jong, and A. Samali, "TRAIL receptor signalling and modulation: are we on

the right TRAIL?" *Cancer Treatment Reviews*, vol. 35, no. 3, pp. 280–288, 2009.

[38] A. Ashkenazi, P. Holland, and S. G. Eckhardt, "Ligand-based targeting of apoptosis in cancer: the potential of recombinant human apoptosis ligand 2/tumor necrosis factor-related apoptosis-inducing ligand (rhApo2L/TRAIL)," *Journal of Clinical Oncology*, vol. 26, no. 21, pp. 3621–3630, 2008.

[39] S. Wang, "The promise of cancer therapeutics targeting the TNF-related apoptosis-inducing ligand and TRAIL receptor pathway," *Oncogene*, vol. 27, no. 48, pp. 6207–6215, 2008.

[40] H. Kumamoto and K. Ooya, "Expression of tumor necrosis factor α, TNF-related apoptosis-inducing ligand, and their associated molecules in ameloblastomas," *Journal of Oral Pathology and Medicine*, vol. 34, no. 5, pp. 287–294, 2005.

[41] L. Licitra, S. Suardi, P. Bossi et al., "Prediction of TP53 status for primary cisplatin, fluorouracil, and leucovorin chemotherapy in ethmoid sinus intestinal-type adenocarcinoma," *Journal of Clinical Oncology*, vol. 22, no. 24, pp. 4901–4906, 2004.

[42] B. Perez-Ordonez, N. N. Huynh, K. W. Berean, and R. C. K. Jordan, "Expression of mismatch repair proteins, β catenin, and E cadherin in intestinal-type sinonasal adenocarcinoma," *Journal of Clinical Pathology*, vol. 57, no. 10, pp. 1080–1083, 2004.

[43] M. T. Kennedy, R. C. K. Jordan, K. W. Berean, and B. Perez-Ordoñez, "Expression pattern of CK7, CK20, CDX-2, and villin in intestinal-type sinonasal adenocarcinoma," *Journal of Clinical Pathology*, vol. 57, no. 9, pp. 932–937, 2004.

[44] A. D. Sanlioglu, E. Dirice, O. Elpek et al., "High TRAIL death receptor 4 and decoy receptor 2 expression correlates with significant cell death in pancreatic ductal adenocarcinoma patients," *Pancreas*, vol. 38, no. 2, pp. 154–160, 2009.

[45] E. Dirice, A. D. Sanlioglu, S. Kahraman et al., "Adenovirus-mediated TRAIL gene (Ad5hTRAIL) delivery into pancreatic islets prolongs normoglycemia in streptozotocin-induced diabetic rats," *Human Gene Therapy*, vol. 20, no. 10, pp. 1177–1189, 2009.

[46] S.-S. C. Cheung, D. L. Metzger, X. Wang et al., "Tumor necrosis factor-related apoptosis-inducing ligand and CD56 expression in patients with type 1 diabetes mellitus," *Pancreas*, vol. 30, no. 2, pp. 105–114, 2005.

[47] A. Trauzold, D. Siegmund, B. Schniewind et al., "TRAIL promotes metastasis of human pancreatic ductal adenocarcinoma," *Oncogene*, vol. 25, no. 56, pp. 7434–7439, 2006.

[48] J. Sträter, U. Hinz, H. Walczak et al., "Expression of TRAIL and TRAIL receptors in colon carcinoma: TRAIL-R1 is an independent prognostic parameter," *Clinical Cancer Research*, vol. 8, no. 12, pp. 3734–3740, 2002.

[49] M. M. McCarthy, M. Sznol, K. A. DiVito, R. L. Camp, D. L. Rimm, and H. M. Kluger, "Evaluating the expression and prognostic value of TRAIL-R1 and TRAIL-R2 in breast cancer," *Clinical Cancer Research*, vol. 11, no. 14, pp. 5188–5194, 2005.

[50] B. Yoldas, C. Ozer, O. Ozen et al., "Clinical significance of TRAIL and TRAIL receptors in patients with head and neck cancer," *Head & Neck*, vol. 33, no. 9, pp. 1278–1284, 2011.

12

Preoperative Localization and Surgical Margins in Conservative Breast Surgery

F. Corsi, L. Sorrentino, D. Bossi, A. Sartani, and D. Foschi

Surgery Division, Department of Clinical Sciences, L. Sacco Hospital, University of Milan, Via G.B. Grassi 74, 20157 Milan, Italy

Correspondence should be addressed to F. Corsi, fabio.corsi@unimi.it

Academic Editor: A. K. Dcruz

Breast-conserving surgery (BCS) is the treatment of choice for early breast cancer. The adequacy of surgical margins (SM) is a crucial issue for adjusting the volume of excision and for avoiding local recurrences, although the precise definition of an adequate margins width remains controversial. Moreover, other factors such as the biological behaviour of the tumor and subsequent proper systemic therapies may influence the local recurrence rate (LRR). However, a successful BCS requires preoperative localization techniques or margin assessment techniques. Carbon marking, wire-guided, biopsy clips, radio-guided, ultrasound-guided, frozen section analysis, imprint cytology, and cavity shave margins are commonly used, but from the literature review, no single technique proved to be better among the various ones. Thus, an association of two or more methods could result in a decrease in rates of involved margins. Each institute should adopt its most congenial techniques, based on the senologic equipe experience, skills, and technologies.

1. Introduction

Breast-conserving surgery (BCS) is the treatment of choice for early breast cancer [1, 2]. Various randomized trials have reported this approach to be safe and effective, thus determining a decrease in the adoption of mastectomy as the treatment of choice for early invasive breast cancer [3, 4]. BCS can almost be considered the gold standard of early stage invasive breast cancer treatment, allowing to achieve adequate surgical margins (SM) with an acceptable cosmetic outcome. Some studies have defined the adequacy of SM by its correlation with the locoregional recurrence rate (LRR) [5–14], but the precise definition of an adequate margins width remains controversial [15–17]. However, there is no doubt that obtaining negative margins decreases the risk of local recurrence [1]. Some clinical trials have demonstrated that systemic therapies may also improve the local control in breast cancer [18, 19]. Thus, there seems to be noted a recent trend of reconsideration of the importance of margin width on the incidence of local recurrences, in favour of other prognostic factors such as the biological behaviour of the tumor [15–19].

A requirement for successful BCS is a careful preoperative planning with proper localization of the lesion, especially in nonpalpable breast lesions [1]. In order to obtain adequate excisions, margins assessment techniques are also available. Wire-guided localization, radio-guided occult lesion localization (ROLL), carbon marking, intraoperative ultrasound-guided localization, cavity shave margins, and biopsy markers are commonly used, with different results in terms of LRR. The aim of this review is to investigate how these techniques may assist the surgeon to obtain adequate resections.

2. What Is an Adequate Surgical Margin?

A negative SM is defined by the absence of ink in any malignant cells on histology, and the distance between the closest malignant cells and the inked surface of the surgical specimen defines the microscopic margin width (Table 1) [1]. Gage et al. and Schnitt et al. have described in 1996 four types of margins status: negative if >1 mm between tumor cells and the inked surface; close if ≤1 mm; positive if presence of carcinoma at the inked margin; and focally positive if carcinoma is present

TABLE 1: Local recurrence rates and corresponding threshold distances for negative margins are indicated for each study.

Study	Surgical margins	Local recurrences
Horiguchi et al., 2002 [9]	5 mm	3.2%
Karasawa et al., 2003 [10]	5 mm	1.7%
Perez, 2003 [11]	3 mm	5.8%
Peterson et al., 1999 [8]	2 mm	12.8% (*)
Santiago et al., 2004 [12]	2 mm	12.2%
Karasawa et al., 2005 [13]	2 mm (2.1–5 mm)	3.4% (6.3%)
Gage et al., 1996 [5]	1 mm	10.5% (*)
Park et al., 2000 [7]	1 mm	16% (*)
Kreike et al., 2008 [14]	1 mm	11.5%

*Average percentage calculated from single LRRs for each type of margins status.

at the margin in 3 or fewer low-power fields. The 5-year rates of local recurrence were 3%, 2%, 28%, and 9%, respectively [5, 6].

Park et al. have analyzed in 2000 the 8-year outcome of a series of 533 stage I or II breast cancers treated by BCS, of which 490 could be classified in one of the four margin status types: for patients with negative or close margins, LRR was 7%. Patients with extensively positive margins had an LRR of 27%, while patients with focally positive margins had an LRR of 14% [7]. In 1999 Peterson showed LRRs of 8%, 10%, and 17%, respectively, for negative, focally positive, and focally close (≤ 2 mm) margins from a series of consecutive 1021 stage I or II breast malignancies [8]. A strong correlation between local recurrence rates and margins status has been demonstrated in a large number of other studies based on follow-up after breast-conserving surgery plus local radiotherapy [9–14], but the adequacy of microscopic margins width remains controversial. Horiguchi has reported 7 local recurrences in a series of 217 breast cancers (3.2%) treated with BCS following a 50 Gy radiation therapy, while Karasawa reported in a retrospective analysis of 348 patients who underwent BCS an LRR of 1.7%. Both of these studies considered negative SM width of 5 mm, and Horiguchi identified the microscopic SM as an independent predictive factor for local recurrence in the conserved breast [9, 10].

In 2003 Perez studied BCS outcomes in 1037 patients with T1 and 308 patients with T2 breast cancer, with a cumulative LRR of 5.8% (78/1345) based on a threshold distance for negative/close margins equal to 3 mm, although margins status was not found to be a predictor of ipsilateral breast relapse. A higher LRR was rather noted in patients younger than 40 years with extensive intraductal component (EIC) [11]. Santiago et al. showed in 937 women with stage I or II breast cancer LRRs of 12.2% (78/639, excluded 298 patients in which the final status of margins was unknown), considering close SM ≤ 2 mm [12]. Another study by Karasawa et al. performed on a Japanese multicentre survey in 2005 demonstrated a crude LRR of 3.4% for patients with equal or less than 2 mm margins and an LRR of 6.3% in those with 2.1–5 mm margins [13]. Other authors, besides Gage and Park, have reported LRRs on a threshold distance for close margins ≤ 1 mm, such

TABLE 2: Most common features associated with positive surgical margins [20–23].

Predicting factors of margin status	
Presence of DCIS	$P < 0.0001$
Multifocal disease	$P = 0.0197$
Tumor size	$P < 0.0001$
Lobular histology	$P = 0.005$
Microcalcifications on mammography	$P < 0.0001$

as Kreike et al. who described in a series of 1024 patients (741 with known SM width) LRRs of 11.5% [14].

Houssami et al. reported in a meta-analysis of 21 retrospective studies that the presence of positive or close SM increases the odds of local recurrences relative to negative margins (OR 2.02, $P < 0.001$), but these odds are not associated with the margins width. Thus, there is not a statistically significant difference on LRR between a margin distance of 5 mm and 1 mm. However an evident association between the odds of local recurrences and the decreasing of threshold distances for negative margins was observed, confirming the influence of SM status on LRR [15].

3. What Influences Margins Status?

Preoperative predicting of the SM status has recently gained a key role in planning BCS, and some predictive factors of positive margins have been described (Table 2). According to Tartter et al., a preoperative diagnosis by fine needle aspiration, a small tumor size, and the absence of DCIS or the absence of an extensive intraductal carcinoma are all associated with a decreased risk of involved margins on surgical specimen [20]. In a study based on data collected from 1648 patients through a breast cancer screening program in Melbourne, Kurniawan has identified mammographic microcalcifications ($P < 0.0001$), presence of DCIS ($P < 0.0001$), high tumor grade, multifocal disease, and lobular histology ($P = 0.005$) as factors correlated with positive margins [21]. Reedijk et al. in a prospective study of 305 patients with nonpalpable breast lesions have reported that stereotactic versus sonographic localization ($P < 0.0001$), presence of DCIS, multifocal disease, and larger tumor size (>2 cm versus <1 cm, $P < 0.0001$) are independent predictors of positive margins in BCS [22]. Shin et al. have developed a nomogram for predicting positive margins based on data collected from 1,034 patients, identifying microcalcifications on mammography, grade of mammographic density, >0.5 cm difference in tumor size between MRI and US, DCIS, and presence of lobular components on preoperative biopsy as independent predictive factors of involved margins [23].

4. What about DCIS?

Ductal carcinoma in situ represents 25–30% of all diagnosed breast malignancies, and its treatment with BCS has increased over the past decades [24]. Since DCIS is frequently a multifocal disease with a difficult surgical evaluation of its limits, the adequacy of SM in DCIS has gained a crucial importance and its definition remains controversial. Silverstein et al. recommended in a retrospective study of 469 specimens of DCIS a margin width of minimum 10 mm if radiotherapy is not performed, but radiotherapy for margins width less than 1 mm can be considered mandatory [25]. Rudloff et al. reported in a retrospective study of 291 women with DCIS who underwent BCS 10-year actuarial LRRs of 28%, 21%, and 19% for SM <1 mm, 1–9 mm, and ≥10 mm, respectively, without radiotherapy; these LRRs were reduced by radiotherapy [26].

Vicini et al. studied in a series of 146 DCIS patients treated with BCS a 10-year actuarial rate of recurrence equal to 12.4% and identified margins of excision >5 mm or negative (>2 mm) on reexcision as factors of decreasing risk for local recurrence, while a total volume of excision <60 cm³ or a tumor size ≥0.7 cm was correlated with higher LRRs. These data suggested that the adequacy of DCIS removal should be based on margins status together with volume of resection and tumor size [27]. In a recent meta-analysis of 21 studies, for a total of 7564 patients affected by DCIS, Wang et al. have demonstrated a reduced risk of ipsilateral local recurrence if tumor resected with at least 10 mm of negative margin, compared with a margin of 2 mm [28]. Therefore, there seems to be noted a general agreement on the need for relatively large margins for DCIS, especially if adjuvant radiotherapy is not performed.

5. Oncoplastic Surgery

Oncoplastic surgery refers to a group of surgical techniques that combine primary tumor excision with plastic surgery techniques, and it allows to achieve good cosmetic outcomes also if wider excision is performed [29]. After resection of a breast cancer a correction of a small defect may be necessary, with basic techniques of local volume replacement, more complex reconstruction techniques and may be needed to correct larger defects [29]. A common oncoplastic technique, ideal for tumors adjacent but not attached to the nipple areolar complex, is the batwing mastopexy lumpectomy, in which two half-circle incisions are made with angled wings to each side of the areola, with subsequent excision of the lesion and advance of the superior breast tissue to close the defect [30].

Another common technique is lumpectomy with reduction mammoplasty, particularly useful for tumors in large and ptotic breasts. Of note, this technique requires a careful preoperative localization of the lesion, with an exact evaluation of its extent [31].

Oncoplastic surgery is linked with a double connection with the question of margins: in fact, it allows to obtain excision with wider margins, but on the other hand, it is often difficult to determine exactly the reexcision site if a positive margin is encountered on histopathological examination, due to the handling of breast tissue to correct volume defects. In these cases, completion mastectomy is often required [29].

Interestingly, Down et al. have recently reported, in a study of comparison between patients who underwent BCS alone with patients treated with BCS and oncoplastic surgery, wider clear margins (6.1 mm versus 14.3 mm), larger specimen volumes (112.3 cm³ versus 484.5 cm³), and a subsequent lower reexcision rate (28.9% versus 5.4%) with the oncoplastic approach, without increase in complication rates [32].

Also Losken et al. have recently highlighted the oncological advantage of the oncoplastic surgery, publishing a meta-analysis of comparison between 3165 patients treated by BCS with oncoplastic surgery and 5495 patients treated by BCS alone. The reported positive margins rate is significantly lower in the oncoplastic group (12% versus 21%), although it should be noted that the rate of completion mastectomy is more common with oncoplastic surgery [33].

6. Preoperative Localization Techniques

6.1. Carbon Marking. Carbon marking technique is based on injection of sterile charcoal powder diluted with saline solution into the site of a nonpalpable breast lesion after a preoperative sonographic or stereotactic localization. A charcoal trail is created from the lesion to the superficial layers of the breast, leaving a tattoo on the skin. The subsequent surgical excision of the tumor is guided by the presence of the carbon suspension, which is removed with the lesion [34]. Because of the stability of the charcoal powder, a delayed surgery after the localization procedure is possible; on the contrary, methylene blue has a fast dispersion in the tissue. A potential disadvantage of carbon marking is obstruction of needle tip due to precipitation of charcoal particles [35]; moreover, foreign-body giant-cell reactions mimicking malignancy have been reported after vacuum-assisted breast biopsy with carbon marking [36]. Rose et al. reported in a comparison study between carbon marking and wire-guided excision a close or involved margins rate of 18.9% (27/143) with the former technique [37].

6.2. Wire-Guided Technique. Wire-guided localization consists of positioning a needle or a flexible wire into or alongside a nonpalpable breast lesion under mammographic, sonographic, or CT guidance. The mammographic approach is based on measurements of distances between the lesion and the nipple (or other reference points) performed on the two projections of the mammogram. In this way an approximative estimate of the lesion localization is made by the radiologist on the patient, who is supine or seated, and the wire is placed anteroposteriorly or parallel to the chest wall. Subsequent mammograms are then obtained in order to reposition the wire more accurately, and a confirmatory mammogram is finally obtained [38]. The sonographic approach is performed with the patient in a supine position, with the aid of a 5 mHz or higher transducer, and the wire is positioned under direct visualization [38, 39]. The CT approach requires a preliminary positioning of a wire on the skin in order to have a reference for measuring the lesion localization on slices, and the wire is then introduced. Various types of wires have been developed, such as standard needle, spinal needle, or curved-end retractable wire [38]. Although wire-guided technique is a relatively simple and cost-effective method for nonpalpable breast lesions localization, some disadvantages have been reported, above all the eventuality of wire dislodgment, which could affect an accurate intraoperative finding of the lesion [40]. It should be also remembered that this technique requires a good compliance from the patient, who has to keep the wire in position all the time long before the surgery. Clear margins obtained with wire-guided excision are reported to be 70.8–87.4% [37, 41–43].

6.3. Clip Marker after a Stereotactic or Sonographic Vacuum-Assisted Breast Biopsy. Positioning a biopsy clip is necessary when an occult breast lesion detected by mammography (i.e., microcalcifications), by ultrasound, or by MRI is completely removed within a breast biopsy procedure. After a vacuum-assisted breast biopsy conducted under stereotactic or sonographic guidance, a clip marker may be placed through the biopsy probe into the biopsy cavity to permit an effective and accurate preoperative or intraoperative localization, or to facilitate a follow-up of the lesion, especially after a neoadjuvant chemotherapy which could lead to a nearly complete tumor regression, with no longer clear visibility on imaging [44]. The first type of biopsy clip introduced was the radiopaque metallic marker of titanium or stainless steel, developed for stereotactic procedures [45]. Metallic markers embedded with a bioresorbable material (collagen plug of bovine origin, polylactic acid, polyglycolic acid) later appeared on market; while the metallic core of titanium guarantees long-term visibility and radiopacity, the packing plug of collagen aids for hemostasis after the biopsy procedure, reduces the risk of clip displacement by its expanding in the biopsy cavity, and allows an easy identification of the clip on ultrasound until its reabsorption in 6–8 weeks [46, 47]. Both of these types of clips may be used preoperatively for localization of the tumor by mammography or ultrasound, with the possibility of positioning a wire or marking the lesion's projections on the skin. An intraoperative localization without a wire is also possible, either with a radiography of the surgical specimen in order to assess the presence of the clip or by its direct visibility on ultrasound during the resection [44–47]. Clear margins obtained with this method are reported in 90–92% of cases [48, 49].

6.4. Radio-Guided Occult Lesion Localization (ROLL). Luini et al. described in 1998 the ROLL technique, which consists of a preoperative injection of particles of colloidal human serum albumin labeled with radioactive technetium (^{99m}Tc) into the tumor under sonographic or mammographic guidance. A scintigraphy scan of the breast is then obtained to check the correct inoculation of the tracer by comparison between its position and the localization of the lesion on mammograms. During the surgery, the tumor can be detected by a gamma probe, directly used by the surgeon to verify the adequacy of excision [50]. In addition, another radioactive tracer can be injected near to the tumor to be drained in the sentinel node, which can be easily identified by the gamma probe and then biopsied during the excision of the primary tumor. This technique was named "sentinel node and occult lesion localization" (SNOLL), and it requires two scintigraphy scans [51]. A potential complication of this procedure is the widespread dispersal of the isotope by accidental intraductal injection, which may cause a failure in identification of the lesion; therefore, this method has to be performed by an experienced breast surgeon [52]. Another concern with ROLL regards its cost: Medina-Franco et al. reported a total cost of $209 (USD) per each procedure versus $132 (USD) with wire-guided excision [53]. Negative margins reported with ROLL range from 75 to 93.5% in some studies [41–43, 51].

7. Margin Assessment Techniques

7.1. Ultrasound-Guided Excision. Many breast lesions are clearly visible on ultrasound (US), and thus an intraoperative sonographic localization with a high frequency (7.5 mHz) probe may be performed with a subsequent immediate positioning of a wire, injection of dye, marking on skin, or directly calibrating the excision. This procedure therefore avoids the need of a preoperative localization. An ultrasound scanning of the surgical specimen can also be done to assess the presence of the lesion and the adequacy of SM [54, 55]. However, it must be remembered that ductal carcinoma in situ rarely has a clear visibility on US [56], and since it represents an increasing number of breast malignancies, some methods for improving its visibility on ultrasound have been developed. The hematoma-directed US-guided technique consists of obtaining from the patient 2–5 mL of blood which is left to clot, and then this blood in injected through a needle near to the lesion or into the biopsy cavity if previously performed. This iatrogenically induced hematoma is visible on a 7.5 mHz probe during the surgery [57, 58]. Another technique used to enhance US visibility is the positioning of a titanium embedded with collagen clip after a breast biopsy. Krekel et al. have showed in a study on 201 excisions for nonpalpable invasive breast cancer that negative margins with US-guided lumpectomy are obtained in 89–96.2% of cases [42, 59].

A recent multicentre randomized trial named cosmetic outcome of the breast after lumpectomy treatment (COBALT) has investigated how US-guided excision of palpable breast lesions can influence the quality of resection, with negative margins and smaller volumes of resection reported in 97% of patients [60]. Subsequently these patients could avoid a reexcision, or a boost of radiotherapy, with a reduced psychological stress and a better cosmesis. The rationale for this better outcome is that sonography allows to visualize directly location and margins of the tumor, while preoperative imaging with mammography or magnetic resonance imaging is obtained with the patient being in a different position compared to that in the operating theatre [60].

7.2. Frozen Sections and Imprint Cytology. Frozen section analysis is performed with freezing and sectioning the surgical specimen with subsequent fixation and staining in order to have an extemporaneous assessment of margins; it takes about 30 minutes. Although this technique is extensively used by many surgeons to avoid the need of a postponed reexcision, some pitfalls have been reported, such as the occurrence of artifacts due to the freezing and thawing of adipose tissue in the specimen [61]. A different intraoperative method for margins evaluation is imprint cytology ("touch prep"), which consists of pressing each of the 6 faces of the specimen on 6 different slides so that any malignant cell on an involved margin is theoretically present on the cytology of the respective slide, because of the tendency of tumor cells to adhere on glass compared to adipocytes [61, 62]. Confusion on cytology interpretation may exist for specimens with irregular surfaces or presence of atypical cells, although some immunofluorescence stains (i.e., anti-MUC-1 or anti-E-cadherin antibodies) may aid the pathologist in identifying cancer cells on slides [63]. With frozen section analysis and imprint cytology, adequate SM is achieved in 89–91% of cases [61].

7.3. Cavity Shave Margins. Excision of cavity shave margins consists of resection of breast tissue from all 6 margins (anterior, posterior, superior, inferior, medial, and lateral) after the excision of the primary specimen, in the same procedure. This approach allows to precisely assess which margin is involved in order to calibrate the resection of the tumor. Kobbermann et al. have demonstrated with this technique 91.3% of negative or close margin if routinely performed. Interestingly, of the patients requiring reexcision of the tumor, no significant difference has been noted in terms of surgical localization technique [64]. Bolger et al. have recently reported with cavity shave margins a reexcision rate of 25%, compared with 34% if no margins assessment is carried out. Thus, cavity shave margins reduced significantly the likelihood of having residual disease ($P = 0.02$). Of note, close margins (<2 mm) are correlated with the presence of residual disease ($P = 0.01$) [65]. Marudanayagam et al. showed negative margins in 94.4% of 394 patients who underwent lumpectomy plus cavity shave margins, compared to 87.5% of 392 patients with lumpectomy only [66]. Although this technique is cost effective and it significantly reduces the rate of positive margins, it may lengthen the operating time, but it is not correlated with a worse cosmetic outcome due to larger final volumes of resection [67].

8. Discussion

The adequacy of SM in BCS still remains a crucial point of controversy, ranging from 10 mm for DCIS to 1–5 mm for invasive cancers [15, 25–28]. Singletary et al. stated in a review published in 2002 that it is not clear how much SM width influences LRR, although it is unacceptable to have involved margins, because the presence of tumor cells directly at the cut edge of the specimen may not be overcome merely by adjuvant therapy [1]. Then, the importance of achieving clear margins on local recurrence rate has been discussed in relation to other clinical factors correlated with the prognosis, such as the biological behaviour of the tumor (i.e., ER+/ER– or HER2) [18, 19, 68]. The NSABP B-14 trial has demonstrated an improved local control in node-negative, ER positive breast cancer patients receiving tamoxifen, with a 10-year LRR of 4.3% compared to 14.7% if tamoxifen was not administered [18]. The NSABP B-13 trial has shown a reduction of LRR from 13.4% to 2.6% in patients with node-negative, ER negative breast cancer if chemotherapy administered [19]. Thus, there seems to be noted a recent trend of reconsideration of the role of surgery in the local control of the malignancy, with a lesser interest in margins width [16, 17]. This more balanced implementation of systemic therapy and surgery is expanding also in the therapeutic strategy for positive sentinel node, and some authors are proposing not to perform the axillary dissection after the detection of micrometastases in the sentinel node [69, 70].

In 2012, Morrow et al. asserted that margins width has no influence on LRR, since systemic therapies reduce both risks of distant metastases and of local recurrence, concluding that LRR could be more correlated with the biological features of the tumor. However, it is also highlighted that adequacy of surgical resection depends on clinical judgement, so that a wider excision could be recommended, for example, in a young woman with an extensive DCIS [16]. Of note, Jatoi has responded that, while systemic therapies may improve control on early local recurrences, late recurrences are more frequent among patients treated with BCS than those treated with mastectomy [71, 72]. Finally, while there is not statistical significance in a margin of 2 mm versus a margin of 5 mm for invasive breast cancer [15], the role of margins width for DCIS, which represents 25–30% of all diagnosed breast malignancies, remains even less clear [28]. In the 13th St. Gallen International Breast Cancer Conference 2013, it was stated that systemic therapy and excellent radiation therapy techniques could make margins width less important, but the best recommendation remains a case-by-case judgement based on clinical and biological features of the tumor [73]. Moreover, a recent position statement by the American Society of Breast Surgeons on breast cancer lumpectomy margins suggests a reexcision in the case of ink positive margins but a case-by-case decision if close (<1 mm) or focally positive margin, evaluating proper adjuvant radiotherapy and systemic therapies [74].

However, since achieving negative margins (independently of the definition of adequate margins width) remains a key point of breast cancer surgery, a precise localization of the lesion is of particular importance, especially for nonpalpable breast lesions or in case of oncoplastic approach (Table 3). Certainly, it should be highlighted that obtaining negative margins depends not only on localization method or margin assessment technique, but also on extent of the lesion, on the surgical procedure, and on the pathological handling of the specimen.

An easy and cost-effective method is carbon marking: Rose et al. reported in a comparison study a close or involved margins rate of 18.9% (27/143) and 2 (0.9%) missed

TABLE 3: Rates of adequate margins and main disadvantages for each technique.

Technique	Rate of adequate margins	Disadvantages
Carbon marking	81.1%	Possible foreign-body reactions mimicking malignancy on follow up; obstruction of needle tip due to charcoal precipitation.
Wire-guided	70.8–87.4%	Wire dislodgment; vasovagal episodes; pneumothorax.
ROLL	75–93.5%	Possible widespread dispersal of the tracer by accidental intraductal injection; nuclear medicine department required; for experienced surgeons; expensive.
Clip marker	90–92%	Clip migration.
US-guided	89–97%	DCIS rarely visible on US if not marked with a clip or hematoma.
Cavity shave	91.3–94.4%	Long operative times.
Imprint cytology and frozen section analysis	89–91%	Sensibility equal to 72–83%; possible difficult interpretation by pathologist due to presence of irregular specimen's surfaces or atypical cells; long operative times.

lesions with carbon marking, while positive margins were encountered in 29.2% (21/72) with 3 (1%) missed lesions with wire-guided localization. These differences have been nonstatistically significant, but carbon marking resulted to be less expensive than wire-guided technique [37]. Wire-guided localization is a widely used and relatively simple technique, but some complications may be encountered, such as wire dislodgment, vasovagal episodes, or pneumothorax, and it requires a good compliance from the patient who has to keep in position the wire all the time long before the surgery. Moreover clear margins obtained with wire-guided excision are reported to be 70.8–87.4%, a lower percentage in comparison with those reported with other methods like ROLL or ultrasound-guided in many systematic reviews [37, 41–43, 53].

Negative margins reported with ROLL range from 75 to 93.5% in some studies [41–43, 51], but a Nuclear Medicine Department is required. Another concern with ROLL is the eventuality of a dispersal of the radioactive tracer causing a failure in the identification of the lesion, and thus an experienced surgeon is required [52]. Clip placement after a vacuum-assisted breast biopsy appears to be effective, especially if the intraoperative localization is performed under sonographic guidance: Nurko et al. have reported clear margins in 90% (37/41) of cases [48]. A US-visible clip marker may be positioned after breast biopsies performed under sonographic or stereotactic guidance, with positive margins encountered in 8% of cases [49]. A disadvantage in clip markers is their possible dislodgment, but the average distance between the target lesion and the clip has been found to be <10 mm in 71.3% of cases [44], with an average distance of 1.1 mm if the biopsy has been performed on US [75]. Krekel et al. have shown in a study on 201 excisions for nonpalpable invasive breast cancer negative margins in 96.2% with the aid of US-guided lumpectomy [42], while Rahusen has reported clear SM in 89% of cases with the same technique [59].

Esbona et al. have demonstrated, in a systematic review on the effectiveness of intraoperative imprint cytology (IC) and frozen section analysis (FSA) versus permanent histopathology (PH), a reexcision rate of 35%, 11% and 10% with PH, IC and FSA, respectively. The pooled sensibility resulted to be 72% for IC and 83% for FSA, with a pooled specificity of 97% and 95% for IC and FSA. An intraoperative assessment permits an immediate correction of the adequacy of excision but with an elongation of the surgery time equal to 13–27 minutes [61].

9. Conclusion

The effectiveness of breast-conserving therapy for treatment of early stage invasive breast malignancies has been established. Surely the adequacy of margins is a crucial issue for adjusting the volume of excision, for avoiding unnecessary resection of healthy breast parenchyma, and for a good cosmetic outcome. Thus the surgical accuracy, together with improved systemic therapy and better radiation techniques, avoids reexcisions which generally are poorly tolerated by the patients. From the literature review, no single technique proved to be better among the various ones described for achieving adequate SM, because all of them have some advantages and disadvantages, although many reviews have stated the wire-guided excision to be probably the less effective method in obtaining clear margins. According to our opinion, each surgeon should adopt his most congenial localization or margin assessment technique, based on the senologic equipe experience and on available skills and technologies. Moreover, an association of two or more methods could result in a decrease in rates of involved margins. Certainly both margins status and the biological behaviour of the malignancy contribute to local recurrence rate, and future studies are needed to ascertain the relevance of both factors.

References

[1] S. E. Singletary, "Surgical margins in patients with early-stage breast cancer treated with breast conservation therapy," *American Journal of Surgery*, vol. 184, no. 5, pp. 383–393, 2002.

[2] E. R. Fisher, S. Anderson, C. Redmond, and B. Fisher, "Ipsilaterial breast tumor recurrence and survival following lumpectomy and irradiation: pathological findings from NSABP protocol B-06," *Seminars in Surgical Oncology*, vol. 8, no. 3, pp. 161–166, 1992.

[3] B. Fisher, S. Anderson, J. Bryant et al., "Twenty-year follow-up of a randomized trial comparing total mastectomy, lumpectomy, and lumpectomy plus irradiation for the treatment of invasive breast cancer," *The New England Journal of Medicine*, vol. 347, no. 16, pp. 1233–1241, 2002.

[4] U. Veronesi, N. Cascinelli, L. Mariani et al., "Twenty-year follow-up of a randomized study comparing breast-conserving surgery with radical mastectomy for early breast cancer," *The New England Journal of Medicine*, vol. 347, no. 16, pp. 1227–1232, 2002.

[5] I. Gage, S. J. Schnitt, A. J. Nixon et al., "Pathologic margin involvement and the risk of recurrence in patients treated with breast-conserving therapy," *Cancer*, vol. 9, pp. 1921–1928, 1996.

[6] S. J. Schnitt, A. Abner, R. Gelman et al., "The relationship between microscopic margins of resection and the risk of local recurrence in patients with breast cancer treated with breast-conserving surgery and radiation therapy," *Cancer*, vol. 74, pp. 1746–1751, 1994.

[7] C. C. Park, M. Mitsumori, A. Nixon et al., "Outcome at 8 years after breast-conserving surgery and radiation therapy for invasive breast cancer: influence of margin status and systemic therapy on local recurrence," *Journal of Clinical Oncology*, vol. 18, no. 8, pp. 1668–1675, 2000.

[8] M. E. Peterson, D. J. Schultz, C. Reynolds, and L. J. Solin, "Outcomes in breast cancer patients relative to margin status after treatment with breast-conserving surgery and radiation therapy: the University of Pennsylvania experience," *International Journal of Radiation Oncology Biology Physics*, vol. 43, no. 5, pp. 1029–1035, 1999.

[9] J. Horiguchi, Y. Koibuchi, H. Takei et al., "Breast-conserving surgery following radiation therapy of 50 Gy in stages I and II carcinoma of the breast: the experience at one institute in Japan," *Oncology Reports*, vol. 9, no. 5, pp. 1053–1057, 2002.

[10] K. Karasawa, T. Obara, T. Shimizu et al., "Outcome of breast-conserving therapy in the Tokyo women's medical university breast cancer society experience," *Breast Cancer*, vol. 10, no. 4, pp. 341–348, 2003.

[11] C. A. Perez, "Conservation therapy in T1-T2 breast cancer: past, current issues, and future challenges and opportunities," *Cancer Journal*, vol. 9, no. 6, pp. 442–453, 2003.

[12] R. J. Santiago, L. Wu, E. Harris et al., "Fifteen-year results of breast-conserving surgery and definitive irradiation for Stage I and II breast carcinoma: the University of Pennsylvania experience," *International Journal of Radiation Oncology Biology Physics*, vol. 58, no. 1, pp. 233–240, 2004.

[13] K. Karasawa, M. Mitsumori, C. Yamauchi et al., "Treatment outcome of breast-conserving therapy in patients with positive or close resection margins: Japanese muiti institute survey for radiation dose effect," *Breast Cancer*, vol. 12, no. 2, pp. 91–98, 2005.

[14] B. Kreike, A. A. M. Hart, T. van de Velde et al., "Continuing risk of ipsilateral breast relapse after breast-conserving therapy at long-term follow-up," *International Journal of Radiation Oncology Biology Physics*, vol. 71, no. 4, pp. 1014–1021, 2008.

[15] N. Houssami, P. Macaskill, M. L. Marinovich et al., "Meta-analysis of the impact of surgical margins on local recurrence in women with early-stage invasive breast cancer treated with breast-conserving therapy," *European Journal of Cancer*, vol. 46, no. 18, pp. 3219–3232, 2010.

[16] M. Morrow, J. R. Harris, and S. J. Schnitt, "Surgical margins in lumpectomy for breast cancer—bigger is not better," *The New England Journal of Medicine*, vol. 367, pp. 79–82, 2012.

[17] J. M. Dixon and N. Houssami, "Bigger margins are not better in breast conserving surgery," *British Medical Journal*, vol. 345, Article ID e5855, 2012.

[18] B. Fisher, J. Dignam, J. Bryant et al., "Five versus more than five years of tamoxifen therapy for breast cancer patients with negative lymph nodes and estrogen receptor-positive tumors," *Journal of the National Cancer Institute*, vol. 88, no. 21, pp. 1529–1542, 1996.

[19] B. Fisher, J. Dignam, E. P. Mamounas et al., "Sequential methotrexate and fluorouracil for the treatment of node-negative breast cancer patients with estrogen receptor-negative tumors: eight-year results from National Surgical Adjuvant Breast and Bowel Project (NSABP) B-13 and first report of findings from NSABP B-19 comparing methotrexate and fluorouracil with conventional cyclophosphamide, methotrexate and fluorouracil," *Journal of Clinical Oncology*, vol. 14, pp. 1982–1992, 1996.

[20] P. I. Tartter, I. J. Bleiweiss, and S. Levchenko, "Factors associated with clear biopsy margins and clear reexcision margins in breast cancer specimens from candidates for breast conservation," *Journal of the American College of Surgeons*, vol. 185, no. 3, pp. 268–273, 1997.

[21] E. D. Kurniawan, M. H. Wong, I. Windle et al., "Predictors of surgical margin status in breast-conserving surgery within a breast screening program," *Annals of Surgical Oncology*, vol. 15, no. 9, pp. 2542–2549, 2008.

[22] M. Reedijk, N. Hodgson, G. Gohla et al., "A prospective study of tumor and technical factors associated with positive margins in breast-conservation therapy for nonpalpable malignancy," *The American Journal of Surgery*, vol. 204, pp. 263–268, 2012.

[23] H. C. Shin, W. Han, H. G. Moon et al., "Nomogram for predicting positive resection margins after breast-conserving surgery," *Breast Cancer Research and Treatment*, vol. 134, pp. 1115–1123, 2012.

[24] B. Cady, M. D. Stone, J. G. Schuler, R. Thakur, M. A. Wanner, and P. T. Lavin, "The new era in breast cancer: invasion, size, and nodal involvement dramatically decreasing as a result of mammographic screening," *Archives of Surgery*, vol. 131, no. 3, pp. 301–308, 1996.

[25] M. J. Silverstein, M. D. Lagios, S. Groshen et al., "The influence of margin width on local control of ductal carcinoma in situ of the breast," *The New England Journal of Medicine*, vol. 340, no. 19, pp. 1455–1461, 1999.

[26] U. Rudloff, E. Brogi, A. S. Reiner et al., "The influence of margin width and volume of disease near margin on benefit of radiation therapy for women with DCIS treated with breast-conserving therapy," *Annals of Surgery*, vol. 251, no. 4, pp. 583–591, 2010.

[27] F. A. Vicini, L. L. Kestin, N. S. Goldstein, K. L. Baglan, J. E. Pettinga, and A. A. Martinez, "Relationship between excision volume, margin status, and tumor size with the development of local recurrence in patients with ductal carcinoma-in-situ

treated with breast-conserving therapy," *Journal of Surgical Oncology*, vol. 76, no. 4, pp. 245–254, 2001.

[28] S.-Y. Wang, H. Chu, T. Shamliyan et al., "Network meta-analysis of margin threshold for women with ductal carcinoma in situ," *Journal of the National Cancer Institute*, vol. 104, no. 7, pp. 507–516, 2012.

[29] J. A. Margenthaler, "Optimizing conservative breast surgery," *Journal of Surgical Oncology*, vol. 103, no. 4, pp. 306–312, 2011.

[30] B. O. Anderson, R. Masetti, and M. J. Silverstein, "Oncoplastic approaches to partial mastectomy: an overview of volume-displacement techniques," *Lancet Oncology*, vol. 6, no. 3, pp. 145–157, 2005.

[31] S. L. Spear, C. V. Pelletiere, A. J. Wolfe, T. N. Tsangaris, and M. F. Pennanen, "Experience with reduction mammaplasty combined with breast conservation therapy in the treatment of breast cancer," *Plastic and Reconstructive Surgery*, vol. 111, no. 3, pp. 1102–1109, 2003.

[32] S. K. Down, P. K. Jha, A. Burger, and M. I. Hussien, "Oncological advantages of oncoplastic breast-conserving surgery in treatment of early breast cancer," *Breast Journal*, vol. 19, pp. 56–63, 2013.

[33] A. Losken, C. S. Dugal, T. M. Styblo, and G. W. Carlson, "A meta-analysis comparing breast conservation therapy alone to the oncoplastic technique," *Annals of Plastic Surgery*, 2013.

[34] G. Canavese, A. Catturich, C. Vecchio et al., "Pre-operative localization of non-palpable lesions in breast cancer by charcoal suspension," *European Journal of Surgical Oncology*, vol. 21, no. 1, pp. 47–49, 1995.

[35] K. Ko, B.-K. Han, M. J. Kyung et al., "The value of ultrasound-guided tattooing localization of nonpalpable breast lesions," *Korean Journal of Radiology*, vol. 8, no. 4, pp. 295–301, 2007.

[36] M. L. Ruiz-Delgado, J. A. Lòpez-Ruiz, and A. Sàiz-Lòpez, "Abnormal mammography and sonography associated with foreign-body giant-cell reaction after stereotactic vacuum-assisted breast biopsy with carbon marking," *Acta Radiologica*, vol. 49, no. 10, pp. 1112–1118, 2008.

[37] A. Rose, J. P. Collins, P. Neerhut, C. V. Bishop, and G. B. Mann, "Carbon localisation of impalpable breast lesions," *Breast*, vol. 12, no. 4, pp. 264–269, 2003.

[38] D. B. Kopans and C. A. Swann, "Preoperative imaging-guided needle placement and localization of clinically occult breast lesions," *American Journal of Roentgenology*, vol. 152, no. 1, pp. 1–9, 1989.

[39] D. B. Kopans, J. E. Meyer, K. K. Lindfors, and S. S. Bucchianeri, "Breast sonography to guide cyst aspiration and wire localization of occult solid lesions," *American Journal of Roentgenology*, vol. 143, no. 3, pp. 489–492, 1984.

[40] D. B. Kopans, "Migration of breast biopsy localization wire," *American Journal of Roentgenology*, vol. 151, no. 3, pp. 614–615, 1988.

[41] M. S. Sajid, U. Parampalli, Z. Haider, and R. Bonomi, "Comparison of radioguided occult lesion localization (ROLL) and wire localization for non-palpable breast cancers: a meta-analysis," *Journal of Surgical Oncology*, 2011.

[42] N. M. A. Krekel, B. M. Zonderhuis, H. B. A. C. Stockmann et al., "A comparison of three methods for nonpalpable breast cancer excision," *European Journal of Surgical Oncology*, vol. 37, no. 2, pp. 109–115, 2011.

[43] P. L. Giacalone, A. Bourdon, P. D. Trinh et al., "Radioguided occult lesion localization plus sentinel node biopsy (SNOLL) versus wire-guided localization plus sentinel node detection: a

case control study of 129 unifocal pure invasive non-palpable breast cancers," *European Journal of Surgical Oncology*, vol. 38, no. 3, pp. 222–229, 2012.

[44] I. Thomassin-Naggara, L. Lalonde, J. David, E. Darai, S. Uzan, and I. Trop, "A plea for the biopsy marker: how, why and why not clipping after breast biopsy?" *Breast Cancer Research and Treatment*, vol. 132, pp. 881–893, 2012.

[45] F. R. Margolin, L. Kaufman, S. R. Denny, R. P. Jacobs, and J. D. Schrumpf, "Metallic marker placement after stereotactic core biopsy of breast calcifications: comparison of two clips and deployment techniques," *American Journal of Roentgenology*, vol. 181, no. 6, pp. 1685–1690, 2003.

[46] F. R. Margolin, R. P. Jacobs, S. R. Denny, and J. D. Schrumpf, "Clip placement after sonographically guided percutaneous breast biopsy," *Breast Journal*, vol. 9, no. 3, pp. 226–230, 2003.

[47] P. R. Eby, K. E. Calhoun, B. F. Kurland et al., "Preoperative and intraoperative sonographic visibility of collagen-based breast biopsy marker clips," *Academic Radiology*, vol. 17, no. 3, pp. 340–347, 2010.

[48] J. Nurko, A. T. Mancino, E. Whitacre, and M. J. Edwards, "Surgical benefits conveyed by biopsy site marking system using ultrasound localization," *American Journal of Surgery*, vol. 190, no. 4, pp. 618–622, 2005.

[49] M. A. Gittleman, "Single-step ultrasound localization of breast lesions and lumpectomy procedure," *American Journal of Surgery*, vol. 186, no. 4, pp. 386–390, 2003.

[50] A. Luini, S. Zurrida, V. Galimberti, and G. Paganelli, "Radioguided surgery of occult breast lesions," *European Journal of Cancer*, vol. 34, no. 1, pp. 204–205, 1998.

[51] S. Monti, V. Galimberti, G. Trifiro et al., "Occult breast lesion localization plus sentinel node biopsy (SNOLL): experience with 959 patients at the European Institute of Oncology," *Annals of Surgical Oncology*, vol. 14, no. 10, pp. 2928–2931, 2007.

[52] R. S. Rampaul, R. D. MacMillan, and A. J. Evans, "Intraductal injection of the breast: a potential pitfall radioisotope occult lesion localization," *British Journal of Radiology*, vol. 76, no. 906, pp. 425–426, 2003.

[53] H. Medina-Franco, L. Abarca-Pérez, M. N. García-Alvarez, J. L. Ulloa-Gómez, C. Romero-Trejo, and J. Sepúlveda-Méndez, "Radioguided occult lesion localization (ROLL) versus wire-guided lumpectomy for non-palpable breast lesions: a randomized prospective evaluation," *Journal of Surgical Oncology*, vol. 97, no. 2, pp. 108–111, 2008.

[54] B. D. Fornage, M. I. Ross, S. E. Singletary, and D. D. Paulus, "Localization of impalpable breast masses: value of sonography in the operating room and scanning of excised specimens," *American Journal of Roentgenology*, vol. 163, no. 3, pp. 569–573, 1994.

[55] I. C. Bennett, J. Greenslade, and H. Chiam, "Intraoperative ultrasound-guided excision of nonpalpable breast lesions," *World Journal of Surgery*, vol. 29, no. 3, pp. 369–374, 2005.

[56] A. J. Potterton, D. J. Peakman, and J. R. Young, "Ultrasound demonstration of small breast cancers detected by mammographic screening," *Clinical Radiology*, vol. 49, no. 11, pp. 808–813, 1994.

[57] L. F. Smith, R. Henry-Tillman, S. Harms et al., "Hematoma-directed ultrasound-guided breast biopsy," *Annals of Surgery*, vol. 233, no. 5, pp. 669–675, 2001.

[58] M. Thompson, R. Henry-Tillman, A. Margulies et al., "Hematoma-directed ultrasound-guided (HUG) breast lumpectomy," *Annals of Surgical Oncology*, vol. 14, no. 1, pp. 148–156, 2007.

[59] F. D. Rahusen, A. H. Taets van Amerongen, P. J. van Diest, P. J. Borgstein, R. P. Bleichrodt, and S. Meijer, "Ultrasound-guided lumpectomy of nonpalpable breast cancers: a feasibility study looking at the accuracy of obtained margins," *Journal of Surgical Oncology*, vol. 72, pp. 72–76, 1999.

[60] N. M. Krekel, M. H. Haloua, A. M. L. Cardozo et al., "Intraoperative ultrasound guidance for palpable breast cancer excision (COBALT trial): a multicentre, randomised controlled trial," *The Lancet Oncology*, vol. 14, pp. 48–54, 2013.

[61] K. Esbona, Z. Li, and L. G. Wilke, "Intraoperative imprint citology and frozen section pathology for margin assessment in breast conservation surgery: a systematic review," *Annals of Surgical Oncology*, vol. 19, no. 10, pp. 3236–3245.

[62] C. E. Cox, M. Hyacinthe, R. J. Gonzalez et al., "Cytologic evaluation of lumpectomy margins in patients with ductal carcinoma in situ: clinical outcome," *Annals of Surgical Oncology*, vol. 4, no. 8, pp. 644–649, 1997.

[63] S. L. Blair, J. Wang-Rodriguez, M. J. Cortes-Mateos et al., "Enhanced touch preps improve the ease of interpretation of intraoperative breast cancer margins," *American Surgeon*, vol. 73, no. 10, pp. 973–976, 2007.

[64] A. Kobbermann, A. Unzeitig, X.-J. Xie et al., "Impact of routine cavity shave margins on breast cancer re-excision rates," *Annals of Surgical Oncology*, vol. 18, no. 5, pp. 1349–1355, 2011.

[65] J. C. Bolger, J. G. Solon, S. A. Khan, A. D. Hill, and C. P. Power, "A comparison of intra-operative margin management techniques in breast-conserving surgery: a standardised approach reduces the likelihood of residual disease without increasing operative time," *Breast Cancer*, 2013.

[66] R. Marudanayagam, R. Singhal, B. Tanchel, B. O'Connor, B. Balasubramanian, and I. Paterson, "Effect of cavity shaving on reoperation rate following breast-conserving surgery," *Breast Journal*, vol. 14, no. 6, pp. 570–573, 2008.

[67] J. Mook, R. Klein, A. Kobbermann et al., "Volume of excision and cosmesis with routine cavity shave margins technique," *Annals of Surgical Oncology*, vol. 19, pp. 886–891, 2012.

[68] E. H. Romond, E. A. Perez, J. Bryant et al., "Trastuzumab plus adjuvant chemotherapy for operable HER2-positive breast cancer," *The New England Journal of Medicine*, vol. 353, no. 16, pp. 1673–1684, 2005.

[69] A. E. Giuliano, L. McCall, P. Beitsch et al., "Locoregional recurrence after sentinel lymph node dissection with or without axillary dissection in patients with sentinel lymph node metastases: The American college of surgeons oncology group z0011 randomized trial," *Annals of Surgery*, vol. 252, no. 3, pp. 426–432, 2010.

[70] V. Galimberti, E. Botteri, C. Chifu et al., "Can we avoid axillary dissection in the micrometastatic sentinel node in breast cancer?" *Breast Cancer Research and Treatment*, vol. 131, no. 3, pp. 819–825, 2012.

[71] I. Jatoi, "Surgical margins in lumpectomy for breast cancer," *The New England Journal of Medicine*, vol. 367, pp. 1269–1270, 2012.

[72] R. Arriagada, M. G. Lê, J.-M. Guinebretière, A. Dunant, F. Rochard, and T. Tursz, "Late local recurrences in a randomised trial comparing conservative treatment with total mastectomy in early breast cancer patients," *Annals of Oncology*, vol. 14, no. 11, pp. 1617–1622, 2003.

[73] G. Curigliano, C. Criscitiello, F. Andrè, M. Colleoni, and A. Di Leo, "Highlights from the 13th St Gallen International Breast Cancer Conference 2013. Access to innovation for patients with breast cancer: how to speed it up?" *Ecancermedicalscience*, vol. 7, article 299, 2013.

[74] The American Society of Breast Surgeons, "Position statement on breast cancer lumpectomy margins," 2013, https://www.breastsurgeons.org/statements/PDF_Statements/Lumpectomy_Margins.pdf.

[75] S. W. Phillips, H. Gabriel, C. E. Comstock, and L. A. Venta, "Sonographically guided metallic clip placement after core needle biopsy of the breast," *American Journal of Roentgenology*, vol. 175, no. 5, pp. 1353–1355, 2000.

13

Optimizing Surgical Margins in Breast Conservation

Preya Ananthakrishnan,[1] Fatih Levent Balci,[1] and Joseph P. Crowe[2]

[1] *Breast Surgery Division, Department of Surgery, Columbia University College of Physicians and Surgeons, New York, NY 10032, USA*
[2] *Department of General Surgery, Cleveland Clinic Foundation, Cleveland, OH 44195, USA*

Correspondence should be addressed to Preya Ananthakrishnan, pa2325@columbia.edu

Academic Editor: Eisuke Fukuma

Adequate surgical margins in breast-conserving surgery for breast cancer have traditionally been viewed as a predictor of local recurrence rates. There is still no consensus on what constitutes an adequate surgical margin, however it is clear that there is a trade-off between widely clear margins and acceptable cosmesis. Preoperative approaches to plan extent of resection with appropriate margins (in the setting of surgery first as well as after neoadjuvant chemotherapy,) include mammography, US, and MRI. Improvements have been made in preoperative lesion localization strategies for surgery, as well as intraoperative specimen assessment, in order to ensure complete removal of imaging findings and facilitate margin clearance. Intraoperative strategies to accurately assess tumor and cavity margins include cavity shave techniques, as well as novel technologies for margin probes. Ablative techniques, including radiofrequency ablation as well as intraoperative radiation, may be used to extend tumor-free margins without resecting additional tissue. Oncoplastic techniques allow for wider resections while maintaining cosmesis and have acceptable local recurrence rates, however often involve surgery on the contralateral breast. As systemic therapy for breast cancer continues to improve, it is unclear what the importance of surgical margins on local control rates will be in the future.

1. Introduction

Breast-conservation therapy (BCT), including lumpectomy and sentinel lymph node biopsy followed by radiation therapy, is the treatment of choice for women with early stage breast cancer. Randomized trials have shown that overall survival of women undergoing BCT is equivalent to mastectomy [1, 2]. The goal of lumpectomy is to completely excise the tumor with negative margins while maintaining acceptable cosmesis. Rates of margin positivity at initial lumpectomy have been reported ranging from 15% to 47% [3–6]. Positive margins are usually addressed with surgical reexcision, since the risk of local recurrence associated with a positive margin is approximately 2 to 3 times that compared with a negative margin [7]. Reexcision can include reoperative lumpectomy or possibly mastectomy. This additional surgical reoperative procedure can result in increased psychological trauma to the patient, delay of adjuvant therapy, worsened cosmesis, and increased cost [7].

It is well accepted that complete removal of tumor is necessary, however, there is aconsiderable debate regarding what margin of normal tissue surrounding the tumor constitutes a negative margin. Definitions range from no ink on tumor surface (NSABP B-06) to 1 cm or more [8]. Blair et al. sent a survey to nearly 1000 breast cancer surgeons, and found that 15% defined a negative margin as no tumor on inked margin, 21% accepted a 1 mm margin, 50% accepted a 2 mm margin, 12% accepted a 5 mm margin, and 3% accepted a 1 cm margin [9]. A meta-analysis by Wang et al. found that wider margins minimize the risk of ipsilateral local recurrence, with lowest recurrence rates achieved with a negative margin larger than 10 mm rather than 2 mm. This finding was independent of whether or not the patient received radiation [10].

In another meta-analysis of 21 retrospective studies which included 14,571 patients, Houssami et al. demonstrated an odds ratio for local recurrence of 2.42 ($P < 0.001$) with positive margins. This meta-analysis did not identify a statistically significant difference in local recurrence associated with margin widths of more than 1 mm, more than 2 mm, or more than 5 mm after adjustment for a radiation boost and endocrine therapy [11]. This suggests that a 2 or 5 mm margin is not necessarily better than a 1 mm margin.

When considering optimal margin width, it is useful to remember that a "negative" margin does not indicate the absence of residual unresected tumor in the breast [12]. It simply suggests that the residual tumor burden is probably low enough to be controlled with radiotherapy. Even the widest margins resulting from mastectomy do not eliminate risk of local recurrence. This indicates that residual disease burden is not totally eliminated by local surgery and that tumor biology, radiation therapy, and systemic therapy may play an important role in controlling local recurrence [13].

In further defining this idea of residual disease burden, Margenthaler et al. have proposed calculating a "margin index" as a predictive tool for residual disease after breast-conservation surgery [14]. This margin index is calculated by dividing the closest margin (in mm) by the tumor size (in mm) $\times$ 100. They found that with a margin index >5, the risk of residual disease was 3.2%. With a margin index of 20, no residual disease was found in the reexcision specimen.

The NSABP B-06 study showed that in 1851 patients who underwent breast conservation, the positive margin rate was 6.8% and the in-breast tumor recurrence rate was 14.2% over 20 years of followup [1]. Other randomized controlled trials described a range of local recurrences rates from 5.9% at 20 years to 19.7% at 13 years [22]. These randomized trials do not explicitly define margin width, which ranged from no ink on tumor to 1 cm gross margin. While the B-06 trial was conducted in the 1970s, several subsequent NSABP trials in the 1990s showed improvement in 10-year local recurrence rates ranging from 3.5% to 6.5% [23]. Although developments in breast imaging and pathological evaluation of lumpectomy specimens probably contributed to these improvements, significant strides were also made in systemic therapy during this time. This suggests that the likelihood of local recurrence is related to not only the surgical margin width as well, but also to the underlying tumor biology as well as the effectiveness of adjuvant therapy.

Multiple retrospective studies have attempted to define predictors of a positive margin at lumpectomy. These studies identified a number of independent predictors of local recurrence including age less than 40 years, microcalcifications on mammography, palpable tumors, large tumors, multi-centricity, presence of DCIS or lobular histology, and lymphovascular invasion [24]. While these studies showed that 1-2 mm margins were associated with decreased local recurrence rates, it is unclear what the impact of improved systemic therapy and boost radiation therapy is on these results. Cabioglu retrospectively assessed patient and tumor characteristics as well as IBTR rates in two cohorts of patients (those treated from 1970 to 1993, and those treated from 1994 to 1996) [25]. Patients treated after 1994 were less likely to have positive or unknown margin status (2.9% compared to 24.1% before 1994,) and the 5-year IBTR rate was lower in patients treated after 1994 (1.3% compared to 5.7% in those treated before 1994). These investigators postulated that

multidisciplinary management, including improvements in pathologic evaluation and systemic therapy, could be credited for the improvement in IBTR.

Further evidence supports the fact that systemic treatments not only reduce the risk of distant metastases but also reduce the risk of local recurrence. In the NSABP B-14 trial, women with node-negative, estrogen-receptor (ER)-positive tumors were randomly assigned to tamoxifen or placebo [26]. The 10-year rate of local recurrence after breast-conserving surgery was reduced from 14.7% in the placebo group to 4.3% in the tamoxifen group. Similarly, in the NSABP B-13 trial, women with node-negative, ER-negative tumors were randomly assigned to methotrexate and fluorouracil or to no treatment [27]. A reduction was noted in the 10-year local recurrence rate from 13.4% in the no-treatment group to 2.6% in the treatment group. In both studies, the NSABP definition of no ink on tumor was used to define a negative margin.

Studies examining the effect of adding trastuzumab to adjuvant chemotherapy in women with human epidermal growth factor receptor 2 (HER2)-overexpressing tumors have shown an additional 40% reduction in the risk of local recurrence over a median follow-up of 1.5 to 2.0 years [28]. Triple negative tumors have the highest risk of local recurrence after both breast-conserving therapy and mastectomy [29–31], and retrospective studies do not show an improvement in local control after mastectomy as compared with lumpectomy and radiation in this subgroup of patients with biologically aggressive tumors [32, 33].

The effect of tumor biology on local recurrence was clearly shown in a study examining the usefulness of the 21-gene recurrence score (Oncotype DX) in predicting local and regional recurrence [34]. The recurrence score was developed to predict the likelihood of distant metastases in patients with ER-positive, node-negative breast cancer who received tamoxifen [35]. Mamounas et al. found that without systemic therapy, 18.4% of patients with a high recurrence score ($\geq$31) had a recurrence of local or regional disease [34]. The addition of tamoxifen had a minimal effect on the rate of local and regional recurrence, with a decrease to 15.8%. In contrast, the combination of chemotherapy and tamoxifen was associated with a reduction in the local recurrence rate to 7.8%.

Interestingly, the majority of the studies describing local recurrence rates do not make the distinction between true local recurrences and new ipsilateral primary tumors. Yi et al. suggested that approximately 50% of IBTRs are actually new primary cancers as differentiated by histologic subtype and receptor status [36]. This would lead us to expect that the true local recurrence rate may be half of what is reported in the above studies, if in fact half of in-breast recurrences are new primaries. These new primary tumors therefore would not be expected to be affected by margin width.

2. Preoperative Imaging and Treatment Strategies

Thorough preoperative imaging is necessary to plan the extent of resection while minimizing positive margins.

Standard preoperative imaging includes mammography and ultrasound, and often MRI. Mammography can delineate tumor size and borders, as well as identify extent of microcalcifications, presence of multifocality, and multicentricity. Mammography is also important for assessment of the contralateral breast. Compared to mammography, ultrasonography can often give more accurate estimation of tumor size and borders, particularly in patients of young age with dense breasts.

MRI is a more sensitive test that can detect additional foci of disease not appreciated on mammogram and ultrasound. Houssami et al., in a metaanalysis of 19 studies, found that MRI detected additional disease in 16% and led to more extended surgery in 5.5% with a change from lumpectomy to mastectomy in 1.1% [37]. Crowe et al. demonstrated that MRI identified occult or separate tumors in 13% of patients [38]. MRI has a high false-positive rate, so it is clear that additional lesions identified on MRI must be biopsied to demonstrate malignancy prior to changes in surgical planning. Of note, the clinical consequence of detecting these additional lesions on MRI is unknown since no study has demonstrated that use of MRI translates into improved local recurrence rates or survival.

Another theoretical advantage of MRI is the potential to better define the extent of the index lesion in order to better plan surgical resection. However, Bleicher et al. in a retrospective review of 577 patients (130 of which had preoperative MRI) failed to demonstrate a difference in margin positivity or the need to convert from breast conservation to mastectomy in the group who had MRI [39]. At this time, preoperative MRI does not improve surgical planning and does not reduce the need for reexcision. Furthermore, Shin et al. in a retrospective analysis showed that breast MRI provided more accurate estimation of tumor size in comparison to ultrasound for both invasive and in situ breast cancer. However, no clear benefit in terms of lower reexcision rate, higher rate of success of breast conservation, or reduced rate of local recurrence emerged with routine use of breast MRI before BCT [40].

There is some suggestion that MRI may be better at assessing DCIS than conventional imaging. Kropcho et al. prospectively evaluated patients diagnosed with DCIS with and without MRI [41]. In this study, the correlation between MRI and tumor size was found to be significantly higher; however, no significant difference was found in betweengroup analysis of the incidence of margin involvement with MRI versus without MRI (30% versus 24.7%, $P = 0.414$, resp.).

Neoadjuvant chemotherapy can often shrink larger tumors to allow for breast conservation. Sweeting et al. demonstrated that over 6-year median followup in young women <age 45, locoregional recurrence rates were no different after breast conservation than mastectomy (13% versus 18%) in patients who underwent neoadjuvant chemotherapy [42]. Higher posttreatment, but not pretreatment, stage was associated with higher locoregional recurrence rates. Recently, Moon et al demonstrated that the accuracy of MRI after neoadjuvant chemotherapy is influenced by the molecular subtype of the tumor. MRI was most accurate in predicting residual tumor extent for triple-negative breast tumors, and least accurate in the Luminal A subtype (Pearson correlation coefficient of 0.754 and 0.531.)

Multivariate analysis suggested that ER status was an independent factor which influenced the accuracy of MRI. In HER2 amplified tumors, the use of HER2-targeted agents was associated with a less accurate MRI prediction of residual tumor extent.

Huang et al. proposed a prognostic index score for patients receiving neoadjuvant chemotherapy composed of four points: (1) clinical N2 to N3 disease, (2) lymphovascular invasion, (3) pathologic size >2 cm, and (4) multifocal residual disease [43]. Patients with an index of 0 or 1 had similar LRR rates between mastectomy and BCT. Patients with a score of 2 had a trend towards less LRR that was not significant (12% after mastectomy versus 28% after BCT), and patients with a score of 3 or 4 had a significant difference (19% after mastectomy versus 61% after BCT.) This index provides a framework in which to guide surgery selection after neoadjuvant chemotherapy, however, does not explicitly address the impact of margin status on LRR rates.

Other novel preoperative imaging strategies include optical spectroscopy and molecular vibrational imaging. Optical spectroscopy uses properties of tissue microstructure and biochemical composition to characterize tissue. It can differentiate normal from malignant tissue by distinguishing deoxy-hemoglobin, oxy-hemoglobin, water, and lipids, and thus is not limited by mammographic tissue density. This has also shown promise in assessing tumor response to neoadjuvant chemotherapy [44]. This technology is limited in distinguishing DCIS from normal tissue. Molecular vibrational imaging is another quantitative imaging technology that uses Coherent anti-Stokes Raman scattering (CARS) microscopy to visualize cellular and tissue features. This technology shows promise in differentiating invasive ductal from invasive lobular lesions, as well as DCIS from normal tissue.

3. Lesion Localization, Margin Assessment, and Intraoperative Techniques

Preoperative tumor localization for nonpalpable lesions was traditionally performed by the radiologist with either a mammographically or sonographically guided wire placement into the tumor. The limitation of this technique is that it identifies the lesion in one plane only, with limited ability to guide a three-dimensional resection of the lesion. Lesion bracketing with multiple guidewires as opposed to a single wire would theoretically improve margin clearance by facilitating complete resection of an imaging abnormality. However, Liberman et al. found that while bracketing a lesion (particularly if the lesion was a large area of calcifications) with multiple wires may help to ensure removal of the entire mammographic lesion, it still did not improve on rates of margin positivity [45].

Intraoperative specimen radiography using the Faxitron can be done immediately after specimen excision. The Faxitron allows the surgeon to visualize an eccentric location of a tumor or clip so that additional tissue can be removed.

Bathla et al. demonstrated a reexcision rate of 14.3% when 2-dimensional Faxitron was used to guide further tissue removal at the time of initial lumpectomy [46]. In this study, 95.8% of patients who would have required subsequent reexcision were spared further surgery since additional margins were taken at the time of lumpectomy based on Faxitron imaging findings.

Intraoperative ultrasonography allows for improved guidance on extent of resection. This technique is quite promising for lesions that can be visualized with ultrasound. This was demonstrated by Rahusen et al. in a randomized clinical study comparing ultrasound guided lumpectomy of nonpalpable breast cancer to wire-guided resection. Using ultrasound to localize the cancer improved rates of margin positivity from 45% with wire guided localization alone to 11% with intraoperative US localization [47]. However, many lesions are not visualized on ultrasound; in particular DCIS lesions which are diagnosed as calcifications on mammography often have no ultrasound correlate. For this reason, it is essential for the surgeon to document presence of the lesion on ultrasound preoperatively to ensure visualization.

For lesions not visible on ultrasound, a hydrogel based-breast biopsy clip can be placed at the time of biopsy. This clip is visible on ultrasound and enables the surgeon to use US guidance rather than preoperative wire localization for excision of sonographically occult lesions. However, this approach has limitations. Klein et al. reported that while the clip was very well visualized with intraoperative US, there was a high rate of clip migration either prior to the procedure (6.4%) or when the biopsy cavity was transected (45.2%) [48].

Another technique to enable use of intraoperative ultrasound for lesion excision involves cryoprobe assisted localization (CAL), in which an ultrasound-guided cryoprobe is placed into the tumor to freeze it. This enables the tumor to be easily palpable and visible on ultrasound. Tafra et al. demonstrated that although similar rates of margin positivity (28% with CAL compared to 31% with wire guided localization) and reexcision (19% and 21%) were noted, the cosmetic outcome was improved with CAL since less healthy surrounding tissue around the tumor was removed [49].

Another technique that is showing promise in improving margin clearance is radioguided occult lesion localization (ROLL). This involves placement of a small radioactive seed under imaging guidance. This seed can be detected with a hand-held gamma probe at the time of surgery. A recent metaanalysis of four randomized controlled trials including 449 patients comparing radioguided seed localization to wire guided localization showed improvement in margin status as well as reoperation rates with the ROLL technique [50]. However, when Krekel et al. compared wire guided localization, intraoperative US localization, and the ROLL technique, the rate of positive margins was the lowest in the intraoperative US group [51].

These studies suggest that the ability to visualize the lesion in multiple dimensions facilitates complete removal, however, rates of margin positivity may still be unchanged. Therefore, efforts have been focused on methods of evaluating the lumpectomy specimen intraoperatively to assess

margin positivity. Traditional margin assessment intraoperatively consists of either frozen section histology or imprint cytology. Frozen section histology, while relatively accurate in reflecting margin status, is limited due to time, cost, and loss of tissue for permanent section evaluation. Furthermore this method is very labor intensive and can only examine a limited amount of tissue, with false negative rates reported in 19% of patients [52]. Imprint cytology or "touch prep" involves touching the lumpectomy margins to a glass slide, then fixing and staining them based on the principle that cancer cells will stick to the slide and fat cells will not. This method only assesses tumor cells at the lumpectomy surface and does not indicate when margins are close. The accuracy is extremely variable and experience dependant, with positive predictive values ranging from 21% to 73.6% [53, 54]. In addition, both of these pathologic techniques are limited in their ability to predict invasive lobular cancer as well as DCIS at the margins [52].

Besides pathologic techniques to assess margins, significant efforts have been directed towards intraoperative margin probes to assess the lumpectomy specimen margins at the time of surgery. The MarginProbe (TM, Dune Medical Devices) uses radiofrequency spectroscopy to assess margin status. Using this probe, Allweis et al. reported a decrease in reexcision rate from 12.7% to 5.6% [55]. High frequency ultrasound probes have also been developed for intraoperative margin assessment [56]. This technology may have the ability to differentiate carcinomas and precancerous lesions such as ADH from normal tissue. It can also differentiate invasive lobular cancer from normal tissue, which is a limitation of other techniques.

Dooley et al. described ductoscopy-assisted lumpectomy based on the "sick lobe" hypothesis, with the idea that the entire lobe of the breast containing disease should be evaluated and all affected areas should be removed in order to minimize local recurrence rates [57]. His nonrandomized series showed a lower rate of local failure in those patients who had ductoscopy assisted surgical excision. Furthermore, 42% of patients were noted to have extensive disease within the affected lobe.

Since a primary drawback of large excisions to achieve negative margins is due to removal of excess volume of tissue and resultant cosmetic deformity, several ablative methods have been investigated to provide a larger perimeter of margin clearance without resecting additional tissue. Manenti et al. demonstrated that cryoablation of unifocal small malignant tumors led to complete necrosis in 14 of 15 patients [58]. Laser ablation has been demonstrated to ablate mammographically detected breast cancer [59]. Klimberg et al. have demonstrated that radiofrequency ablation at the time of surgical excision (eRFA) creates a 5–10 mm zone of ablation around the resected tumor, without removing excess of volume of tissue to achieve the same result [60]. These technologies hold promise in achieving wider margins without compromising cosmesis.

Since most true in-breast recurrences occur at or near the initial lumpectomy cavity, partial breast intraoperative radiation has been investigated as an alternative to traditional external beam. The use of a single dose of intraoperative radiation using a spherical applicator placed in the surgical cavity was compared to traditional external beam radiation in the TARGIT-A trial [61]. This trial showed that at 4 years of followup in selected patients, a single intraoperative radiation dose is an acceptable alternative to external beam radiotherapy.

4. Pathologic Assessment

There is no universally accepted pathology standard for assessing breast specimens, and translation of intraoperative findings to the pathology lab can be quite difficult. After a lumpectomy specimen is removed from the breast, there may be distortion of the margins due to compression of the specimen for radiographic lesion confirmation. The breast tissue is fatty, and often with compression of the tissue for specimen radiograph to confirm lesion excision, the specimen flattens out or "pancakes," resulting in distortion of the specimen and spurious positive margins [62]. Furthermore, even with minimal handling, the breast tissue is fatty and often slides off a tumor which remains firm.

Therefore, in addition to assessing the lumpectomy specimen margins, surgeons often submit additional tissue from the cavity margins once the primary specimen has been removed (cavity shave margins). Assessing the cavity margins rather than lumpectomy margins is likely a better indicator of presence of residual disease in the cavity since it avoids the issues of compression and specimen processing artifact. The technique involves resecting thin samples of tissue from all 6 margins (superior, inferior, medial, lateral, anterior, and posterior) for pathology evaluation. This technique can direct the surgeon to the exact location of a positive margin in the event that reexcision is necessary; however, the drawback is that it further increases resection volume [63]. Although the volume of tissue resected is increased, Rizzo et al. demonstrated a higher rate of pathologic margin negativity and therefore a lower rate of reoperation with this technique [64]. While there is a cost savings associated with fewer reoperations, there is additional time required by pathology to assess the extra tissue removed and may adversely impact cosmesis.

Another challenge as the lumpectomy specimen moves from the operating room to the pathology lab is specimen orientation. Marking sutures have traditionally been placed on 2 or more of the 6 surfaces of a lumpectomy specimen by the surgeon in the operating room, followed by inking of all 6 margins done by the pathologist in the lab. Molina et al. demonstrated that with 2 marking sutures placed by the surgeon, there was a 20% rate of discordance between surgeon and pathologist interpretation of the margins in specimens larger than 20 square cm [65]. In smaller specimens less than 20 square cm, the discordance was as high as 78%.

Particularly disturbing for the surgeon are cases where a positive margin is noted on pathology from the initial lumpectomy, and no further disease is evident on reexcision, since it is unclear whether the reexcision removed the correct area. Dooley and Parker demonstrated that when a single margin was close or positive, reexcision showed tumor in only 35% of cases [66]. When multiple margins were close or positive, reexcision showed tumor in 47% of cases.

Pathologic processing includes inking with close attention so that ink does not run into cut surfaces. Multiple samples are taken perpendicular to each inked surface, with additional samples taken based on gross appearance of the tissue [67]. In order to more accurately orient the specimen for the pathologist and to help guide reexcision, Singh et al. compared standard inking by the pathologist after lumpectomy versus intraoperative inking with surgeon input [68]. This study demonstrated a decrease in margin positivity rate from 46% to 23%, as well as a decrease in reexcision rates from 38% to 19% when the surgeon was responsible for inking the margin. Importantly, residual disease at the time of reexcision was noted to be 67% in the group inked by the surgeon (as opposed to 23% in the group inked by the pathologist). This simple technique of surgeon staining the lumpectomy specimen with 6 different ink colors at the time of lumpectomy can enable orientation to be maintained when evaluating the margins. Furthermore, directed reexcision also decreases the volume of tissue excised when compared to the whole cavity reexcision [69].

5. Oncoplastic Surgery to Achieve Wider Margins

Oncoplastic breast surgery combines the principles of cancer resection with plastic surgery to achieve wide tumor-free margins in such a manner as to maximize resection volume while optimizing cosmetic outcome. The two main techniques used involve volume displacement and volume replacement. Volume displacement techniques combine resection with a variety of different breast-reshaping and breast-reduction techniques and include radial ellipse segmentectomy and circumareolar approach. Lesions in the upper or central breast can be resected with the crescent mastopexy, batwing incision, donut mastopexy, and central quadrantectomy. Lesions of the lower breast can be resected with the triangle incision, inframammary incision, and reduction mastopexy [70].

These procedures can be done by the breast surgeon and/or plastic surgeon at the time of cancer resection. Of note, the three dimensional orientation of the tumor bed is frequently altered with these techniques so that identification of the initial resection cavity for postoperative radiation therapy is not possible. At the very least, placement of surgical clips after tumor resection and before oncoplastic reconstruction may be the most accurate method to localize the RT local boost field. Additionally, oncoplastic techniques commonly prevent a simple further excision in the event of positive margins, so that most patients with involved margins will need a mastectomy [71]. Oncoplastic procedures for cancer often result in the need for a contralateral symmetry procedure. The contralateral procedure can be done at the same time as the cancer resection, or at a later time.

Volume replacement techniques are performed less frequently, and involve autologous tissue flap placement when there is insufficient tissue for a satisfactory cosmetic result. These procedures can retain the volume and shape of the breast and avoid contralateral breast surgery. However, these

Table 1: Oncoplastic surgery and margin involvement, local recurrence rates, and survival rates.

Author	Year	Number of patients	Weight (g)/volume of specimen	Close/involved margins (reexcision/mastectomy)	Local recurrence rate	Survival rate	Median followup (months)
Clough et al. [15]	2003	101	222		9.4%	95.7%	44
Kaur et al. [16]	2005	30	200	16%			
Rietjens et al. [17]	2007	148	198	2.02%	3%	92.47%	74
Giacalone et al. [18]	2006	31	190	21%			
Meretoja et al. [19]	2010	90		12.2%	0%		26
Fitoussi et al. [20]	2010	540	187.7	18.9%	6.8%	92.6%	49
Chakravorty et al. [21]	2012	146	67 (11–1050)	2.7%	4.3%		28

techniques are more complex, require a donor site, and lead to increased recovery time following autologous tissue harvesting. Autologous flaps for volume replacement include transverse rectus abdominus (TRAM), adipofascial flap, a lateral thoracodorsal flap, a thoracoepigastric flap, an intercostal artery perforator (ICAP) flap, a thoracodorsal artery perforator (TDAP) flap, and a latissimus dorsi (LD) myocutaneous flap [72].

Oncoplastic breast conserving surgery (oBCS) has the potential to improve the aesthetic outcome of BCS as well as extending the role of BCS in situations previously considered unsuitable for conservation (large tumors relative to breast size, central and lower pole tumor location, or multifocality). While tumor size, or more precisely tumor-to-breast volume, is a key indication for oBCS, tumor location is an equally important consideration. However, the application of aesthetic techniques for therapeutic purposes must never compromise the main objective of breast cancer surgery: clear margins with good local disease control [72].

There is now agrowing evidence through prospective series that oncoplastic techniques offer patients a safe oncological outcome (Table 1). Clough et al. from Institute Curie published their first evaluation of 101 patients and concluded that oncoplastic techniques allow larger resections, however a recurrence rate of 9% was reported with median followup of 5 years [15]. Kaur et al. found that a larger volume excision is possible in a subset of patients treated by oncoplastic techniques however; this series reported a re-excision rate of 16% [16]. Giacalone et al. concluded in their study on 74 patients comparing oncoplastic surgery with quadrantectomy that oBCS extends the indications for breast conserving surgery [73]. Asgeirsson et al. from the European Institute of Oncology have reported long-term results with a 5-year local recurrence rate of 3% [74]. A recent Institute Curie review of 540 oncoplastic conservation procedures between 1986 and 2008 revealed a local recurrence rate of 6.8%: they also noted involved or close margins in 18.9% with 9.4% requiring further surgery as a mastectomy [20]. It is possible that oBCS using reduction mammoplasty techniques may be oncologically superior to sBCS by allowing larger excision volumes and wider margins without compromising cosmesis [18, 19, 21, 74, 75].

It appears that oncoplastic breast surgery extends the indications of breast conservation and allows for achievement of large resection volumes with good cosmesis. However, drawbacks include frequent necessity to operate on the contralateral healthy breast, increased cost, and increased possibility of complications delaying adjuvant therapy. While there has been some concern that oncoplastic surgery could confound subsequent mammographic imaging, Roberts et al. demonstrated that in patients who underwent reduction mammoplasty, no increase in subsequent imaging or diagnostic interventions was noted [76].

6. Looking Forward

Trends in breast cancer care continue to progress towards less invasive surgical treatment. Recent data from the ACOSOG Z11 trial suggests that axillary dissection may not be of benefit in node positive patients who receive maximal systemic therapy and radiation. As systemic therapy improves, and individualized and targeted approaches evolve, it is unclear what role surgery will play in achieving local control. Primary ablative therapies may make questions of margins obsolete, in that if a tumor is ablated and resolves on imaging, then surgical excision may not be necessary.

References

[1] B. Fisher, S. Anderson, J. Bryant et al., "Twenty-year follow-up of a randomized trial comparing total mastectomy, lumpectomy, and lumpectomy plus irradiation for the treatment of invasive breast cancer," New England Journal of Medicine, vol. 347, no. 16, pp. 1233–1241, 2002.

[2] U. Veronesi, N. Cascinelli, L. Mariani et al., "Twenty-year follow-up of a randomized study comparing breast-conserving surgery with radical mastectomy for early breast cancer," New England Journal of Medicine, vol. 347, no. 16, pp. 1227–1232, 2002.

[3] P. J. Lovrics, S. D. Cornacchi, F. Farrokhyar et al., "The relationship between surgical factors and margin status after breast-conservation surgery for early stage breast cancer," American Journal of Surgery, vol. 197, no. 6, pp. 740–746, 2009.

[4] J. A. Acosta, J. A. Greenlee, K. Dean Gubler, C. J. Goepfert, and J. J. Ragland, "Surgical margins after needle-localization breast

biopsy," *American Journal of Surgery*, vol. 170, no. 6, pp. 643–646, 1995.

[5] C. Gajdos, P. Ian Tartter, I. J. Bleiweiss et al., "Mammographic appearance of nonpalpable breast cancer reflects pathologic characteristics," *Annals of Surgery*, vol. 235, no. 2, pp. 246–251, 2002.

[6] M. Z. Papa, E. Klein, B. Davidson et al., "The effect of anesthesia type on needle localization breast biopsy: another point of view," *American Journal of Surgery*, vol. 171, no. 2, pp. 242–243, 1996.

[7] R. Mullen, E. J. Macaskill, A. Khalil et al., "Involved anterior margins after breast conserving surgery: is re-excision required?" *European Journal of Surgical Oncology*, vol. 38, no. 4, pp. 302–306, 2012.

[8] A. Goldhirsch, J. N. Ingle, R. D. Gelber, A. S. Coates, B. Thürlimann, and H. J. Senn, "Thresholds for therapies: highlights of the St Gallen international expert consensus on the primary therapy of early breast cancer 2009," *Annals of Oncology*, vol. 20, no. 8, pp. 1319–1329, 2009.

[9] S. L. Blair, K. Thompson, J. Rococco, V. Malcarne, P. D. Beitsch, and D. W. Ollila, "Attaining negative margins in breast-conservation operations: is there a consensus among breast surgeons?" *Journal of the American College of Surgeons*, vol. 209, no. 5, pp. 608–613, 2009.

[10] S. Y. Wang, H. Chu, T. Shamliyan et al., "Network meta-analysis of margin threshold for women with ductal carcinoma in situ," *Journal of the National Cancer Institute*, vol. 104, no. 7, pp. 507–516, 2012.

[11] N. Houssami, P. MacAskill, M. L. Marinovich et al., "Meta-analysis of the impact of surgical margins on local recurrence in women with early-stage invasive breast cancer treated with breast-conserving therapy," *European Journal of Cancer*, vol. 46, no. 18, pp. 3219–3232, 2010.

[12] R. Holland, S. H. J. Veling, M. Mravunac, and J. H. C. L. Hendriks, "Histologic multifocality of Tis, T1-2 breast carcinomas: implications for clinical trials of breast-conserving surgery," *Cancer*, vol. 56, no. 5, pp. 979–990, 1985.

[13] M. Morrow, J. R. Harris, and S. J. Schnitt, "Surgical margins in lumpectomy for breast cancer-bigger is not better," *New England Journal of Medicine*, vol. 367, no. 1, pp. 79–82, 2012.

[14] J. A. Margenthaler, F. Gao, and V. S. Klimberg, "Margin index: a new method for prediction of residual disease after breast-conserving surgery," *Annals of Surgical Oncology*, vol. 17, no. 10, pp. 2696–2701, 2010.

[15] K. B. Clough, J. S. Lewis, B. Couturaud, A. Fitoussi, C. Nos, and M. C. Falcou, "Oncoplastic techniques allow extensive resections for breast-conserving therapy of breast carcinomas," *Annals of Surgery*, vol. 237, no. 1, pp. 26–34, 2003.

[16] N. Kaur, J. Y. Petit, M. Rietjens et al., "Comparative study of surgical margins in oncoplastic surgery and quadrantectomy in breast cancer," *Annals of Surgical Oncology*, vol. 12, no. 7, pp. 539–545, 2005.

[17] M. Rietjens, C. A. Urban, P. C. Rey et al., "Long-term oncological results of breast conservative treatment with oncoplastic surgery," *Breast*, vol. 16, no. 4, pp. 387–395, 2007.

[18] P. L. Giacalone, P. Roger, O. Dubon, N. El Gareh, J. P. Daurés, and F. Laffargue, "Lumpectomy versus oncoplastic surgery for breast-conserving therapy of cancer. A prospective study about 99 patients," *Annales de Chirurgie*, vol. 131, no. 4, pp. 256–261, 2006.

[19] T. J. Meretoja, C. Svarvar, and T. A. Jahkola, "Outcome of oncoplastic breast surgery in 90 prospective patients," *American Journal of Surgery*, vol. 200, no. 2, pp. 224–228, 2010.

[20] A. D. Fitoussi, M. G. Berry, F. Famà et al., "Oncoplastic breast surgery for cancer: analysis of 540 consecutive cases," *Plastic and Reconstructive Surgery*, vol. 125, no. 2, pp. 454–462, 2010.

[21] A. Chakravorty, A. K. Shrestha, and N. Sanmugalingam, "How safe is oncoplastic breast conservation? Comparative analysis with standard breast conserving surgery," *European Journal of Surgical Oncology*, vol. 38, no. 5, pp. 395–398, 2012.

[22] S. C. Fisher, S. V. Klimberg, and K. Seema, "Margin index is not a reliable tool for predicting residual disease after breast-conserving surgery for DCIS," *Annals of Surgical Oncology*, vol. 18, pp. 3155–3159, 2011.

[23] S. J. Anderson, I. Wapnir, J. J. Dignam et al., "Prognosis after ipsilateral breast tumor recurrence and locoregional recurrences in patients treated by breast-conserving therapy in five national surgical adjuvant breast and bowel project protocols of node-negative breast cancer," *Journal of Clinical Oncology*, vol. 27, no. 15, pp. 2466–2473, 2009.

[24] M. Reedijk, N. Hodgson, G. Gohla et al., "A prospective study of tumor and technical factors associated with positive margins in breast-conservation therapy for non-palpable malignancy," *American Journal of Surgery*, pp. 263–268, 2012.

[25] N. Cabioglu, K. K. Hunt, A. A. Sahin et al., "Role for intra-operative margin assessment in patients undergoing breast-conserving surgery," *Annals of Surgical Oncology*, vol. 14, no. 4, pp. 1458–1471, 2007.

[26] B. Fisher, J. Dignam, J. Bryant et al., "Five versus more than five years of tamoxifen therapy for breast cancer patients with negative lymph nodes and estrogen receptor-positive tumors," *Journal of the National Cancer Institute*, vol. 88, no. 21, pp. 1529–1542, 1996.

[27] B. Fisher, J. Dignam, and E. P. Mamounas, "Sequential methotrexate and fluorouracil for the treatment of node-negative breast cancer patients with estrogen receptor-negative tumors: eight-year results from National Surgical Adjuvant Breast and Bowel Project (NSABP) B-13 and first report of findings from NSABP B-19 comparing methotrexate and fluorouracil with conventional cyclophosphamide, methotrexate, and fluorouracil," *Journal of Clinical Oncology*, vol. 14, pp. 1982–1992, 1996.

[28] E. H. Romond, E. A. Perez, J. Bryant et al., "Trastuzumab plus adjuvant chemotherapy for operable HER2-positive breast cancer," *New England Journal of Medicine*, vol. 353, no. 16, pp. 1673–1684, 2005.

[29] M. Kyndi, F. B. Sørensen, H. Knudsen, M. Overgaard, H. M. Nielsen, and J. Overgaard, "Estrogen receptor, progesterone receptor, HER-2, and response to postmastectomy radiotherapy in high-risk breast cancer," *Journal of Clinical Oncology*, vol. 26, no. 9, pp. 1419–1426, 2008.

[30] E. K. A. Millar, P. H. Graham, S. A. O'Toole et al., "Prediction of local recurrence, distant metastases, and death after breast-conserving therapy in early-stage invasive breast cancer using a five-biomarker panel," *Journal of Clinical Oncology*, vol. 27, no. 28, pp. 4701–4708, 2009.

[31] P. L. Nguyen, A. G. Taghian, M. S. Katz et al., "Breast cancer subtype approximated by estrogen receptor, progesterone receptor, and HER-2 is associated with local and distant recurrence after breast-conserving therapy," *Journal of Clinical Oncology*, vol. 26, no. 14, pp. 2373–2378, 2008.

[32] B. S. Abdulkarim, J. Cuartero, J. Hanson, J. Deschênes, D. Lesniak, and S. Sabri, "Increased risk of locoregional recurrence for women with T1-2N0 triple-negative breast cancer treated with modified radical mastectomy without adjuvant radiation therapy compared with breast-conserving therapy," *Journal of Clinical Oncology*, vol. 29, no. 21, pp. 2852–2858, 2011.

[33] A. Y. Ho, G. Gupta, T. A. King et al., "Favorable prognosis in patients with T1a/bN0 triple-negative breast cancers treated with multimodality therapy," *Cancer*, vol. 118, no. 20, pp. 4944–4952, 2012.

[34] E. P. Mamounas, G. Tang, B. Fisher et al., "Association between the 21-gene recurrence score assay and risk of locoregional recurrence in node-negative, estrogen receptor-positive breast cancer: results from NSABP B-14 and NSABP B-20," *Journal of Clinical Oncology*, vol. 28, no. 10, pp. 1677–1683, 2010.

[35] S. Paik, G. Tang, S. Shak et al., "Gene expression and benefit of chemotherapy in women with node-negative, estrogen receptor-positive breast cancer," *Journal of Clinical Oncology*, vol. 24, no. 23, pp. 3726–3734, 2006.

[36] M. Yi, T. A. Buchholz, F. Meric-Bernstam et al., "Classification of ipsilateral breast tumor recurrences after breast conservation therapy can predict patient prognosis and facilitate treatment planning," *Annals of Surgery*, vol. 253, no. 3, pp. 572–579, 2011.

[37] N. Houssami, S. Ciatto, P. Macaskill et al., "Accuracy and surgical impact of magnetic resonance imaging in breast cancer staging: systematic review and meta-analysis in detection of multifocal and multicentric cancer," *Journal of Clinical Oncology*, vol. 26, no. 19, pp. 3248–3258, 2008.

[38] J. P. Crowe, R. J. Patrick, and A. Rim, "The importance of preoperative breast MRI for patients newly diagnosed with breast cancer," *Breast Journalournal*, vol. 15, no. 1, pp. 52–60, 2009.

[39] R. J. Bleicher, R. M. Ciocca, B. L. Egleston et al., "Association of routine pretreatment magnetic resonance imaging with time to surgery, mastectomy rate, and margin status," *Journal of the American College of Surgeons*, vol. 209, no. 2, pp. 180–187, 2009.

[40] H. C. Shin, W. Han, H. G. Moon et al., "Limited value and utility of breast MRI in patients undergoing breast-conserving cancer surgery," *Annals of Surgical Oncology*, vol. 19, no. 8, pp. 2572–2579, 2012.

[41] L. C. Kropcho, S. T. Steen, and A. P. Chung, "Preoperative breast MRI in the surgical treatment of ductal carcinoma in situ," *Breast Journal*, vol. 18, no. 2, pp. 151–156, 2012.

[42] R. S. Sweeting, N. Klauber-Demore, and M. O. Meyers, "Young women with locally advanced breast cancer who achieve breast conservation after neoadjuvant chemotherapy have a low local recurrence rate," *American Surgeon*, vol. 77, no. 7, pp. 850–855, 2011.

[43] E. H. Huang, E. A. Strom, G. H. Perkins et al., "Comparison of risk of local-regional recurrence after mastectomy or breast conservation therapy for patients treated with neoadjuvant chemotherapy and radiation stratified according to a prognostic index score," *International Journal of Radiation Oncology Biology Physics*, vol. 66, no. 2, pp. 352–357, 2006.

[44] O. Falou, H. Soliman, A. Sadeghi-Naini et al., "Diffuse optical spectroscopy evaluation of treatment response in women with locally advanced breast cancer receiving neoadjuvant chemotherapy," *Translational Oncology*, vol. 5, no. 4, pp. 238–246, 2012.

[45] L. Liberman, J. Kaplan, K. J. Van Zee et al., "Bracketing wires for preoperative breast needle localization," *American Journal of Roentgenology*, vol. 177, no. 3, pp. 565–572, 2001.

[46] L. Bathla, A. Harris, M. Davey et al., "High resolution intra-operative two-dimensional specimen mammography and its impact on second operation for re-excision of positive margins at final pathology after breast conservation surgery," *American Journal of Surgery*, vol. 202, no. 4, pp. 387–394, 2011.

[47] F. D. Rahusen, A. J. A. Bremers, H. F. J. Fabry, A. H. M. Taets van Amerongen, R. P. A. Boom, and S. Meijer, "Ultrasound-guided lumpectomy of nonpalpable breast cancer versus wire-guided resection: a randomized clinical trial," *Annals of Surgical Oncology*, vol. 9, no. 10, pp. 994–998, 2002.

[48] R. L. Klein, J. A. Mook, and D. M. Euhus, "Evaluation of a hydrogel based breast biopsy marker (HydroMARK) as an alternative to wire and radioactive seed localization for non-palpable breast lesions," *Journal of Surgical Oncology*, vol. 105, no. 6, pp. 591–594, 2012.

[49] L. Tafra, R. Fine, P. Whitworth et al., "Ultrasound-guided lumpectomy of nonpalpable breast cancer versus wire-guided resection: a randomized clinical trial," *Annals of Surgical Oncology*, vol. 9, no. 10, pp. 994–998, 2002.

[50] M. S. Sajid, U. Parampalli, Z. Haider et al., "Comparison of radioguided occult lesion localization (ROLL) and wire localization for non-palpable breast cancers: a meta-analysis," *Journal of Surgical Oncology*, vol. 105, no. 8, pp. 852–858, 2012.

[51] N. M. A. Krekel, B. M. Zonderhuis, H. B. A. C. Stockmann et al., "A comparison of three methods for nonpalpable breast cancer excision," *European Journal of Surgical Oncology*, vol. 37, no. 2, pp. 109–115, 2011.

[52] J. C. Cendan, D. Coco, and E. M. Copeland III, "Accuracy of intra-operative touch prep frozen-section analysis of breast cancer lumpectomy bed margins," *Journal of the American College of Surgeons*, vol. 201, pp. 194–198, 2005.

[53] F. D'Halluin, P. Tas, S. Rouquette et al., "Intra-operative touch preparation cytology following lumpectomy for breast cancer: a series of 400 procedures," *Breast*, vol. 18, no. 4, pp. 248–253, 2009.

[54] E. K. Valdes, S. K. Boolbol, J. M. Cohen, and S. M. Feldman, "Intra-operative touch preparation cytology; does it have a role in re-excision lumpectomy?" *Annals of Surgical Oncology*, vol. 14, no. 3, pp. 1045–1050, 2007.

[55] T. M. Allweis, Z. Kaufman, S. Lelcuk et al., "A prospective, randomized, controlled, multicenter study of a real-time, intraoperative probe for positive margin detection in breast-conserving surgery," *American Journal of Surgery*, vol. 196, no. 4, pp. 483–489, 2008.

[56] T. E. Doyle, R. E. Factor, C. L. Ellefson et al., "High-frequency ultrasound for intraoperative margin assessments in breast conservation surgery: a feasibility study," *BMC Cancer*, vol. 11, article 444, 2011.

[57] W. Dooley, J. Bong, and J. Parker, "Redefining lumpectomy using a modification of the "sick lobe" hypothesis and ductal anatomy," *International Journal of Breast Cancer*, vol. 2011, pp. 7263–7284, 2011.

[58] G. Manenti, T. Perretta, E. Gaspari et al., "Percutaneous local ablation of unifocal subclinical breast cancer: clinical experience and preliminary results of cryotherapy," *European Radiology*, vol. 21, no. 11, pp. 2344–2353, 2011.

[59] K. Dowlatshahi, D. S. Francescatti, and K. J. Bloom, "Laser therapy for small breast cancers," *American Journal of Surgery*, vol. 184, no. 4, pp. 359–363, 2002.

[60] V. S. Klimberg, J. Kepple, G. Shafirstein et al., "eRFA: excision followed by RFA—a new technique to improve local control in breast cancer," *Annals of Surgical Oncology*, vol. 13, no. 11, pp. 1422–1433, 2006.

[61] J. S. Vaidya, D. J. Joseph, and J. S. Tobias, "Targeted intra-operative radiotherapy versus whole breast radiotherapy for breast cancer (TARGIT-A trial): an international, prospective, randomised, noninferiority phase 3 trial," *The Lancet*, vol. 376, no. 9735, pp. 91–102, 2010.

[62] R. A. Graham, M. J. Homer, J. Katz, J. Rothschild, H. Safaii, and S. Supran, "The pancake phenomenon contributes to the inaccuracy of margin assessment in patients with breast cancer," *American Journal of Surgery*, vol. 184, no. 2, pp. 89–93, 2002.

[63] T. L. Huston, R. Pigalarga, M. P. Osborne, and E. Tousimis, "The influence of additional surgical margins on the total specimen volume excised and the reoperative rate after breast-conserving surgery," *American Journal of Surgery*, vol. 192, no. 4, pp. 509–512, 2006.

[64] M. Rizzo, R. Iyengar, S. G. A. Gabram et al., "The effects of additional tumor cavity sampling at the time of breast-conserving surgery on final margin status, volume of resection, and pathologist workload," *Annals of Surgical Oncology*, vol. 17, no. 1, pp. 228–234, 2010.

[65] M. A. Molina, S. Snell, D. Franceschi et al., "Breast specimen orientation," *Annals of Surgical Oncology*, vol. 16, no. 2, pp. 285–288, 2009.

[66] W. C. Dooley and J. Parker, "Understanding the mechanisms creating false positive lumpectomy margins," *American Journal of Surgery*, vol. 190, no. 4, pp. 606–608, 2005.

[67] S. M. Feldman, E. K. Valdes, S. K. Boolbol, J. M. Cohen, and J. Gross, "Excisional breast specimen orientation/processing: a multidisciplinary approach for breast conservation," *Seminars in Breast Disease*, vol. 8, no. 3, pp. 121–126, 2006.

[68] M. Singh, G. Singh, K. T. Hogan, K. A. Atkins, and A. T. Schroen, "The effect of intraoperative specimen inking on lumpectomy re-excision rates," *World Journal of Surgical Oncology*, vol. 8, article 4, 2010.

[69] G. R. Gibson, B. A. Lesnikoski, J. Yoo, L. A. Mott, B. Cady, and R. J. Barth, "A comparison of ink-directed and traditional whole-cavity re-excision for breast lumpectomy specimens with positive margins," *Annals of Surgical Oncology*, vol. 8, no. 9, pp. 693–704, 2001.

[70] D. R. Holmes, W. Schooler, and R. Smith, "Oncoplastic approaches to breast conservation," *International Journal of Breast Cancer*, vol. 2011, pp. 303–379, 2011.

[71] L. A. Newman, H. M. Kuerer, M. D. McNeese et al., "Reduction mammoplasty improves breast conservation therapy in patients with macromastia," *American Journal of Surgery*, vol. 181, no. 3, pp. 215–220, 2001.

[72] J. D. Yang, J. W. Lee, Y. K. Cho et al., "Surgical techniques for personalized oncoplastic surgery in breast cancer patients with small- to moderate-sized breasts (part 2): volume replacement," *Journal of Breast Cancer*, vol. 15, no. 1, pp. 7–14, 2012.

[73] P. L. Giacalone, P. Roger, O. Dubon et al., "Comparative study of the accuracy of breast resection in oncoplastic surgery and quadrantectomy in breast cancer," *Annals of Surgical Oncology*, vol. 14, no. 2, pp. 605–614, 2007.

[74] K. S. Asgeirsson, T. Rasheed, S. J. McCulley, and R. D. Macmillan, "Oncological and cosmetic outcomes of oncoplastic breast conserving surgery," *European Journal of Surgical Oncology*, vol. 31, no. 8, pp. 817–823, 2005.

[75] O. C. Iwuchukwu, J. R. Harvey, M. Dordea, A. C. Critchley, and P. J. Drew, "The role of oncoplastic therapeutic mammoplasty in breast cancer surgery—a review," *Surgical Oncology*, vol. 21, no. 2, pp. 133–141, 2012.

[76] J. M. Roberts, C. J. Clark, M. J. Campbell, and K. T. Paige, "Incidence of abnormal mammograms after reduction mammoplasty: implications for oncoplastic closure," *American Journal of Surgery*, vol. 201, no. 5, pp. 608–610, 2011.

14

Reoperation following Pancreaticoduodenectomy

J. R. Reddy, R. Saxena, R. K. Singh, B. Pottakkat, A. Prakash, A. Behari, A. K. Gupta, and V. K. Kapoor

Department of Surgical Gastroenterology, Sanjay Gandhi Postgraduate Institute of Medical Sciences (SGPGIMS), Rae Bareily Road, Lucknow 226014, India

Correspondence should be addressed to R. Saxena, rajan@sgpgi.ac.in

Academic Editor: Michael Hünerbein

Introduction. The literature on reoperation following pancreaticoduodenectomy is sparse and does not address all concerns. *Aim.* To analyze the incidence, causes, and outcome of patients undergoing reoperations following pancreaticoduodenectomy. *Methods.* Retrospective analysis of 520 consecutive patients undergoing pancreaticoduodenectomy from May 1989 to September 2010. *Results.* 96 patients (18.5%) were reoperated; 72 were early, 18 were late, and 6 underwent both early and late reoperations. Indications for early reoperation were post pancreatectomy hemorrhage in 53 (68%), pancreatico-enteric anastomotic leak in 10 (13%), hepaticojejunostomy leak in 3 (3.8%), duodenojejunostomy leak in 4 (5%), intestinal obstruction in 1 (1.2%) and miscellaneous causes in 7 (9%). Patients reoperated early did not fare poorly on long-term follow up. Indications for late reoperations were complications of index surgery ($n = 12$), recurrence of the primary disease ($n = 8$), complications of adjuvant radiotherapy ($n = 3$), and gastrointestinal bleed ($n = 1$). The median survival of 16 patients reoperated late without recurrent disease was 49 months. *Conclusion.* Early reoperations following pancreaticoduodenectomy, commonly for post pancreatectomy hemorrhage, carries a high mortality due to associated sepsis, but has no impact on long-term survival. Long-term complications related to pancreaticoduodenectomy and adjuvant radiotherapy can be managed successfully with good results.

1. Introduction

Descriptions of post pancreaticoduodenectomy (PD) reoperations have largely addressed relaparotomy for early complications such as postpancreatectomy hemorrhage (PPH) and pancreaticoenteric anastomotic leak (PEA) with associated intraabdominal collection [1, 2]. The literature on other indications is very limited. Quite a number of studies have addressed the long-term survival of patients undergoing PD and the need for readmission in them on long-term follow up [3, 4]. However, there is very limited data that specifically addresses the need for and the outcome of surgical reintervention in these patients on long-term follow up. The aim of this study was to analyze the following.

(i) The incidence and causes of early and late reoperations following PD.

(ii) Factors predicting the need for early reoperation and its related mortality.

(iii) The outcome of patients undergoing early and late reoperations.

2. Patients and Methods

Five hundred and twenty patients underwent PD between May 1989 and September 2010 at the Department of Surgical Gastroenterology, Sanjay Gandhi Postgraduate Institute of Medical Sciences, a tertiary referral institute in the northern part of India. Data was retrieved from a prospectively maintained database which included variables recorded during the index hospitalization and further readmissions if any. Information about patient follow up was obtained from follow up cards and telephonic follow up interviews.

All pancreaticoduodenectomies at our institute were performed by or under the direct supervision of consultant surgeons. Preoperatively all these patients underwent routine blood counts, liver and renal function tests, abdominal sonography, and an abdominal computed tomography (CT) scan for tumour staging. A side viewing endoscopic examination with biopsy was contemplated in almost all patients as a predominant number of patients who undergo PD at our hospital have periampullary carcinoma. In patients with a negative biopsy and a demonstrable CT scan evidence of a periampullary mass, decision to proceed with PD was taken. Endoscopic ultrasound was selectively used in those patients with a negative biopsy and no evidence of a mass lesion on CT scan. A preoperative endoscopic biliary drainage procedure with stenting was carried out in those patients with cholangitis, high preoperative bilirubin (>15 mg/dL), or poor nutritional status and surgery was then performed 4–6 weeks after stenting. All patients received preoperative antibiotic dose of cefoperazone and sulbactam 2 g and amikacin 500–750 mg at the time of induction. An equal number of patients underwent a pylorus preserving PD or a classical Whipple procedure according to the surgeon's preference. Pancreatic reconstruction was performed first by an end to end or end to side pancreatico-jejunostomy in 514 patients. Of the remaining, 3 patients underwent pancreatico-gastrostomy and 3 had no pancreatico-enteric reconstruction due to underlying acute pancreatitis and necrosis. Duct to mucosa and pancreatic dunking or invagination was performed equally based on surgeon preference and pancreatic duct stenting was used selectively. This was followed by an end to side hepaticojejunostomy and antecolic duodenojejunostomy or gastrojejunostomy. Nasojejunal tube was used preferentially over feeding jejunostomy as a feeding access. Intraoperative octreotide (100 ug stat) was used selectively in those patients with a soft pancreas and continued for 5 days postoperatively. Abdomen was closed with drainage. A nasogastric tube was placed for gastric decompression. Postoperatively drain fluid and serum amylase levels were estimated on postoperative days 4 and 7.

Reoperations were classified into early and late. Reoperations performed during index hospital admission following PD were classified as early while those reoperations performed any time after the index hospitalization were classified as late. Patients operated for indications unrelated to complications of index surgery (PD), tumour recurrence, or adjuvant radiotherapy were excluded. The reoperation data was retrieved from the database. Patients requiring early reoperations due to complications of index surgery were compared with those who did not need reoperation. The parameters evaluated were demographic factors, clinical presenting symptoms, intra-operative parameters, pathology, and postoperative complications. A univariate analysis was done to determine factors predictive of early reoperation. Chi-square test was used for categorical variables and Mann-Whitney U test for continuous variables. A multivariate logistic regression analysis was done to identify the variables independently predicting reoperation within this group. A similar analysis was done to identify the factors predictive of in-hospital mortality in patients undergoing early reoperation. Patients requiring late reoperations were classified into four groups: reoperation for complications of index surgery (group 1), tumour recurrence (group 2), complications of radiotherapy (group 3), and miscellaneous indications (group 4). To analyze the impact of early reoperations on survival, a Kaplan Meier survival curve was constructed including patients undergoing pancreatico-duodenectomy till September 2007, and statistical significance was tested using log-rank test. Median survival of patients undergoing

late reoperation was analyzed after excluding patients being reoperated for tumour recurrence. P value < 0.05 was considered as significant. Statistical analysis was performed using SPSS version 15 (SPSS, Chicago, IL, USA).

3. Results

Between May 1989 and September 2010, 520 patients underwent PD. Of these, 26 patients (5%) underwent PD for benign disease and 494 patients (95%) for malignant disease. The median age was 52 years (range 14–82 years). The in-hospital mortality rate was 8.1 percent (42 of 520), the overall morbidity rate was 62% per cent (322 of 520), and the median hospital stay was 14 days (range 5–112 days). 96 of these 520 patients (18.5%) were reoperated upon. 72 (75%) of these were early, 18 (18.8%) were late reoperations, and 6 patients (6.2%) had both early and late reoperations. For the purpose of analysis, the 6 patients who underwent both early and late reoperation were included in both the groups, thereby accounting for 78 patients (72 + 6) who underwent early reoperation and 24 patients (18+6) who underwent late reoperation. Among patients undergoing early reoperations, there were 53 males and 25 females with a median age of 52 years (range 23–72 years). Median time to reoperation was 8 days (range 0–59 days), 42% of patients were reoperated within 5 days, 63% within 10 days, and 89% within 20 days following PD.

3.1. Early Reoperations. The indications for early reoperation were postpancreatectomy hemorrhage (PPH) in 53 patients (68%), pancreatico-enteric anastomotic leak (PEA) with intra-abdominal collection in 10 (13%), hepatico-jejunostomy (HJ) leak in 3 (3.8%), duodeno-jejunostomy (DJ) leak in 4 (5%), intestinal obstruction in 1 (1.2%), and miscellaneous causes in 7 (9%) such as wound dehiscence ($n = 4$), feeding jejunostomy or T-tube related complications ($n = 2$), and afferent loop obstruction ($n = 1$). 70 patients were reoperated once, 7 patients twice and 1 patient thrice. The surgical indications and the interventions performed are enumerated in Figure 1.

Of the 53 patients undergoing reoperation for PPH, 41 patients (77.3%) had late bleeds (>24 hours) and 32 patients (60.4%) had extra luminal bleeds. The commonest surgery for PPH was suture ligation of the pancreatic cut surface bleeder which was done in 23 (43%) patients. Nearly 10% of patients operated for PPH had a negative laparotomy as no active source of bleed was identified. The median time to surgery in patients being reoperated for PPH was 5 days (range 0–59 days). 10 of these 53 patients (18.8%) presented with rebleed following first relaparotomy. Among these 10 patients, 4 patients required a second relaparotomy and in 6 patients angiographic embolization was done for gastroduodenal artery ($n = 4$) or right hepatic artery pseudoaneurysm ($n = 2$). The 10 patients reoperated for PEA leak with intra-abdominal collection were done so due to failure of percutaneous drainage or lack of radiological access for the same. 3 patients were reoperated for HJ leak, of which 2 were within 48–72 hours due to right

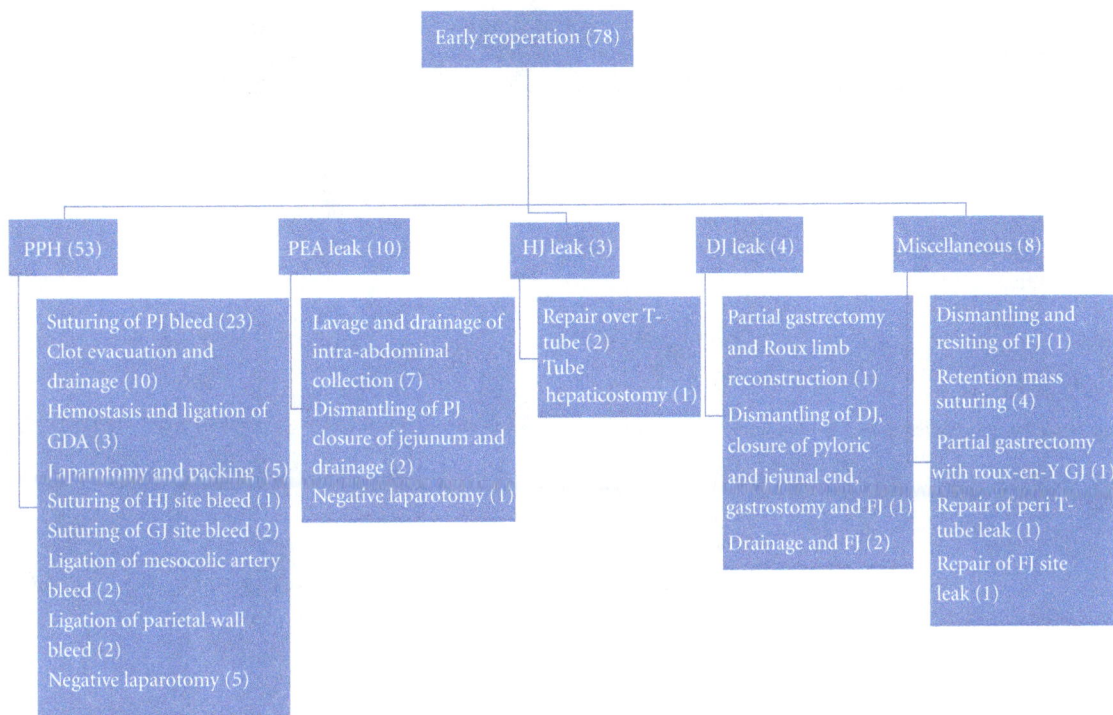

FIGURE 1: Indications of early reoperations and surgeries performed.

TABLE 1: Changes over time.

	1989–2000	2000–2005	2006–2010
Number of pancreaticoduodenectomies	160	132	228
Incidence of PPH	20% (32/160)	24.2% (32/132)	13.1% (30/228)
reoperation rate	17.5% (28/160)	21.2% (28/132)	9.6% (22/228)
Indications for reoperation			
(i) PPH	20	21	12
(ii) PJ leak with intra-abdominal collection	4	4	2
(iii) HJ leak		1	2
(iv) DJ/GJ leak	2		2
(v) Miscellaneous	2	2	4
Overall in-hospital mortality	11.9% (19/160)	9% (12/132)	4.8% (11/228)
In-hospital mortality following early reoperation	42.8% (12/28)	28.5% (8/28)	27.2% (6/22)
In-hospital mortality in patients not undergoing early reoperation	5.3% (7/132)	3.8% (4/104)	2.4% (5/206)

PPH: post pancreatectomy hemorrhage; PJ: pancreaticojejunostomy; HJ: hepaticojejunostomy; DJ: duodenojejunostomy; GJ: gastrojejunostomy.

subhepatic drain showing bile effluent and a third patient was reoperated on postoperative day 24 for persistent bile leak for which a tube hepaticostomy was done. Median postoperative stay following index surgery was significantly longer in patients undergoing early reoperation (25.5 days versus 13 days; $P = 0.000$). The in-hospital mortality was also significantly more in patients undergoing early reoperation (33.3% versus 3.6%; $P = 0.000$). Over the years, the number of pancreaticoduodenectomies performed at our institute has significantly increased. With experience thereby, there has been a reduction in our overall in-hospital mortality rate, incidence of PPH, reoperation rate, and mortality rate following reoperation and this is enumerated in Table 1.

Factors predictive of early reoperation on univariate analysis were preoperative factors such as longer duration of jaundice (>3 months) ($P = 0.051$) and total bilirubin > 10 mg% ($P = 0.010$), intra-operative parameters such as blood loss ($P = 0.001$) and requirement of intra-operative blood transfusion ($P = 0.010$), and occurrence of postoperative complications in the form of PPH ($P = 0.000$), PEA leak ($P = 0.001$), HJ leak ($P = 0.000$), DJ leak ($P = 0.000$), intra-abdominal collection ($P = 0.000$), delayed gastric emptying (DGE) ($P = 0.007$), acute renal failure ($P = 0.000$), and septicemia ($P = 0.000$) Table 2.

On multivariate analysis using the logistic regression model, preoperative duration of jaundice > 3 months

TABLE 2: Univariate analysis of factors predicting the need for early reoperation.

Parameters	Early reoperations ($N = 78$)	Not reoperated early ($N = 442$)	P value
Age in years (median)	52	51.5	0.850
Gender (M/F)	53/25	318/124	0.498
Duration of jaundice > 3 months	21 (27%)	69 (15.6%)	0.051
Comorbidities	17 (21.8%)	111 (25.1%)	0.572
Preoperative hemoglobin (median)	11.0	11.2	0.425
Preoperative albumin (median)	3.5	3.5	0.643
Total bilirubin > 10 mg%	18 (23.1%)	51 (11.5%)	0.010
Preoperative biliary drainage	41 (52.6%)	276 (62.4%)	0.103
Duration of surgery (hours)	7.35	7.0	0.096
Blood loss (mL) (median)	750 mL	500 mL	0.001
Blood transfusion	50 (64.1%)	213 (48.2%)	0.010
Pathology	Malignancy (94%) Ampullary Ca (74%) Benign (6%)	Malignancy (93%) Ampullary Ca (71%) Benign (7%)	0.844
PPH	67.9%	9.3%	0.000
PEA leak	34.6%	14.3%	0.001
HJ leak	24.3%	6.3%	0.000
DJ/GJ leak	14.1%	2.5%	0.000
DGE	21.8%	10.2%	0.007
Intraabdominal collection	43.6%	10.2%	0.000
ARF	11.5%	1.6%	0.000
Septicemia	32%	6.3%	0.000
Postoperative hospital stay (Mean)	25.5 days	13 days	0.000
In-hospital mortality	26 (33.1%)	16 (3.6%)	0.000

PPH: post pancreatectomy hemorrhage; PEA: pancreaticoenteric anastamosis; HJ: hepaticojejunostomy; DJ: duodenojejunostomy; GJ: gastrojejunostomy; DGE: delayed gastric emptying; ARF: acute renal failure.

TABLE 3: Multivariate analysis of factors predicting the need for early reoperation.

Parameter	P value	Exp. (B)	95% CI for Exp. (B)
Duration of jaundice > 3 months	0.019	3.532	1.23–10.147
PPH	0.000	0.101	0.052–0.198
Intraabdominal collection	0.020	0.426	0.200–0.908
DJ/GJ leak	0.041	0.307	0.099–0.0951

PPH: post pancreatectomy hemorrhage; PEA: pancreaticoenteric anastamosis; HJ: hepaticojejunostomy; DJ: duodenojejunostomy; GJ: gastrojejunostomy; DGE: delayed gastric emptying; ARF: acute renal failure.

($P = 0.019$), occurrence of postoperative complications such as PPH ($P = 0.000$), intra-abdominal collection ($P = 0.027$), and DJ/GJ leak ($P = 0.041$) were independently predictive of the need for early reoperations (Table 3).

Of the 26 patients who had postoperative mortality following early reoperation, the underlying cause was PPH in 17 patients, PEA leak and intra-abdominal collection in 6 patients, DJ leak, feeding jejunostomy site leak with peritonitis and acute renal failure in 1 patient each. In the 17 patients who expired following reoperation for PPH, 15 (88%) of them were reoperated for late bleeds (>24 hours following PD). Septic shock with supervening multiorgan failure was the main cause of death in all these patients. Analysis of factors affecting mortality in patients undergoing early reoperation showed that the only significant factor on multivariate analysis was development of postoperative acute renal failure ($P = 0.014$; Exp. (B) = 0.109, 95% CI = 0.020–0.596) defined as an increase in serum creatinine level × 1.5 of the patients baseline or urine output <0.5 mL/kg/h for at least 6 hours.

3.2. Late Reoperations. Twenty four patients underwent late reoperations (16 males; 8 females, median age 47.5 years (range 20–68 years)). Of these 6 patients had also undergone early reoperations, 4 for PPH and 2 for PEA leak with intra-abdominal collection. The indications for late reoperations were complications of index surgery (group 1) ($n = 12$), recurrence of primary disease (group 2) ($n = 8$), complications related to adjuvant radiotherapy (group 3), ($n = 3$) and miscellaneous causes (group 4) ($n = 1$) Table 4. Among the 12 patients in group 1, the predominant number were incisional hernias (4 patients), 2 patients presented

TABLE 4: Indications for late reoperations.

Indications	Number of patients	Surgery performed	Interval between PD and re-operation
Group 1			
Incisional hernia	4	Mesh hernioplasty	8–68 months
Pancreatico-jejunostomy stricture	2	Revision PJ/PG	31/36 months
Adhesive SAIO	2	Band release	16/96 months
HJ stricture	1	Revision HJ	29 months
Persistent gastroparesis	1	Distal gastrectomy	26 months
Enterocutaneous fistula (ECF)	1	Repair of ECF	8 months
Afferent limb perforation with intraabdominal collection	1	Abscess drainage, external drainage of afferent limb perforation, lavage and FJ	21 months
Group 2			
Peritoneal dissemination with SAIO	4	Peritoneal nodule biopsy: 2 Jejunojejunal by pass: 2	5–19 months
Liver metastasis			
(i) Metastatic GIST-2	3	Nonanatomical resection: 1 Right hepatectomy: 1	12/30 months
(ii) Ruptured liver metastasis-1		Lavage and drainage: 1	9 months
Scar site recurrence	1	Wide local excision with mesh repair	16 months
Group 3			
Radiation enteritis, jejunal stricture with SAIO	1	Jejuno-jejunal by pass	9 months
Colonic and afferent loop necrosis	1	Excision of afferent loop, right hemicolectomy, revision roux-en-Y hepaticojejunostomy	21 months
DJ stricture	1	Gastrojejunostomy	128 months
Group 4			
Vascular ectasia of jejunum with upper gastrointestinal bleed	1	Partial gastrectomy, revision gastrojejunostomy, side to side jejunojejunostomy	40 months

SAIO: sub-acute intestinal obstruction; GIST: gastrointestinal stromal tumour; PJ: pancreatico-jejunostomy; PG: pancreatico-gastrostomy; HJ: hepatico-jejunostomy; DJ: duodeno-jejunostomy; FJ: feeding jejunostomy.

with symptoms suggestive post-PD chronic pancreatitis and required a revision pancreatico-enteric anastamosis and are symptom free on long-term follow up. In group 2, 4 patients presented with peritoneal dissemination with subacute intestinal obstruction and of these 2 patients were amenable for a bypass procedure to relieve obstruction. 2 patients with duodenal gastro-intestinal stromal tumours on long-term follow up presented with liver metastasis, in spite of continued imatinib therapy and required a right hepatectomy and a nonanatomic liver resection, respectively. The patient who underwent right hepatectomy expired 5 months later due to extensive metastasis in the remnant liver and the other is alive and disease free 29 months following nonanatomic resection of liver metastasis. One patient in the disease recurrence group presented with intraabdominal hemorrhage following intraperitoneal rupture of liver metastasis and expired in the postoperative period. In group 3, two patients were reoperated for radiation enteritis induced jejunal stricture and DJ stricture and one patient required an emergency relaparotomy for a colonic and afferent jejunal limb necrosis.

The median time to reoperation was 21 months (range 5–128 months) and the median hospital stay was 13 days.

To analyze the impact of reoperation on survival, patients with a minimum follow up of 3 years were included and Kaplan Meier survival curves were generated. 3 year survival of patients undergoing early reoperations ($n = 38$) was compared to those patients not requiring reoperation ($n = 297$). The median survival of patients undergoing reoperation was 20 months and that of those not undergoing reoperation was 23 months. There was no statistical difference in survival between the two groups $P = 0.993$ on log rank analysis (Figure 2). In the late reoperation group ($n = 24$), excluding the 8 patients reoperated for disease recurrence the median survival was 49 months.

4. Discussion

Experience from high volume tertiary care centers around the world has shown a significant decrease in mortality

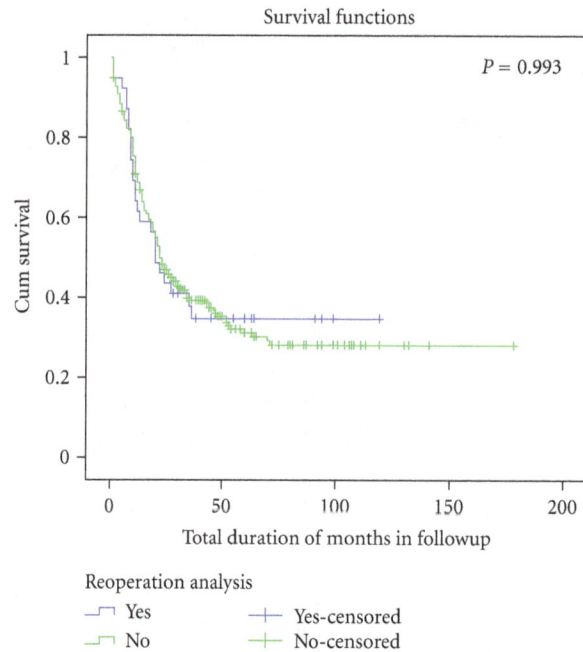

FIGURE 2: Kaplan Meier survival curve. Comparison of 3 year survival of patients undergoing early reoperation versus those patients not requiring reoperation.

following PD over the last couple of decades. Despite a significant decrease in postoperative mortality, PD is still associated with a fairly high postoperative morbidity as reported by various centers in the range of 30–60% [5, 6]. Some of these common postoperative complications including PPH and PEA leak with intra-abdominal collection and associated septic complications may require surgical intervention, despite the widespread availability of endovascular and radiological interventions. This morbidity prolongs hospital stay and results in mortality in a significant proportion of patients. Reoperative surgery after PD is a difficult undertaking and the reoperation itself may be the cause of further morbidity and mortality [7]. Due to increasing long-term survival of patients undergoing PD for periampullary carcinoma, some may on long-term follow up develop complications that may need intervention. These complications may be related to the complications of primary surgical procedure, recurrence of the primary disease per se, and/or complications of adjuvant radiotherapy.

Reoperation rates in series dealing with pancreatic head resection have varied from 4–11% [7]. Recent studies by Standop et al. and Shukla et al. dealing specifically with operative reinterventions have also shown similar rates [7, 8]. In the present series, we had an overall reoperation rate of 18.5%. With increasing experience and better access to interventional radiological expertise, our reoperation rate has significantly decreased to 7.4% over the last 5 years.

PPH is one of the grave complications following PD and occurs in 2–20% of patients as reported by various series [9–11]. Our overall incidence of PPH following PD is 18% but this has decreased to 13% over the past 5 years. Although an uncommon occurrence, hemorrhage following PD has been associated with high mortality ranging from 14% to 56% [12–14]. Indeed, hemorrhage is an important predictor of prognosis and mortality in patients with PEA leak. According to the International Study Group of Pancreatic Surgery classification, the management of PPH depends on various factors like time of onset of bleed (early versus late), location (intraluminal versus extra-luminal), and severity of bleed (mild versus severe) [15].

PPH was the predominant cause of early reoperation in our subset of patients similar to that reported by the other series [7, 8]. Overall 56% (53 of 94) of our patients with PPH underwent relaparotomy for the same. The number of reoperations for PPH in our series has reduced by 25% (from 65% to 40%) in the past 5 years due to better use of endovascular coil embolization. Our higher overall reoperation rate for PPH is due to the fact that all patients with early PPH and hemodynamic instability undergo relaparotomy and lower threshold for reoperation in delayed presentation of PPH in event of delay in the interventional radiology back up because of pre-occupation. The aggressive use of surgical intervention for management of delayed presentation of PPH in our study is similar to that reported by de Castro et al. [9], who preferred surgical intervention over embolization for management for the delayed massive hemorrhage following major pancreatic or biliary surgery. The basic principles of relaparotomy surgery are hemostasis and wide drainage. One of the important causes of hemorrhage in our experience as previously published and also in the present series has been a bleeding pancreatic stump following an intact or a disrupted pancreatic anastomosis [13]. Bleeding from the pancreatic stump can present as intra-abdominal bleed manifesting through the intra-abdominal drains due to secondary disruption of the PEA or can present as intra-luminal bleed in the form of hematemesis or hemorrhagic aspirate in the nasogastric tube. This can be localized preoperatively by evidence of brisk bleeding from afferent loop of jejunum on endoscopy. A significant proportion of our patients who present with an intraluminal bleed have a pancreatic cut surface bleeder and hence are not amenable for endoscopic management thereby requiring relaparotomy. The management options are variable depending upon whether the PEA is intact or not. In a wide anastomotic disruption with a bleeding pancreatic stump, direct suturing should be done to achieve hemostasis. In an occasional patient without significant disruption of the anastomosis serial jejunal clamping may indicate the segment of the bowel from which the bleeding is originating and hemostasis can then be achieved by suturing through an appropriately placed enterotomy [16]. If at surgery the site of hemorrhage is not found and the stumps of ligated vessels have been carefully inspected, then enterotomy should be considered to look at one or more of the several suture lines, which may be the source of bleeding. In addition to local hemostasis, it is of utmost importance to drain all the adjacent collections and abscesses, as these may lead to further episodes of rebleed due to erosion of adjacent vascular structures. It may not always be possible to achieve adequate surgical control due to diffuse nature of the ooze from the operative site raw area or retroperitoneum. In such cases, abdominal packing can be done as temporizing measure and planned relaparotomies can be done once the patient has stabilized and the coagulation abnormalities have been corrected. The problems encountered with surgery for rebleed are two-fold; first intraoperatively it may not be always possible to identify the site of bleed due to difficult access in the presence of dense adhesion, friable, and inflamed tissues and secondly a small percentage of patients may require a second relaparotomy or a prophylactic embolization of the common hepatic or splenic artery after surgery to prevent the occurrence of rebleed [10, 13].

The second commonest cause of reoperation after PPH was PEA leak with intra-abdominal collection. Majority of these collections can be managed successfully by percutaneously placed drains under image guidance [17]. Relaparotomy is occasionally required in some patients due to failure of percutaneous drainage or lack of radiological access for the same in the presence of persisting sepsis. Disrupted PEA can be dealt with in one of the following ways. Resuturing has been attempted by some but it invariably fails in the presence of edematous friable tissues. Others, including us, are in favour of dismantling the anastamosis completely, closing the

jejunal loop and providing drainage of the pancreatic duct, often with a laparostomy to ensure free drainage [13, 18]. This invariably leads to a pancreatic fistula but free drainage helps in controlling the sepsis. Still others have successfully opted for a completion total pancreatectomy to remove the focus of sepsis altogether [19]. Regardless of the surgical procedure chosen, it is of utmost importance to drain all collections and abscesses. Preoperative CT scan is a good guide to locate these collections in the presence of adjacent inflamed and friable tissues.

Bilioenteric anastomotic leak is very uncommon following PD and the management is usually conservative [20]. Surgery is indicated in those patients presenting with bilious effluent in the drain early in the postoperative period, that is, within 48 hours. This is usually due to a technical problem and surgical correction of the same would lead to faster recovery and avoid the development of a strictured HJ. Deficiency of gastro-jejunostomy or duodeno-jejunostomy is very rare following PD. Some of these patients can present with an enterocutaneous fistula, which can be very difficult to manage due to the high output, persistent nature of the fistula, and associated pancreatic enzymatic leak. Revision surgery in the form of a revision roux- en-Y reconstruction or just a simple drainage with a feeding access can be done in these patients. Other infrequent indications of relaparotomy after PD are complete dehiscence of the laparotomy wound with evisceration which would need meticulous closure with interrupted sutures accompanied by retention mass sutures. Feeding jejunostomy related complications requiring relaparotomy were seen in a couple of patients in the present series. Albeit a simple procedure, FJ related complications can be catastrophic in some patients and hence the feeding access of choice in our patients is an intraoperatively placed nasojejunal tube.

Various surgical series have looked into the factors predictive of the occurrence of complications following PD. Some of them are presence of associated medical risk factors, need for preoperative biliary drainage, texture of remnant pancreas, and size of pancreatic duct [21–23]. The factors that were more frequently associated with early reoperation on multivariate analysis in the present study were longer preoperative duration of jaundice (>3 months), postoperative occurrence of complications such as PPH, presence of intra-abdominal collections, and leakage of alimentary tract reconstructions. Patients with longer duration of preoperative jaundice are more nutritionally depleted due to prolonged poor oral intake which thereby leads to increased postoperative complications [24].

Overall mortality following PD significantly increases after early reoperation, and is in the range of 13–60% as shown by Standop et al. [7], which included pooled data from various studies. Recent single institution series from Standop et al. [7] and Shukla et al. [8] dealing specifically with early reoperation have shown a significantly decreased mortality rate of 11.7% and 13%, respectively. Although our overall mortality rate is 33.3% following reoperation, this has decreased from 35.7% in the initial 16 years to 27.2% in the past 5 years. This can be attributed to the lower overall incidence of PPH, lesser number of patients being reoperated for PPH, and increased use of interventional radiology techniques for management of post-PD complications. Though non-surgical management options for PPH like endovascular coiling or stenting and endoscopic interventions cause lesser physiological insult, they have not been conclusively shown to be better than relaparotomy in terms of the success rate for management of delayed PPH [25, 26]. de Castro et al. [9] who favored surgical reintervention over embolization for the management of patients presenting with delayed hemorrhage following PD, reported an overall mortality of 22% but 5 of the 16 patients (31%) who underwent surgical re-intervention in their series expired in the postoperative period due to sepsis. A recent meta-analysis and a systematic review on the management of delayed PPH by Limongelli et al. [25] and Roulin et al. [26] have shown high mortality rates of 43% and 47%, respectively, following relaparotomy for PPH. This is similar to our study where the mortality rate following reoperation for late presentation of PPH was 36% (15 of 41). Roulin et al. [26] in their systematic review in addition showed that there was a statistically significant difference in favour of interventional radiology in term of mortality after PPH compared to relaparotomy. Although surgical intervention is very successful for the management of PPH, most of the patients presenting with late bleeds have underlying sepsis which contributes to the increased incidence of morbidity and mortality in them.

Due to improved long-term survival of patients with nonpancreatic periampullary carcinoma as compared to pancreatic cancer, quite a few patients present on long-term follow up with complications related to the index surgery or disease recurrence which may be amenable to surgical intervention. With the increasing use of adjuvant radiotherapy to gain better local control and thereby improve disease-free survival, patients may require intervention for complications of the same. Excluding patients with malignant pancreatic neuroendocrine tumours, this issue has been very sparsely addressed in the literature with most of them being occasional case reports or short case series [27, 28].

The indications for late reoperations are varied. Patients undergoing second surgery for complications related to recurrence of primary disease following PD other than those with malignant neuroendocrine tumours usually have a relatively poor outcome even after resectional surgery for local or distant recurrences as shown by Nakano et al. and Fujii et al. [28, 29]. Excluding these patients, those presenting with late complications related to PD or complications of adjuvant radiotherapy can be managed successfully with good long-term outcome.

Early reoperation had no impact on 3 year survival of patients in our series. This is in contrast to that reported by Yeo et al. in the 1990s, in which they showed that in addition to the tumour pathologic characteristics, the addition of reoperation had a negative impact on long-term survival of patients undergoing PD for periampullary carcinoma [30]. The detrimental effect of postoperative complications on the long-term survival of patients undergoing PD for pancreatic cancer has been a matter of controversy [31, 32]. In the present study-patients surviving the initial insult of early reoperations had similar long-term survival rates to those who did not undergo an early reoperation.

5. Conclusion

In this study, 18.5% of patients were reoperated following PD. The two main indications for early reoperation were PPH (68%) and PEA leak with associated intra-abdominal collection (13%). Reoperation for PPH is usually indicated in patients with early presentation of PPH (<24 hours) or delayed presentation of PPH where angiographic embolization is not feasible or successful. Early reoperation when used judiciously in conjunction with arterial coil embolization continues to be an important tool in the armamentarium for the management of PPH in the present era. Although in-hospital mortality in this subset of patients was high (33.3%), this is largely due to the associated sepsis rather than insult of the reoperation. Early reoperation did not have a bearing on long-term survival ($P = 0.993$). On long-term follow up patients presenting with complications related to PD or adjuvant radiotherapy can be managed with good outcome.

Disclosure

This paper was presented as a poster at the joint conference of the International Association of Pancreatology and the Indian Pancreas Club, February 10th–13th, 2011, Cochin, India.

References

[1] C. M. Halloran, P. Ghaneh, L. Bosonnet, M. N. Hartley, R. Sutton, and J. P. Neoptolemos, "Complications of pancreatic cancer resection," *Digestive Surgery*, vol. 19, no. 2, pp. 138–146, 2002.

[2] S. Connor, "Haemorrhage following pancreatoduodenectomy: the importance of surgery," *Digestive Surgery*, vol. 23, no. 4, pp. 201–202, 2006.

[3] R. C. I. van Geenen, T. M. van Gulik, O. R. C. Busch, L. T. de Wit, H. Obertop, and D. J. Gouma, "Readmissions after pancreatoduodenectomy," *British Journal of Surgery*, vol. 88, no. 11, pp. 1467–1471, 2001.

[4] D. M. Emick, T. S. Riall, J. L. Cameron et al., "Hospital readmission after pancreaticoduodenectomy," *Journal of Gastrointestinal Surgery*, vol. 10, no. 9, pp. 1243–1253, 2006.

[5] C. Gouillat and J. F. Gigot, "Pancreatic surgical complications—the case for prophylaxis," *Gut*, vol. 49, supplement 4, pp. iv32–iv39, 2001.

[6] J. P. Simons, S. A. Shah, S. C. Ng, G. F. Whalen, and J. F. Tseng, "National complication rates after pancreatectomy: beyond mere mortality," *Journal of Gastrointestinal Surgery*, vol. 13, no. 10, pp. 1798–1805, 2009.

[7] J. Standop, T. Glowka, V. Schmitz et al., "Operative re-intervention following pancreatic head resection: indications and outcome," *Journal of Gastrointestinal Surgery*, vol. 13, no. 8, pp. 1503–1509, 2009.

[8] P. J. Shukla, S. G. Barreto, K. M. Mohandas, and S. V. Shrikhande, "Defining the role of surgery for complications after pancreatoduodenectomy," *ANZ Journal of Surgery*, vol. 79, no. 1-2, pp. 33–37, 2009.

[9] S. M. M. de Castro, K. F. D. Kuhlmann, O. R. C. Busch et al., "Delayed massive hemorrhage after pancreatic and biliary surgery: embolization or surgery?" *Annals of Surgery*, vol. 241, no. 1, pp. 85–91, 2005.

[10] E. F. Yekebas, L. Wolfram, G. Cataldegirmen et al., "Post-pancreatectomy hemorrhage: diagnosis and treatment—an analysis in 1669 consecutive pancreatic resections," *Annals of Surgery*, vol. 246, no. 2, pp. 269–280, 2007.

[11] P. Limongelli, S. E. Khorsandi, M. Pai et al., "Management of delayed postoperative hemorrhage after pancreaticoduodenectomy: a meta-analysis," *Archives of Surgery*, vol. 143, no. 10, pp. 1001–1007, 2008.

[12] S. H. Choi, H. J. Moon, J. S. Heo, J. W. Joh, and Y. I. Kim, "Delayed hemorrhage after pancreaticoduodenectomy," *Journal of the American College of Surgeons*, vol. 199, no. 2, pp. 186–191, 2004.

[13] P. Balachandran, S. S. Sikora, R. V. Raghavendra Rao, A. Kumar, R. Saxena, and V. K. Kapoor, "Haemorrhagic complications of pancreaticoduodenectomy," *ANZ Journal of Surgery*, vol. 74, no. 11, pp. 945–950, 2004.

[14] I. Koukoutsis, R. Bellagamba, G. Morris-Stiff et al., "Haemorrhage following pancreaticoduodenectomy: risk factors and the importance of sentinel bleed," *Digestive Surgery*, vol. 23, no. 4, pp. 224–228, 2006.

[15] M. N. Wente, J. A. Veit, C. Bassi et al., "Postpancreatectomy hemorrhage (PPH): an International Study Group of Pancreatic Surgery (ISGPS) definition," *Surgery*, vol. 142, no. 1, pp. 20–25, 2007.

[16] M. N. Wente, S. V. Shrikhande, J. Kleeff et al., "Management of early hemorrhage from pancreatic anastomoses after pancreaticoduodenectomy," *Digestive Surgery*, vol. 23, no. 4, pp. 203–208, 2006.

[17] D. A. Gervais, C. Fernandez-Del Castillo, M. J. O'Neill, P. F. Hahn, and P. R. Mueller, "Complications after pancreato-duodenectomy: imaging and imaging-guided interventional procedures," *Radiographics*, vol. 21, no. 3, pp. 673–690, 2001.

[18] Y. W. Tien, P. H. Lee, C. Y. Yang, M. C. Ho, and Y. F. Chiu, "Risk factors of massive bleeding related to pancreatic leak after pancreaticoduodenectomy," *Journal of the American College of Surgeons*, vol. 201, no. 4, pp. 554–559, 2005.

[19] M. I. van Berge Henegouwen, L. T. de Wit, T. M. van Gulik, H. Obertop, and D. J. Gouma, "Incidence, risk factors, and treatment of pancreatic leakage after pancreaticoduodenectomy: drainage versus resection of the pancreatic remnant," *Journal of the American College of Surgeons*, vol. 185, no. 1, pp. 18–24, 1997.

[20] S. M. M. de Castro, K. F. D. Kuhlmann, O. R. C. Busch et al., "Incidence and management of biliary leakage after hepatico-jejunostomy," *Journal of Gastrointestinal Surgery*, vol. 9, no. 8, pp. 1163–1173, 2005.

[21] J. W. Lin, J. L. Cameron, C. J. Yeo, T. S. Riall, and K. D. Lillemoe, "Risk factors and outcomes in postpancreaticoduodenectomy pancreaticocutaneous fistula," *Journal of Gastrointestinal Surgery*, vol. 8, no. 8, pp. 951–959, 2004.

[22] N. A. van der Gaag, E. A. J. Rauws, C. H. J. van Eijck et al., "Preoperative biliary drainage for cancer of the head of the pancreas," *New England Journal of Medicine*, vol. 362, no. 2, pp. 129–137, 2010.

[23] Y. M. Yang, X. D. Tian, Y. Zhuang, W. M. Wang, Y. L. Wan, and Y. T. Huang, "Risk factors of pancreatic leakage after pancreaticoduodenectomy," *World Journal of Gastroenterology*, vol. 11, no. 16, pp. 2456–2461, 2005.

[24] T. S. Yeh, Y. Y. Jan, L. B. Jeng et al., "Pancreaticojejunal anastomotic leak after pancreaticoduodenectomy—multivariate analysis of perioperative risk factors," *Journal of Surgical Research*, vol. 67, no. 2, pp. 119–125, 1997.

[25] P. Limongelli, S. E. Khorsandi, M. Pai et al., "Management of delayed postoperative hemorrhage after pancreaticoduodenectomy: a meta-analysis," *Archives of Surgery*, vol. 143, no. 10, pp. 1001–1007, 2008.

[26] D. Roulin, Y. Cerantola, N. Demartines, and M. Schäfer, "Systematic review of delayed postoperative hemorrhage after pancreatic resection," *Journal of Gastrointestinal Surgery*, vol. 15, no. 6, pp. 1055–1062, 2011.

[27] D. Jaeck, E. Oussoultzoglou, P. Bachellier et al., "Hepatic metastases of gastroenteropancreatic neuroendocrine tumors: safe hepatic surgery," *World Journal of Surgery*, vol. 25, no. 6, pp. 689–692, 2001.

[28] H. Nakano, T. Asakura, S. Koizumi et al., "Second surgery after a pancreaticoduodenectomy in patients with periampullary malignancies," *Hepato-Gastroenterology*, vol. 55, no. 82-83, pp. 687–691, 2008.

[29] K. Fujii, J. Yamamoto, K. Shimada, T. Kosuge, S. Yamasaki, and Y. Kanai, "Resection of liver metastases after pancreatoduodenectomy: report of seven cases," *Hepato-Gastroenterology*, vol. 46, no. 28, pp. 2429–2433, 1999.

[30] C. J. Yeo, J. L. Cameron, T. A. Sohn et al., "Six hundred fifty consecutive pancreaticoduodenectomies in the 1990s: pathology, complications, and outcomes," *Annals of Surgery*, vol. 226, no. 3, pp. 248–260, 1997.

[31] C. M. Kang, D. H. Kim, G. H. Choi, K. S. Kim, J. S. Choi, and W. J. Lee, "Detrimental effect of postoperative complications on oncologic efficacy of R0 pancreatectomy in ductal adenocarcinoma of the pancreas," *Journal of Gastrointestinal Surgery*, vol. 13, no. 5, pp. 907–914, 2009.

[32] F. Ausania, N. Cook, N. Jamieson, E. Huguet, A. Jah, and R. Praseedom, "Impact of pancreatic leaks on survival following pancreaticoduodenectomy," *Journal of the Pancreas*, vol. 11, no. 3, pp. 226–229, 2010.

15

Ductal Carcinoma In Situ of the Breast: A Surgical Perspective

Mohammed Badruddoja

Department of Surgical Oncology, Rehabilitation Associates of Northern Illinois, Rockford, IL 61111, USA

Correspondence should be addressed to Mohammed Badruddoja, badruddoja@hotmail.com

Academic Editor: Bernando Bonanni

Ductal carcinoma in situ (DCIS) of the breast is a heterogeneous neoplasm with invasive potential. Risk factors include age, family history, hormone replacement therapy, genetic mutation, and patient lifestyle. The incidence of DCIS has increased due to more widespread use of screening and diagnostic mammography; almost 80% of cases are diagnosed with imaging with final diagnosis established by biopsy and histological examination. There are various classification systems used for DCIS, the most recent of which is based on the presence of intraepithelial neoplasia of the ductal epithelium (DIN). A number of molecular assays are now available that can identify high-risk patients as well as help establish the prognosis of patients with diagnosed DCIS. Current surgical treatment options include total mastectomy, simple lumpectomy in very low-risk patients, and lumpectomy with radiation. Adjuvant therapy is tailored based on the molecular profile of the neoplasm and can include aromatase inhibitors, anti-estrogen, anti-progesterone (or a combination of antiestrogen and antiprogesterone), and HER2 neu suppression therapy. Chemopreventive therapies are under investigation for DCIS, as are various molecular-targeted drugs. It is anticipated that new biologic agents, when combined with hormonal agents such as SERMs and aromatase inhibitors, may one day prevent all forms of breast cancer.

1. Introduction

Ductal carcinoma in situ (DCIS) of the breast is a noninvasive carcinoma with a wide spectrum of disease, ranging from low-grade to high-grade malignancy with foci of invasive malignancy. Histologically, DCIS is characterized by a proliferation of malignant cells in the ductal epithelium that are confined to the basement membrane and are not invading the normal breast parenchyma.

2. Epidemiology

Prior to advent of mammography, the diagnosis of DCIS was established only after excision of palpable lumps and histological examination of the tissue. Egan et al. [1], a radiologist based at the MD Anderson Cancer Center in Houston, Texas, is credited as the inventor of mammography in the late 1960s. By 1975, the widespread use of this imaging technique not only resulted in early detection of lesions in the breast but also led to a 60–70% reduction in morbidity and mortality from malignant diseases of breast [2]. The adoption of screening and diagnostic mammography resulted in an increase in the incidence of DCIS worldwide, with 80% of DCIS diagnosed by mammography. Currently, DCIS accounts for 20–25% of all newly diagnosed cases of breast cancer [3] and 17–34% of mammographically detected breast neoplasms [4, 5]. Approximately 1 of every 1300 screening mammograms results in a diagnosis of DCIS, and over 62,000 new cases of DCIS were diagnosed in 2009 [6].

Between 1983 and 2000 in the United States, there was a 500% increase in DCIS among women ≥50 years of age, though the incidence decreased by 2005 [7, 8]. Among women <50 years of age, DCIS incidence increased 290%

from 1983 to 2003, followed by a continuous decline that was most likely due to a reduction in the use of hormone replacement therapy [9]. Virnig et al. [10] showed that the incidence of DCIS markedly increased from 5.8 per 100,000 women in the 1970s to 32.5 per 100,000 women in 2004, but then plateaued. DCIS is not common in younger women (<30 years of age). The risk of DCIS is 0.6 per 100,000 women 49–60 years of age, and increases to 1.4 per 100,000 women 70–84 years of age.

The risk of death from DCIS is very low; for women who were diagnosed between 1984 and 1989, the 10-year risk was 1.9% based on data from the National Cancer Institute (NCI) Surveillance, Epidemiology, and End Results (SEER) database [11]. The estimated incidence of DCIS was 32.5 per 100,000 women in 2004, based on NCI SEER data from 1975–2004. This is considerably higher than that reported in 1975 (5.8% per 100,000), but is consistent with the findings of the Swedish Two-County trial [12].The same trend is noted in numerous studies [13, 14]. In summary, there has been an overall increase in the incidence of DCIS in women after the age of 50 around the globe. This increase could be due to a greater awareness among women about breast malignancy, an increase in screening or diagnostic mammograms, the selective use of magnetic resonance imaging (MRI) in high-risk patients, or the use of genetic markers to identify high-risk patients, which will be discussed in detail below.

3. Risk Factors for DCIS

There are multiple risk factors for development of DCIS, including demographic, reproductive, biological, and behavioral risk factors. It is clear that the incidence of DCIS, like invasive carcinoma, is related to age. Incidence increases after the age of 50 years; several studies have shown that the incidence is 2.5 per 100,000 for women 30–40 years of age and steadily increases to a peak of 96.7 per 100,000 women 65–69 years of age. The incidence of DCIS is highest in Caucasian women compared with African American and Asians and Pacific Islanders, with the lowest incidence in Hispanics [15]. Prior to 1973, there were no data on the incidence of DCIS in urban and rural populations; however, one study showed that while the incidence of DCIS was increasing in both populations, the incidence was higher in urban women compared with rural women [16]. Another study showed that DCIS is also more prevalent in women who are less educated, particularly those with no high school degree [17]. One Australian study showed that the incidence of DCIS was 7.3% in those with relatively higher incomes compared to 4.5% in those with lower incomes.

Older age at menopause was associated with a higher incidence of DCIS [19]. One study showed that peri- and postmenopausal women had higher incidences of DCIS compared with premenopausal women [20]. The study, which was based on the Connecticut Tumor Registry, showed that there was a significant relationship between an increased risk of developing DCIS and older age at menopause; women who reached menopause after the age of 50 years had a higher risk of developing DCIS compared to those who reached menopause before the age of 45 years [20]. These

findings are consistent with the likely role that hormone status plays in determining DCIS risk. A large prospective study from the United Kingdom reported a 56% increase in the risk of developing DCIS in women taking hormone replacement therapy (HRT), with the risk increasing with the duration of HRT [21]. Compared to those who never received HRT, women who took HRT for less than 5 years had significantly lower risk of DCIS. While the Iowa Women's Health Study found that there was no increased risk of DCIS in women who received HRT compared with those who did not [22], a subsequent metaanalysis found that women who had previously taken HRT had a higher risk of developing DCIS [22]. However, women who had used oral contraceptives (OCs) or were current users were found to have the same risk of DCIS as those who had never used OCs [23]. Nulliparity or women who had a late pregnancy (after 30 years of age) also had a higher incidence of DCIS [24]. Similar results were reported in a Danish cohort study [25]. Recently, the National Research Council of Australia published a summary of the evidence on HRT and the risk of breast cancer [26]. Only estrogen, combined estrogen-progesterone, combined estrogen-testosterone, and Tibolone are used for HRT. In women 50–79 years of age, the absolute risk of breast cancer is 38 per 100,000 for those taking combined estrogen and progestin (average over 5 years) compared with 30 per 100,000 for those who have never used combined HRT. It is not possible to accurately determine the duration of HRT after which breast cancer risk is increased; however, HRT for more than 3 years appears to be associated with an increased risk [27]. The Women's Health Initiative trial also showed that there is significant risk of developing breast cancer in women who had prior exposure to combined HRT for more than 6 years, while there is no overall increase in the incidence of breast cancer in women who were never exposed to HRT [28]. There are only inconsistent reports regarding the risk of breast cancer and the use of estrogen-only HRT. In one study, short-term use of estrogen-only HRT did not increase the risk of breast cancer [29]. In the Nurses Health Study, the risk of breast cancer was increased significantly in women with prior hysterectomy after 20 years or more of HRT, and the relative risk was higher for estrogen receptor (ER)+/progesterone receptor (PR)+ cancers [30]. One prospective study reported that combined use of estrogen and testosterone HRT in postmenopausal women increases the risk of breast cancer by 17% per year [31]. In the LIFT study of older postmenopausal women with low bone mineral density, breast cancer risk was decreased in the group receiving Tibolone compared with placebo; however, the study was terminated early due to an increased incidence of stroke [32]. There does not appear to be a significant difference in the risk of breast cancer based on the route of HRT administration (e.g., transdermal, oral, implant [33]).

A history of benign biopsied breast disease is associated with a higher risk of breast cancer [34]. In addition, the same study indicated that high intake of vitamin A and alcohol increases the risk of breast cancer. Obesity and increases in BMI by 25% are also risk factors for breast cancer. In a study conducted in Alberta, Canada, by Friedenreich and colleagues, increased physical activity decreased the serum levels of all sex hormones [35], previously sedentary post-menopausal women who adhered to a moderate-to-vigorous intensity exercise program showed decreases in serum levels of estrogen, progesterone, testosterone, and sex hormone binding globulin and had a lower risk of postmenopausal breast cancer. In addition, the exercise program led to weight loss which also contributed to the decrease in breast cancer risk.

Mammographic detection of increased density of breast tissue is also a risk factor for breast cancer. In a recent study by Boyd and colleagues, women with 75% or higher density on a mammogram had an increased risk of breast cancer compared with women with mammograms with less than 10% density [36]. Women with extensive mammographic density detected between screening tests are also at high risk of developing DCIS, and considerable number of DCIS cases are associated with this single risk factor. Thus, high-risk patients who have dense breast tissue detected by mammogram should have a follow-up MRI of the breast so that lesions are not missed.

Observational studies have suggested that beta carotene, vegetables, fruits, and antioxidants may have protective effects against breast cancer. However, a recent randomized controlled trial found no such protective effects of a diet supplemented with beta carotene, vitamin C and E, fruits, and other antioxidants [37]. This trial followed 624 women for a period of 9.4 years and found that compared to placebo group, the relative risks of developing breast cancer were 1.11% in vitamin C group, 0.79% in vitamin E group, and 1% in beta carotene group. The Iowa Study showed that aspirin and nonsteroidal anti-inflammatory drugs (NSAIDs) have a protective effect against breast cancer [38]. An animal and in vitro study also showed that aspirin not only prevents breast cancer, but also prevents metastasis in breast cancer [39].This was a prospective observational study in which 4164 female patients with stage I, II, or III breast carcinoma were followed for 26 years [39]. The relative adjusted risk of metastasis in those who took aspirin for 1 day, 2 to 5 days, and 6 to 7 days per week compared with those who did not take aspirin were 1.07 (95% CI, 0.70 to 1.63), 0.29 (95% CI, 0.16 to 0.52), and 0.36 (95% CI, 0.24 to 0.54), respectively. The most recent study, based on a systematic comparison of evidence from observational studies, indicated that daily aspirin intake not only prevents colorectal cancer, but also prevents breast, esophageal, biliary, and gastric cancer [40]. The study also showed that aspirin prevents and delays metastasis from breast, esophageal, gastric, and hepatobiliary cancer.

4. Diagnosis

Diagnosis of DCIS is primarily based on imaging results in developed countries of the world, while developing and or underdeveloped countries of the world continue to rely on excision and histologic analysis of the tissue biopsy. This disparity is due to the lack of screening facilities and imaging equipment, lack of funding, and cultural barriers in certain developing and underdeveloped countries [41]. In these

countries, only 20% of ductal carcinomas are diagnosed on clinical examination and 80% of patients present to the clinician with a palpable lump, nipple discharge, or skin change over the breast [42]. Very recently, the US Cancer Prevention Task Force made a very cautionary remark regarding the overuse of imaging studies (i.e., mammography) for evaluation of diseases of breast [43]; however, even with such cautionary remarks, mammography remains the gold standard for diagnosis of breast diseases. Clinicians continue to advocate for yearly screening mammography in low-risk or non-risk patients after the age of 50 years and in high-risk patients before age of 40 years. Nevertheless, there is concern about radiation exposure during screening mammography. Advances in digital mammography have led to a 22% reduction in radiation exposure compared with film mammography [44]. While digital mammography is more expensive than film mammography, some claim that digital mammography is able to detect more lesions. In one study [45], the detection rate of each modality is same, but the sensitivity and specificity of digital versus film mammography vary with age, tumor characteristics, breast density, and menopausal status. The detection rate was higher with digital mammography than film mammography in women between the ages of 60 and 69 years (89.5% versus. 83%; $P = 0.014$) and in those with ER+ cancers. Clinicians and radiologists will have to decide which imaging study is appropriate for an individual patient.

MRI is used frequently after the detection of lesions by digital or screening mammography, primarily because MRI can help guide surgical decision making among the possible options—breast conserving surgery, mastectomy, or bilateral mastectomy. Surgical decision making is based on the multicentricity of the disease, tumor size, status of the contralateral breast, and family history. The accuracy of MRI over mammography in evaluating the first 3 factors defines its clinical value. In addition, MRI has a higher diagnostic accuracy for DCIS compared with either film or digital mammography. Riedl and colleagues [46] studied 672 imaging rounds in a high-risk population and found that the detection rate of DCIS by mammography, ultrasound (US), and MRI were 50%, 42.9%, and 85.7%, respectively. This detection rate is similarly high for both in invasive cancer and preinvasive cancer (DCIS). Based on their findings, the authors recommended that MRI should be included in the imaging of high-risk patients. Kuhl and colleagues [47] performed a retrospective study and found that the detection rate of DCIS is 92% by MRI and 56% by mammography, and that 48% of high-grade DCIS are missed on mammography but detected by MRI.

Collectively, the literature reports that MRI is able to detect multicentric lesions, estimate the size of the tumor, and predict the invasive nature of the lesion. Hwang and colleagues [48] found that MRI has 94% sensitivity in detecting multicentric lesions compared to mammography, which has 38% sensitivity. In a similar study, Menell and colleagues [49] found that the sensitivity of MRI and mammography for detecting multicentric lesions in DCIS are 94% and 38%, respectively. However, in another study of 86 women, Santamaría and colleagues [50] did not find any difference in sensitivity between MRI and mammography for detecting multicentric lesions in DCIS, but did report a higher performance of MRI than mammography. Hollingsworth and Stough [51] reported that the incidence of occult multicentric disease in DCIS was 6.3% and could be detected by MRI. Multicentricity is defined as a lesion 5.0 cm from the index lesion or discontinuous growth into another quadrant of the breast [52]. Assessment of the growth patterns of DCIS during tissue processing and histologically based tumor measurements are difficult, as the three-dimensional (3-D) extent of the disease must be reconstructed using 2-D pathology slides. For this reason, MRI measurements of tumor size may be more accurate than pathologic measurements. Uematsu and colleagues [53] found that MRI measurement of DCIS is more accurate than mammographic measurement of the extent of disease, and Lehman and colleagues [54] reported that the sensitivity rate of MRI in detecting contralateral DCIS is 77%. Interestingly, MRI results led to biopsy of the contralateral breast in 18 patients, of which only 28% were positive.

Ultrasound (US) also plays a significant role in diagnosis of DCIS. Gwak et al. [55] conducted a retrospective study of US for detecting DCIS and found that US is more accurate than mammography. In a similar study by Moon et al. [56], DCIS detected by US that has speculated margins, marked hypoechogenicity, thick echogenic margin, and posterior acoustic shadowing is highly suggestive of invasion.

The literature shows that each and every imaging technique available for detecting DCIS has pitfalls and limitations, but each technique also complements one other. Clinicians and radiologists will need to decide which imaging technique is appropriate for their particular patient, taking into consideration her age, family history, and other risk factors. It must be pointed out, however, that MRI is very expensive; in the United States, the average cost of a breast MRI is $5000.00 [57]. For this reason, the indications for preoperative MRI for the diagnosis of breast diseases are clearly stated in the literature and guidelines and ensure that only selected patients undergo breast MRI [58].

Complete physical examination is mandatory after discovery of a possible lesion or lesions on an imaging study; however, the ultimate diagnosis of the lesion still depends on the histology of a biopsy specimen. Currently, the 3 most popular methods of biopsy are needle biopsy, core needle biopsy (CNB), and vacuum-assisted biopsy. Fine-needle aspiration (FNA) is not adequate to establish a diagnosis of DCIS [59]. With advances in imaging, CNB can now be performed as a US-guided or stereotactic procedure by the radiologist. CNB is the best method for establishing the histologic diagnosis of DCIS. Vacuum-assisted biopsy has a high specificity and sensitivity, but may still miss a diagnosis of DCIS in 17% of cases [60].

Prior to image-guided biopsy, needle localization excisional biopsy was a very common practice for treating DCIS. This technique has the advantages of completion of therapy, provided a negative margin is obtained, and is therefore highly cost effective [61]. However, this method is rarely used today for treating DCIS.

Preoperative variables of CNB for diagnosis of DCIS are significantly associated with under-staging of the disease and include experience of the operator, biopsy device, guidance method, size, mammographic features, and palpability of the neoplasm [62]. Based on these variables, 25% of DCIS may have invasive carcinoma and the treatment plan may change. The best approach is to take multiple samples during CNB in order to establish an appropriate histologic diagnosis. CNB specimens must have adequate tissue so that the pathologist can determine the prognostic factors, degree of invasiveness based on nuclear grading, presence or absence of necrosis, mitotic figure, hormonal status of the lesion, and the presence of molecular markers.

5. Pathologic Classification

DCIS is not a single entity, but rather a spectrum of disease; in essence, it refers to malignant change in the ductal epithelium. Because of the heterogenicity of DCIS lesions, no single satisfactory pathological classification system has been adopted. The traditional classification system is based on morphology, architecture, and nuclear grading of the lesion [63], as well as on the presence or absence of necrosis. Silverstein et al. [64] proposed the division of DCIS into 3 groups: high grade, non-high grade with comedonecrosis, and non-high grade without comedonecrosis. One study [65] reported that 23 pathologists were in complete agreement using 5 different classification systems, including that proposed by Silverstein. The International Consensus Conference has failed to endorse any classification, but recommended that pathology reports must include information on nuclear grading, necrosis, polarization, and architectural pattern [66]. Allred [67] proposed the following clarification.

(A) Comedo group—large cell: more aggressive form also referred to as comedocarcinoma.

(B) Noncomedo group—small cell: less aggressive and is further divided into:

    (a) cribriform,
    (b) micropapillary,
    (c) solid.

DCIS can also be classified depending on the presence of central necrosis [68]:

(1) DCIS with no central necrosis (noncomedo group).

(2) Low grade with no central necrosis:

    (a) low grade DCIS,
    (b) intermediate grade DCIS: well differentiated, cribriform, micropapillary, solid- and small-cell type.

(2) DCIS with central necrosis:

    (a) poorly differentiated,
    (b) comedo type,
    (c) large-cell type.

Such classifications may be clinically meaningful in terms of describing the invasive potential of the neoplasm and informing the treatment plan to avoid overtreatment. In the past, nuclear grading using microscopy could not predict which DCIS would develop into invasive carcinoma. Chapman and colleagues [69] found that nuclear grading by image analysis does have prognostic value, with quantitative nuclear image features able to predict which DCIS will transform into invasive cancer. While the traditional classification is probably going to be changed based on hyperplasia of the duct or epithelium, because an element of subjectivity in the microscopic interpretation of these hyperplastic lesions persists, it is very unlikely that this issue will be resolved soon. A new classification system was proposed based on the presence of mammary intraepithelial neoplasia (MIN) of epithelium either in the duct or lobule, followed by grading in accordance with the trend in many other sites [70]. Most recently, Tavassoli [18] proposed a completely new classification system with some modifications as proposed by Rosai [70]. These classification systems are based on the presence of ductal intraepithelial neoplasia (DIN; Table 1).

Such new classifications have certain advantages and obvious merits, and it is possible that a modified version of the DIN classification will eventually be adopted, though not in the near future. Recently, Costa and Zanini [71] have questioned whether DIN is really a malignant lesion. Guerrieri-Gonzaga and colleagues [72] published their experience in treating 1267 cases of DIN and showed that it is a potentially malignant lesion and should be treated either by BCS or by chemopreventive therapy. These authors have accepted the new pathological classification.

Recently, considerable efforts have been made in evaluating potential molecular markers of DCIS. However, most studies have shown that candidate molecular markers of DCIS have little prognostic value [73, 74]. Approximately 70% of DCIS express ER [75], which is normally expressed by luminal epithelium. Almost 50% of DCIS express HER2/neu [76]. Mutated p53 (a tumor suppressor gene) is expressed by about 25% of DCIS [77]. DCIS of solid, flat or micropapillary type exists in the basal phenotype of breast cancer and demonstrates the same immunophenotype as invasive breast cancer [78]. Androgen receptor (AR) has been detected in female breast cancer and is often associated with apocrine differentiation. Inherited differences in AR CAG length might influence the transition from DCIS to invasive carcinoma, perhaps by modulating the function of AR in breast tissue [79]. All DCIS express E-cadherin, but lobular carcinoma shows focal loss of E-cadherin or complete lack of membrane staining. It is sometimes difficult to differentiate histologically between lobular carcinoma and ductal carcinoma, and E-cadherin immunohistochemical studies can be used to differentiate between the 2 groups of in situ carcinoma of breast [80]. In the future, molecular markers may help to predict which group of DCIS will become invasive carcinoma.

New technologies, such as array-based CGH, RNA expression profiling, have proven to be of great value in distinguishing between poorly differentiated and well-differentiated DCIS by detecting quantitative difference in gene expression. Proteomic analysis also may be able to predict which DCIS will become invasive carcinoma and will help inform the appropriate treatment [81]. Kerlikowske and colleagues [82] conducted standardized pathology reviews and immunohistochemistry staining for ER, PR, Ki67 (tumor proliferating index) antigen, p53, p16, epidermal growth factor receptor-2 (ERBB2, HER2 neu oncoprotein), and cyclooxygenase-2 (COX-2) in paraffin-embedded DCIS tissue. They found that DCIS lesions positive for p16, COX-2, and Ki67, or those detected by palpation are more likely to develop into invasive cancer. Radisky and colleagues [83] examined the significance of p16 INK4a expression in women with atypical hyperplasia and found that expression was not a risk for breast cancer. Most recently, a study by Adler and colleagues [84] found that the vascular pattern is not a predictor of aggressive behavior of DCIS, suggesting that DCIS biology is independent of angiogenesis. We do not yet know whether this also means that vascular endothelial growth factor (VEGF) does not control the aggressive nature of DCIS.

6. Treatment Plan

The goal of DCIS treatment is complete removal of the neoplasm, if possible, and prevention of recurrence. Local treatment of DCIS is simple mastectomy, lumpectomy (though there is usually no lump when DCIS is diagnosed by imaging), lumpectomy with post lumpectomy radiation, quadrantectomy without or with postquadrantectomy adjuvant treatment, followed by chemopreventive therapy. Traditionally, simple mastectomy is the curative treatment for 98% of cases of DCIS, and the local recurrence rate is very low [85]. However, even after simple mastectomy there may be local recurrence. The causes of such local recurrence are either a missed diagnosis of invasive carcinoma during the original surgery or incomplete removal of breast tissue, especially from the skin flap in nipple-sparing mastectomy. Such recurrence occurs only in 1% to 2% of cases [86].

This traditional treatment of DCIS has been challenged by Fisher and colleagues [87] who conducted a randomized trial that demonstrated that total mastectomy and breast conservative surgery for DCIS are associated with equivalent outcomes. Nevertheless, there are certain indications for complete mastectomy for DCIS, beyond the preference of the patient and/or the physician. The indications for total mastectomy as determined by a joint committee of the American College of Surgeons, American College of Radiology, and the American College of Pathologists are women with 2 lesions in the same breast; diffuse malignant appearing lesion in the breast; persistent positive margin after lumpectomy and cavity shaving with multiple attempts; inability to give radiation due to prior radiation or presence of SLE; radiation treatment is not available, especially in underdeveloped countries; extensive DCIS where the tumor is removed with a very small negative margin; tumor size and breast size will produce poor cosmetic result; pregnancy.

Currently, lumpectomy with no radiation in the low-risk patient or with radiation following surgery is the standard of care in the United States and other developed countries

TABLE 1: Classification of Tavassoli [18].

Proposed classification	Current designation	Necrosis	Excised margin
DIN 1a	IDH	None	Negative
DIN 1b	AIDH, flat monomorphic	−	? Negative
	DCIS, grade 1 (crib/micropap)	−	Positive
	DCIS, grade 2	+	Positive
	(crib/micropap + necrosis or atypia)	+	
	Special type—specify		
DIN 3b	DCIS Grade 3	+ + +	Positive
	(Anaplastic DCIS)	±	

[88]. However, this standard of care is not possible in underdeveloped countries where DCIS is detected by the patient or by the physician as either palpable lump, discharge from nipple, or skin dimpling, rather than by screening or diagnostic imaging studies due to lack of resources [41]. In addition, there are also limited capabilities for radiation treatment following local excision of resectable tumors in developing and underdeveloped countries. Therefore, in these areas, the standard of care is simple mastectomy for all stages of DCIS.

Studies have shown that there is a low recurrence rate of DCIS with excision alone as compared to excision and radiation, especially in low-risk patients [89, 90]. For this reason, it is worthwhile to further explore the possibility of breast conserving surgery alone, especially in patients with low risk. Three randomized trials have compared the outcomes with excision alone versus excision and radiotherapy [91–93]. These trials showed that addition of radiation therapy significantly reduces the risk of recurrence by 40% in the ipsilateral breast. Multiple observational studies, though less powerful than the NSABP-17 trial, also showed lower rates of local recurrence of DCIS or invasive cancer for women undergoing breast conserving surgery followed by radiation, although not all reported statistically significant differences [94–96]. Observational studies from Sweden indicate no mortality benefit associated with breast conserving surgery with radiation compared to breast conserving surgery alone [97]; these results were echoed in one other study [98]. Though these results are from observational studies, taken together, there is no evidence that conservative surgery plus radiation is more or less effective than breast conserving surgery alone. This lack of differential effect can be seen across all of the most important prognostic factors, including grade, tumor size, involved margins, and comedonecrosis.

It is felt that an involved margin is one of the most important prognostic factors for recurrence, yet it is still not agreed what should be the safe margin of lumpectomy [99]. In their review, Revesz and Khan do not provide any specific safe margin; rather, they state that until better data are available, the desirable margin will vary depending on individual factors, including age, histology, and patient preference. It is likely that a safe margin is "ink should not touch the margin of the excised mass and should be at least 2 mm from the surgical margin," as stated by Ruggiero et al. in [42]. The margin varies in the literature, from 1 mm to 3 mm

[42]. Blair et al. [100] reported that in the United States, only 48% of surgeons perform cavity and bed shaving, very few undertake frozen section analysis or imprint cytology, and 57% never reexcise with positive margins. The literature suggests that there is still controversy as to whether all patients should be treated with radiation after lumpectomy. Jiveliouk and colleagues [101] recently reported their experiences with the treatment of pure DCIS using lumpectomy and postoperative external beam radiation in an Israeli population; during an 8-year follow-up period, the overall survival, disease-free survival, and event-free survival were 100%, 100%, and 87%, respectively. This is a unique result and may be due to early initiation of treatment or that the biological behavior of DCIS in Israeli women is different from that in women from other Western countries. Kayani and Bhurgri [102] also reviewed their experience with 38 women with DCIS in Karachi, Pakistan; they found that, if untreated, only 40% of cases were aggressive and 60% were very indolent. Most likely, the biological behavior of DCIS is different in Pakistani women such that they do not develop the more aggressive types of DCIS. The Eastern Cooperative Oncology Group recently reviewed their experiences with local excision without radiation for DCIS [103]. Patients with either low or intermediate risk, with tumors measuring 2.5 cm or smaller or high-grade or DCIS 1 cm or smaller who had microscopic margins of 3 mm or wider, were eligible for study. During the 6.2 years of followup, the 5-year rate of cancer recurrence and related morbidity was 6.1% in patients with low or intermediaterisk, and 15.3% in the high-grade DCIS group. This study proves that all patients with DCIS do not need radiation after lumpectomy. Very recently, similar study has been carried out by Ruggiero et al. [42] in 161 patients who were followed for 5 years; the recurrence rate was 6.2% in the group of patients who had only quadrantectomy without radiation therapy. According to these authors, the risk factors for local recurrence were age <45 years, positive margin <2 mm, and grade 3 neoplasm. Based on their findings, the authors recommended adjuvant radiotherapy in patients who had these risk factors for local recurrence.

Taken together, the current trend is that only high-risk patient should undergo adjuvant radiotherapy after lumpectomy. Typically, 50 Gy of external beam radiation is administered in 25 fractions. There is also growing interest in balloon brachytherapy for treatment of DCIS following lumpectomy, which would allow for accelerated breast radiation therapy. The literature contains reports of satisfactory results with balloon brachytherapy in DCIS in terms of disease-free survival and cosmoses [104, 105]. However, a recent report about the long-term result of brachytherapy for treatment of DCIS was presented at the San Antonio Breast Cancer Symposium (2011) and published by the American Association for Cancer Research [106]. In this study, Smith et al. at MD Anderson Cancer Center reviewed the medical records of 130,535 patients who underwent brachytherapy for DCIS and then were followed for 5 years. Surprisingly, 50% of the patients eventually underwent complete mastectomy, either due to complications of the brachytherapy or recurrence of the tumor. Multiple studies have demonstrated that MRI detects multiple foci in 10%–30% of patients with DCIS, and that neither mammography nor US can detect these metacentric lesions [107]. When these patients are treated with balloon brachytherapy, they are inadequately treated; this may explain why there is such a high recurrence rate of DCIS after brachytherapy. It is therefore appropriate that patients undergo MRI evaluation prior to brachytherapy, and if multiple foci are present, then either these patients should undergo total mastectomy or total breast radiation.

Controversy exists regarding the treatment of micrometastasis in DCIS. Micrometastasis should be treated either with axillary dissection, chemotherapy, or radiotherapy [108]. DCIS is a part of breast and ovarian cancer syndrome [109], and the BRCA1 and BRCA2 mutation rate in invasive carcinoma is same as that in DCIS. These findings suggest that a patient with personal and family history of breast cancer and or ovarian cancer should be followed very closely as per the risk protocol for breast cancer.

The value of genetic testing for BRCA1 and BRCA 2 mutation is its ability to reduce the number of women who develop breast cancer and the number of women who die of disease. Patients with BRCA1 and BRCA2 mutations have several options for breast cancer prevention. These options include prophylactic total mastectomy, prophylactic bilateral oophorectomy and chemoprevention with SERM, third generation aromatase inhibitors, or raloxifene. Statistical analyses indicate that total mastectomy reduces the risk of developing breast cancer by 89% [110]. Though prophylactic total mastectomy offers the best protection against developing breast cancer in BRCA1 and BRCA 2 mutation carriers, one study in Canada showed that the majority of women with BRCA1/2 mutations are unwilling to undergo such a radical surgical procedure [111].

The NSABP-24 trial assessed the value of tamoxifen following the diagnosis of DCIS and found that treatment reduces the recurrence rate of DCIS or invasive carcinoma in the ipsilateral breast. The effect of tamoxifen is highly significant for patients with ER+ DCIS, whereas the effect in reducing recurrence DCIS in the ipsilateral breast is not significant in ER− DCIS [112]. The same trial also found that tamoxifen therapy was associated with a 50% reduction of DCIS or invasive carcinoma in the contralateral breast, but had no impact on all-cause mortality. Combined treatment (lumpectomy, radiation, and tamoxifen) compared with lumpectomy and tamoxifen reduced the overall rate of cancer 29% [113]. This study also showed that tamoxifen is less effective in patients without comedonecrosis or who have smaller tumors. The unwanted effects of tamoxifen include hot flashes, fluid retention, vaginal discharge, osteoporosis, thromboembolic disease, and endometrial carcinoma. A study by Cuzick and colleagues [114] reported that the risk reduction of breast cancer with tamoxifen persists for at least 10 years, but that most side effects do not continue after 5 years. However, an observational study by Warren and colleagues [115] found that women with DCIS who receive tamoxifen had the same hazard of local recurrence of DCIS or invasive cancer as women who did not receive tamoxifen.

In addition to tamoxifen, other SERMs such as raloxifene and lasofoxifene are also used as chemoprevention agents. The STAR trial, MORE trial, and CORE trial have studied the role of raloxifene for prevention of breast cancer and have shown positive results [116]. However, a recent study by Viring and colleagues [117] reported that while raloxifene reduced the risk of invasive breast cancer, it was not associated with decreased incidence of DCIS.

Currently, third-generation aromatase inhibitors (anastrozole, letrozole, and exemestane) are also used as chemoprevention agents with greater specificity and fewer side effects [118]. However, all of these chemopreventive drugs have no impact on ER-tumors and this remains a challenging area for breast cancer prevention. Possible agents for prevention of ER-neoplasms include cyclooxygenase-2 inhibitors, statins, and vitamin D analogs. Yet none of these drugs has been tested in humans in a randomized controlled trial, which is necessary to prove the efficacy of these drugs for prevention of breast cancer. There is one laboratory study in progress that is evaluating inhibition of p38 kinase as a chemopreventive measure for ER-breast tumors [119]. The p38 kinase causes cell proliferation, and most ER-negative breast neoplasms overexpress p38 kinase. This preliminary study will provide the foundation for new approaches to the treatment or prevention of ER-breast neoplasms.

Rexinoid LG100268 [120] has been shown in animal models to be an effective chemopreventive agent for prevention of preinvasive neoplasm of the breast with minimal toxicity [121]. Future trials are needed in humans to assess the clinical translation of this chemopreventive agent. PPAR-α and PPAR-γ ligands induce apoptotic and antiproliferative responses, respectively, in human breast cancer cells, and their activation is associated with specific changes in gene expression [122]. Therefore, PPAR-selective retinoids may also be potential chemopreventive agents.

The issue of sentinel lymph node (SLN) biopsy in DCS has been extensively studied by various investigators. Tada and colleagues [123] have found that the incidence of positive SLN is 1.25% and 6.8% in DCIS and intraductal carcinoma (IDC), respectively. Intra et al. [124] studied the incidence of positive SLN in 854 patients with DCIS. They found the incidence of positive SLN was 4%, or 12 cases. Of these 12 cases, 7 had micrometastases with tumor size <2 mm and 5 had macrometastases with tumor size >2 mm. Four additional cases had isolated tumor cells (ITC). Julian and colleagues [125] reviewed the records of 813 patients with DCIS. These patients were studied under the auspices of the NSABP B-17 and B-24 projects. The NSABP B-17 investigators found that 7 patients developed ipsilateral nodal recurrence (INR) and the overall INR rate was 0.83 per 1000 patient-years. In NSABP B-24, the overall INR rate was 0.36 per 1000 patient-years. It was concluded that INR can be considered a surrogate for axillary involvement at the time of diagnosis of DCIS. These findings suggest that the rate of positive SLN in DCIS is so low that there is generally no indication for performing SLN biopsies in patients with DCIS. However, if at any time the patient undergoes complete mastectomy, then the patient must also have an SLN biopsy. Other relative indications of SLN biopsy are perineural invasion and high grade with comedonecrosis.

Various treatment options should be discussed with the patient with DCIS. Patients should be told in detail about the biological behavior of the DCIS, with special reference to the natural history of the disease, the outcomes of various types of treatment, the recurrence rate after treatment, the results of salvage treatment in the event of recurrence, the risks and benefits of the various treatment options, and the disease-free survival and overall survival rates of the various treatments. The patient and possibly family members should be actively involved in treatment decision making. Katz and colleagues [126, 127] conducted a population-based cohort study of 659 women from the Detroit and Los Angeles areas who were diagnosed with DCIS in 2002 to examine the role of the patient in treatment decision making and how the patient's input affected the treatment. In the study, greater patient involvement in the decision-making process led to larger number of mastectomies. Furthermore, the Katz study showed that only 13.1% of women were not influenced by their physicians concerns about recurrence and underwent mastectomy compared to 48.5% who were greatly influenced by the possibility of recurrence. This finding suggests that the engagement of a knowledgeable surgeon in the treatment discussion can be a very powerful tool in guiding the treatment of a particular patient. The surgeon must consider all the risk factors of recurrence after the definitive curative treatment of DCIS and must work with the oncologist to select adjuvant treatment, if needed, and chemopreventive treatment.

7. Conclusion

DCIS is a heterogeneous neoplasm whose biological behavior is still incompletely understood. Epidemiologic studies show that with the advent of various imaging techniques, the incidence of DCIS increased and has reached a plateau in past decade. Approximately 80% of DCIS cases are diagnosed by imaging studies in developing countries, whereas the majority of cases in developing or underdeveloped countries present as palpable lumps, nipple discharge, and comedonecrosis. Each of the imaging modalities has advantages and limitation, but they can complement each other to achieve an accurate diagnosis of DCIS. Definite histological diagnosis of nonpalpable DCIS is established by either needle- or US-guided CNB or stereotactic biopsy or vacuum-assisted biopsy. Currently, CNB is best technique to obtain

an accurate histologic diagnosis. Various treatment options are available. The gold standard of treatment of DCIS in developed countries is wide local excision of the tumor with negative margins followed by external beam radiation. Such treatment options may not be available in underdeveloped countries, where total mastectomy is the treatment of choice. Surgery and radiation are superior to surgery alone with regard to recurrence, but there is no benefit in terms of overall survival for either of these approaches. Long-term survival is possible, even in underdeveloped countries without treatment. Additional research is needed to determine the role of balloon brachytherapy as an adjuvant treatment. Tamoxifen is a beneficial adjuvant therapy. Further research to understand the biological nature DCIS will resolve some of the remaining controversy about the best treatment for DCIS. Various preventive measures are available to protect against the development or progression of DCIS, including surgical and nonsurgical interventions. Investigations are ongoing regarding molecularly targeted drug development for prevention and treatment of DCIS.

Acknowledgments

The author thanks Roksana Badruddoja, Ph.D., and Farzana Badruddoja, M.S., for their advice in the preparation of this paper. He would also like to thank Ronda Brown, M.S., for typing the paper and correcting typographical errors and Dr. Stacey C. Tobin, Ph.D., for final editing of the paper.

References

[1] M. A. Shampo and R. A. Kyle, "Pioneers of mammography—Warren and Egan," *Mayo Clinic Proceedings*, vol. 72, no. 1, article 32, 1997.

[2] D. Rosner, R. N. Bedwani, and J. Vana, "Noninvasive breast carcinoma. Results of a national survey by the American College of Surgeons," *Annals of Surgery*, vol. 192, no. 3, pp. 139–147, 1980.

[3] L. A. Brinton, M. E. Sherman, J. D. Carreon, and W. F. Anderson, "Recent trends in breast cancer among younger women in the United States," *Journal of the National Cancer Institute*, vol. 100, no. 22, pp. 1643–1648, 2008.

[4] V. L. Ernster, R. Ballard-Barbash, W. E. Barlow et al., "Detection of ductal carcinoma in situ in women undergoing screening mammography," *Journal of the National Cancer Institute*, vol. 94, no. 20, pp. 1546–1554, 2002.

[5] D. S. May, N. C. Lee, L. C. Richardson, A. G. Giustozzi, and J. K. Bobo, "Mammography and breast cancer detection by race and Hispanic ethnicity: results from a national program (United States)," *Cancer Causes and Control*, vol. 11, no. 8, pp. 697–705, 2000.

[6] A. Jemal, R. Siegel, E. Ward, Y. Hao, J. Xu, and M. J. Thun, "Cancer statistics, 2009," *CA: A Cancer Journal for Clinicians*, vol. 59, no. 4, pp. 225–249, 2009.

[7] C. I. Li, J. R. Daling, and K. E. Malone, "Age-specific incidence rates of in situ breast carcinomas by histologic type,

1980 to 2001," *Cancer Epidemiology Biomarkers and Prevention*, vol. 14, no. 4, pp. 1008–1011, 2005.

[8] V. L. Ernster, J. Barclay, K. Kerlikowske, D. Grady, and I. C. Henderson, "Incidence of and treatment for ductal carcinoma in situ of the breast," *JAMA*, vol. 275, no. 12, pp. 913–918, 1996.

[9] M. Horner, L. Rice, M. Krapcho et al., *SEER Cancer Statistics Review, 1975–2006*, National Cancer Institute, Bethesda, Md, USA, 2009.

[10] B. A. Virnig, T. M. Tuttle, T. Shamliyan, and R. L. Kane, "Ductal carcinoma in Situ of the breast: a systematic review of incidence, treatment, and outcomes," *Journal of the National Cancer Institute*, vol. 102, no. 3, pp. 170–178, 2010.

[11] L. Tabar, G. Fagerberg, H.-H. Chen et al., "Efficacy of breast cancer screening by age: new results from the Swedish two-county trial," *Cancer*, vol. 75, no. 10, pp. 2507–2517, 1995.

[12] L. Tabár, B. Vitak, H. H. Chen et al., "The Swedish two-county trial twenty years later: updated mortality results and new insights from long-term follow-up," *Radiologic Clinics of North America*, vol. 38, no. 4, pp. 625–651, 2000.

[13] N. G. Coburn, M. A. Chung, J. Fulton, and B. Cady, "Decreased breast cancer tumor size, stage, and mortality in Rhode Island: an example of a well-screened population," *Cancer Control*, vol. 11, no. 4, pp. 222–230, 2004.

[14] J. Fracheboud, S. J. Otto, J. A. M. M. Van Dijck, M. J. M. Broeders, A. L. M. Verbeek, and H. J. De Koning, "Decreased rates of advanced breast cancer due to mammography screening in The Netherlands," *British Journal of Cancer*, vol. 91, no. 5, pp. 861–867, 2004.

[15] W. F. Anderson, K. C. Chu, and S. S. Devesa, "Distinct incidence patterns among in situ and invasive breast carcinomas, with possible etiologic implications," *Breast Cancer Research and Treatment*, vol. 88, no. 2, pp. 149–159, 2004.

[16] C. Y. Chen, L. M. Sun, and B. O. Anderson, "Paget disease of the breast: changing patterns of incidence, clinical presentation, and treatment in the U.S," *Cancer*, vol. 107, no. 7, pp. 1448–1458, 2006.

[17] D. L. Weaver, P. M. Vacek, J. M. Skelly, and B. M. Geller, "Predicting biopsy outcome after mammography: what is the likelihood the patient has invasive or in situ breast cancer?" *Annals of Surgical Oncology*, vol. 12, no. 8, pp. 660–673, 2005.

[18] F. Tavassoli, "Ductal intraepithelial neoplasia of the breast," *Virchows Archiv*, vol. 438, no. 3, pp. 221–227, 2001.

[19] A. Kricker, C. Goumas, and B. Armstrong, "Ductal carcinoma in situ of the breast, a population-based study of epidemiology and pathology," *British Journal of Cancer*, vol. 90, no. 7, pp. 1382–1385, 2004.

[20] E. B. Claus, M. Stowe, and D. Carter, "Breast carcinoma in situ: risk factors and screening patterns," *Journal of the National Cancer Institute*, vol. 93, no. 23, pp. 1811–1817, 2001.

[21] G. K. Reeves, V. Beral, J. Green, T. Gathani, and D. Bull, "Hormonal therapy for menopause and breast-cancer risk by histological type: a cohort study and meta-analysis," *The Lancet Oncology*, vol. 7, no. 11, pp. 910–918, 2006.

[22] S. M. Gapstur, M. Morrow, and T. A. Sellers, "Hormone replacement therapy and risk of breast cancer with a favorable histology: results of the Iowa Women's Health Study," *JAMA*, vol. 281, no. 22, pp. 2091–2141, 1999.

[23] E. B. Claus, M. Stowe, and D. Carter, "Oral contraceptives and the risk of ductal breast carcinoma in situ," *Breast Cancer Research and Treatment*, vol. 81, no. 2, pp. 129–136, 2003.

[24] K. Kerlikowske, J. Barclay, D. Grady, E. A. Sickles, and V. Ernster, "Comparison of risk factors for ductal carcinoma in

situ and invasive breast cancer," *Journal of the National Cancer Institute*, vol. 89, no. 1, pp. 77–82, 1997.

[25] J. Wohlfahrt, F. Rank, N. Kroman, and M. Melbye, "A comparison of reproductive risk factors for CIS lesions and invasive breast cancer," *International Journal of Cancer*, vol. 108, no. 5, pp. 750–753, 2004.

[26] National and Medical Research Council, *Hormone Replacement Therapy: A Summary of the Evidence for General Practitioners and oOther Health Professionals*, National Health and Medical Council, Canberra, Australia, 2005.

[27] J. E. Rossouw, G. L. Anderson, R. L. Prentice et al., "Risks and benefits of estrogen plus progestin in healthy postmenopausal women: principal results from the women's health initiative randomized controlled trial," *JAMA*, vol. 288, no. 3, pp. 321–333, 2002.

[28] G. L. Anderson, R. T. Chlebowski, J. E. Rossouw et al., "Prior hormone therapy and breast cancer risk in the Women's Health Initiative randomized trial of estrogen plus progestin," *Maturitas*, vol. 55, no. 2, pp. 103–115, 2006.

[29] M. L. Stefanick, G. L. Anderson, K. L. Margolis et al., "Effects of conjugated equine estrogens on breast cancer and mammography screening in postmenopausal women with hysterectomy," *JAMA*, vol. 295, no. 14, pp. 1647–1657, 2006.

[30] W. Y. Chen, J. E. Manson, S. E. Hankinson et al., "Unopposed estrogen therapy and the risk of invasive breast cancer," *Archives of Internal Medicine*, vol. 166, no. 9, pp. 1027–1032, 2006.

[31] R. M. Tamimi, S. E. Hankinson, W. Y. Chen, B. Rosner, and G. A. Colditz, "Combined estrogen and testosterone use and risk of breast cancer in postmenopausal women," *Archives of Internal Medicine*, vol. 166, no. 14, pp. 1483–1489, 2006.

[32] S. R. Cummings, B. Ettinger, P. D. Delmas et al., "The effects of tibolone in older postmenopausal women," *The New England Journal of Medicine*, vol. 359, no. 7, pp. 697–708, 2008.

[33] Australian Bureau of Statistics, *National Health Survey, Australia (2004-2005)*, Australian Bureau of Statistics, Canberra, Australia, 2006.

[34] A. Trentham-Dietz, P. A. Newcomb, B. E. Storer, and P. L. Remington, "Risk factors for carcinoma in situ of the breast," *Cancer Epidemiology Biomarkers and Prevention*, vol. 9, no. 7, pp. 697–703, 2000.

[35] C. M. Friedenreich, C. G. Woolcott, A. McTiernan et al., "Alberta physical activity and breast cancer prevention trial: sex hormone changes in a year-long exercise intervention among postmenopausal women," *Journal of Clinical Oncology*, vol. 28, no. 9, pp. 1458–1466, 2010.

[36] N. F. Boyd, H. Guo, L. J. Martin et al., "Mammographic density and the risk and detection of breast cancer," *The New England Journal of Medicine*, vol. 356, no. 3, pp. 227–236, 2007.

[37] J. Lin, N. R. Cook, C. Albert et al., "Vitamins C and E and beta carotene supplementation and cancer risk: a randomized controlled trial," *Journal of the National Cancer Institute*, vol. 101, no. 1, pp. 14–23, 2009.

[38] T. W. Johnson, K. E. Anderson, D. Lazovich, and A. R. Folsom, "Association of aspirin and nonsteroidal anti-inflammatory drug use with breast cancer," *Cancer Epidemiology Biomarkers and Prevention*, vol. 11, no. 12, pp. 1586–1591, 2002.

[39] M. D. Holmes, W. Y. Chen, L. Li, E. Hertzmark, D. Spiegelman, and S. E. Hankinson, "Aspirin intake and survival after breast cancer," *Journal of Clinical Oncology*, vol. 28, no. 9, pp. 1467–1472, 2010.

[40] A. M. Algra and P. M. Roth, "Effects of aspirin on long-term cancer incidence and metastasis: a systemic comparison of evidence from observational studies versus randomized trial," *The Lancet Oncology*, vol. 13, no. 5, pp. 518–527, 2012.

[41] N. S. Nair, N. Pandey, P.V. Vanmali et al., *Journal of Clinical Oncology*, vol. 29, no. 27, p. 146, 2001.

[42] R. Ruggiero, E. Procaccini, A. Sanguinetti et al., "Ductal carcinoma in situ of the breast: our experience," *Il Giornale di Chirurgia*, vol. 30, no. 3, pp. 121–124, 2009.

[43] H. D. Nelson, K. Tyne, A. Naik et al., "Screening for breast cancer: US preventive task force recommendation statement," *Annals of International Medicine*, vol. 151, no. 10, pp. 716–726, 2009.

[44] R. E. Hendrick, E. D. Pisano, A. Averbukh et al., "Comparison of acquisition parameters and breast dose in digital mammography and screen-film mammography in the American College of Radiology imaging network digital mammographic imaging screening trial," *American Journal of Roentgenology*, vol. 194, no. 2, pp. 362–369, 2010.

[45] K. Kerlikowske, R. A. Hubbard, D. L. Miglioretti et al., "Comparative effectiveness of digital versus film-screen mammography in community practice in the United States: a cohort study," *Annals of Internal Medicine*, vol. 155, no. 8, pp. 493–502, 2011.

[46] C. C. Riedl, L. Ponhold, D. Flöry et al., "Magnetic resonance imaging of the breast improves detection of invasive cancer, preinvasive cancer, and premalignant lesions during surveillance of women at high risk for breast cancer," *Clinical Cancer Research*, vol. 13, no. 20, pp. 6144–6152, 2007.

[47] C. K. Kuhl, S. Schrading, H. B. Bieling et al., "MRI for diagnosis of pure ductal carcinoma in situ: a prospective observational study," *The Lancet*, vol. 370, no. 9586, pp. 485–492, 2007.

[48] E. S. Hwang, K. Kinkel, L. J. Esserman, Y. Lu, N. Weidner, and N. M. Hylton, "Magnetic resonance imaging in patients diagnosed with ductal carcinoma-in-situ: value in the diagnosis of residual disease, occult invasion, and multicentricity," *Annals of Surgical Oncology*, vol. 10, no. 4, pp. 381–388, 2003.

[49] J. H. Menell, E. A. Morris, D. D. Dershaw, A. F. Abramson, E. Brogi, and L. Liberman, "Determination of the presence and extent of pure ductal carcinoma in situ by mammography and magnetic resonance imaging," *Breast Journal*, vol. 11, no. 6, pp. 382–390, 2005.

[50] G. Santamaría, M. Velasco, B. Farrús, G. Zanón, and P. L. Fernández, "Preoperative MRI of pure intraductal breast carcinoma-A valuable adjunct to mammography in assessing cancer extent," *Breast*, vol. 17, no. 2, pp. 186–194, 2008.

[51] A. B. Hollingsworth and R. G. Stough, "Preoperative breast MRI for locoregional staging," *The Journal of the Oklahoma State Medical Association*, vol. 99, no. 10, pp. 505–515, 2006.

[52] A. B. Hollingsworth, R. G. Stough, C. A. O'Dell, and C. E. Brekke, "Breast magnetic resonance imaging for preoperative locoregional staging," *American Journal of Surgery*, vol. 196, no. 3, pp. 389–397, 2008.

[53] T. Uematsu, S. Yuen, M. Kasami, and Y. Uchida, "Comparison of magnetic resonance imaging, multidetector row computed tomography, ultrasonography, and mammography for tumor extension of breast cancer," *Breast Cancer Research and Treatment*, vol. 112, no. 3, pp. 461–474, 2008.

[54] C. D. Lehman, C. Gatsonis, C. K. Kuhl et al., "MRI evaluation of the contralateral breast in women with recently diagnosed breast cancer," *The New England Journal of Medicine*, vol. 356, no. 13, pp. 1295–1303, 2007.

[55] Y. J. Gwak, H. J. Kim, J. Y. Kwak et al., "Ultrasonographic detection and characterization of asymptomatic ductal carcinoma in situ with histopathologic correlation," *Acta Radiologica*, vol. 52, no. 4, pp. 364–371, 2011.

[56] W. K. Moon, J. S. Myung, Y. J. Lee, I. A. Park, D. Y. Noh, and J. G. Im, "US of ductal carcinoma in situ," *Radiographics*, vol. 22, no. 2, pp. 269–281, 2002.

[57] M. Badruddoja and J. H. Yang, "Size of breast cancer tumor after core-needle biopsy and fine-needle aspiration does not affect patient treatment plan," *Archives of Surgery*, vol. 140, no. 10, pp. 1008–1009, 2005.

[58] M. Badruddoja, "Image-guided treatment of breast cancer," *Journal of the American College of Surgeons*, vol. 210, no. 3, pp. 372–374, 2010.

[59] M. Badruddoja, "Routine preoperative MRI for breast carcinoma," *Journal of the American College of Surgeons*, vol. 210, no. 2, pp. 253–255, 2010.

[60] C. H. Lee, D. Carter, L. E. Philpotts et al., "Ductal carcinoma in situ diagnosed with stereotactic core needle biopsy: can invasion be predicted?" *Radiology*, vol. 217, no. 2, pp. 466–470, 2000.

[61] R. M. Golub, C. L. Bennett, T. Stinson, L. Venta, and M. Morrow, "Cost minimization study of image-guided core biopsy versus surgical excisional biopsy for women with abnormal mammograms," *Journal of Clinical Oncology*, vol. 22, no. 12, pp. 2430–2437, 2004.

[62] M. E. Brennan, R. M. Turner, S. Ciatto et al., "Ductal carcinoma in situ at core-needle biopsy: meta-analysis of underestimation and predictors of invasive breast cancer," *Radiology*, vol. 260, no. 1, pp. 119–128, 2011.

[63] P. P. Rosen and H. Oberman, *Tumors of Mammary Gland*, Armed Forces Institute of Pathology, Washington, DC, USA, 1993.

[64] M. J. Silverstein, D. N. Poller, J. R. Waisman et al., "Prognostic classification of breast ductal carcinoma-in-situ," *The Lancet*, vol. 345, no. 8958, pp. 1154–1157, 1995.

[65] J. P. Sloane, I. Amendoeira, N. Apostolikas et al., "Consistency achieved by 23 European pathologists in categorizing ductal carcinoma in situ of the breast using five classifications," *Human Pathology*, vol. 29, no. 10, pp. 1056–1062, 1998.

[66] The Census Conference Committee, "Consensus conference of the classification of ductal carcinoma in situ," *Cancer*, vol. 80, no. 9, pp. 1798–1802, 1997.

[67] D. C. Allred, "Ductal carcinoma in situ: terminology, classification, and natural history," *Journal of the National Cancer Institute. Monographs*, vol. 2010, no. 41, pp. 134–138, 2010.

[68] G. Cardenosa, *Clinical Breast Imaging, a Patient Focused Teaching File*, Lippincott Williams & Wilkins, Philadelphia, Pa, USA, 2006.

[69] J. A. Chapman, N. A. Miller, H. L. Lickley et al., "Ductal carcinoma in situ of the breast (DCIS) with heterogeneity of nuclear grade: prognostic effects of quantitative nuclear assessment," *BMC Cancer*, vol. 7, article 174, 2007.

[70] J. Rosai, "Borderline epithelial lesions of the breast," *American Journal of Surgical Pathology*, vol. 15, no. 3, pp. 209–221, 1991.

[71] A. Costa and V. Zanini, "Precancerous lesions of the breast," *Nature Clinical Practice Oncology*, vol. 5, no. 12, pp. 700–704, 2008.

[72] A. Guerrieri-Gonzaga, E. Botteri, N. Rotmensz et al., "Ductal intraepithelial neoplasia: postsurgical outcome for 1,267 women cared for in one single institution over 10 years," *Oncologist*, vol. 14, no. 3, pp. 201–212, 2009.

[73] A. J. Guidi, L. Fischer, J. R. Harris, and S. J. Schnitt, "Micro-vessel density and distribution in ductal carcinoma in situ of the breast," *Journal of the National Cancer Institute*, vol. 86, no. 8, pp. 614–619, 1994.

[74] A. J. Evans, S. E. Pinder, I. O. Ellis et al., "Correlations between the mammographic features of ductal carcinoma in situ (DCIS) and C-erbB-2 oncogene expression," *Clinical Radiology*, vol. 49, no. 8, pp. 559–562, 1994.

[75] H. J. Burstein, K. Polyak, J. S. Wong, S. C. Lester, and C. M. Kaelin, "Ductal carcinoma in situ of the breast," *The New England Journal of Medicine*, vol. 350, no. 14, pp. 1430–1441, 2004.

[76] D. C. Allred, G. M. Clark, R. Molina et al., "Overexpression of HER-2/neu and its relationship with other prognostic factors change during the progression of in situ to invasive breast cancer," *Human Pathology*, vol. 23, no. 9, pp. 974–979, 1992.

[77] M. Rudas, R. Neumayer, M. F. X. Gnant, M. Mittelböck, R. Jakesz, and A. Reiner, "p53 Protein expression, cell prolifer-ation and steroid hormone receptors in ductal and lobular in situ carcinomas of the breast," *European Journal of Cancer Part A*, vol. 33, no. 1, pp. 39–44, 1997.

[78] D. J. Dabbs, M. Chivukula, G. Carter, and R. Bhargava, "Basal phenotype of ductal carcinoma in situ: recognition and immunohistologic profile," *Modern Pathology*, vol. 19, no. 11, pp. 1506–1511, 2006.

[79] M. Kasami, H. Gobbi, W. D. Dupont, J. F. Simpson, D. L. Page, and C. L. Vnencak-Jones, "Androgen receptor CAG repeat lengths in ductal carcinoma in situ of breast, longest in apocrine variety," *Breast*, vol. 9, no. 1, pp. 23–27, 2000.

[80] G. Acs, T. J. Lawton, T. R. Rebbeck, V. A. LiVolsi, and P. J. Zhang, "Differential expression of E-cadherin in lobular and ductal neoplasms of the breast and its biologic and diagnostic implication," *American Journal of Clinical Pathology*, vol. 115, no. 1, pp. 85–98, 2001.

[81] L. Wiechmann and H. M. Kuerer, "The molecular journey from ductal carcinoma in situ to invasive breast cancer," *Cancer*, vol. 112, no. 10, pp. 2130–2142, 2008.

[82] K. Kerlikowske, A. M. Molinari, and M. L. Gauthier, "Biomarker expression and risk of subsequent tumors after initial ductal carcinoma in situ diagnosis," *Journal of the National Cancer Institute*, vol. 102, no. 9, pp. 627–637, 2010.

[83] D. C. Radisky, M. Santisteban, H. K. Berman et al., "p16 ^{INK4a} expression and breast cancer risk in women with atypical hyperplasia," *Cancer Prevention Research*, vol. 4, no. 12, pp. 1953–1960, 2011.

[84] E. H. Adler, J. Sunkara, A. S. Patchefsky et al., "Predictor of disease progression in ductal carcinoma in situ of the breast and vascular pattern," *Human Pathology*, vol. 43, no. 4, pp. 550–556, 2012.

[85] V. L. Ernster, J. Barclay, K. Kerlikowske, H. Wilkie, and R. Ballard-Barbash, "Mortality among women with ductal car-cinoma in situ of the breast in the population-based surveil-lance, epidemiology and end results program," *Archives of Internal Medicine*, vol. 160, no. 7, pp. 953–958, 2000.

[86] L. G. Arnesson, S. Smeds, G. Fagerberg, and O. Grontoft, "Follow-up of two treatment modalities for ductal cancer in situ of the breast," *British Journal of Surgery*, vol. 76, no. 7, pp. 672–675, 1989.

[87] B. Fisher, M. Bauer, and R. Margolese, "Five-year results of a randomized clinical trial comparing total mastectomy and segmental mastectomy with or without radiation in the treatment of breast cancer," *The New England Journal of Medicine*, vol. 312, no. 11, pp. 665–673, 1985.

[88] D. J. Winchester, H. R. Menck, and D. P. Winchester, "National treatment trends for ductal carcinoma in situ of the breast," *Archives of Surgery*, vol. 132, no. 6, pp. 660–665, 1997.

[89] E. R. Fisher, R. Sass, and B. Fisher, "Pathologic findings from the National Adjuvant Breast Project (protocol 6). I. Intraductal carcinoma (DICS)," *Cancer*, vol. 57, no. 2, pp. 197–208, 1986.

[90] A. Recht, B. S. Danoff, and L. J. Solin, "Intraductal carcinoma of the breast: results of treatment with excisional biopsy and irradiation," *Journal of Clinical Oncology*, vol. 3, no. 10, pp. 1329–1343, 1985.

[91] B. Fisher, J. Costantino, C. Redmond et al., "Lumpectomy compared with lumpectomy and radiation therapy for the treatment of intraductal breast cancer," *The New England Journal of Medicine*, vol. 328, no. 22, pp. 1581–1586, 1993.

[92] J. P. Julien, N. Bijker, I. S. Fentiman et al., "Radiotherapy in breast-conserving treatment for ductal carcinoma in situ: first results of the EORTC randomised phase III trial 10853," *The Lancet*, vol. 355, no. 9203, pp. 528–533, 2000.

[93] J. Houghton, "Radiotherapy and tamoxifen in women with completely excised ductal carcinoma in situ of the breast in the UK, Australia, and New Zealand: randomised controlled trial," *The Lancet*, vol. 362, no. 9378, pp. 95–102, 2003.

[94] B. D. Smith, B. G. Haffty, T. A. Buchholz et al., "Effectiveness of radiation therapy in older women with ductal carcinoma in situ," *Journal of the National Cancer Institute*, vol. 98, no. 18, pp. 1302–1310, 2006.

[95] C. Vargas, L. Kestin, N. Go et al., "Factors associated with local recurrence and cause-specific survival in patients with ductal carcinoma in situ of the breast treated with breast-conserving therapy or mastectomy," *International Journal of Radiation Oncology Biology Physics*, vol. 63, no. 5, pp. 1514–1521, 2005.

[96] E. W. L. Chuwa, V. H. S. Tan, P. H. Tan, W. S. Yong, G. H. Ho, and C. Y. Wong, "Treatment for ductal carcinoma in situ in an Asian population: outcome and prognostic factors," *ANZ Journal of Surgery*, vol. 78, no. 1-2, pp. 42–48, 2008.

[97] F. Wärnberg, J. Bergh, M. Zack, and L. Holmberg, "Risk factors for subsequent invasive breast cancer and breast cancer death after ductal carcinoma in situ: a population-based case-control study in Sweden," *Cancer Epidemiology Biomarkers and Prevention*, vol. 10, no. 5, pp. 495–499, 2001.

[98] S. A. Joslyn, "Ductal carcinoma in situ: trends in geographic, temporal, and demographic patterns of care and survival," *Breast Journal*, vol. 12, no. 1, pp. 20–27, 2006.

[99] E. Revesz and S. A. Khan, "What are the safe margins of resection for invasive and in situ breast cancer," *Oncology*, vol. 25, no. 10, pp. 1–5, 2011.

[100] S. L. Blair, K. Thompson, J. Rococco, V. Malcarne, P. D. Beitsch, and D. W. Ollila, "Attuning negative margins in breast-conversion operation: is there a consensus among breast surgeons," *Journal of the American College of Surgeons*, vol. 209, no. 5, pp. 608–613, 2009.

[101] I. Jivel]iouk, B. Corn, M. Inbar, and O. Merimsky, "Ductal carcinoma in situ of the breast in Israeli women treated by breast-conserving surgery followed by radiation therapy," *Oncology*, vol. 76, no. 1, pp. 30–35, 2008.

[102] N. Kayani and Y. Bhurgri, "Ductal carcinoma in situ (DCIS) in Karachi," *Journal of the Pakistan Medical Association*, vol. 55, no. 5, pp. 199–202, 2005.

[103] L. L. Hughes, M. Wang, D. L. Page et al., "Local excision alone without irradiation for ductal carcinoma in situ of the breast:

a trial of the Eastern Cooperative Oncology Group," *Journal of Clinical Oncology*, vol. 27, no. 32, pp. 5319–5324, 2009.

[104] P. R. Benitez, O. Streeter, F. Vicini et al., "Preliminary results and evaluation of MammoSite balloon brachytherapy for partial breast irradiation for pure ductal carcinoma in situ: a phase II clinical study," *American Journal of Surgery*, vol. 192, no. 4, pp. 427–433, 2006.

[105] M. Trombetta, T. B. Julian, D. E. Werts et al., "Long-term Cosmesis after lumpectomy and brachytherapy in the management of carcinoma of the previously irradiated breast," *American Journal of Clinical Oncology*, vol. 32, no. 3, pp. 314–318, 2009.

[106] American Association of Cancer Research, "Brachytherapy was associated with two-fold increase risk for mastectomy and complications," *American Association of Cancer Research*, 2011.

[107] L. Liberman, E. A. Morris, D. D. Dershaw, A. F. Abramson, and L. K. Tan, "MR imaging of the ipsilateral breast in women with percutaneously proven breast cancer," *American Journal of Roentgenology*, vol. 180, no. 4, pp. 901–910, 2003.

[108] M. Badruddoja, "Micrometastasis and axillary dissection in breast cancer," *Archives of Surgery*, vol. 145, no. 10, pp. 1022–1023, 2010.

[109] E. B. Claus, S. Petruzella, E. Matloff, and D. Carter, "Prevalence of BRCA1 and BRCA2 mutations in women diagnosed with ductal carcinoma in situ," *JAMA*, vol. 293, no. 8, pp. 964–969, 2005.

[110] L. C. Hartmann, T. A. Sellers, D. J. Schaid et al., "Efficacy of bilateral prophylactic mastectomy in BRCA1 and BRCA2 gene mutation carriers," *Journal of the National Cancer Institute*, vol. 93, no. 21, pp. 1633–1637, 2001.

[111] K. A. Metcalf, P. Ghadirian, B. Rosen et al., "Variation in rates of uptake of preventive options in Canadian women carrying the BRCA 1 or BRCA 2 genetic mutation," *Open Medicine*, vol. 1, no. 2, pp. e92–e98, 2007.

[112] D. C. Allred, J. Bryant, S. Land et al., "Estrogen receptor expression as a predictive marker of effectiveness of tamoxifen in the treatment of DCIS: findings from NSABP B-24," *Breast Cancer Research and Treatment*, vol. 76, supplement 1, article S36, 2002.

[113] N. Bijker, P. Meijnen, J. L. Peterse et al., "Breast-conserving treatment with or without radiotherapy in ductal carcinoma-in-situ: ten-year results of european organisation for research and treatment of cancer randomized phase III trial 10853— A study by the EORTC breast cancer cooperative group and EORTC radiotherapy group," *Journal of Clinical Oncology*, vol. 24, no. 21, pp. 3381–3387, 2006.

[114] J. Cuzick, J. F. Forbes, I. Sestak et al., "Long-term results of tamoxifen prophylaxis for breast cancer-96-month follow-up of the randomized IBIS-I trial," *Journal of the National Cancer Institute*, vol. 99, no. 4, pp. 272–282, 2007.

[115] J. L. Warren, D. L. Weaver, T. Bocklage et al., "The frequency of ipsilateral second tumors after breast-conserving surgery for DCIS: a population-based analysis," *Cancer*, vol. 104, no. 9, pp. 1840–1848, 2005.

[116] J. A. Cauley, L. Norton, M. E. Lippmann et al., "Continued breast risk reduction in postmenopausal women with raloxefine: 4-year results from the MORE trial. Multiple outcomes of raloxifene evaluation," *Breast Cancer Research and Treatment*, vol. 65, no. 2, pp. 125–134, 2001.

[117] B. A. Viring, T. Samliyan, and T. M Tuttle, "Diagnosis and management of ductal carcinoma in situ (DCIS)," Evidence Report/Technology Assessment 09-E018, AHRQ, 2009.

[118] P. E. Goss, K. Strasser-Weippl, M. Brown, R. Santen, J. Ingle, and M. Bissell, "Prevention strategies with aromatase inhibitors," *Clinical Cancer Research*, vol. 10, no. 1, part 2, pp. 372S–379S, 2004.

[119] L. Chen, J. A. Mayer, T. I. Krisko et al., "Inhibition of the p38 kinase suppresses the proliferation of human ER-negative breast cancer cells," *Cancer Research*, vol. 69, no. 23, pp. 8853–8861, 2009.

[120] Y. Li, Y. Zhang, J. Hill et al., "The rexinoid LG100268 prevents the development of preinvasive and invasive estrogen receptor-negative tumors in MMTV-erbB2 mice," *Clinical Cancer Research*, vol. 13, no. 20, pp. 6224–6231, 2007.

[121] L. R. Howe, "Rexinoids and breast cancer prevention," *Clinical Cancer Research*, vol. 13, no. 20, pp. 5983–5987, 2007.

[122] D. L. Crowe and R. A. Chandraratna, "A retinoid X receptor (RXR)-selective retinoid reveals that RXR-alpha is potentially a therapeutic target in breast cancer cell lines, and that it potentiates antiproliferative and apoptotic responses to peroxisome proliferator-activated receptor ligands," *Breast Cancer Research*, vol. 6, no. 5, pp. R546–R555, 2004.

[123] K. Tada, A. Ogiya, K. Kimura et al., "Ductal carcinoma in situ and sentinel lymph node metastasis in breast cancer," *World Journal of Surgical Oncology*, vol. 8, article 6, 2010.

[124] M. Intra, N. Rotmensz, P. Veronesi et al., "Sentinel node biopsy is not a standard procedure in ductal carcinoma in situ of the breast: the experience of the European institute of oncology on 854 patients in 10 years," *Annals of Surgery*, vol. 247, no. 2, pp. 315–319, 2008.

[125] T. B. Julian, S. R. Land, V. Fourchotte et al., "Is sentinel node biopsy necessary in conservatively treated DCIS?" *Annals of Surgical Oncology*, vol. 14, no. 8, pp. 2202–2208, 2007.

[126] S. J. Katz, P. M. Lantz, N. K. Janz et al., "Patient involvement in surgery treatment decisions for breast cancer," *Journal of Clinical Oncology*, vol. 23, no. 24, pp. 5526–5533, 2005.

[127] S. J. Katz, P. M. Lantz, N. K. Janz et al., "Patterns and correlates of local therapy for women with ductal carcinoma-in-situ," *Journal of Clinical Oncology*, vol. 23, no. 13, pp. 3001–3007, 2005.

16

Clinical Characteristics and Prognosis of Incidentally Detected Lung Cancers

S. Quadrelli,[1] G. Lyons,[1] H. Colt,[2] D. Chimondeguy,[1] and A. Buero[1]

[1]*Thoracic Oncology Centre, Buenos Aires British Hospital, Perdriel 74, C1280AEB Buenos Aires, Argentina*
[2]*University of California, Irvine, CA 92697, USA*

Correspondence should be addressed to S. Quadrelli; silvia.quadrelli@gmail.com

Academic Editor: S. Curley

Objective. To evaluate clinical characteristics and outcomes in incidentally detected lung cancer and in symptomatic lung cancer. *Material and Methods.* We designed a retrospective study including all patients undergoing pulmonary resection with a curative intention for NSCLC. They were classified into two groups according to the presence or absence of cancer-related symptoms at diagnosis in asymptomatic (ASX)—incidental diagnosis—or symptomatic. *Results.* Of the 593 patients, 320 (53.9%) were ASX. In 71.8% of these, diagnosis was made by chest X-ray. Patients in the ASX group were older ($P = 0.007$), had a higher prevalence of previous malignancy ($P = 0.002$), presented as a solitary nodule more frequently ($P < 0.001$), and were more likely to have earlier-stage disease and smaller cancers ($P = 0.0001$). A higher prevalence of incidental detection was observed in the last ten years ($P = 0.008$). Overall 5-year survival was higher for ASX ($P = 0.001$). Median survival times in pathological stages IIIB-IV were not significantly different. *Conclusion.* Incidental finding of NSCLC is not uncommon even among nonsmokers. It occurred frequently in smokers and in those with history of previous malignancy. Mortality of incidental diagnosis group was lower, but the better survival was related to the greater number of patients with earlier-stage disease.

1. Introduction

Lung cancer is the most common cause of cancer mortality in the western world, accounting for approximately 5% of all deaths in many countries [1]. Currently less than 25–30% of patients present with localised, potentially curable disease. Five-year survival for those with pathological stage IA nonsmall cell lung cancer (NSCLC) is 73% whereas metastatic disease has a dismal prognosis (13% 5-year survival) [2].

Results from several studies suggest that frequent chest radiographic screening does not result in reduced lung cancer mortality, a conclusion reinforced by the Prostate, Lung, Colorectal, and Ovarian (PLCO) Cancer Screening Trial [3, 4]. *In fact, some* studies suggest that frequent chest radiographic screening is associated with an 11% relative increase in lung cancer mortality compared with less frequent screening [3].

Randomized trials of screening low-dose computed tomography (LDCT) scans demonstrate that computed tomography (CT) is far more sensitive than chest radiography. CT is now considered the most suitable imaging screening modality. The National Lung Screening Trial (NLST) showed that, in heavy (30 pack-years or more) current or former (within 15 years) smokers between the ages of 55 and 75, three annual LDCT screens reduced lung cancer-specific mortality from 309 to 247 deaths per 100,000 person-years [5].

There are still many unanswered questions about the benefits and harms of those programs that could determine the ultimate success of the mass screening implementation. Additionally, despite expert guidelines for screening high-risk populations, most national health service providers have not implemented (and probably will not implement in the near future) mass lung cancer screening programs. One of the main concerns is that the extrapolation of findings from tightly controlled trials to real-life mass screening programs requires uniform standards and high quality controls not easily achievable in most institutions [6]. Consequently, the current practice is that the patients themselves or their physicians may choose early lung cancer detection on an individual basis. There is little information, however, on the clinical characteristics and outcomes of patients with incidentally detected early stage lung cancer from strictly controlled randomized trials.

The objective of this study was to analyze the clinical records of lung cancer patients who underwent surgical resection to evaluate the clinical characteristics and outcomes of patients with incidentally detected lung cancer and patients with symptomatic lung cancer.

2. Material and Methods

All patients undergoing pulmonary resection with a curative intention for non-small cell lung cancer (NSCLC) in the British Hospital in Buenos Aires between January 1986 and July 2009 were eligible for inclusion in this retrospective study. Our Thoracic Oncology Centre keeps a database of all patients evaluated, with data entered prospectively at the time of their initial evaluation. Patients were excluded if they had exhibited small cell lung cancer or a rare histological result.

Preoperative data included methods of diagnosis and a symptoms questionnaire, tobacco exposure history, and medical history. Only patients with complete and accurate preoperative data about indications for imaging were eligible. Patients were included only after institutional review board approval.

Preoperative staging was performed according to the 7th TNM classification system of the International Association for the Study of Lung Cancer [2] using chest computed tomography (CT) and abdominal CT or ultrasonography in all patients. Brain computed tomography or magnetic resonance imaging was done only in case of clinical suspicion of brain metastases. In cases of uncertain clinical or radiologic findings, further examinations were performed to exclude extrapulmonary metastases. PET was included only during the last 3 years and not on a routine basis. Mediastinoscopy has not been performed routinely in this series unless the CT scan demonstrated mediastinal lymph node enlargement, PET suggested a malignant involvement of hilar or mediastinal nodes, or high-risk criteria of N2 were present. Bronchopulmonary, hilar, and mediastinal lymph nodes were systematically sampled. After surgery a final pathologic stage was determined based on operative findings.

Patients were classified into two groups: Group 1 (asymptomatic): patients who had no symptoms attributable to lung cancer at the time of imaging (patients whose cancer was detected by a medical checkup or under evaluation for other diseases), and Group B (symptomatic): patients with lung cancer-related symptoms. The charts of patients classified as having asymptomatic incidentally detected lung cancers were reviewed to check if the indications for imaging really were not based on any potentially cancer-related symptom.

Postoperative follow-up included office visits, quarterly chest X-rays, and yearly chest-CT. Operative or in-hospital mortality was defined as death occurring within 30 days after the operation or during hospitalization, respectively.

TABLE 1: Indications for imaging in symptomatic (SX) patients.

Leading symptom	n	%
Cough	113	41.39
Pneumonia	50	18.32
Hemoptysis	35	12.82
Dyspnea	21	7.69
Chest wall pain	13	4.76
Shoulder pain	6	2.20
Weight loss	9	3.30
Other symptoms	26	9.52
	273	100

TABLE 2: Indications for imaging in symptomatic (SX) patients.

Indication of imaging	n	%
Routine checkup	108	33.75
Preoperative CXR	42	13.12
Surveillance for cancer	42	13.12
Evaluation of chronic respiratory conditions	44	13.75
Evaluation of nonchest conditions or symptoms	66	20.62
Unknown	18	5.62
	320	100

All patients with postoperative or in-hospital mortality were included in this study.

2.1. Statistical Analysis. Statistical analysis was performed using SPSS 13.0 statistical software. The analysis of differences in categorical outcomes was determined using the Chi-squared test or Fisher's exact test. Probabilities of survival rates were estimated using the Kaplan-Meier method and ASX and SX patients were compared by using the log-rank test.

3. Results

Of 593 patients included in this study (68.3% male, median age 60.9, and range 23–86 years) 320 patients were asymptomatic (ASX) (53.9%). Two hundred and thirty (71.8% of the ASX patients) were diagnosed incidentally on chest X-ray and the remaining on CT scan. Amongst the patients with symptoms, the leading complaints that resulted in the indication for imaging were the appearance of new cough or the increase of a previously manifested clinical picture suggestive of pneumonia and haemoptysis (Table 1). Amongst the 320 ASX patients, the main reason for the imaging was a routine checkup (Table 2). Once the initial chest-X ray (71.8%) or CT scan (28.2%) showed an abnormal image, the usual workup for pulmonary nodules was started.

Patients in the ASX group were older than patients in SX group (median age 61.9 ± 9.9 versus 59.51 years/old ± 10.2, $P = 0.007$), without differences in sex (men 66 versus 73.5%, $P = 0.084$). They had a higher prevalence of previous

TABLE 3: Characteristics of patients diagnosed after an incidental finding and patients with symptoms.

	Incidental finding $n = 320$		Symptomatic patients $n = 273$		P
Age (mean, SD)	61.93	9.8	59.51	10.1	0.007
Male (*n*, %)	212	66%	200	73%	0.054
Never smoker	50	15.6%	18	6.6%	0.003
Previous malignancy	41	13%	13	5%	0.002
Pathological staging (*n*, %)					
IA	121	37.81	36	13.19	
IB	71	22.19	52	19.05	
IIA	16	5.00	10	3.66	
IIB	40	12.50	50	18.32	0.0001
IIIA	46	14.38	86	31.50	
IIIB	15	4.69	24	8.79	
IV	11	3.44	15	5.49	
Squamous cell	51	16%	63	23.1%	0.031
Adenocarcinoma	214	66.9%	147	53.8%	0.025
Pneumonectomy	10	3.1%	28	11%	0.005
Tumor size >3 cm	149	46.5	200	73%	0.0001
Central tumor location	60	18.75	99	36.20%	0.001
Resection considered curative	288	90%	220	81%	0.007
Postoperative complication rate	57	17.8%	73	26.7%	0.022
ICU stay days (mean, SD)	1.73	3.209	1.44	4.388	0.38
Operative mortality	11	3.6%	17	6.2%	0.355

malignancy (13.2 versus 4.8%, $P = 0.002$). The frequency of presentation as SPN (49.5 versus 19.4%, $P < 0.001$) or peripheral location (80.3 versus 63.7%, $P < 0.001$) was higher in this group, without differences in clinical suspicion of N2 (8.8 versus 12.9%, $P = 0.146$). Patients with incidentally detected lung cancer were more likely to have earlier-stage disease, smaller cancers (3.00 ± 2.2 versus 4.3 ± 2.9 cm, $P = 0.0001$). The incidence of adenocarcinoma (66.9% versus 53.8%; $P = 0.025$) was significantly higher in the ASX group. Clinical characteristics of both groups are shown in Table 3.

When the last ten years were analyzed, a higher prevalence of incidental detection compared to previous years was observed (51.7 versus 39.8%, $P = 0.008$).

The overall 5-year survival rates were higher for ASX patients: 66.2% and 46.0% for ASX and symptomatic patients, respectively ($P = 0.001$) (Figure 1). Amongst the stage I patients, the 5-year survival rates were 81.2% in ASX patients and 58.6% in SX patients ($P = 0.014$) (Figure 2). When only stage IA was considered, 5-year survival rates were not different (71.2 versus 84.1%, $P = 0.191$) (Figure 3). When analysis was restricted to T1a tumors there were no differences either in 5-year survival (94.7 versus 93.2, $P = 0.489$). Median survival times in pathological stages IIIB (41.6 m in ASX versus 22.0 m in SX patients, $P = 0.065$) and IV (13.7 versus 12.7 m, $P = 0.964$) were not significantly different.

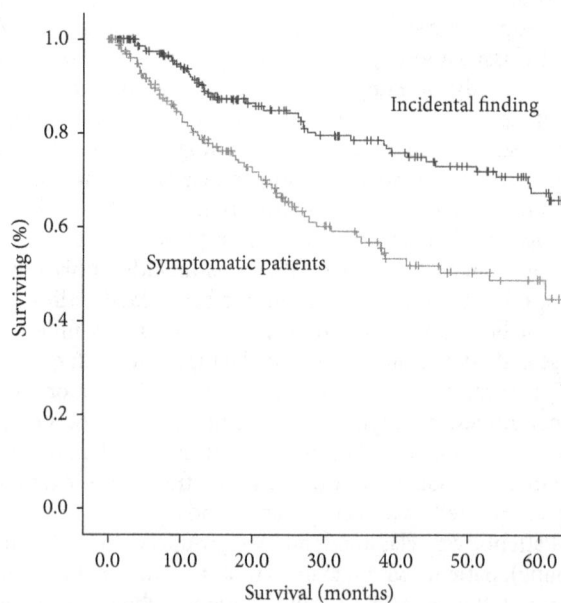

FIGURE 1: Overall survival curves of patients with lung cancer. The 5-year survival rates were 66.2% and 46.0% in ASX and symptomatic patients, respectively. Group I (ASX) had significantly more favorable prognoses ($P = 0.001$).

4. Discussion

Our study shows that the incidental finding of non-small cell lung cancer occurred more frequently in smokers and in patients with a history of previous malignancy. There were a higher proportion of solitary nodules in stage I patients. The mortality of patients with NSCLC as an incidental diagnosis was lower, and this difference persisted into stage I.

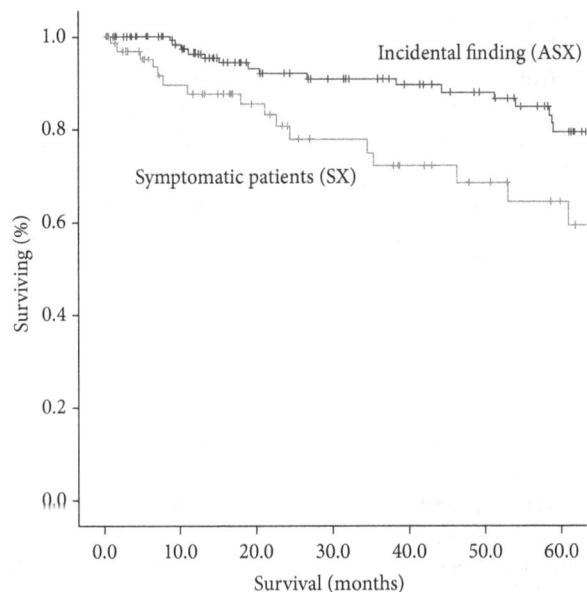

FIGURE 2: Overall survival curves of patients with pathologic stage I disease. Amongst the stage I patients, the 5-year survival rates were 81.2% in ASX patients and 58.6% in SX patients ($P = 0.014$).

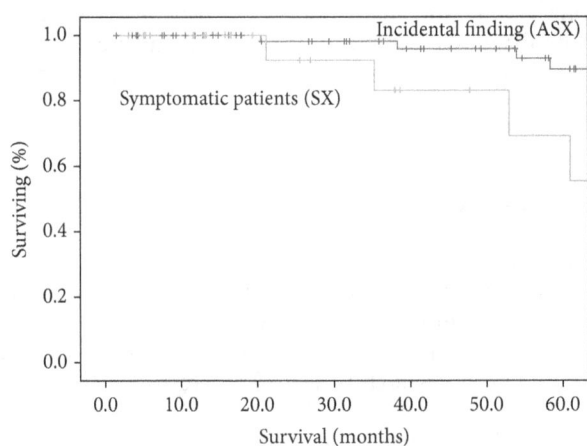

FIGURE 3: Overall survival curves of patients with pathologic stage IA disease. Amongst the stage IA patients, the 5-year survival rates were not different (89.2% in ASX patients and 71.8% in SX patients, $P = 0.191$).

More than a half of patients who underwent surgical resection of lung cancer at our institution had incidentally detected cancers and the most common indication for the initial imaging was a routine checkup. That proportion of ASX patients is higher than that reported by Raz et al. in San Francisco [7] but far lower than that published by Hanagiri et al. in Japan [8]. In the absence of a uniform policy appertaining to the role for screening in clinical practice, the indication of imaging asymptomatic patients relies on the preferences and beliefs of both patients and physicians. Different levels of awareness and access to healthcare may justify differences amongst different studied populations. Also, our ASX patients were slightly older (contrary to the study by Raz et al. [7]) and more frequently smokers which

may mean a higher degree of awareness of their risk for lung cancer as the higher prevalence of previous malignancy may have been one of the reasons for routine radiological surveillance. However, it is noticeable that more than 70% of patients in our group (as in other series) were studied by chest-X-ray, a method that has proved to be ineffective and that is not recommended as a screening tool by any major medical organizations.

The proportion of early stages of lung cancer was higher amongst our patients with incidental findings. It has been also shown in the early report by Shimizu et al. that stage I cases accounted for 65.3% and stage III cases for 22% in their mass screened group, while, in the symptom group, there was only half that percentage of stage I cases (32.2%) [9]. Similarly, in the two more recently published series [7, 8] and in the Korean Lung Cancer Registry Study [10] asymptomatic patients had higher proportions of stages I-II. However, there were still 20% of our patients that did not have any symptom and had a stage III or IV lung cancer. Interestingly, in a retrospective review of coronial autopsies even when the median tumor size of previously undetected cancers was 3 cm, the range was 1–10 cm and there were several tumours over 5 cm and even some large endobronchial and hilar tumours undetected before death [11].

We found that survival time in symptomatic cases was worse than in incidentally detected lung cancer patients. The 5-year overall survival was lower for the whole group and for pathological stage I. That better outcome has been consistently demonstrated in all the previous reports; however, the causes for those differences are still unclear. The Korean registry [10] has shown that absence of symptoms at diagnosis significantly reduced the risk of death from NSCLC, regardless of age, gender, stage, smoking history, or whether treatment was performed. Similarly, Hanagiri and colleagues [8] showed that their patients with incidentally diagnosed NSCLC had significantly better prognoses than the symptomatic group even in stage II–IV disease cases. Even when they had a larger proportion of stage IV amongst asymptomatic patients than our series (6.7 versus 3.4%) they were still a small number of patients ($n = 18$) and exact figures of survival rates for those advanced patients were not provided. In our series, whilst pathological stage I patients had a better survival in ASX patients, median survival times in stages IIIB and IV were similar. It resembles the results of Raz et al. who found that their patients with completely resected incidental lung cancer had similar long-term survival rates as patients with symptomatic lung cancer, after adjusting for stage [7].

In the present study, stage IA disease was diagnosed less frequently in the symptomatic group, similar to what has been reported in other studies [7, 8, 10]. A study by Kashiwabara et al. [12] (published in 2002, before the publication of the 7th TNM edition) compared the outcomes in patients with one-year delayed detection of lung cancer on mass screening with chest-X-ray and in patients with no delay (patients with tumours which could versus could not be detected on past chest roentgenograms). They found that one-year delayed detection of lung cancer on mass screening did not affect outcome, but that, according to the maximum dimension of the tumours on the overlooked chest roentgenogram, the 5-year survival rates in patients with missed tumours were different and that survival in early stages (I-II) for missed tumours >20 mm was worse than that in patients with missed tumours <10 mm. We had previously shown that tumors over 15 mm are associated with shorter 5-year survival in all TNM stages [13] and several studies have reported tumor size may have an independent predictive value on survival in stage I patients [14, 15]. The impact of the tumor size was finally made evident by the analyses of the database of the IASLC and generated the reclassification of T1 in T1a and T1b and T2 in T2a and T2b [16]. When we analyzed separately the pathological stage IA cases, differences in survival in stage I between the two groups disappeared, suggesting that the size was the most important factor in determining survival.

Our study shows that patients with incidentally detected lung cancer had a better survival because they had smaller cancers and earlier-stage disease. The *clinical significance* of *these results* is difficult to interpret. The conclusions of clinical studies like this or any of the previously published studies should not be extrapolated to the potential value of mass screening. This sort of study design does not allow demonstrating if there is a survival benefit of treatments in asymptomatic patients or how large the proportion of invasive procedures for benign lesions is performed. One of the main concerns about any screening program is that a proportion of screen-detected cases will be "overdiagnosed" simply because of competing mortality [17], a hypothesis that cannot be excluded by a population study like this one. On the other hand, many of the patients in this and the other clinical series were not represented in the clinical trials about mass screening programs: 15% of our asymptomatic patients were never smokers and many of them were under 55 years old and would have not filled criteria for being included in a screening program. This study shows the importance of identifying risk at an individual level as many subjects different from the NLST participants may have a risk similar to or greater than the level of risk observed in NLST. Several studies have previously recognized that there is wide variation in lung cancer risk even amongst those who are smokers [18, 19] and we do not know yet how to identify other risk factors for lung cancer that could potentially justify extending screening to those individuals. Future research to develop clinically useful risk model might include molecular or genetic indicators of risk in order to answer these questions [20].

The National Lung Screening Trial (NLST) showed that, in heavy (30 pack-years or more) current or former (within 15 years) smokers between the ages of 55 and 75, three annual low-dose computed tomographic (LDCT) screens reduced lung cancer-specific mortality from 309 to 247 deaths per 100,000 person-years (relative risk of 0.8) [5]. But at the moment to make individual decisions (such as screening of certain nonsmokers) it is necessary to take into account the potential effectiveness of such measures. Whilst the number needed to screen (NNS) to prevent one death for the entire NLST population was calculated as 320, according to Bach and Gould for very low risk individuals (defined by the authors as a 40-year-old former smoker) the NNS was over 35,000 to prevent one lung cancer death [21]. In order

to minimise the potential for harm when screening large populations for a condition that is very rare (derived not only from the costs [22] associated with screening but also from the impact on quality of life of the potential for invasive procedures for incidental findings) but at the same time not to miss other high-risk subjects out of the NSLT criteria, better risk models must be developed to have the greatest predictive accuracy for lung cancer risk.

This study has some limitations. Firstly, the classification of a cancer as incidentally detected is a potential bias, once the spontaneous patient consultation may not exclude the presence of some nonspecific symptom that prompted the patient to seek medical consultation. Secondly, the results from a single institution might not be generalizable.

It is remarkable that, in the study by Kashiwabara et al. [23] about patients that did not consult a physician after the discovery of a shadow in a radiological screening (almost 25% of the asymptomatic screened patients in their series), when asked about the reason why patients did not consult a doctor, two-thirds answered that it was because they did not have any respiratory symptoms. It shows that a screening program must assure that the health care system can provide all the necessary resources to treat the incidental findings and also the education to guarantee the availability of well-qualified primary care providers trained to encourage patients to follow diagnosis and treatment recommendations once a suspicion of lung cancer is raised from the imaging studies.

5. Conclusion

In summary, our study shows that lung cancer as an incidental finding is not uncommon even amongst nonsmokers and that the better survival of patients with asymptomatic NSCLC is related to the greater number of patients with earlier-stage disease. Future research is needed to prospectively identify those patients not represented in the NSLT who might benefit from LDCT screening.

References

[1] A. Lopez, "The lung cancer epidemic in developed countries," in *Adult Mortality in Developed Countries: From Description to Explanation*, A. D. Lopez, G. Caselli, and T. Valkonen, Eds., pp. 111–134, Oxford University Press, Oxford, UK, 1995.

[2] P. Goldstraw, J. Crowley, K. Chansky et al., "The IASLC lung cancer staging project: proposals for the revision of the TNM stage groupings in the forthcoming (seventh) edition of the TNM classification of malignant tumours," *Journal of Thoracic Oncology*, vol. 2, no. 8, pp. 706–714, 2007.

[3] R. L. Manser, L. B. Irving, G. Byrnes, M. J. Abramson, C. A. Stone, and D. A. Campbell, "Screening for lung cancer: a systematic review and meta-analysis of controlled trials," *Thorax*, vol. 58, no. 9, pp. 784–789, 2003.

[4] M. M. Oken, W. G. Hocking, P. A. Kvale et al., "Screening by chest radiograph and lung cancer mortality: the Prostate, Lung,

Colorectal, and Ovarian (PLCO) randomized trial," *The Journal of the American Medical Association*, vol. 306, no. 17, pp. 1865–1873, 2011.

[5] D. R. Aberle, A. M. Adams, C. D. Berg et al., "Reduced lung-cancer mortality with low-dose computed tomographic screening," *The New England Journal of Medicine*, vol. 365, no. 5, pp. 395–409, 2011.

[6] J. K. Field, R. A. Smith, D. R. Aberle et al., "International association for the study of lung cancer computed tomography screening workshop 2011 report," *Journal of Thoracic Oncology*, vol. 7, no. 1, pp. 10–19, 2012.

[7] D. J. Raz, D. V. Glidden, A. Y. Odisho, and D. M. Jablons, "Clinical characteristics and survival of patients with surgically resected, incidentally detected lung cancer," *Journal of Thoracic Oncology*, vol. 2, no. 2, pp. 125–130, 2007.

[8] T. Hanagiri, K. Sugio, M. Mizukami et al., "Postoperative prognosis in patients with non-small cell lung cancer according to the method of initial detection," *Journal of Thoracic Oncology*, vol. 2, no. 10, pp. 907–911, 2007.

[9] N. Shimizu, A. Ando, S. Teramoto, Y. Moritani, and K. Nishii, "Outcome of patients with lung cancer detected via mass screening as compared to those presenting with symptoms," *Journal of Surgical Oncology*, vol. 50, no. 1, pp. 7–11, 1992.

[10] K.-H. In, Y.-S. Kwon, I.-J. Oh et al., "Lung cancer patients who are asymptomatic at diagnosis show favorable prognosis: a Korean Lung Cancer Registry Study," *Lung Cancer*, vol. 64, no. 2, pp. 232–237, 2009.

[11] R. L. Manser, M. Dodd, G. Byrnes, L. B. Irving, and D. A. Campbell, "Incidental lung cancers identified at coronial autopsy: implications for overdiagnosis of lung cancer by screening," *Respiratory Medicine*, vol. 99, no. 4, pp. 501–507, 2005.

[12] K. Kashiwabara, S.-I. Koshi, K. Ota, M. Tanaka, and M. Toyonaga, "Outcome in patients with lung cancer found retrospectively to have had evidence of disease on past lung cancer mass screening roentgenograms," *Lung Cancer*, vol. 35, no. 3, pp. 237–241, 2002.

[13] G. Lyons, S. Quadrelli, C. Silva et al., "Analysis of survival in 400 surgically resected non-small cell lung carcinomas: towards a redefinition of the T factor," *Journal of Thoracic Oncology*, vol. 3, no. 9, pp. 989–993, 2008.

[14] Ö. Birim, A. P. Kappetein, J. J. M. Takkenberg, R. J. van Klaveren, and A. J. J. C. Bogers, "Survival after pathological stage IA nonsmall cell lung cancer: tumor size matters," *The Annals of Thoracic Surgery*, vol. 79, no. 4, pp. 1137–1141, 2005.

[15] M. Riquet, D. Manac'h, F. le Pimpec Barthes, A. Dujon, D. Debrosse, and B. Debesse, "Prognostic value of T and N in non small cell lung cancer three centimeters or less in diameter," *European Journal of Cardio-thoracic Surgery*, vol. 11, no. 3, pp. 440–444, 1997.

[16] R. Rami-Porta, D. Ball, J. Crowley et al., "The IASLC lung cancer staging project: proposals for the revision of the T descriptors in the forthcoming (seventh) edition of the TNM classification for lung cancer," *Journal of Thoracic Oncology*, vol. 2, no. 7, pp. 593–602, 2007.

[17] W. C. Black, "Overdiagnosis: an underrecognized cause of confusion and harm in cancer screening," *Journal of the National Cancer Institute*, vol. 92, no. 16, pp. 1280–1282, 2000.

[18] A. Cassidy, J. P. Myles, M. van Tongeren et al., "The LLP risk model: an individual risk prediction model for lung cancer," *British Journal of Cancer*, vol. 98, no. 2, pp. 270–276, 2008.

[19] M. R. Spitz, W. K. Hong, C. I. Amos et al., "A risk model for prediction of lung cancer," *Journal of the National Cancer Institute*, vol. 99, no. 9, pp. 715–726, 2007.

[20] D. Arenberg, "Lung cancer screening," *Seminars in Respiratory and Critical Care Medicine*, vol. 34, no. 6, pp. 727–737, 2013.

[21] P. B. Bach and M. K. Gould, "When the average applies to no one: personalized decision making about potential benefits of lung cancer screening," *Annals of Internal Medicine*, vol. 157, no. 8, pp. 571–573, 2012.

[22] L. Dominioni, N. Rotolo, A. Poli et al., "Cost of a population-based programme of chest x-ray screening for lung cancer," *Monaldi Archives for Chest Disease*, vol. 79, no. 2, pp. 67–72, 2013.

[23] K. Kashiwabara, S.-I. Koshi, K. Itonaga, O. Nakahara, M. Tanaka, and M. Toyonaga, "Outcome in patients with lung cancer found on lung cancer mass screening roentgenograms, but who did not subsequently consult a doctor," *Lung Cancer*, vol. 40, no. 1, pp. 67–72, 2003.

17

The Role of Para-Aortic Lymphadenectomy in the Surgical Staging of Women with Intermediate and High-Risk Endometrial Adenocarcinomas

Taymaa May,[1,2] Melina Shoni,[1] Allison F. Vitonis,[3] Charles M. Quick,[4]
Whitfield B. Growdon,[5] and Michael G. Muto[1,2]

[1] Department of Obstetrics and Gynecology, Division of Gynecologic Oncology, Brigham and Women's Hospital,
  Harvard Medical School, Boston, MA 02115, USA
[2] Division of Gynecologic Oncology, Dana-Farber Cancer Institute, Boston, MA 02115, USA
[3] Department of Obstetrics and Gynecology, Epidemiology Center, Brigham and Women's Hospital, Boston, MA 02115, USA
[4] Department of Pathology, University of Arkansas for Medical Sciences, Little Rock, AR 72205, USA
[5] Department of Obstetrics and Gynecology, Division of Gynecologic Oncology, Massachusetts General Hospital,
  Harvard Medical School, Boston, MA 02214, USA

Correspondence should be addressed to Taymaa May; tmay1@partners.org

Academic Editor: Masaki Mori

Objectives. To characterize clinical outcomes in patients with intermediate or high-risk endometrial carcinoma who underwent surgical staging with or without para-aortic lymphadenectomy. *Methods.* This is a retrospective cohort study of patients with intermediate or high-risk endometrial adenocarcinoma who underwent surgical staging with (PPALN group) or without (PLN) para-aortic lymphadenectomy. Data were collected, Kaplan-Meier curves were generated, and univariate and multivariate analyses performed to compare differences in adjuvant therapy, disease recurrence, disease-free survival (DFS), and overall survival (OS). *Results.* 118 patients were included in the PPALN group and 139 in the PLN group. Patients in the PPALN group were more likely to receive adjuvant vaginal brachytherapy (25.4% versus 11.5%, OR = 2.5, $P = 0.03$) and less likely to receive adjuvant multimodal combination therapy (17.81% versus 28.8%, OR = 0.28, $P = 0.002$). DFS was improved in the PLN group as compared to PPALN (80% versus 62%, $P = 0.02$). OS was equivalent ($P = 0.93$). Patients in the PPALN group who had less than 10 para-aortic nodes removed were twice as likely to recur than patients who had 10 or more para-aortic nodes or patients in the PLN group (HR 2.08, CI 1.20–3.60, $P = 0.009$). *Conclusions.* Patients in the PLN group were more likely to receive multimodal adjuvant therapy and had better DFS than the PPALN group. Pelvic lymphadenectomy followed by adjuvant radiation and chemotherapy may represent an effective treatment option for patients with intermediate or high-risk disease. If systematic para-aortic lymphadenectomy is performed and less than 10 para-aortic lymph nodes are obtained, multimodality adjuvant therapy should be considered to improve DFS.

1. Introduction

The landmark study GOG 33 described the patterns of spread in endometrial carcinoma and concluded that clinical staging is inaccurate as 22% of clinical stage I patients were assigned a higher surgical stage [1]. As such, the International Federation of Gynecology and Obstetrics (FIGO) changed the endometrial cancer staging system from clinical to surgical [2]. Conventionally, surgical staging includes a total hysterectomy, bilateral salpingooophorectomy, and retroperitoneal pelvic and para-aortic lymphadenectomy. Although pelvic washings are no longer part of the 2009 FIGO surgical staging system, they are still collected at time of surgery [2].

Multivariate analysis of GOG 33 indicated 3 uterine factors as independent predictors of nodal metastasis, including tumor grade, depth of myometrial invasion, and the presence of intraperitoneal disease [3]. Using these factors as predictors of disease aggressive behavior, endometrial carcinoma is often divided into low, intermediate, and high-risk diseases [3]. Typically, patients with intermediate and high-risk diseases undergo surgical staging. However, the beneficial effect of complete, systematic lymphadenectomy is debatable. Several studies reported increased morbidity associated with the addition of retroperitoneal lymphadenectomy to the surgical procedure including increased mean blood loss, increased risk of blood transfusion, increased operative time and longer hospital stay [4, 5]. Additionally, lymphadenectomy increases the risk of postoperative fever, incision site infection, lymphocyst formation, lower-extremity edema, embolic events, gastrointestinal obstruction, and perioperative mortality [6]. Notably, the addition of para-aortic lymph node dissection further increases the surgical morbidity. Cragun et al. reported increased blood loss, transfusion rates, and length of hospital stay in patients undergoing both pelvic and para-aortic lymphadenectomy as compared to patients undergoing pelvic lymphadenectomy alone [7].

We designed a study examining the role of para-aortic lymphadenectomy in the surgical staging of patients with intermediate and high-risk endometrial adenocarcinomas. Our objectives were to assess whether or not para-aortic lymphadenectomy impacts administration of adjuvant therapy, disease recurrence, disease-free survival (DFS), and overall survival (OS).

2. Materials and Methods

2.1. Study Design. This a retrospective cohort study investigating patients who underwent surgical staging for newly diagnosed high-grade endometrioid, serous, or clear cell endometrial adenocarcinoma at Brigham and Women's Hospital and Massachusetts General Hospital, Harvard Medical School, Boston, MA, USA, between January 2000 and December 2010. Institutional review board (IRB) approval was obtained from the hospitals' ethics board. Eligible patients were identified using the hospitals' pathology data base and data points were obtained from the patients' electronic medical records.

2.2. Study Population. The first study group included patients who underwent primary surgical staging including total abdominal, laparoscopic or robotic hysterectomy, bilateral salpingooophorectomy, washings, and pelvic and para-aortic lymphadenectomy (PPALN group). The second study group included patients who underwent a similar staging procedure with the exception of the para-aortic lymphadenectomy (PLN group). Data were collected from the patients' hospital charts and analyzed using appropriate statistical tests.

2.3. Outcome Measures. The primary outcome measure of this study was to compare overall survival (OS) between the two study groups to evaluate the impact that para-aortic lymphadenectomy has on OS. The secondary outcome measures were to examine whether the absence of a para-aortic lymphadenectomy impacts administration of adjuvant therapy, disease recurrence, or disease-free survival (DFS).

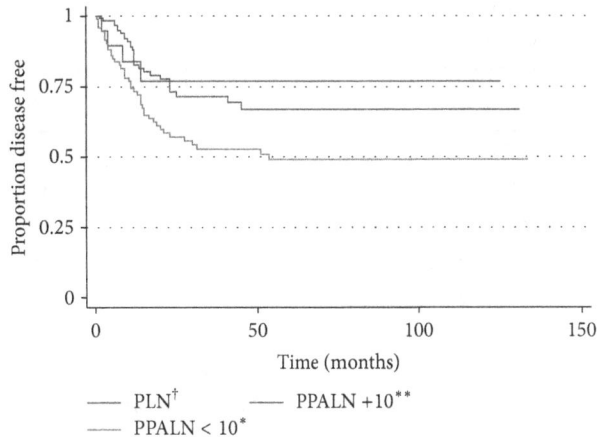

FIGURE 1: Kaplan-Meier disease-free survival estimate. PPALN < 10* versus PLN[†] or PPALN+10** logrank test: HR 2.34, CI 1.36–4.02, P = 0.002. *Patients in the pelvic and para-aortic Lymph node (PPALN) group with less than 10 para-aortic lymph nodes retrieved at time of dissection. **Patients in the pelvic and para-aortic lymph node (PPALN) group with 10 or more para-aortic lymph nodes retrieved at time of dissection. [†]Patients in the pelvic lymph node (PLN) group.

2.4. Statistical Analysis. Chi-square, Fisher's exact tests, and *t*-tests were used to compare the characteristics of patients in the two study groups. Kaplan-Meier curves and Cox proportional hazards models were used to compare OS and DFS between the groups. Models were adjusted for age, year of surgery, histology, lymphovascular invasion, myometrial invasion, and adjuvant therapy. All analyses were performed using SAS version 9.2 (SAS Institute Inc., Cary, NC, USA).

3. Results

3.1. Population Characteristics. Of all women diagnosed with endometrial carcinoma at Brigham and Women's Hospital and Massachusetts General Hospital, Boston, MA, USA, between January 2000 and December 2010, 257 met our inclusion criteria and were subjected to our final analysis. The PPALN group was composed of 118 patients, while 139 patients underwent PLN. The mean age at time of diagnosis in the PPALN group was 63.1, and in the PLN group it was 67.1 (P = 0.002). Importantly, survival was not significantly altered when controlling for the difference in age. Demographic and clinical characteristics of the study cohort are provided in Table 1.

3.2. Clinical and Surgical Characteristics. The surgical stages were similar between the PPALN group and the PLN group (Table 1). Patients in the PLN group had higher rates of papillary serous histology (32.4% versus 19.7%, P = 0.02) and lower rates of grade 3 endometrioid carcinoma (23.7% versus 44.4%) than patients in the PPALN group. Risks of recurrence and DFS were not affected when controlling for the differences in histology using multivariate analysis (Table 2). The other histological subtypes were similar between the two groups. Patients in the PPALN group had significantly

TABLE 1: Demographic and clinical characteristics of patients in the PPALN and the PLN groups.

	PPALN* N = 118	PLN** N = 139	P value
Age			
Mean (SD)	63.1 (10.7)	67.1 (9.5)	0.002
Histology			
Grade 3 endometrioid	52 (44.4%)	33 (23.7%)	0.002
Papillary serous	23 (19.7%)	45 (32.4%)	
Clear cell	9 (7.7%)	15 (10.8%)	
Grade 2 endometrioid	4 (3.4%)	2 (1.4%)	
Mixed	25 (21.4%)	43 (30.9%)	
Stage			
I	66 (55.9%)	74 (53.2%)	0.33
II	7 (5.9%)	12 (8.6%)	
III	35 (29.7%)	33 (23.7%)	
IV	10 (8.5%)	20 (14.4%)	
Lymphovascular invasion			
No	52 (47.7%)	83 (64.8%)	0.008
Yes	57 (52.3%)	45 (35.2%)	
Myometrial invasion			
No	60 (52.6%)	88 (64.7%)	0.05
Yes	54 (47.4%)	48 (35.3%)	
Intraoperative complications			
None	99 (86.1%)	124 (89.9%)	0.44
1 or more	16 (13.9%)	14 (10.1%)	
Postoperative complications			
None	54 (46.6%)	79 (57.2%)	0.09
1 or more	62 (53.4%)	59 (42.8%)	

*Pelvic and para-aortic lymph node group.
**Pelvic lymph node group.

higher lymphovascular space invasion (52.3% versus 35.2%, $P = 0.008$) and higher outer half myometrial invasion (47.4% versus 35.3%, $P = 0.05$). Risks of recurrence and DFS were not significantly affected when controlling for these variables by multivariate analysis (Table 2). The intraoperative complications studied included cystotomy, enterotomy, vascular injury, ureteral injury, and intraoperative blood transfusion. Postoperative complications studied included fever, blood transfusion, paralytic ileus, small bowel obstruction, wound cellulitis, deep wound infection, and reoperation within 28 days of original surgery. Intraoperative and postoperative complication rates were equivalent between the groups ($P = 0.36$ and $P = 0.09$, resp.). The mean number of pelvic nodes removed per patient in the PLN group was 10.7 (range 1–35). The mean numbers of pelvic and para-aortic nodes in the PPALN group were 16.1 (range 2–40) and 5.3 (range 1–19), respectively. Forty-one patients (29.4%) in the PLN group had positive pelvic lymph nodes (Table 3). In the PPALN group,

34 patients (28.8%) had positive pelvic lymph nodes, and 26 patients (22.03%) had positive para-aortic lymph nodes. Of the 26 patients with positive para-aortic lymph nodes, 20 (16.9%) had concurrent positive pelvic lymph nodes, and 6 (5.08%) had negative pelvic lymph nodes (Table 3).

3.3. Treatment and Recurrence. Patients in the PPALN group were more likely to receive adjuvant vaginal brachytherapy (25.4% versus 11.5%, OR = 2.5, $P = 0.03$) and less likely to receive adjuvant multimodal therapy consisting of combined vaginal brachytherapy, pelvic radiation and chemotherapy (17.8% versus 28.8%, OR = 0.28, $P = 0.0019$) (see Table 1(a) in Supplementary Material available online at http://dx.doi.org/10.1155/2013/858916). Patients in the PPALN group were more likely to experience disease recurrence than patients in the PLN group (38.9% versus 20.14%, $P = 0.003$). Variation in adjuvant therapy was not an independent predictor of recurrence, DFS or OS (see Tables 1(b) and 1(c) in Supplementary Material). The number of para-aortic nodes removed at time of surgery was associated with disease recurrence. Patients in the PPALN group who had less than 10 para-aortic nodes removed were twice more likely to recur than patients who had 10 or more para-aortic nodes or patients in the PLN group (HR 2.34, CI 1.36–4.02, $P = 0.002$) (Figure 1). As such, the number of para-aortic lymph nodes obtained at time of surgery was an independent factor associated with disease recurrence and DFS (Table 2). Abdominal recurrences represented a significantly increased portion of recurrences in the PLN group compared to the PPALN group (53.6% versus 28.3%, $P = 0.03$) (Table 4(a)). Recurrence patterns at other sites including vagina, pelvis, pelvic lymph nodes, para-aortic lymph nodes and extra-peritoneal sites were similar between the groups (Table 4(a)). Cox proportional hazards model for overall survival showed no association between recurrence site and survival (Table 4(b)). These analyses were adjusted for age (continuous), year of surgery (continuous), lymph nodes (PLN and PALN), histology (endometrioid, mixed, clear cell, and papillary serous), lymphovascular invasion, and myometrial invasion.

3.4. Disease Free and Overall Survival. OS was similar between the PLN and the PPALN groups ($P = 0.93$) (Figure 2(a)). Patients in the PLN group had better DFS than patients in the PPALN group (80% versus 62%, $P = 0.02$) (Figure 2(b)). The mean followup time was 32.4 months.

4. Discussion

Our study investigates the role and extent of retroperitoneal lymphadenectomy in the management of women with intermediate and high-risk endometrial adenocarcinomas. Women who underwent para-aortic lymph node dissections had an overrepresentation of deep myometrial invasion, lymphovascular invasion, and grade 3 endometrioid histology, and they were less likely to undergo postoperative multimodality adjuvant therapy. Cox proportional hazards models as well as multivariate analysis were adjusted for age, year

TABLE 2: Disease-free survival analysis adjusting for the following variables: tumor histology, lymphovascular invasion, myometrial invasion, and number of para-aortic lymph nodes.

	No recurrence $N = 183$	Recurrence $N = 74$	Age-adjusted HR (95% CI)	Fully adjusted* HR (95% CI)	P
Histology					
Endometrioid/mixed	112 (61.5%)	52 (70.3%)	1.00	1.00	
Clear cell	17 (9.3%)	7 (9.5%)	0.95 (0.42, 2.14)	1.33 (0.58, 3.05)	0.50
Papillary serous	53 (29.1%)	15 (20.3%)	0.64 (0.36, 1.15)	0.68 (0.37, 1.26)	0.23
Lymphovascular invasion					
No	112 (67.1%)	23 (32.9%)	1.00	1.00	
Yes	55 (32.9%)	47 (67.1%)	2.99 (1.82, 4.93)	1.67 (0.91, 3.07)	0.10
Myometrial invasion					
No	121 (67.6%)	27 (38.0%)	1.00	1.00	
Yes	58 (32.4%)	44 (62.0%)	2.76 (1.70, 4.45)	1.69 (0.93, 3.06)	0.08
Lymph nodes					
PLN	111 (60.7%)	28 (37.8%)	1.00	1.00	
PPALN < 10*	56 (30.6%)	42 (56.8%)	2.16 (1.33, 3.52)	2.34 (1.36, 4.02)	0.002
PPALN ≥ 10**	16 (8.7%)	4 (5.4%)	1.06 (0.37, 3.01)	1.36 (0.44, 4.24)	0.59

*PPALN patients with less than 10 para-aortic nodes dissected.
**PPALN patients with 10 or more dissected para-aortic nodes.

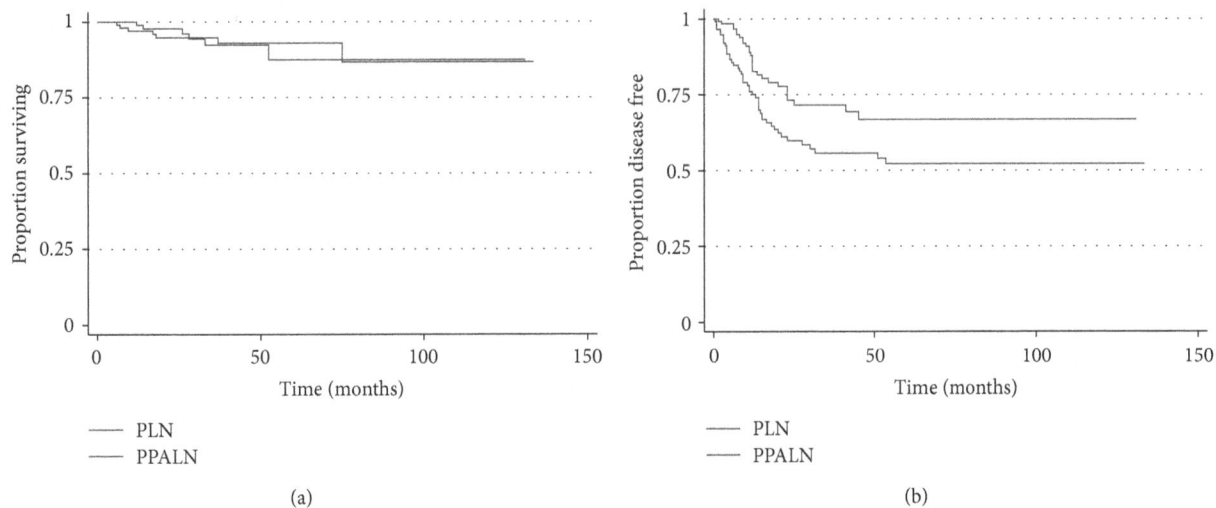

FIGURE 2: (a) Kaplan-Meier overall survival estimate. Logrank test PLN versus PPALN P value = 0.93. (b) Kaplan-Meier Disease-Free survival estimate. PLN versus PPALN Logrank test P value = 0.02.

of surgery, histology, lymphovascular invasion, myometrial invasion and adjuvant therapy to control for the variations within the groups. Multivariate analysis incorporating these significant variables along with the extent of lymphadenectomy confirmed that only para-aortic lymphadenectomy yielding less than 10 nodes was associated with an increased risk of recurrence and decreased PFS. No difference in OS was observed between the groups. These data suggest that limited para-aortic lymph node dissection may not obviate the need for aggressive, multimodality adjuvant therapy based on clinical risk factors.

The role of para-aortic lymph node dissection in the staging of endometrial carcinoma is debatable. At our center, the decision to perform systematic para-aortic nodal

dissection is largely surgeon dependent. Moreover, the necessity of systematic para-aortic lymphadenectomy is being challenged by some surgeons as they believe it increases morbidity without added benefit. Notably, lymphatic drainage of uterine lesions confined to the corpus is primarily to the external iliac and the obturator lymph nodes [8]. In advanced disease, para-aortic nodal involvement may occur via spread through the common iliac lymphatic channels [8]. As such, para-aortic involvement often follows pelvic nodal involvement. Abu-Rustum et al. examined the incidence of isolated para-aortic nodal metastasis in the setting of negative pelvic lymph nodes and found it was approximately 1% in both low and high-grade diseases [9]. In our study, 6 of 118 patients (5.08%) in the PPALN group

TABLE 3: (a) Number of positive lymph nodes in the PLN and PPALN groups. (b) Breakdown of pelvic and para-aortic nodal metastasis in the PPALN group.

(a)

	PPALN			PLN
	All	<10	≥10	
Positive pelvic lymph nodes				
None	84 (71.2)	68 (69.4)	16 (80.0)	98 (70.5)
1 or more	34 (28.8)	30 (30.6)	4 (20.0)	41 (29.5)
Mean (SD)	1.0 (2.4)	1.1 (2.6)	0.4 (1.1)	0.5 (1.1)
Positive para-aortic lymph nodes				
None	92 (78.0)	75 (76.5)	17 (85.0)	—
1 or more	26 (22.0)	23 (23.5)	3 (15.0)	—
Mean (SD)	0.4 (0.9)	0.4 (1.0)	0.2 (0.4)	—

(b)

PPALN (P < 0.0001)	Negative pelvic and para-aortic nodes	Positive pelvic and para-aortic nodes	Positive pelvic nodes only	Positive para-aortic nodes only
118 (100)	78 (66.1)	20 (16.9)	14 (11.8)	6 (5.08)

had positive para-aortic nodal metastasis with negative pelvic lymph nodes.

The therapeutic effects of lymphadenectomy are an issue of great debate in the gynecologic oncology literature. Findings from two large prospective randomized trials of pelvic lymphadenectomy failed to demonstrate a clear therapeutic benefit [10, 11]. Conversely, Mariani et al. showed that patients with poorly differentiated endometrial adenocarcinoma who underwent retroperitoneal lymphadenectomy had an associated survival advantage [12]. However, this advantage did not extend to the addition of para-aortic lymphadenectomy to the lymph node dissection [12]. Recently, the survival effect of para-aortic lymphadenectomy in endometrial cancer (SEPAL) study aimed to examine whether complete, systematic para-aortic lymphadenectomy would have a survival effect in patients with intermediate and high-risk endometrial carcinomas [13]. The results of this retrospective cohort study showed an increased overall survival in patients who had both pelvic and para-aortic lymph node dissection compared to patients who underwent pelvic lymphadenectomy alone. Notably, the average number of lymph nodes in this study was 34 nodes in patients who had pelvic lymph node dissection and 59 nodes in patients who had pelvic and para-aortic lymph nodes dissection with an average of 24 para-aortic nodes [13]. These numbers are significantly higher than the average nodal dissection quoted in most studies.

Interestingly, our results indicate that patients in the PPALN group had an increased disease recurrence compared to patients in the PLN group. The number of para-aortic lymph nodes retrieved at dissection was a significant variable in predicting DFS. Abu-Rustum et al. showed that removal of 10 or more regional lymph nodes was indicative of adequate surgical staging [14]. Furthermore, Chan et al. noted an improved DFS in patients with intermediate and high-risk diseases who underwent extensive lymph node dissection [15]. These data show that patients with 10 or more para-aortic nodes had improved DFS compared to those who had less than 10 nodes removed. Furthermore, patients in the PPALN group who had 10 or more para-aortic nodes had similar DFS to patients in the PLN group, while those with less than 10 nodes had a worse DFS than patients in the PLN group. These data suggest that limited para-aortic nodal sampling may not provide survival advantage and may negatively impact DFS.

Adjuvant treatment is an important consideration in the management of women with endometrial carcinoma. The SEPAL study indicated that adjuvant chemotherapy improves survival in intermediate and high-risk diseases [13]. The majority of these cancers are comprised of aggressive histopathological types including high-grade endometrioid, clear cell, and serous carcinomas. It is well established that clear cell and serous endometrial carcinomas are highly malignant, estrogen-independent tumors and are thus classified as type 2 carcinomas [16, 17]. These subtypes account for 10% of endometrial malignancies but are responsible for approximately 50% of relapses [16, 17]. Similarly, high-grade endometrioid cancers often have an aggressive clinical course. Voss et al. examined the immunohistochemical patterns of grade 3 endometrioid carcinoma and found them to be similar to those of clear cell and papillary serous carcinomas [18]. The authors concluded that grade 3 endometrioid cancer may be better characterized as type 2 cancer and should be treated with similar adjuvant therapy to serous and clear cell carcinoma [18]. Given the aggressive tumor biology of type 2 carcinoma, some authorities believe patients should be managed with a limited staging procedure followed by systemic therapy irrespective of stage. In our series, patients in the PLN group were more likely to receive systemic therapy as compared to patients of similar stage in the PPALN group. Given the presumed comprehensive surgical staging, patients in the PPALN group were less likely to receive comprehensive adjuvant therapy consisting of vaginal cuff brachytherapy, pelvic radiation, and systemic chemotherapy.

Patients in the PPALN group experienced a decreased DFS than patients in the PLN group. Recurrences in the vagina, pelvis, pelvic lymph nodes, para-aortic lymph nodes, and extraperitoneal sites were similar between the groups. Interestingly, the absence of a para-aortic lymph node dissection in the PLN group did not impact the risk of para-aortic recurrence. Isolated para-aortic lymph node recurrence usually occurs in approximately 6% of women with endometrial carcinoma [8]. Our results revealed 17 patients (6.6%) with para-aortic recurrence-5 in the PLN group (3.59%) and 12 in the PPALN group (10.16%) (P = 0.39). Importantly, patients who experienced disease recurrence were successfully salvaged as the OS was similar between the study groups.

The limitations of this study are inherent to its retrospective nature. Patients underwent surgical staging with or without para-aortic lymph node dissection based on

TABLE 4: (a) Disease recurrence patterns in the PPALN and the PLN groups. (b) Overall survival analysis adjusting for recurrence site amongst patients who experienced a recurrence[*].

(a)

	PPALN N = 118	PLN N = 139	Chi-square P value
Vagina			
No	39 (84.8%)	24 (85.7%)	0.91
Yes	7 (15.2%)	4 (14.3%)	
Pelvic lymph node			
No	38 (82.6%)	24 (85.7%)	0.72
Yes	8 (17.4%)	4 (14.3%)	
Pelvis			
No	34 (73.9%)	22 (78.6%)	0.65
Yes	12 (26.1%)	6 (21.4%)	
Para-aortic lymph node			
No	33 (71.7%)	23 (82.1%)	0.31
Yes	13 (28.3%)	5 (17.9%)	
Extraperitoneal			
No	21 (45.7%)	12 (42.9%)	0.81
Yes	25 (54.3%)	16 (57.1%)	
Abdomen			
No	33 (71.7%)	13 (46.4%)	0.03
Yes	13 (28.3%)	15 (53.6%)	

(b)

	Alive N = 63	Dead N = 11	Age-adjusted HR (95% CI)	Fully adjusted[*] HR (95% CI)	P
Vagina					
No	52 (82.5%)	11 (100.0%)			
Yes	11 (17.5%)	0 (0%)			
Pelvic lymph node					
No	53 (84.1%)	9 (81.8%)	1.00	1.00	
Yes	10 (15.9%)	2 (18.2%)	0.64 (0.12, 3.31)	0.22 (0.02, 2.43)	0.22
Pelvis					
No	48 (76.2%)	8 (72.7%)	1.00	1.00	
Yes	15 (23.8%)	3 (27.3%)	1.06 (0.28, 4.02)	1.41 (0.15, 13.1)	0.76
Para-aortic lymph node					
No	48 (76.2%)	8 (72.7%)	1.00	1.00	
Yes	15 (23.8%)	3 (27.3%)	0.46 (0.11, 1.93)	0.37 (0.04, 3.16)	0.36
Extraperitoneal					
No	31 (49.2%)	2 (18.2%)	1.00	1.00	
Yes	32 (50.8%)	9 (81.8%)	3.26 (0.69, 15.4)	10.9 (0.42, 285)	0.15
Abdomen					
No	39 (61.9%)	7 (63.6%)	1.00	1.00	
Yes	24 (38.1%)	4 (36.4%)	1.46 (0.39, 5.43)	1.19 (0.16, 8.87)	0.86

[*]Adjusted for age (continuous), year of surgery (continuous), lymph nodes (PLN and PALN), histology (endometrioid/mixed, clear cell, and papillary serous), lymphovascular invasion, and myometrial invasion.

recommendations by the attending surgeon. This decision may have been influenced by preoperative biopsy results, medical or surgical co-morbidities, and surgeon preferences and practice. Patients in the PLN group were older, and tumors in that group were less likely to invade the outer myometrium or the lymphovascular space. To control for the heterogeneity between the groups, multivariate statistical analyses were preformed. Importantly, the heterogeneous variables had no impact on DFS or OS. As such, the results were statistically significant and consequently have clinical relevance.

In conclusion, patients in the PLN group had improved DFS than patients in the PPALN group. DFS was equivalent between patients in the PLN group and patients in the PALN group who had more than 10 para-aortic lymph nodes removed. Notably, intermediate and high-risk endometrial malignancies often exhibit aggressive tumor biology and may require adjuvant therapy to decrease the risk of recurrence. Importantly, patients in the PLN group were more likely to receive multimodality adjuvant therapy than patients in the PALN group, which may have contributed to their improved survival. Thus, operative staging with pelvic lymphadenectomy alone followed by adjuvant radiation and chemotherapy may represent a safe and effective treatment option for women with this disease. Alternatively, if systematic pelvic and para-aortic lymphadenectomy is performed, thorough nodal dissection is advocated with the goal of obtaining 10 or more nodes per lymphatic chain. If less than 10 para-aortic lymph nodes are sampled, the dissection may be an inadequate triage tool for adjuvant therapy. Hence, adjuvant radiation therapy and chemotherapy should be considered to improve DFS.

Acknowledgment

The authors wish to thank Dr. Dan Cramer, Department of Obstetrics and Gynecology, Epidemiology Center, Brigham and Women's Hospital, Boston, MA, USA, for his assistance in statistical analysis and for critically reviewing the paper.

References

[1] W. T. Creasman, C. P. Morrow, B. N. Bundy, H. D. Homesley, J. E. Graham, and P. B. Heller, "Surgical pathologic spread patterns of endometrial cancer. A gynecologic oncology group study," *Cancer*, vol. 60, supplement 8, pp. 2035–2041, 1987.

[2] S. Pecorelli, "Revised FIGO staging for carcinoma of the vulva, cervix, and endometrium," *International Journal of Gynaecology and Obstetrics*, vol. 105, no. 2, pp. 103–104, 2009.

[3] C. P. Morrow, B. N. Bundy, R. J. Kurman et al., "Relationship between surgical-pathological risk factors and outcome in clinical stage I and II carcinoma of the endometrium: a gynecologic oncology group study," *Gynecologic Oncology*, vol. 40, no. 1, pp. 55–65, 1991.

[4] T. Hidaka, K. Kato, R. Yonezawa et al., "Omission of lymphadenectomy is possible for low-risk corpus cancer," *European Journal of Surgical Oncology*, vol. 33, no. 1, pp. 86–90, 2007.

[5] D. M. Larson, K. Johnson, and K. A. Olson, "Pelvic and para-aortic lymphadenectomy for surgical staging of endometrial cancer: morbidity and mortality," *Obstetrics and Gynecology*, vol. 79, no. 6, pp. 998–1001, 1992.

[6] J. W. Orr, R. W. Holloway, P. F. Orr, and J. L. Holimon, "Surgical staging of uterine cancer: an analysis of perioperative morbidity," *Gynecologic Oncology*, vol. 42, no. 3, pp. 209–216, 1991.

[7] J. M. Cragun, L. J. Havrilesky, B. Calingaert et al., "Retrospective analysis of selective lymphadenectomy in apparent early-stage endometrial cancer," *Journal of Clinical Oncology*, vol. 23, no. 16, pp. 3668–3675, 2005.

[8] A. Mariani, M. J. Webb, G. L. Keeney, and K. C. Podratz, "Routes of lymphatic spread: a study of 112 consecutive patients with endometrial cancer," *Gynecologic Oncology*, vol. 81, no. 1, pp. 100–104, 2001.

[9] N. R. Abu-Rustum, J. D. Gomez, K. M. Alektiar et al., "The incidence of isolated paraaortic nodal metastasis in surgically staged endometrial cancer patients with negative pelvic lymph nodes," *Gynecologic Oncology*, vol. 115, no. 2, pp. 236–238, 2009.

[10] ASTEC study group, H. Kitchener, A. M. Swart, Q. Qian, C. Amos, and M. K. Parmar, "Efficacy of systematic pelvic lymphadenectomy in endometrial cancer (MRC ASTEC trial): a randomized study," *The Lancet*, vol. 373, no. 9658, pp. 125–136, 2009.

[11] P. B. Panici, S. Basile, F. Maneschi et al., "Systematic pelvic lymphadenectomy vs no lymphadenectomy in early-stage endometrial carcinoma: randomized clinical trial," *Journal of the National Cancer Institute*, vol. 100, no. 23, pp. 1707–1716, 2008.

[12] A. Mariani, M. J. Webb, G. L. Keeney, M. G. Haddock, G. Calori, and K. C. Podratz, "Low-risk corpus cancer: is lymphadenectomy or radiotherapy necessary?" *American Journal of Obstetrics and Gynecology*, vol. 182, no. 6, pp. 1506–1519, 2000.

[13] Y. Todo, H. Kato, M. Kaneuchi, H. Watari, M. Takeda, and N. Sakuragi, "Erratum: survival effect of para-aortic lymphadenectomy in endometrial cancer (SEPAL study): a retrospective cohort analysis," *The Lancet*, vol. 376, no. 9741, p. 594, 2010.

[14] N. R. Abu-Rustum, A. Iasonos, Q. Zhou et al., "Is there a therapeutic impact to regional lymphadenectomy in the surgical treatment of endometrial carcinoma?" *American Journal of Obstetrics and Gynecology*, vol. 198, no. 4, pp. 457.e1–457.e6, 2008.

[15] J. K. Chan, M. K. Cheung, W. K. Huh et al., "Therapeutic role of lymph node resection in endometrioid corpus cancer: a study of 12,333 patients," *Cancer*, vol. 107, no. 8, pp. 1823–1830, 2006.

[16] P. Singh, C. L. Smith, G. Cheetham, T. J. Dodd, and M. L. J. Davy, "Serous carcinoma of the uterus-determination of HER-2/neu status using immunohistochemistry, chromogenic in situ hybridization, and quantitative polymerase chain reaction techniques: its significance and clinical correlation," *International Journal of Gynecological Cancer*, vol. 18, no. 6, pp. 1344–1351, 2008.

[17] S. M. Ueda, D. S. Kapp, M. K. Cheung et al., "Trends in demographic and clinical characteristics in women diagnosed with corpus cancer and their potential impact on the increasing number of deaths," *American Journal of Obstetrics and Gynecology*, vol. 198, no. 2, pp. 218.e1–218.e6, 2008.

[18] M. A. Voss, R. Ganesan, L. Ludeman et al., "Should grade 3 endometrioid endometrial carcinoma be considered a type 2 cancer—a clinical and pathological evaluation," *Gynecologic Oncology*, vol. 124, no. 1, pp. 15–20, 2012.

18

Pancreatogastrostomy versus Pancreatojejunostomy: An Up-to-Date Meta-Analysis of RCTs

Konstantinos Perivoliotis,[1,2] Eleni Sioka,[2] Athina Tatsioni,[2,3,4] Ioannis Stefanidis,[2,5] Elias Zintzaras,[2,6] and Dimitrios Zacharoulis[1]

[1] Department of Surgery, University Hospital of Larissa, Mezourlo, 41110 Larissa, Greece
[2] Postgraduate Programme (MSc): Research Methodology in Biomedicine, Biostatistics and Clinical Bioinformatics, University of Thessaly, Larissa, Greece
[3] Research Unit for General Medicine and Primary Health Care, Faculty of Medicine, School for Health Sciences, University of Ioannina, Ioannina, Greece
[4] Tufts University School of Medicine, Boston, MA, USA
[5] Department of Nephrology, Medical School, University of Thessaly, Larissa, Greece
[6] Department of Biomathematics, University of Thessaly School of Medicine, Larissa, Greece

Correspondence should be addressed to Konstantinos Perivoliotis; kperi19@gmail.com

Academic Editor: George H. Sakorafas

Background. A meta-analysis was conducted in order to provide an up-to-date comparison of pancreatogastrostomy (PG) and pancreatojejunostomy (PJ), after pancreatoduodenectomy (PD), in terms of clinically significant postoperative pancreatic fistula (POPF) and other postoperative complications. *Methods.* This meta-analysis was conducted according to the PRISMA guidelines and the Cochrane Handbook for Systematic Reviews of Interventions. A systematic literature search in MEDLINE and Cochrane Central Register of Controlled Clinical Trials was performed. Fixed Effects or Random Effects model was used, based on the Cochran Q test. *Results.* In total, 10 studies (1629 patients) were included. There was no statistical significance between PG and PJ regarding the rate of clinically significant POPF (OR: 0.70, 95%CI: 0.46–1.06). PG was associated with a higher rate of postpancreatoduodenectomy haemorrhage (PPH) (OR: 1.52, 95%CI: 1.08–2.14). There was no difference between the two techniques in terms of clinically significant PPH (OR: 1.35, 95%CI: 0.95–1.93) and clinically significant postoperative delayed gastric emptying (DGE) (OR: 0.98, 95%CI: 0.59–1.63). *Discussion.* There is no difference between the two anastomotic techniques regarding the rate of clinically significant POPF. Given several limitations, more large scale high quality RCTs are required.

1. Introduction

1.1. Rationale. Pancreatoduodenectomy (PD) is still the gold standard of treatment for patients with resectable benign and malignant lesions of the head of the pancreas and the periampullary region. Although PD is considered a safe operative technique, with 30-day mortality rates in specialized, high volume centers currently estimated below 3% [1, 2], complications, such as postoperative pancreatic fistula (POPF), delayed gastric emptying (DGE), and postpancreatoduodenectomy haemorrhage (POPH), increase the overall morbidity to the rate of 45%, despite the application of enhanced recovery approaches after surgery [3].

Given the fact that the frequency of POPF, the most notorious postpancreatoduodenectomy complication, remains as high as 40% [4], researchers have focused on factors that may influence this rate, with the pancreatoenteric anastomosis being one of them. The anastomosis between the pancreatic stump and the GI is regarded as prone to leakage, due to exposure of the suture line to pancreatic juice. The two most widely adopted postpancreaticoduodenectomy anastomotic techniques are the pancreatogastrostomy (PG) and the pancreatojejunostomy (PJ), which combined with anastomotic reinforcing techniques, such as glue and intraductal stenting, are designed to provide a sealed and stable pancreatoenteric junction. In the current literature, a series of retrospective and prospective studies [5–10] have compared PG and PJ with inconclusive results. Keck et al. [11], in a large multicenter randomized controlled trial, reported no difference between the two techniques in terms of clinically significant POPF, which is in contrast with results from previous meta-analyses [12–14], where it was suggested that PG was a safer and more effective method of reconstruction, with lower rates of POPF and other intra-abdominal complications and shorter length of hospital stay (LOS).

1.2. Objectives. In light of these conflicting evidences, we conducted a meta-analysis, in order to provide an up-to-date comparison of PG and PJ after PD, for benign or malignant diseases of the head of the pancreas and the periampullary region, in terms of clinically significant POPF and other postoperative complications.

2. Methods

2.1. Study Protocol. The conduction of this meta-analysis was completed according to the PRISMA [15] guidelines and the Cochrane Handbook for Systematic Reviews of Interventions. The present study was not registered in any database.

2.2. Primary Endpoint. The primary endpoint of this study was the rate of clinically significant postoperative pancreatic fistula (grade B/C according to ISGPF). POPF was defined by ISGPF [16] as a drain output of any measurable volume of fluid on or after POD 3 with an amylase content > 3 times the serum amylase activity. Classification to grades A, B, and C is based on the impact of POPF on the overall clinical course.

2.3. Secondary Endpoints. Secondary endpoints included overall postoperative POPF, postoperative delayed gastric emptying (DGE) [17], clinically significant DGE (grade B/C), postpancreatectomy haemorrhage (PPH) [18], clinically significant PPH (grade B/C), biliary fistula, intra-abdominal fluid collection, overall morbidity, mortality, reoperation rate, wound infection, intraoperative blood transfusion, operative time, and the length of hospital stay (LOS).

2.4. Eligibility Criteria. Eligible trials were prospective human studies with a RCT design, comparing PG and PJ after PD for benign or malignant diseases of the head of the pancreas and the periampullary region, whose outcome data were reported in English and could be retrieved. Excluded studies included those not written in English or studies with no outcome of interest and no comparison group and observational, nonhuman, or nonrandomized studies. Moreover, studies reported in the form of editorials, letters, conference abstracts, expert opinion, or duplicate studies were excluded.

2.5. Literature Search. A systematic literature search in electronic databases (MEDLINE and Cochrane Central Register of Controlled Clinical Trials) was performed (search date: 20 July 2016) in order to identify the eligible RCTs.

In order to perform the literature search the following keywords were used:

(i) *MEDLINE*: (Pancreaticoduodenectomy OR Pancreatoduodenectomy OR Whipple OR "pancreatoduodenal resection" OR "pancreaticoduodenal resection" OR pancreaticojejunostomy OR pancreatojejunostomy OR "pancreaticoenteric anastomosis" OR "pancreatoenteric anastomosis" OR pancreaticogastrostomy OR pancreatogastrostomy OR "pancreaticogastric anastomosis" OR "pancreatogastric anastomosis" OR "pancreaticojejunal anastomosis" OR "pancreatojejunal anastomosis") AND ("Clinical Trials as Topic" OR "randomized controlled trial" OR "controlled clinical trial" OR randomized OR placebo OR randomly OR trial)

(ii) *Cochrane Central Register of Controlled Clinical Trials (Wiley)*: (Pancreaticoduodenectomy OR Pancreatoduodenectomy OR Whipple OR "pancreatoduodenal resection" OR "pancreaticoduodenal resection" OR pancreaticojejunostomy OR pancreatojejunostomy OR "pancreaticoenteric anastomosis" OR "pancreatoenteric anastomosis" OR pancreaticogastrostomy OR pancreatogastrostomy OR "pancreaticogastric anastomosis" OR "pancreatogastric anastomosis" OR "pancreaticojejunal anastomosis" OR "pancreatojejunal anastomosis")

2.6. Study Selection and Data Collection. After duplicate removal, titles and abstracts of the studies were screened according to eligibility criteria. The next step included the full text review of the articles in order to assess that they are consistent with the inclusion criteria.

All electronic database search, study selection, data extraction, and methodological assessment of the studies were performed blindly and in duplicate by two independent investigators (PK and SE). Disagreements were resolved by mutual revision and discussion, in order to reach a consensus. In case of not resolving the discrepancies, the opinion of a third investigator (TA) was considered.

From all eligible studies, the data extracted included author's name, study location and year, RCT type, sample size, the age and gender of the participants, primary outcome, follow-up duration, overall morbidity, underlying disease, operation type, rate of PD/pylorus preserving PD (PPPD), anastomotic technique, operative time, postoperative hospital stay, use of intraductal stent, glue and drains, postoperative administration of somatostatin, and information regarding the diameter of pancreatic duct and the texture of pancreas. Only results reported in the article of the studies were extracted.

All studies imported in this meta-analysis were submitted to rigorous quality and methodological evaluation for bias appraisal according to Cochrane's risk of bias assessing tool [19]. Validity checkpoints included assessment of random sequence allocation, allocation concealment, blinding of participants and personnel and blinding of outcome assessment, incomplete outcome data, and selective reporting. Cohen's *k* statistic was also calculated.

2.7. Statistical Analysis. Data analysis was performed using the Cochrane Collaboration RevMan version 5.3. Dichotomous variables were reported in the form of Odds Ratio (OR), while for continuous variables Weighted Mean Differences (WMD) were used. Results of the analyses were presented with the corresponding 95% Confidence Interval (95% CI).

In the case of continuous variables, if the article did not provide the mean and the Standard Deviation (SD), these were calculated from the median and the Interquartile Range (IR), based on the formula by Hozo et al. [20]. To be more specific, if the sample size was >25, then the mean was considered equal to the median. For sample sizes <70, SD was regarded as IR/4. If the sample size was >70, then SD was equal to IR/6. For dichotomous variables, the statistical method used was the Mantel-Haenszel (MH) and for continuous variables the Inverse Variance (IV). Both Fixed Effects (FE) and Random Effects (RE) model were calculated and reported. The decision of which model to finally estimate was based on the Cochran Q test. If statistically significant heterogeneity was present (Q test $P < 0.1$), then RE model was applied. Moreover, heterogeneity was quantified with the use of I^2. The studies were weighted on the basis of sample size. Statistical significance was considered at the level of $P < 0.05$.

2.8. Risk of Bias across Studies. The funnel plot of the primary outcome was also visually inspected, in order to determine the possible presence of publication bias. An Egger's test was also performed for the primary outcome.

3. Results

3.1. Study Selection. From the literature search, 1240 citations (Figure 1) were retrieved, published up to 20 July 2016. After the removing of 236 duplicate records, the screening of the titles and the abstracts begun. From the 1004 studies submitted to the first phase of the screening, 993 were excluded. More specific, 10 were comments or conference abstracts, 5 did not have a RCT design, 5 did not have a comparison group, 18 were reviews of the current literature, 20 were meta-analysis, 3 articles were not written in English, 23 compared different techniques of PG or PJ instead, and 909 were irrelevant to the subject records. In full text review, 11 articles were submitted [9, 11, 21–29]. At this step, 1 trial [9] was rejected due to a no RCT design. Finally, 10 studies [11, 21–29] were included in qualitative and quantitative analysis.

3.2. Study Characteristics. Table 1 summarizes the characteristics of the included studies. The publication date ranges from 1995 up to 2016. Four studies were multicentered while the other six were single-centered. Fernàndez-Cruz et al. [24] were the first to adopt the ISGPS definition and classification of POPF. Since then, heterogeneity existed in the definition and diagnosis of POPF. The overall amount of patients included in this meta-analysis is 1629 (Table 2). A total of 826 PGs and 803 PJs were performed. The age of the participants extended from 12 to 87 years. Regarding the gender allocation between the two comparison groups,

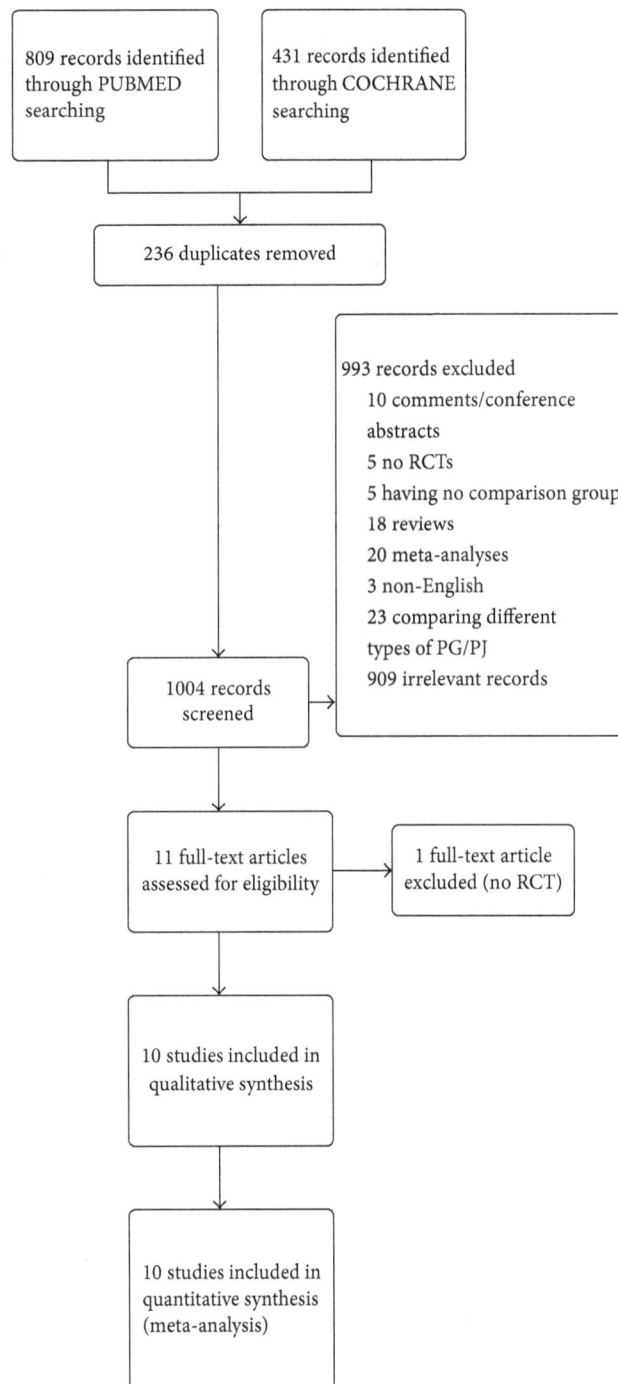

FIGURE 1: Study flow diagram.

data are shown in Table 2. El Nakeeb et al. [23] compared the results of PG and an isolated Roux loop pancreatojejunostomy while Fernàndez-Cruz et al. [24], respectively, compared PJ and PG with gastric partition. In the rest of the studies, PG was considered the intervention and PJ the control. All studies, except Duffas et al. [22], had the rate of POPF as primary outcome. Four studies [21, 24, 26, 29] did not report the duration of follow-up. In the other six studies, follow-up varied from 30 days to 12 months. Regarding the

TABLE 1: Included studies.

PMID	First author	Country	Publication year	RCT type	POPF definition
26135690	Keck	Germany	2016	Multicenter, randomized, controlled, observer- and patient-blinded trial	ISGPS (grade B/C)
25799130	Grendar	Canada	2015	Single-center, randomized, controlled trial	Radiologically proven anastomotic leak or continued drainage of lipase-rich fluid on PoD 10. Classification by ISGPS
24467711	El Nakeeb	Egypt	2014	Single-center, prospective, randomized study	ISGPS (grade A/B/C)
24264781	Figueras	Spain	2013	Multicenter, prospective, randomized study	ISGPS (grade B/C)
23643139	Topal	Belgium	2013	Multicenter, randomised, superiority trial	ISGPS (grade B/C)
22744638	Wellner	Germany	2012	Single-center, open, randomized, controlled study	ISGPS (grade B/C)
19092337	Fernàndez-Cruz	Spain	2008	Single-center, prospective, randomized study	ISGPS (grade B/C)
16327486	Bassi	Italy	2005	Single-center, prospective, randomized study	Any clinical significant output of fluid, rich in amylase, confirmed by fistulography
15910726	Duffas	France	2005	Multicenter, single blind, controlled, randomized trial	Fluid obtained through drains or percutaneous aspiration, containing at least 4 times normal serum values of amylase for 3 days or as anastomotic leaks shown by fistulography
7574936	Yeo	USA	1995	Single-center, prospective, randomized trial	Drainage of greater than 50 mL of amylase rich fluid (greater than threefold elevation above upper limit of normal in serum) through the operatively placed drains on or after

underlying disease, carcinoma of the pancreatic head was the most frequent (Table 3). The PD and PPPD ratio is shown in Table 3. There was a lack of uniformity between the studies regarding the technique of PG and PJ anastomoses. Both PG and PJ could be performed in either a telescoped or a duct-to-mucosa manner. Table 4 reports a summary of the studies implementing the use of stents in the pancreatic duct, anastomotic glue reinforcement, and the overall drain use. Postoperative octreotide was administered in 7 studies [21–23, 25–28]. All studies reported data regarding the main pancreatic duct diameter. Similarly, only Topal et al. [27] did not provide the allocation of the patients regarding pancreatic texture.

3.3. Risk of Bias within Studies.

Figure 2 represents a summary of the included studies quality assessment. More specifically, as shown in Figure 3, all studies included a random sequence generation procedure in their protocol. Allocation concealment was also applied in all studies except one [29]. Only two trials [11, 22] reported the blinding of participants and personnel and the blinding of outcome assessment. Only in the study of Grendar et al. [26], incomplete outcome data and possible selective reporting were detected. There was almost perfect agreement between the two investigators (Cohen's k statistic: 82.3% $P < 0.001$).

3.4. Primary Endpoint

(i) All ten studies (Figure 4(a)) compared the two anastomotic techniques regarding the clinically significant POPF. More specifically, 108 patients from a total of 826 in the PG group developed clinically significant POPF, whereas in the PJ group the same ratio was 144/803. Meta-analysis of these data showed no statistically significant ($P = 0.09$) difference between the two groups regarding clinically significant POPF (OR:

TABLE 2: Study characteristics.

First author	Sample size PG	Sample size PJ	Age PG	Age PJ	Gender (M/F) PG	Gender (M/F) PJ	Intervention	Comparator	Primary outcome	Follow-up	Morbidity PG	Morbidity PJ
Keck	171	149	68 (35–86)	66 (29–87)	95/76	93/56	PG	PJ	Clinically relevant POPF, grade B or C	12 months	N/A	
Grendar	48	50	63.6 ± 13.1	68.1 ± 10.7	20/28	29/21	PG	PJ	Rate of pancreatic anastomotic leak/fistula	N/A	29	24
El Nakeeb	45	45	58 (12–73)	54 (15–73)	23/22	27/18	PG	Isolated Roux loop pancreaticojejunostomy	Rate of POPF	12 months	17	14
Figueras	65	58	67 (35–80)	65.5 (42–80)	44/21	37/21	PG	PJ	Rate of POPF	6 months	41	38
Topal	162	167	67.0 (60.6–73.5)	66.1 (59.4–74.6)	100/62	91/76	PG	PJ	Clinically relevant POPF, grade B or C	2 months	100	99
Wellner	59	57	67 (34–84)	64 (23–81)	27/32	29/28	PG	PJ	Clinically relevant POPF, grade B or C	90 days	N/A	
Fernàndez-Cruz	53	55	63 ± 13	63 ± 14	29/24	38/17	PG with gastric partition	PJ	Rate of POPF	N/A	12	24
Bassi	69	82	59.3 (58.2–60.4)	55.5 (54.5–56.6)	44/25	35/33	PG	PJ	Rate of POPF	N/A	20	32
Duffas	81	68	58.2 ± 11	58.6 ± 12	51/30	35/33	PG	PJ	Rate of one or more postoperative IACs	30 days	37	32
Yeo	73	72	61.5 ± 1.7	62.4 ± 1.4	33/40	38/34	PG	PJ	Rate of POPF	N/A	36	31

TABLE 3: Operative characteristics.

First author	Disease (PDAC/DD/AMP/DBD/OTHER) PG	PJ	Operation type	pd/pppd PG	PJ	Technique PG	PJ	Operative time PG	PJ	Postoperative hospital stay PG	PJ
Keck	104/-/10/-/14	98/-/11/-/14	pd or pppd	37/134	28/121	Dunking, pursestring, or interrupted or combination suture	Duct to mucosa or dunking, running, or interrupted or combination suture	332 (165–600)	337 (165–565)	15 (5–208)	16 (3–129)
Grendar	N/A	N/A	pd or pppd	N/A		Posterior gastrostomy, 2-layer anastomosis	2-layer end-to-side anastomosis	349 ± 70	356 ± 65	17.4 ± 11.6	14.0 ± 5.4
El Nakeeb	26/2/17/0/0	20/4/19/2/0	pd	45/0	45/0	Posterior gastrostomy, 2-layer anastomosis	Two-layer end-to-side pancreaticojejunostomy	300 (210–420)	320 (240–480)	9 (4–34)	8 (5–41)
Figueras	33/6/8/8/10	29/10/7/3/19	pd or pppd	35/30	30/28	Posterior gastrostomy double-layer invaginated	Duct-to-mucosa pancreaticojejunostomy	330 (235–620)	305 (240–510)	12 (1–52)	15,5 (6–55)
Topal	98/11/23/28/2	107/14/28/15/3	pd or pppd	65/98	65/102	End-to-side telescoped antecolic posterior gastrostomy	End-to-side telescoped pancreaticojejunostomy	250 (210–320)	250 (210–310)	19 (14–25)	18 (14–25)
Wellner	26/3/9/2/8	30/2/7/2/10	pd or pppd	7/52	2/55	Invagination, posterior pancreatogastrostomy with pursestring suture	Duct-to-mucosa pancreaticojejunostomy	404 (280–629)	443 (230–683)	15 (7–135)	17 (10–60)
Fernàndez-Cruz	26/1/12/8/9	28/1/10/7/9	pppd	0/53	0/55	End-to-side duct-to-mucosa pancreatogastrostomy	End-to-side duct mucosa anastomosis PPPD-PJ	300 ± 50	310 ± 60	12 ± 2	16 ± 3
Bassi	32/1/13/1/22	28/1/11/2/40	pd or pppd	3/66	12/70	Posterior single-layer telescoped gastrostomy	Single-layer pancreaticojejunal or duct to mucosa	337.2 (336.1–338.2)	359.3 (352.9–354.9)	14.2 (13.1–15.3)	15.4 (14.3–16.5)
Duffas	34/3/17/8/19	25/3/19/11/10	pd or pppd	63/18	50/18	Depending on surgeon's preference	Depending on surgeon's preference	6.5 ± 2.6 (h)	6.4 ± 2.2 (h)	20 (1–98)	21 (7–97)
Yeo	40/4/7/6/16	40/5/11/7/9	pd or pppd	13/60	13/59	Posterior gastrostomy	End-to-end or end-to-side pancreaticojejunostomy	7.4 ± 0.2 (h)	7.2 ± 0.2 (h)	17.1 ± 1.6	17.7 ± 1.5

TABLE 4: Intraoperative characteristics.

First author	Stent		Postoperative octreotide		Anastomotic glue reinforcement		Drains		Pancreatic parenchyma (soft/hard)		Pancreatic duct diameter	
	PG	PJ	PG	PJ	PG	PJ	PG	PJ	PG	PJ	PG	PJ
Keck	N/A		N/A		N/A		N/A		95/66	83/62	94 (<3 mm)	78
Grendar	10	39	42	39	N/A		38	44	25/23	18/32	3.8 ± 2.4 (mm)	4.3 ± 2.6
El Nakeeb	0	0	45	45	N/A		N/A		26/19	22/23	22 (<3 mm)	21
Figueras	N/A		65	58	N/A		65	58	34/31	33/25	4 (1–15) (mm)	4 (1–11)
Topal	0	0	162	167	0	0	162	167	N/A		98 (<3 mm)	102
Wellner	0	57	22	13	N/A		59	57	35/23	29/28	26 (<3 mm)	18
Fernàndez-Cruz	53	55	0	0	N/A		53	55	24/29	25/30	3.0 ± 1.7 (mm)	3.0 ± 1.6
Bassi	0	0	69	82	N/A		69	82	69/0	82/0	<5 mm	
Duffas	15	15	22	22	17	12	81	68	49/32	41/27	32 (<3 mm)	31
Yeo	0	0	0	0	0	0	73	72	16/21	17/28	3.4 ± 0.2 (mm)	2.9 ± 0.2

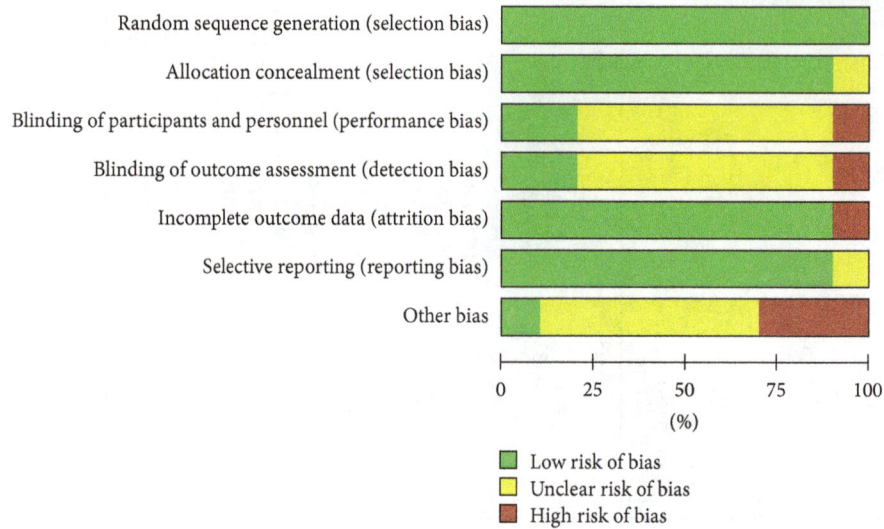

FIGURE 2: Risk of bias graph: review authors' judgments about each risk of bias item presented as percentages across all included studies.

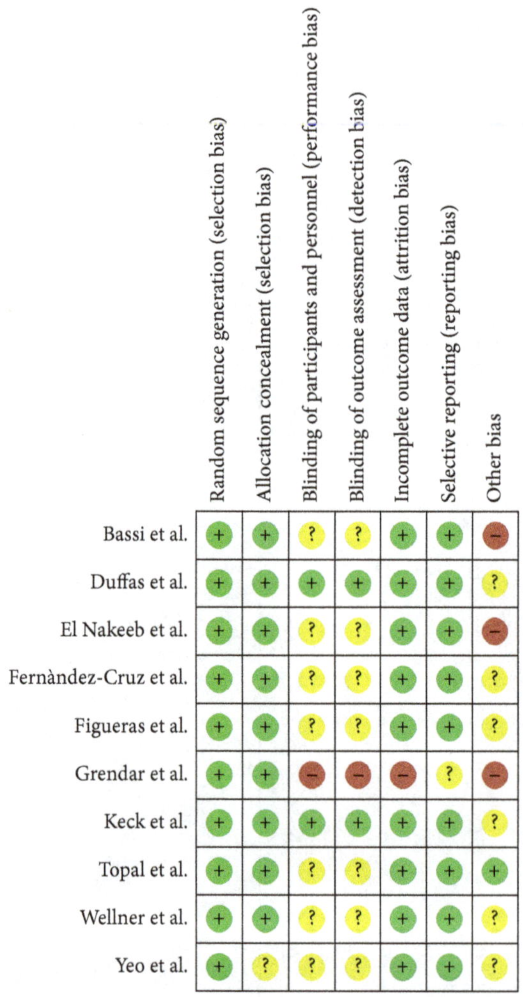

FIGURE 3: Risk of bias summary: review authors' judgments about each risk of bias item for each included study.

0.70, 95% CI: 0.46–1.06). Since there was significant heterogeneity between the studies (Q test P: 0.04,

I^2: 48% (95% CI: 0–75%)), a RE model was applied. Estimation of FE model did not wield consistent results (OR: 0.68, 95% CI: 0.51–0.89) with the RE model.

3.5. Secondary Endpoints

(i) All the included studies (Figure 4(b)) provided comparison between the two anastomotic techniques regarding POPF. In summary, 138 patients from a total of 826 submitted to PG developed POPF, instead of 175 and 803, respectively, in the PJ group. Meta-analysis of these data showed a statistically significant (P = 0.008) lower ratio of POPF (OR: 0.71, 95% CI: 0.55–0.91) for the PG group. Since there was no significant heterogeneity between the studies (Q test P: 0.27, I^2: 19% (95% CI: 0–59.8%)), a FE model was applied. Estimation of RE model wielded consistent results (OR: 0.73, 95% CI: 0.54–0.98) with the FE model.

(ii) Eight studies (Figure 4(c)) provided data for DGE. Meta-analysis of the data showed no statistically significant (P = 0.75) difference between the two groups regarding DGE (OR: 1.08, 95% CI: 0.68–1.70). Heterogeneity was significant between the studies (Q test P: 0.04, I^2: 53% (95% CI: 0–78.9%)), so a RE model was used. Estimation of FE model wielded consistent results (OR: 1.07, 95% CI: 0.81–1.40) with the RE model.

(iii) Eight studies (Figure 4(d)) provided data for clinically significant DGE. Meta-analysis of the data showed no statistically significant (P = 0.93) difference between the two groups regarding clinically significant DGE (OR: 0.98, 95% CI: 0.59–1.63). Heterogeneity was significant between the studies (Qtest P: 0.03, I^2: 55% (95% CI: 1.7%–79.8%)), so a RE model was used.

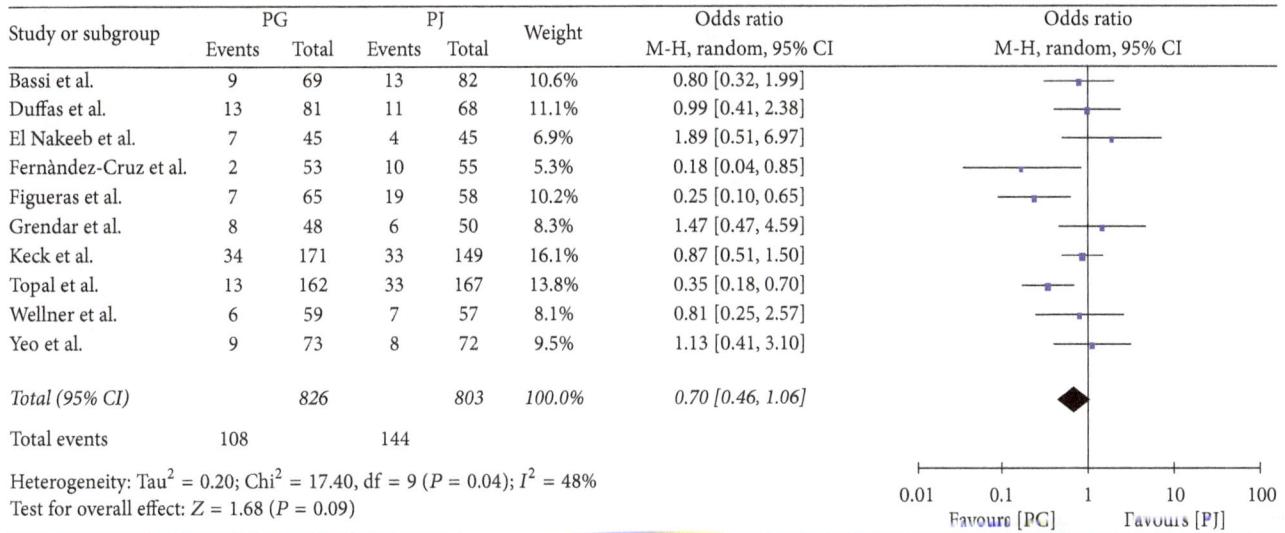

(a)

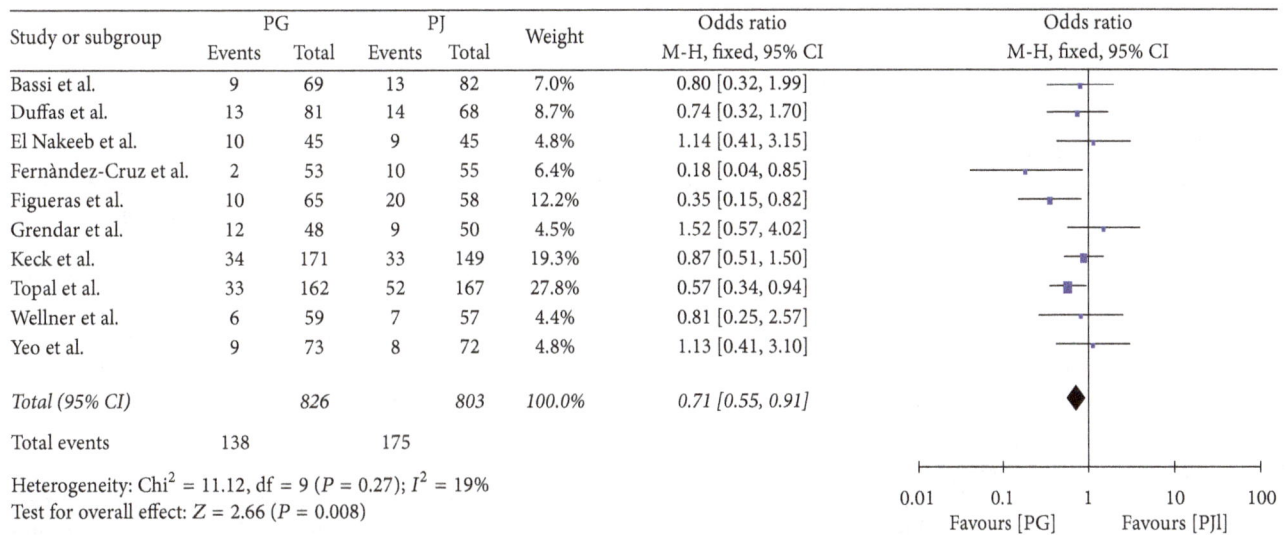

(b)

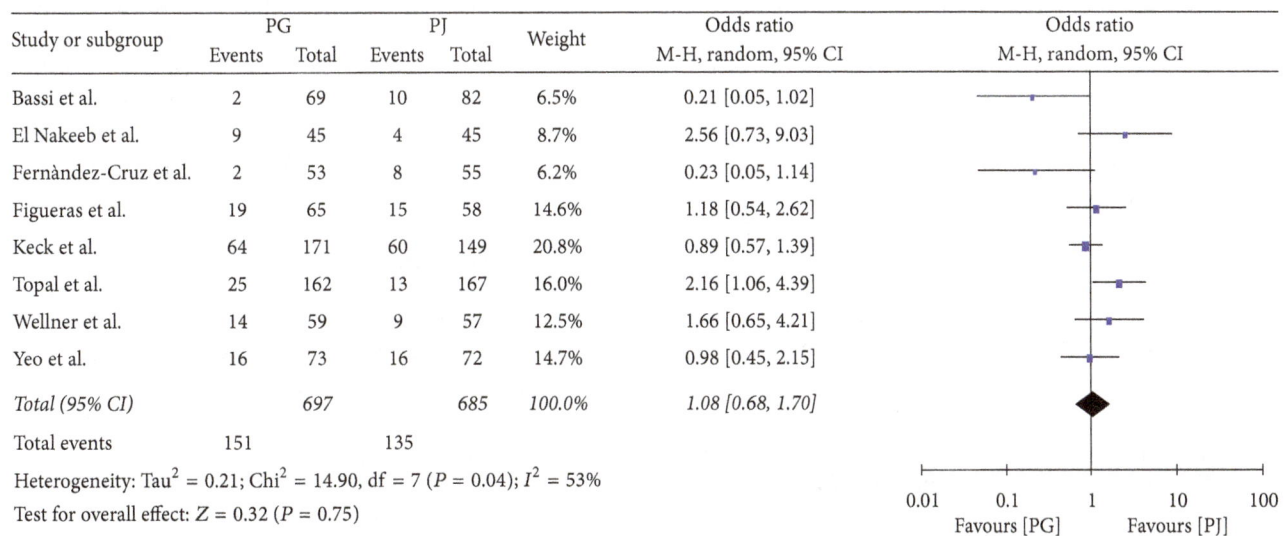

(c)

Figure 4: Continued.

Study or subgroup	PG Events	PG Total	PJ Events	PJ Total	Weight	Odds ratio M-H, random, 95% CI	Odds ratio M-H, random, 95% CI
Bassi et al.	2	69	10	82	7.5%	0.21 [0.05, 1.02]	
El Nakeeb et al.	9	45	4	45	9.8%	2.56 [0.73, 9.03]	
Fernàndez-Cruz et al.	2	53	8	55	7.2%	0.23 [0.05, 1.14]	
Figueras et al.	9	65	11	58	13.0%	0.69 [0.26, 1.80]	
Keck et al.	20	171	21	149	17.3%	0.81 [0.42, 1.56]	
Topal et al.	25	162	13	167	16.5%	2.16 [1.06, 4.39]	
Wellner et al.	14	59	9	57	13.4%	1.66 [0.65, 4.21]	
Yeo et al.	16	73	16	72	15.4%	0.98 [0.45, 2.15]	
Total (95% CI)		697		685	100.0%	0.98 [0.59, 1.63]	
Total events	97		92				

Heterogeneity: Tau^2 = 0.28; Chi^2 = 15.73, df = 7 (P = 0.03); I^2 = 55%

Test for overall effect: Z = 0.08 (P = 0.93)

0.01   0.1   1   10   100

Favours [PG]   Favours [PJ]

(d)

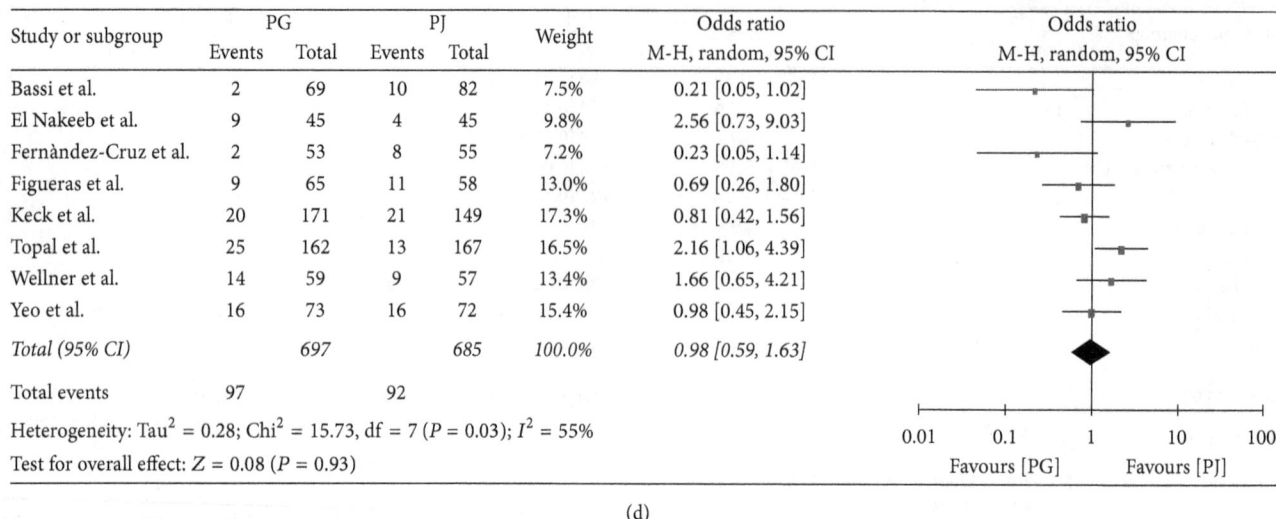

FIGURE 4: (a) Clinically significant postoperative pancreatic fistula, (b) postoperative pancreatic fistula, (c) delayed gastric emptying, and (d) clinically significant delayed gastric emptying.

Estimation of FE model wielded consistent results (OR: 1.03, 95% CI: 0.76–1.40) with the RE model.

(iv) Eight studies (Figure 6(a)) provided data for PPH. Meta-analysis of the data showed statistically significant (P = 0.02) difference between the two groups regarding PPH (OR: 1.52, 95% CI: 1.08–2.14) in favor of PJ group. Heterogeneity was not significant between the studies (Q test P: 0.85, I^2: 0% (95% CI: 0–80.3%)), so a FE model was used. Estimation of RE model wielded consistent results (OR: 1.52, 95% CI: 1.08–2.14) with the FE model.

(v) Eight studies (Figure 6(b)) provided data for clinically significant PPH. Meta-analysis of the data showed no statistically significant (P = 0.10) difference between the two groups regarding clinically significant PPH (OR: 1.35, 95% CI: 0.95–1.93). Heterogeneity was not significant between the studies (Q test P: 0.96, I^2: 0% (95% CI: 0–75.9%)), so a FE model was used. Estimation of RE model wielded consistent results (OR: 1.35, 95% CI: 0.94–1.94) with the FE model.

(vi) Seven studies (Figure 6(c)) provided data for biliary fistula. Meta-analysis of the data showed no statistically significant (P = 0.08) difference between the two groups regarding biliary fistula (OR: 0.58, 95% CI: 0.31–1.06). Heterogeneity was not significant between the studies (Q test P: 0.14, I^2: 38% (95% CI: 0–73.7%)), so a FE model was used. Estimation of RE model wielded consistent results (OR: 0.58, 95% CI: 0.23–1.48) with the FE model.

(vii) Nine studies (Figure 6(d)) provided data for intra-abdominal fluid collection. Meta-analysis of the data showed no statistically significant (P = 0.06) difference between the two groups regarding intra-abdominal fluid collection (OR: 0.64, 95% CI: 0.40–1.02). Heterogeneity was significant between the studies (Q test P: 0.07, I^2: 45% (95% CI: 0–74.6%)), so

a RE model was used. Estimation of FE model wielded consistent results (OR: 0.64, 95% CI: 0.47–0.87) with the RE model.

(viii) Eight studies (Figure 7(a)) provided data for morbidity. Meta-analysis of the data showed no statistically significant (P = 0.82) difference between the two groups regarding morbidity (OR: 0.97, 95% CI: 0.77–1.23). Heterogeneity was not significant between the studies (Q test P: 0.21, I^2: 28% (95% CI: 0–67.5%)), so a FE model was used. Estimation of RE model wielded consistent results (OR: 0.97, 95% CI: 0.73–1.28) with the FE model.

(ix) Ten studies (Figure 7(b)) provided data for mortality. Meta-analysis of the data showed no statistically significant (P = 0.94) difference between the two groups regarding mortality (OR: 0.98, 95% CI: 0.60–1.61). Heterogeneity was not significant between the studies (Q test P: 0.94, I^2: 0% (95% CI: 0–76.8%)), so a FE model was used. Estimation of RE model wielded consistent results (OR: 0.99, 95% CI: 0.60–1.64) with the FE model.

(x) Eight studies (Figure 7(c)) provided data for reoperation rate. Meta-analysis of the data showed no statistically significant (P = 0.33) difference between the two groups regarding reoperation rate (OR: 0.84, 95% CI: 0.59–1.20). Heterogeneity was not significant between the studies (Q test P: 0.79, I^2: 0% (95% CI: 0–83%)), so a FE model was used. Estimation of RE model wielded consistent results (OR: 0.83, 95% CI: 0.58–1.20) with the FE model.

(xi) Four studies (Figure 7(d)) provided data for wound infection. Meta-analysis of the data showed no statistically significant (P = 0.77) difference between the two groups regarding wound infection (OR: 1.08, 95% CI: 0.66–1.76). Heterogeneity was not significant between the studies (Q test P: 0.86, I^2: 0% (95%

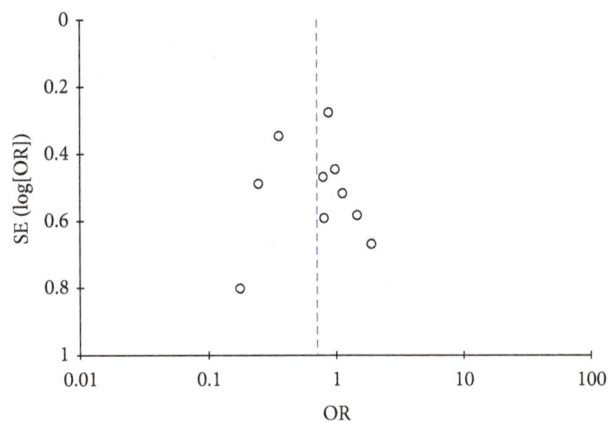

FIGURE 5: Funnel plot of comparison: postoperative pancreatic fistula.

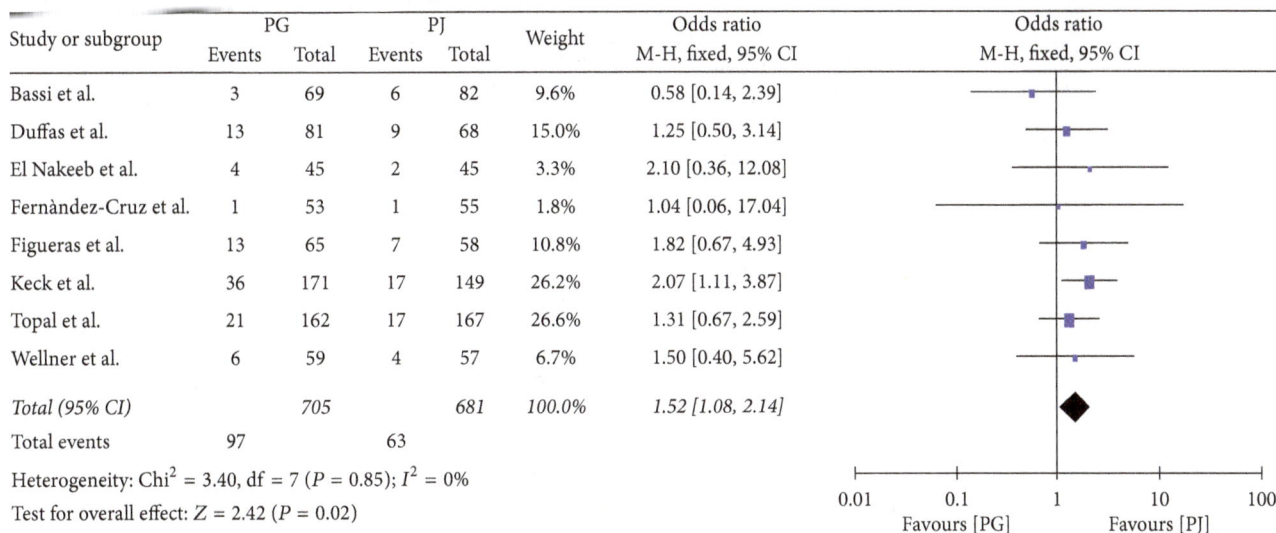

(a)

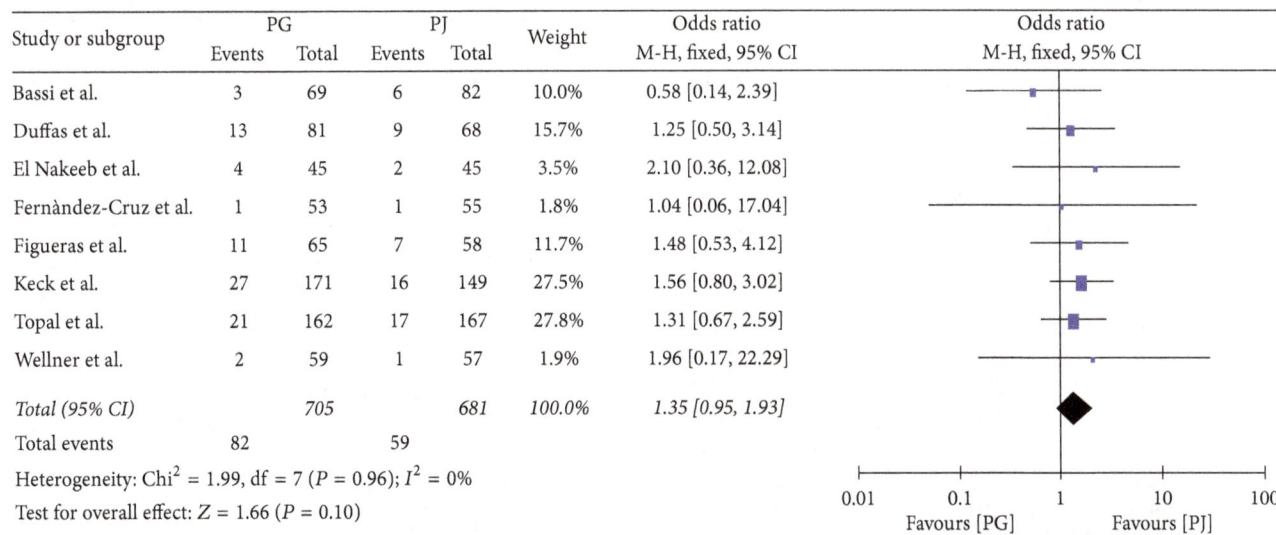

(b)

FIGURE 6: Continued.

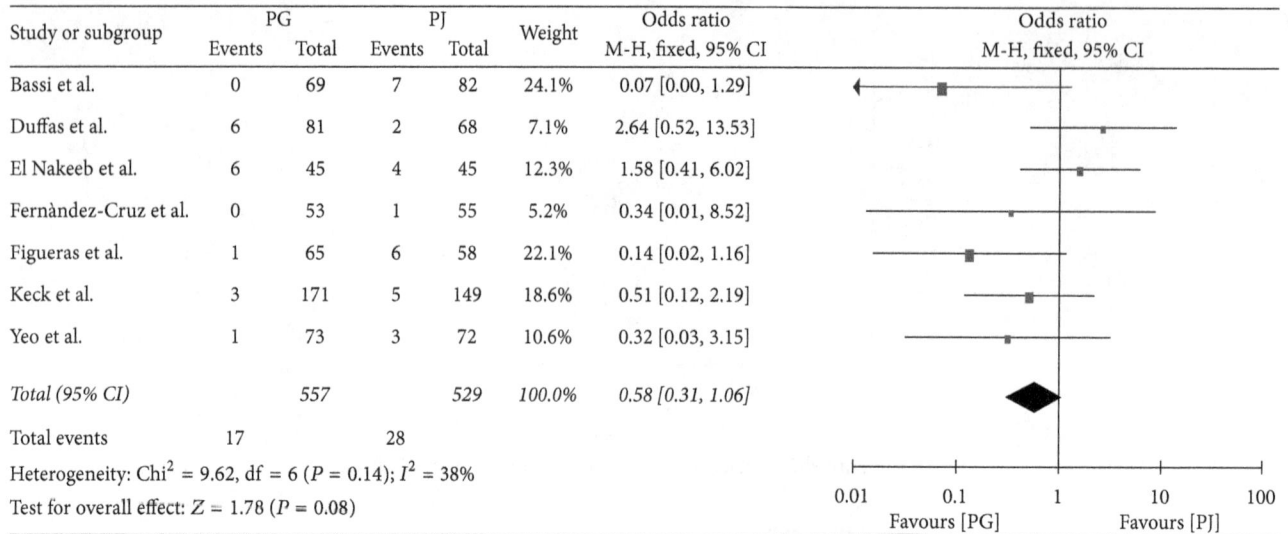

(c)

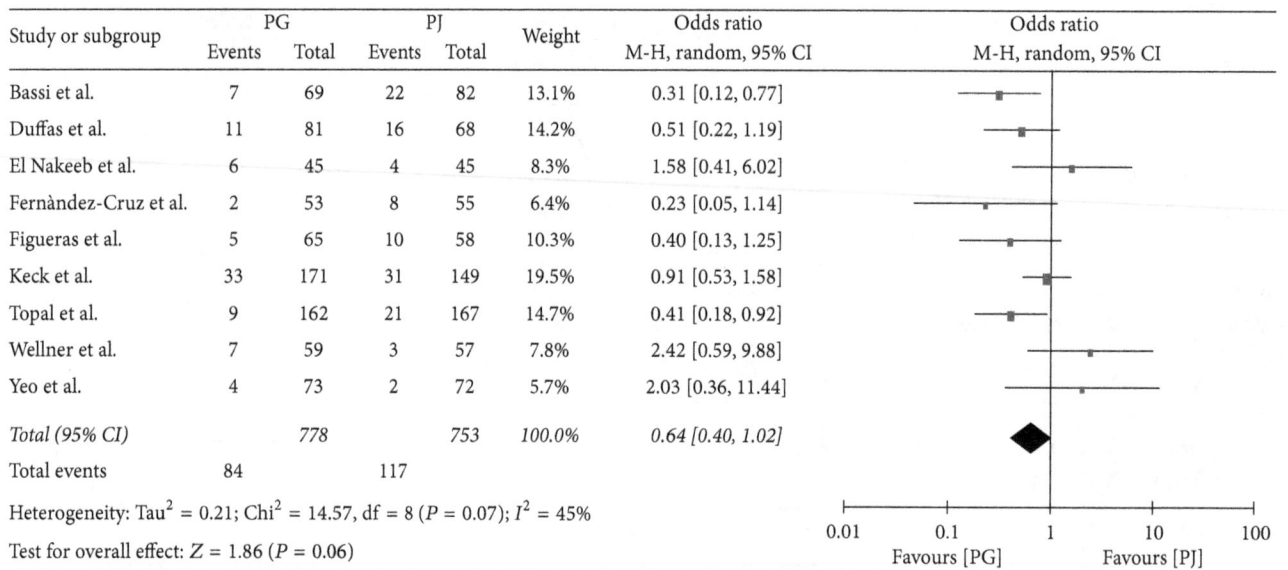

(d)

FIGURE 6: (a) Postpancreatectomy haemorrhage, (b) clinically significant postpancreatectomy haemorrhage, (c) biliary fistula, and (d) intra-abdominal fluid collection.

CI: 0–90%)), so a FE model was used. Estimation of RE model wielded consistent results (OR: 1.08, 95% CI: 0.66–1.76) with the FE model.

(xii) Six studies (Figure 8(a)) provided data for blood transfusion. Meta-analysis of the data showed no statistically significant ($P = 0.86$) difference between the two groups regarding blood transfusion (OR: 1.03, 95% CI: 0.72–1.47). Heterogeneity was not significant between the studies (Q test P: 0.39, I^2: 5% (95% CI: 0–91.4%)), so a FE model was used. Estimation of RE model wielded consistent results (OR: 1.04, 95% CI: 0.72–1.51) with the FE model.

(xiii) Ten studies (Figure 8(b)) provided data for operative time. Meta-analysis of the data showed no statistically significant ($P = 0.41$) difference between the two

groups regarding operative time (MWD: −5.73, 95% CI: −19.3, 7.85). Heterogeneity was significant between the studies (Q test P: <0.001, I^2: 97% (95% CI: 0–98.1%)), so a RE model was used. Estimation of FE model did not wield consistent results (MWD: −16, 95% CI: −17.24, −14.76) with the RE model.

(xiv) Ten studies (Figure 8(c)) provided data for LOS. Meta-analysis of the data showed no statistically significant ($P = 0.33$) difference between the two groups LOS (MWD: −0.74, 95% CI: −2.24, 0.76). Heterogeneity was significant between the studies (Q test P: <0.001, I^2: 91% (95% CI: 0–94.6%)), so a RE model was used. Estimation of FE model wielded consistent results (MWD: −0.06, 95% CI: −0.35, 0.23) with the RE model.

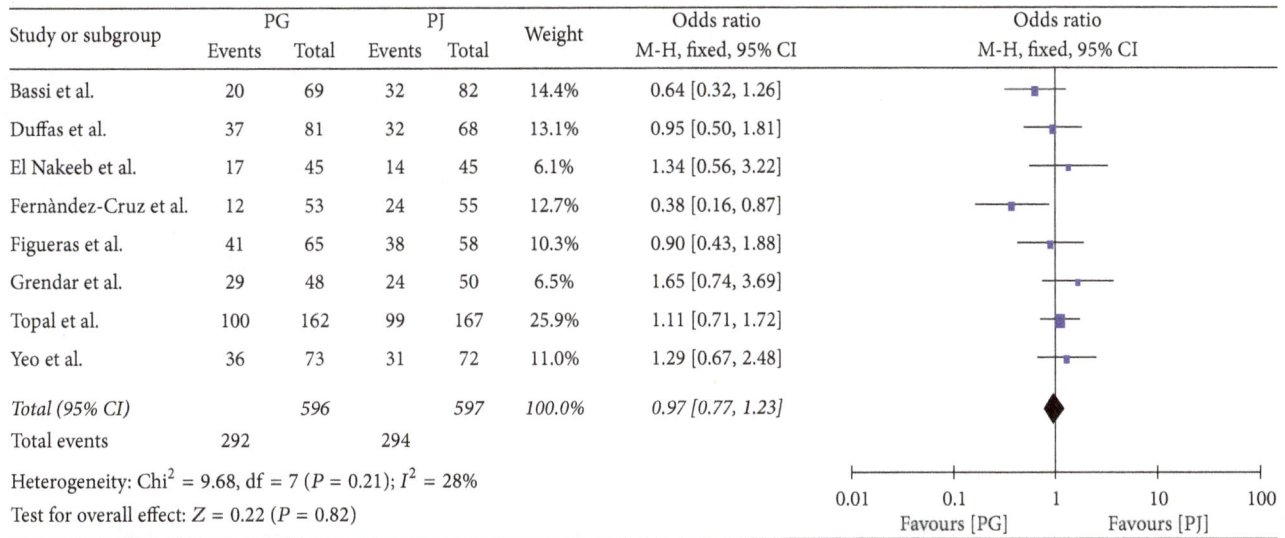

(a)

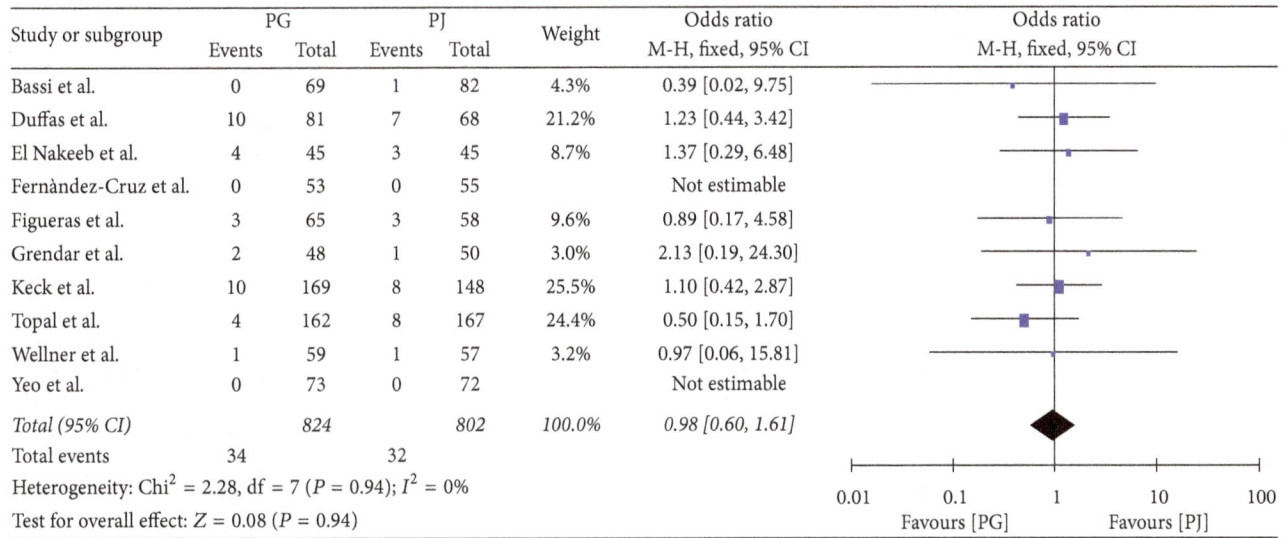

(b)

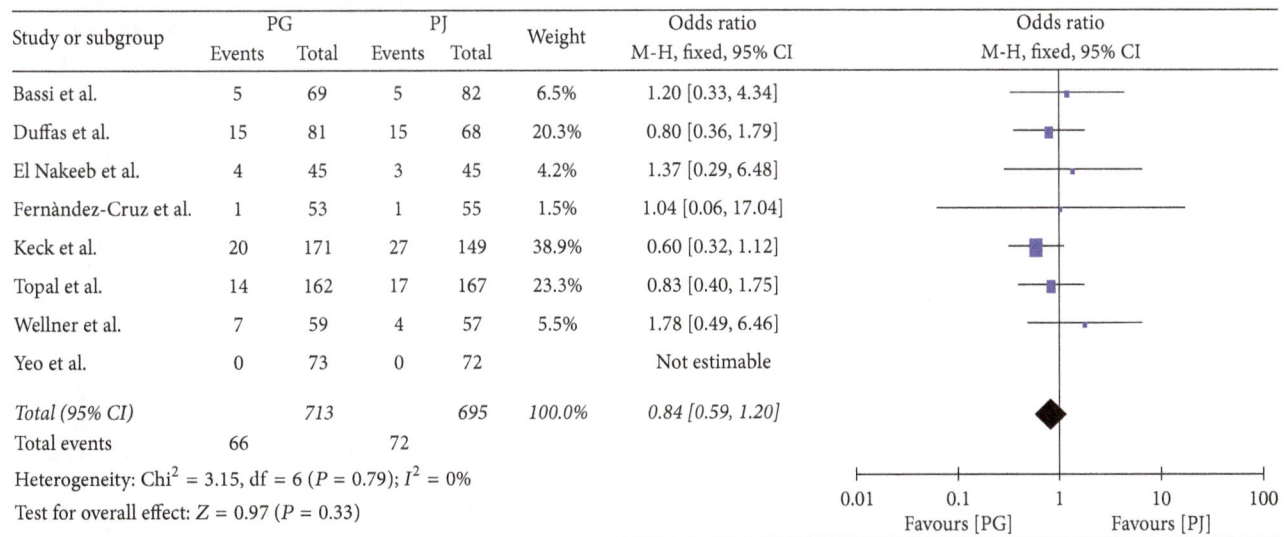

(c)

FIGURE 7: Continued.

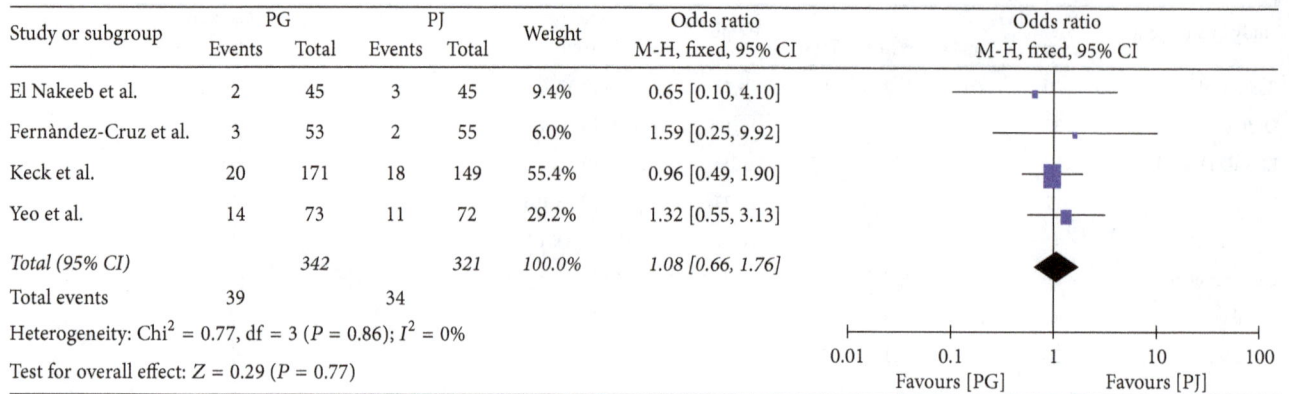

Study or subgroup	PG		PJ		Weight	Odds ratio M-H, fixed, 95% CI	Odds ratio M-H, fixed, 95% CI
	Events	Total	Events	Total			
El Nakeeb et al.	2	45	3	45	9.4%	0.65 [0.10, 4.10]	
Fernàndez-Cruz et al.	3	53	2	55	6.0%	1.59 [0.25, 9.92]	
Keck et al.	20	171	18	149	55.4%	0.96 [0.49, 1.90]	
Yeo et al.	14	73	11	72	29.2%	1.32 [0.55, 3.13]	
Total (95% CI)		342		321	100.0%	1.08 [0.66, 1.76]	
Total events	39		34				

Heterogeneity: Chi^2 = 0.77, df = 3 (P = 0.86); I^2 = 0%

Test for overall effect: Z = 0.29 (P = 0.77)

0.01 0.1 1 10 100
Favours [PG]   Favours [PJ]

(d)

FIGURE 7: (a) Morbidity, (b) mortality, (c) reoperation, and (d) wound infection.

3.6. Risk of Bias across Studies. Funnel plot of primary outcome (POPF) is shown in Figure 5. No study resides beyond the limits of 95% CI. Egger's test showed that there was no statistically significant publication bias (P = 0.951).

4. Discussion

4.1. Summary of Evidence. Pancreaticoduodenectomy remains the most widely used surgical modality for the treatment of pancreatic head and periampullary tumors. Failure of the pancreatic anastomosis resulting in POPF has been identified as one of the most important factors of postoperative morbidity. It must also be mentioned that POPF is assumed to have a close relationship with other post-PD complications, such as IAC, DGE, and PPH [30, 31]. As a result, surgeons, in an attempt to minimize post-PD complications have meticulously compared the available anastomotic techniques.

In our study, after a systematic literature search, a meta-analysis of available RCTs was performed. In the qualitative and quantitative analysis, 10 studies with a total of 1629 patients were included. Regarding the primary outcome, PG was not superior to PJ. However, this result was different when the two techniques were compared on the basis of overall POPF, where a significant difference was found. Heterogeneity in clinically significant POPF could possibly be the result of nonuniformity in the definition of POPF. Although the included studies after 2005 were consistent with the 2005 ISGPS POPF definition, the remaining defined POPF in an inconsistent way. DGE and clinically significant DGE were found to have no difference between PG and PJ, with a high level of heterogeneity though. As the operation type was not determined in most eligible studies, surgeons performed either PD or PPPD. The above-mentioned heterogeneity could be explained in the light of lack of stratification regarding the operation type.

Respectively, results from pooled data showed a lower rate of PPH for PJ, but no difference for clinically significant PPH. Heterogeneity for both of them was 0%, increasing thus the validity of these findings. The rate of biliary fistula and the intra-abdominal fluid collection was not significantly different between PG and PJ, which diverges from the results

of previous studies [32–35], due to inclusion of the recent RCTs [11, 26]. Moreover, overall postoperative morbidity for both techniques was estimated at the level of 49%, complying with current literature [4]. Similarly, no difference was found in terms of mortality, reoperation rate, wound infection, and perioperative blood transfusion. Finally, PG was not superior to PJ in terms of operative time and LOS. Heterogeneity was significantly high in these comparisons, possibly due to the approximate calculation of the mean and SD.

Risk factors for development of POPF are the age, gender of the patient, preoperative jaundice and malnutrition, underlying pathology, cirrhotic liver, BMI, soft pancreas, pancreatic diameter, pancreatic duct size, operative time, resection type, anastomotic technique, and intraoperative blood loss [36]. El Nakeeb et al. [31], however, in a retrospective study of 471 patients, suggested that risk factors for POPF include the cirrhotic liver, BMI, soft pancreas, pancreatic diameter < 3 mm, and pancreatic duct near the posterior border.

The superiority of PG over PJ in terms of POPF can be justified by some theoretical advantages. Firstly, due to the fact that the posterior wall of the stomach lies just above the pancreatic remnant, the tension between the stomach and the pancreatic stump is minimized. Secondly, the acidic gastric content prevents the activation of pancreatic enzymes and consequently the anastomotic lysis. Moreover, compared to a jejunum loop, the stomach wall is thicker, thus stabilizing the anastomosis. Finally, the abundant stomach wall vascularization decreases the chance of an anastomotic ischaemia. This may also be the reason of increased post-PD PPH in the PG group, rendering perioperative meticulous haemostasis of utmost importance.

As far as postoperative exocrine pancreatic function is concerned, data are scarce and inconsistent, thus making further analysis very difficult. More specifically, a higher stool elastase level and a significant lesser weight loss were reported in the PG group [25]. Comparing PG and IRPJ, El Nakeeb et al. [23] concluded that postoperative steatorrhea and need for pancreatic enzyme supplements were higher in the PG group, while post-PD serum albumin was in a lower level in patients submitted to PG. On the contrary, the need for oral

Study or subgroup	PG Events	PG Total	PJ Events	PJ Total	Weight	Odds ratio M-H, fixed, 95% CI
Bassi et al.	5	69	5	82	7.0%	1.20 [0.33, 4.34]
Duffas et al.	19	81	12	68	16.6%	1.43 [0.64, 3.21]
Fernàndez-Cruz et al.	15	53	16	55	18.7%	0.96 [0.42, 2.22]
Grendar et al.	5	48	13	50	19.0%	0.33 [0.11, 1.02]
Keck et al.	25	171	17	149	25.8%	1.33 [0.69, 2.57]
Wellner et al.	9	59	9	57	12.9%	0.96 [0.35, 2.62]
Total (95% CI)		481		461	100.0%	1.03 [0.72, 1.47]
Total events	78		72			

Heterogeneity: Chi^2 = 5.25, df = 5 (P = 0.39); I^2 = 5%
Test for overall effect: Z = 0.17 (P = 0.86)

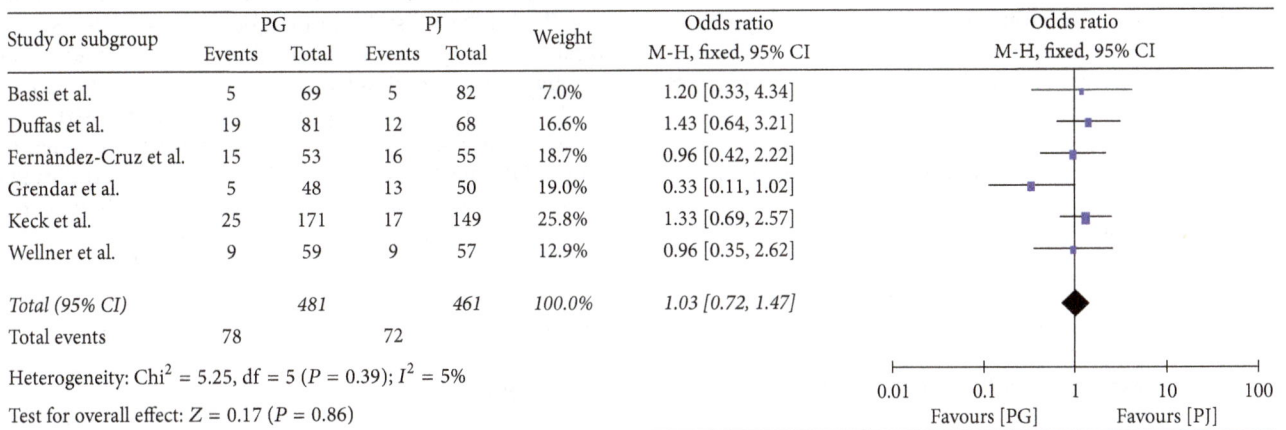

(a)

Study or subgroup	PG Mean	PG SD	PG Total	PJ Mean	PJ SD	PJ Total	Weight	Mean difference IV, random, 95% CI
Bassi et al.	337.2	4.23	69	359.3	4.61	82	13.3%	−22.10 [−23.51, −20.69]
Duffas et al.	390	156	81	384	132	68	5.2%	6.00 [−40.24, 52.24]
El Nakeeb et al.	300	52.5	45	320	60	45	9.6%	−20.00 [−43.29, 3.29]
Fernàndez-Cruz et al.	300	50	53	310	60	55	10.2%	−10.00 [−30.80, 10.80]
Figueras et al.	330	96.25	65	305	67.5	58	8.3%	25.00 [−4.14, 54.14]
Grendar et al.	349	70	48	356	65	50	8.8%	−7.00 [−33.77, 19.77]
Keck et al.	332	72.5	171	337	66.6	149	11.4%	−5.00 [−20.25, 10.25]
Topal et al.	250	18.3	162	250	16.6	167	13.2%	0.00 [−3.78, 3.78]
Wellner et al.	404	87.25	59	443	113.25	57	6.7%	−39.00 [−75.88, −2.12]
Yeo et al.	444	12	73	432	12	72	13.2%	12.00 [8.09, 15.91]
Total (95% CI)			826			803	100.0%	−5.73 [−19.30, 7.85]

Heterogeneity: Tau^2 = 359.13; Chi^2 = 350.82, df = 9 (P < 0.00001); I^2 = 97%
Test for overall effect: Z = 0.83 (P = 0.41)

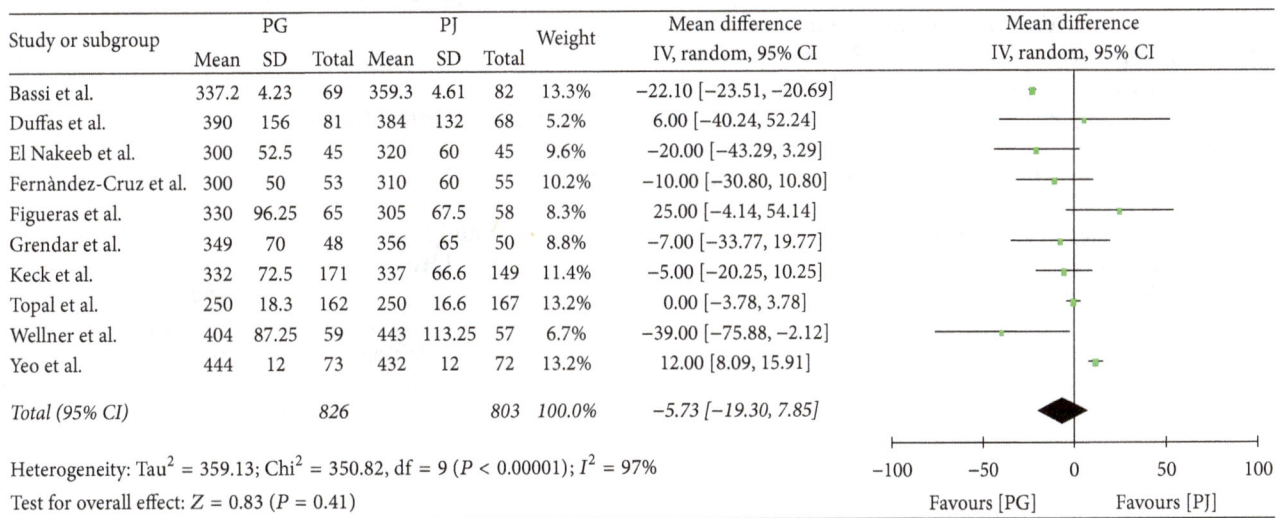

(b)

Study or subgroup	PG Mean	PG SD	PG Total	PJ Mean	PJ SD	PJ Total	Weight	Mean difference IV, random, 95% CI
Bassi et al.	14.2	4.65	69	15.4	5.07	82	14.5%	−1.20 [−2.75, 0.35]
Duffas et al.	20	16.16	81	21	22.5	68	4.2%	−1.00 [−7.40, 5.40]
El Nakeeb et al.	9	7.5	45	8	9	45	9.1%	1.00 [−2.42, 4.42]
Fernàndez-Cruz et al.	12	2	53	16	3	55	16.0%	−4.00 [−4.96, −3.04]
Figueras et al.	12	12.75	65	15.5	12.25	58	6.9%	−3.50 [−7.92, 0.92]
Grendar et al.	17.4	11.6	48	14	5.4	50	8.6%	3.40 [−0.21, 7.01]
Keck et al.	15	33.8	171	16	21	149	4.5%	−1.00 [−7.09, 5.09]
Topal et al.	19	1.83	162	18	1.83	167	16.9%	1.00 [0.60, 1.40]
Wellner et al.	15	32	59	17	12.5	57	2.5%	−2.00 [−10.79, 6.79]
Yeo et al.	17.1	1.6	73	17.7	1.5	72	16.8%	−0.60 [−1.10, −0.10]
Total (95% CI)			826			803	100.0%	−0.74 [−2.24, 0.76]

Heterogeneity: Tau^2 = 3.43; Chi^2 = 105.57, df = 9 (P < 0.00001); I^2 = 91%
Test for overall effect: Z = 0.97 (P = 0.33)

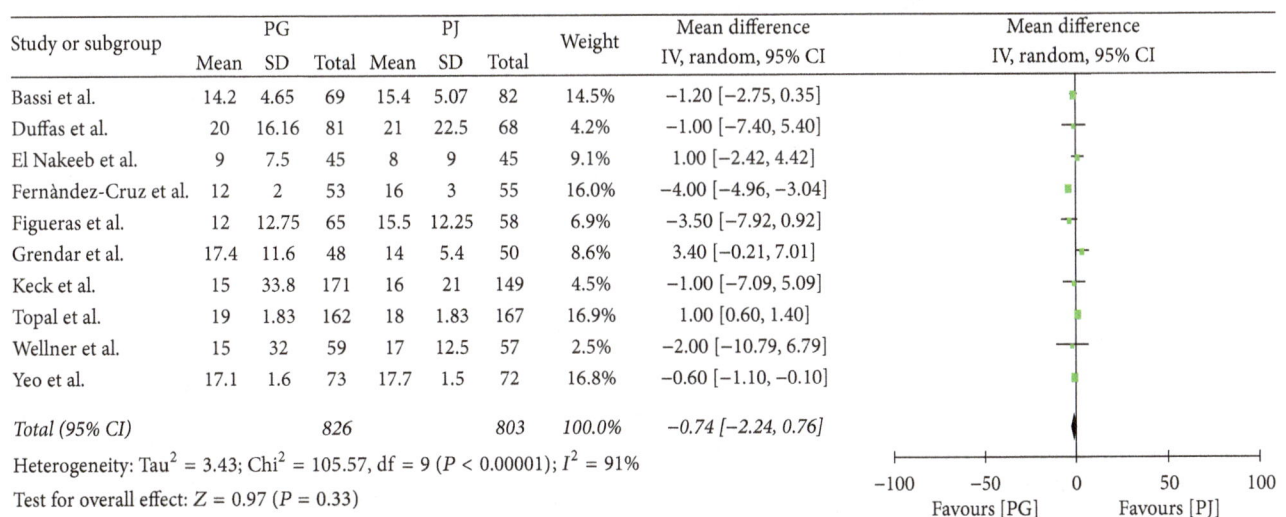

(c)

FIGURE 8: (a) Blood transfusion, (b) operative time, and (c) length of hospital stay.

enzyme supplements, six months after surgery, was lower in the PG group, with the rate of reported steatorrhea further decreasing after 12 months [11]. In a study of 99 patients, Hirono et al. [37] identified hard texture of pancreas and PG reconstruction as individual risk factors for postoperative pancreatic exocrine function insufficiency.

Regarding the pancreatic endocrine function, El Nakeeb et al. [23] showed that, although there was no difference in the overall rate of postoperative diabetes mellitus between PG and IRPJ, postoperative fasting blood sugar was higher in the PG group. Furthermore, fasting blood sugar increased postoperatively in the PG group, unlike IRPJ, where fasting blood sugar was significantly lower after surgery. However, two studies claimed that there was no statistically significant difference between PG and PJ in the rate of de novo diabetes mellitus [11, 25].

Morphological outcomes were not systematically provided and therefore a pooled analysis could not be reported. Data show that pancreatic duct tended to be more dilated in the PG group, even after a median of 32 months and the pancreatic parenchyma density is significantly decreased [38, 39]. A significant higher impact of postoperative atrophy of the pancreatic parenchyma was recorded in the PG group [39]. However, in a study by Fang et al. [40], no significant differences between PG and PJ regarding postoperative pancreatic duct diameter were reported.

Our meta-analysis provides an up-to-date pooled, published only data, estimation of the rate of POPF, and other postoperative complications between the two most popular anastomotic techniques. Compared to other recent studies [12, 41], it reports results not only in overall morbidity but also in clinically significant complications, such as DGE and PPH.

4.2. Limitations. Several limitations should be taken into account before appraising the results of this meta-analysis. First of all, the between studies heterogeneity was substantial, limiting, in this way, the significance of the results. Furthermore, there is a diversity in the POPF definition among the included studies. It must be noted, though, that all studies after 2005 use the ISGPS definition. The included trials have also incorporated both PD and PPPD in their study groups and there was, also, no stratification on the basis of the underlying pathology. Moreover, a lack of uniformity exists, regarding the surgical anastomotic technique that may possibly result in biased results. Factors like the texture of pancreas and the pancreatic duct diameter might also influence the results. Another source of bias could be the perioperative use of glue and stents and the postoperative administration of somatostatin, since not all studies reported this information. Another factor that contributes to heterogeneity is the surgical experience in the applied anastomotic technique. Last literature search was performed 20 July 2016. The new refinement of the ISGPS POPF definition [42] was published later; thus, it was not incorporated.

4.3. Conclusions. The present meta-analysis of RCTs demonstrates that there is no difference between the two anastomotic techniques regarding clinically significant POPF. PG has lower overall incidence of POPF and higher rate of PPH

against PJ. Moreover, PG and PJ did not differ in terms of overall DGE, clinically significant DGE, clinically significant PPH, biliary fistula, intra-abdominal fluid collection, overall morbidity, mortality, reoperation rate, wound infection, intraoperative blood transfusion, operative time, and LOS. Therefore, selection of proper pancreatic reconstruction should be according to the risk of patients, in order to reduce POPF, postoperative complications, and mortality. PG is superior to PJ regarding short term outcomes, while PJ provides better pancreatic function. Given several limitations, more large scale high quality RCTs are required for the effect of the anastomotic technique on the incidence of POPF to be clarified.

Disclosure

This research did not receive any specific grant from funding agencies in the public, commercial, or not-for-profit sectors.

Authors' Contributions

Konstantinos Perivoliotis, Eleni Sioka, Athina Tatsioni, Ioannis Stefanidis, Elias Zintzaras, and Dimitrios Zacharoulis contributed study conception and design. Konstantinos Perivoliotis and Eleni Sioka were responsible for acquisition of data. Konstantinos Perivoliotis and Eleni Sioka performed analysis and interpretation of data. Konstantinos Perivoliotis, Eleni Sioka, and Athina Tatsioni drafted the manuscript. Athina Tatsioni, Ioannis Stefanidis, Elias Zintzaras, and Dimitrios Zacharoulis conducted critical revision.

References

[1] M. E. Lidsky, Z. Sun, D. P. Nussbaum, M. A. Adam, P. J. Speicher, and D. G. Blazer, "Going the Extra Mile: Improved Survival for Pancreatic Cancer Patients Traveling to High-volume Centers," *Annals of Surgery*, 2016.

[2] E. M. Gleeson, M. F. Shaikh, P. A. Shewokis et al., "WHipple-ABACUS, a simple, validated risk score for 30-day mortality after pancreaticoduodenectomy developed using the ACS-NSQIP database," *Surgery*, vol. 160, no. 5, pp. 1279–1287, 2016.

[3] J. Xiong, P. Szatmary, W. Huang et al., "Enhanced recovery after surgery program in patients undergoing pancreaticoduodenectomy a prisma-compliant systematic review and meta-analysis," *Medicine (United States)*, vol. 95, no. 18, Article ID e3497, 2016.

[4] G. Conzo, C. Gambardella, E. Tartaglia et al., "Pancreatic fistula following pancreatoduodenectomy. Evaluation of different surgical approaches in the management of pancreatic stump. Literature review," *International Journal of Surgery*, vol. 21, no. 1, pp. S4–S9, 2015.

[5] J. A. Khalil, N. Mayo, S. Dumitra et al., "Pancreatic fistulae after a pancreatico-duodenectomy: Are pancreatico-gastrostomies safer than pancreatico-jejunostomies? An expertise-based trial and propensity-score adjusted analysis," *HPB*, vol. 16, no. 12, pp. 1062–1067, 2014.

[6] J. P. Arnaud, J. J. Tuech, C. Cervi, and R. Bergamaschi, "Pancreaticogastrostomy compared with pancreaticojejunostomy after pancreaticoduodenectomy," *European Journal of Surgery*, vol. 165, no. 4, pp. 357–362, 1999.

[7] K. Heeger, V. Fendrich, J. Waldmann, P. Langer, V. Kanngießer, and D. K. Bartsch, "Reduced complication rate after modified binding purse-string-mattress sutures pancreatogastrostomy versus duct-to-mucosa pancreaticojejunostomy," *Surgeon*, vol. 11, no. 5, pp. 246–252, 2013.

[8] E. Oussoultzoglou, P. Bachellier, J.-M. Bigourdan, J.-C. Weber, H. Nakano, and D. Jaeck, "Pancreaticogastrostomy decreased relaparotomy caused by pancreatic fistula after pancreaticoduodenectomy compared with pancreaticojejunostomy," *Archives of Surgery*, vol. 139, no. 3, pp. 327–335, 2004.

[9] S. Takano, Y. Ito, Y. Watanabe, T. Yokoyama, N. Kubota, and S. Iwai, "Pancreaticojejunostomy versus pancreaticogastrostomy in reconstructions following pancreaticoduodenectomy," *British Journal of Surgery*, vol. 87, no. 4, pp. 423–427, 2000.

[10] J. J. Tuech, P. Pessaux, R. Duplessis, F. Villapadierna, J. Ronceray, and J. P. Arnaud, "Pancreatico-jejunal vs pancreatico-gastric anastomosis after pancreatico-duodenectomy. A retrospective comparative study," *Chirurgie*, vol. 123, no. 5, pp. 450–455, 1998.

[11] T. Keck, U. F. Wellner, and M. Bahra, "Pancreatogastrostomy versus pancreatojejunostomy for RECOnstruction After PANCreatoduodenectomy (RECOPANC, DRKS 00000767)," *Annals of Surgery*, vol. 263, no. 3, pp. 440–449, 2015.

[12] G. P. Guerrini, P. Soliani, G. D'Amico et al., "Pancreaticojejunostomy versus pancreaticogastrostomy after pancreaticoduodenectomy: an up-to-date meta-analysis," *Journal of Investigative Surgery*, vol. 29, no. 3, pp. 175–184, 2016.

[13] F.-B. Liu, J.-M. Chen, W. Geng et al., "Pancreaticogastrostomy is associated with significantly less pancreatic fistula than pancreaticojejunostomy reconstruction after pancreaticoduodenectomy: A meta-analysis of seven randomized controlled trials," *HPB*, vol. 17, no. 2, pp. 123–130, 2015.

[14] W. Que, H. Fang, B. Yan et al., "Pancreaticogastrostomy versus pancreaticojejunostomy after pancreaticoduodenectomy: a meta-analysis of randomized controlled trials," *American Journal of Surgery*, vol. 209, no. 6, pp. 1074–1082, 2015.

[15] D. Moher, A. Liberati, J. Tetzlaff, and D. G. Altman, "Preferred reporting items for systematic reviews and meta-analyses: the PRISMA statement," *PLoS Medicine*, vol. 6, no. 7, Article ID e1000097, 2009.

[16] C. Bassi, C. Dervenis, G. Butturini et al., "Postoperative pancreatic fistula: an international study group (ISGPF) definition," *Surgery*, vol. 138, no. 1, pp. 8–13, 2005.

[17] M. N. Wente, C. Bassi, C. Dervenis et al., "Delayed gastric emptying (DGE) after pancreatic surgery: a suggested definition by the International Study Group of Pancreatic Surgery (ISGPS)," *Surgery*, vol. 142, no. 5, pp. 761–768, 2007.

[18] M. N. Wente, J. A. Veit, C. Bassi et al., "Postpancreatectomy hemorrhage (PPH): an International Study Group of Pancreatic Surgery (ISGPS) definition," *Surgery*, vol. 142, no. 1, pp. 20–25, 2007.

[19] J. P. T. Higgins, D. G. Altman, P. C. Gøtzsche et al., "The Cochrane Collaboration's tool for assessing risk of bias in randomised trials," *The British Medical Journal*, vol. 343, no. 7829, Article ID d5928, 2011.

[20] S. P. Hozo, B. Djulbegovic, and I. Hozo, "Estimating the mean and variance from the median, range, and the size of a sample," *BMC Medical Research Methodology*, vol. 5, article 13, 2005.

[21] C. Bassi, M. Falconi, E. Molinari et al., "Reconstruction by pancreaticojejunostomy versus pancreaticogastrostomy following pancreatectomy: results of a comparative study," *Annals of Surgery*, vol. 242, no. 6, pp. 767–773, 2005.

[22] J.-P. Duffas, B. Suc, S. Msika et al., "A controlled randomized multicenter trial of pancreatogastrostomy or pancreatojejunostomy after pancreatoduodenectomy," *American Journal of Surgery*, vol. 189, no. 6, pp. 720–729, 2005.

[23] A. El Nakeeb, E. Hamdy, A. M. Sultan et al., "Isolated Roux loop pancreaticojejunostomy versus pancreaticogastrostomy after pancreaticoduodenectomy: a prospective randomized study," *HPB*, vol. 16, no. 8, pp. 713–722, 2014.

[24] L. Fernàndez-Cruz, R. Cosa, L. Blanco, M. A. López-Boado, and E. Astudillo, "Pancreatogastrostomy with gastric partition after pylorus-preserving pancreatoduodenectomy versus conventional pancreatojejunostomy a prospective randomized study," *Annals of Surgery*, vol. 248, no. 6, pp. 930–937, 2008.

[25] J. Figueras, L. Sabater, P. Planellas et al., "Randomized clinical trial of pancreaticogastrostomy versus pancreaticojejunostomy on the rate and severity of pancreatic fistula after pancreaticoduodenectomy," *British Journal of Surgery*, vol. 100, no. 12, pp. 1597–1605, 2013.

[26] J. Grendar, J.-F. Ouellet, F. R. Sutherland, O. F. Bathe, C. G. Ball, and E. Dixon, "In search of the best reconstructive technique after pancreaticoduodenectomy: pancreaticojejunostomy versus pancreaticogastrostomy," *Canadian Journal of Surgery*, vol. 58, no. 3, pp. 154–159, 2015.

[27] B. Topal, S. Fieuws, R. Aerts et al., "Pancreaticojejunostomy versus pancreaticogastrostomy reconstruction after pancreaticoduodenectomy for pancreatic or periampullary tumours: a multicentre randomised trial," *The Lancet Oncology*, vol. 14, no. 7, pp. 655–662, 2013.

[28] U. F. Wellner, O. Sick, M. Olschewski, U. Adam, U. T. Hopt, and T. Keck, "Randomized controlled single-center trial comparing pancreatogastrostomy versus pancreaticojejunostomy after partial pancreatoduodenectomy," *Journal of Gastrointestinal Surgery*, vol. 16, no. 9, pp. 1686–1695, 2012.

[29] C. J. Yeo, J. L. Cameron, M. M. Maher et al., "A prospective randomized trial of pancreaticogastrostomy versus pancreaticojejunostomy after pancreaticoduodenectomy," *Annals of Surgery*, vol. 222, no. 4, pp. 580–592, 1995.

[30] B. Topal, R. Aerts, T. Hendrickx, S. Fieuws, and F. Penninckx, "Determinants of complications in pancreaticoduodenectomy," *European Journal of Surgical Oncology*, vol. 33, no. 4, pp. 488–492, 2007.

[31] A. El Nakeeb, T. Salah, A. Sultan et al., "Pancreatic anastomotic leakage after pancreaticoduodenectomy. Risk factors, clinical predictors, and management (single center experience)," *World Journal of Surgery*, vol. 37, no. 6, pp. 1405–1418, 2013.

[32] P. Lei, J. Fang, Y. Huang, Z. Zheng, B. Wei, and H. Wei, "Pancreaticogastrostomy or pancreaticojejunostomy? Methods of digestive continuity reconstruction after pancreaticodudenectomy: a meta-analysis of randomized controlled trials," *International Journal of Surgery*, vol. 12, no. 12, pp. 1444–1449, 2014.

[33] B. Menahem, L. Guittet, A. Mulliri, A. Alves, and J. Lubrano, "Pancreaticogastrostomy is superior to pancreaticojejunostomy for prevention of pancreatic fistula after pancreaticoduodenectomy: an updated meta-analysis of randomized controlled trials," *Annals of Surgery*, vol. 261, no. 5, pp. 882–887, 2015.

[34] J. J. Xiong, C. L. Tan, P. Szatmary et al., "Meta-analysis of pancreaticogastrostomy versus pancreaticojejunostomy after

pancreaticoduodenectomy," *British Journal of Surgery*, vol. 101, no. 10, pp. 1196–1208, 2014.

[35] Y. Zhou, J. Yu, L. Wu, and B. Li, "Meta-analysis of pancreatico-gastrostomy versus pancreaticojejunostomy on occurrences of postoperative pancreatic fistula after pancreaticoduodenec-tomy," *Asian Journal of Surgery*, vol. 38, no. 3, article no. 199, pp. 155–160, 2015.

[36] N. O. MacHado, "Pancreatic fistula after pancreatectomy: def-initions, risk factors, preventive measures, and manage-ment—review," *International Journal of Surgical Oncology*, vol. 2012, Article ID 602478, 10 pages, 2012.

[37] S. Hirono, Y. Murakami, M. Tani et al., "Identification of risk factors for pancreatic exocrine insufficiency after pancreatico-duodenectomy using a13C-labeled mixed triglyceride breath test," *World Journal of Surgery*, vol. 39, no. 2, pp. 516–525, 2015.

[38] E. Lemaire, D. O'Toole, A. Sauvanet, P. Hammel, J. Belghiti, and P. Ruszniewski, "Functional and morphological changes in the pancreatic remnant following pancreaticoduodenectomy with pancreaticogastric anastomosis," *British Journal of Surgery*, vol. 87, no. 4, pp. 434–438, 2000.

[39] Y. Tomimaru, Y. Takeda, S. Kobayashi et al., "Comparison of postoperative morphological changes in remnant pancreas be-tween pancreaticojejunostomy and pancreaticogastrostomy after pancreaticoduodenectomy," *Pancreas*, vol. 38, no. 2, pp. 203–207, 2009.

[40] W. Fang, C. Su, Y. Shyr et al., "Functional and morphological changes in pancreatic remnant after pancreaticoduodenec-tomy," *Pancreas*, vol. 35, no. 4, pp. 361–365, 2007.

[41] S. Crippa, R. Cirocchi, J. Randolph et al., "Pancreaticojejunos-tomy is comparable to pancreaticogastrostomy after pancre-aticoduodenectomy: an updated meta-analysis of randomized controlled trials," *Langenbeck's Archives of Surgery*, vol. 401, no. 4, pp. 427–437, 2016.

[42] C. Bassi, G. Marchegiani, C. Dervenis et al., "The 2016 update of the International Study Group (ISGPS) definition and grading of postoperative pancreatic fistula: 11 Years After," *Surgery*, vol. 161, no. 3, pp. 584–591, 2017.

19

The Treatment of Peritoneal Carcinomatosis in Advanced Gastric Cancer: State of the Art

Giulia Montori,[1] Federico Coccolini,[2] Marco Ceresoli,[2] Fausto Catena,[3]
Nicola Colaianni,[2] Eugenio Poletti,[2] and Luca Ansaloni[2]

[1] General Surgery Department, Spedali Civili, Chirurgia Generale 3, Piazzale Spedali Civili, 25121 Brescia, Italy
[2] General Surgery Department, Papa Giovanni XXIII Hospital, 42121 Bergamo, Italy
[3] Emergency Surgery Department, Ospedale Maggiore, 43121 Parma, Italy

Correspondence should be addressed to Giulia Montori; giulia.montori@gmail.com

Academic Editor: George H. Sakorafas

Gastric cancer (GC) is the fourth most common cancer and the second leading cause of cancer death in the world; 53–60% of patients show disease progression and die of peritoneal carcinomatosis (PC). PC of gastric origin has an extremely inauspicious prognosis with a median survival estimate at 1–3 months. Different studies presented contrasting data about survival rates; however, all agreed with the necessity of a complete cytoreduction to improve survival. Hyperthermic intraperitoneal chemotherapy (HIPEC) has an adjuvant role in preventing peritoneal recurrences. A multidisciplinary approach should be empowered: the association of neoadjuvant intraperitoneal and systemic chemotherapy (NIPS), cytoreductive surgery (CRS), HIPEC, and early postoperative intraperitoneal chemotherapy (EPIC) could increase the rate of completeness of cytoreduction (CC) and consequently survival rates, especially in patients with Peritoneal Cancer Index (PCI) ≤6. Neoadjuvant chemotherapy may improve survival also in PC from GC and adjuvant chemotherapy could prevent recurrence. In the last decade an interesting new drug, called Catumaxomab, has been developed in Germany. Two studies showed that this drug seems to improve progression-free survival in patients with GC; however, final results for both studies have still to be published.

1. Introduction

Gastric cancer (GC) is the fourth most common cancer and the second leading cause of cancer death in the world [1, 2]. The principal risk factors in development of GC are helicobacter pylori infection, atrophic gastritis, intestinal metaplasia, dysplasia, male gender, cigarette smoking, partial gastrectomy, Menetrier's disease, and genetic factors [3].

Global incidence of primary tumour locations and the histological types are constantly changing: in United States and in Western Europe the incidence of esophagogastric junction (Barrett's type) and gastric cardia adenocarcinoma is increasing [4] while there has been a reduction of incidence of distal GC since the 1970s, especially in Western countries [5].

Although GC mortality has been reduced, it remains a disease with poor prognosis and high mortality, second only to lung tumour. The prognosis of GC depends on stage and location: proximal gastric tumours (i.e., cardia tumor) have poorer prognosis compared to those in the pyloric antrum and when the disease is confined to the stomach mucosa, 5-year survival is near to 95%, while the reported 5-year survival rate for advanced GC varies from 10 to 20% [5].

Metastatic dissemination in GC may occur through the hematic torrent or by dissemination to the peritoneal cavity; this last condition is called peritoneal carcinomatosis (PC) [6], and it is considered a stage IV of GC. Recent studies show that peritoneal dissemination is more frequent than hematogenous metastases. Only 40% of GC deaths have hepatic metastases, while in 53–60% disease evolves through PC [3].

2. Epidemiology of Peritoneal Carcinomatosis

PC is considered the end stage of primary peritoneal malignant disorders (such as peritoneal mesothelioma) and a common manifestation of digestive-tract and gynaecological advanced cancers (such as appendicle tumour, ovarian cancer, colorectal cancer, or gastric cancer). It is generally associated with a poor prognosis; patients with PC of gastric origin have an extremely bad prognosis with a median survival estimate at 1–3 months [3, 14].

Data from the literature show that 15% of patients present PC *ab initio* and 35% of patients die of intraperitoneal recurrence for PC confined exclusively into the peritoneum [15]. Systemic chemotherapy improves median survival in metastatic gastric cancer to 7–10 months [16], but in patients with PC from GC the same improvement has not been reported [17].

Currently, at the intraoperative abdominal examination, peritoneal seeding is found in 10–20% of patients scheduled for potentially curative resection and in 40% of those at stage II-III [15, 18, 19]; 20–50% of patients treated with radical surgery will develop postoperatory peritoneal recurrence [20], and intraperitoneal spread of tumour cells is observed in 54% of patients who died of recurrence after surgery in advanced GC [21].

During the last 30 years multimodal therapeutic approaches on PC improved, resulting in a modified role of surgery: not a simple debulking operation anymore but a complete tumour cytoreduction with no macroscopic residual disease.

Sugarbaker investigated the synergism of the effects of hyperthermia and intraperitoneal anticancer chemotherapy against tumour cells; he found the existence of PC originating by low grade malignancy tumours without invasion capacity (like pseudomyxoma peritonei) that can be treated with cytoreductive surgery (CRS) and hyperthermic intraperitoneal chemotherapy (HIPEC).

In 1995 Sugarbaker definitively codified, in terms of rationale and surgical technique, the procedure of peritonectomy [22]. Following these innovative studies, a growing number of authors have been investigating this procedure [19]. Furthermore, same authors start to test these techniques in more aggressive tumours.

3. Pathophysiology of Peritoneal Carcinomatosis

Peritoneal dissemination of free cancer cells happens through exfoliation and leads to direct invasion of the serosa. Surgical manipulation or trauma can facilitate the mechanism [19]. Tumour cells can also diffuse passing through the "stomata": big communicating orifices present in the peritoneal surface, between peritoneal cavity and lymphatic vessels [15]. Cells distribution into peritoneal cavity is also conditioned by physical factors: tumour primary site, effects of gravity, presence or presence of fluids (ascites, mucus, etc.), and intrinsic biological aggressiveness [23–25]. Some studies showed that there are tumours with a distinct capability to give peritoneal metastases, without giving distant metastases.

4. Diagnosis of Peritoneal Carcinomatosis

For preoperative diagnosis of PC, useful imaging techniques are ultrasound (US), computerized tomography (CT), magnetic resonance imaging (MRI), and 18F-Fluorodeoxyglucose Positron Emission Tomography-CT (FDG PET-CT) [15], but all these imaging techniques have major limitations in diagnosing PC because of the low-volume density of peritoneal nodules. CT and MRI are important mainly in evaluating unresectable disease and cancer staging [26, 27]. PET-CT seem to be a good option, but are expensive and have drawbacks for lesions smaller than 5 mm in diameter [14]. Concerning PC from GC, Yang et al. [28] report an accuracy of PET-CT of 87%, with a sensitivity and specificity of 72.7% and 93.6%, respectively, with a sensitivity better than CT, while for primary GC and lymph node metastases the accuracy for PET-CT is 54%. CT is not accurate (8–17% of sensitivity) particularly for malignant granulations less than 5 mm in diameter and for small bowel nodulations.

Due to the low accuracy given by the imaging, the main diagnosing methods currently used to evaluate peritoneal surface are diagnostic laparoscopy or laparotomy and peritoneal cytological examination that show a greater accuracy in diagnosing PC [14]. Diagnostic laparoscopy, with or without peritoneal washing for malignant cells, has only a III B degree of recommendation; it is used to exclude metastatic disease in tumours that are considered potentially resectable [3]. A standardized technique minimizes the risk of tumour contamination of the trocars insertion sites; this method, compared with laparotomy, is also free from risks related to the complications of diagnostic laparotomy [15] and allows staging before and after CRS + HIPEC and during the follow-up. Moreover, exploratory laparoscopy could be used in order to evaluate the efficacy of neoadjuvant chemotherapy [3].

The three main different scoring systems for intraperitoneal cancer dissemination that have been published until today are as follows.

(i) Japanese rules of GC [14, 29] is a classification into five categories that only considers the presence of cancerous implants and/or of malignant cells in the peritoneal washing fluid, without considering the size of malignant nodules.

(ii) Gilly staging system for PC [14, 19], also called the Lyon score, is based on the size and distribution of malignant granulations (localized or diffused). It demonstrates that the use of complete (R0-R1) or incomplete (R2) cytoreduction, in order to assess the entirety of surgical clearance of cancer, is successful. It is difficult to confirm a R0 resection in patients with carcinomatosis. R0 and R1 can be grouped together as the outcome of these two groups is very similar. This system was also revealed to be an important prognostic indicator, as the median survival of patients with stage I or II is significantly higher than those with stage III or IV, and they can be candidates for CRS and HIPEC. However, this system does not clearly indicate the potential resectability of PC [5].

(iii) Jacquet and Sugarbaker Peritoneal Cancer Index (PCI) [30] is based on quantitative distribution and size of peritoneal nodules. The abdomen cavity is divided into 13 regions and the lesion size is scored in each region. After a meticulous intraoperative inspection, the extent of the disease can be summed as a numerical score (0 to 39). The PCI has a prognostic value, allowing for an estimate of the probability of complete cytoreduction; it is the only method that shows in detail the nodules localization.

The completeness of cytoreduction (CCR) could be evaluated using the Sugarbaker and the Lyon scores combined, as they indicate a direct relation between CCR, prognosis, and survival.

5. Rationale and Technique of Cytoreduction and HIPEC

Pharmacokinetic and peritoneal permeability studies demonstrate a higher intraperitoneal concentration of drugs with chemotherapy administered intraperitoneally than with systemic administration [23, 24]. The peritoneal plasma barrier maintains a positive gradient of chemotherapy in the peritoneum, increasing the local effects of the drugs and reducing the systemic toxicity [3]. Moreover, when chemotherapy treatment is associated with hyperthermia, the locoregional effects are considerably extended, with an increased penetration up to 3–6 mm into malignant nodules and an increased antimitotic effect. Several studies confirm that hyperthermia (42-43°C) enhances the effects of antitumoral drugs, especially of oxaliplatin, mitomycin C, doxorubicin, cisplatin, paclitaxel, and irinotecan [19], also increasing the chemosensibility of neoplastic cells. The intraabdominal temperature, however, should not exceed the temperature of 43°C, in order to avoid the risk of bowel perforation [12].

According to surgical-oncologic principles, the treatment of non-metastatic GC consists of resection with total gastrectomy and D1 and/or D2 lymphadenectomy [3]. Different trials proposed multiple chemotherapy protocols using drugs like Epirubicine, Cisplatin and 5-Fluorouracil (ECF), or Epirubicin, Cisplatin and Capecitabina (ECX), that do not need a central venous access device [3].

S-1, a new drug recently introduced in Japan, combined with Cisplatinum, Paclitaxel, Docetaxel or Irinotecan has become the standard treatment for PC from GC [14].

6. Cytoreductive Surgery and HIPEC for Advanced Gastric Cancer

Correct radiological, clinical, and cytological stadiation is essential requirement for a better prognosis after HIPEC in GC. It is necessary to distinguish PC in early or advanced GC from PC as a recurrence of already operated GC. In fact, in the former case it is easier to succeed with a complete cytoreduction (CCR-0, R0), while in the latter, previous surgical treatment and adhesion development decrease the possibility to achieve a complete cytoreduction.

Common contraindications for HIPEC are age >70 yrs, important comorbidities, clinical aggravation with systemic chemotherapy, malnutrition, extra abdominal metastases, liver metastases when unresectable, and massive retroperitoneal bulk disease or lymph node involvement. Other minor exclusion criteria are Body Mass Index (BMI) >40, history of pelvic irradiation, carcinomatosis extended at the CT or clinically significant, more than 4 surgical procedures, occlusion, and no drop markers with neoadjuvant chemotherapy [19].

Different studies presented contrasting data about survival rates; however, they all agreed with the necessity of a complete (Tables 1 and 2) cytoreduction to improve survival. HIPEC has an adjuvant role to prevent peritoneal recurrences [19]. Gill et al. show that in patients with a CC (completeness of cytoreduction) score of 0 or 1 overall median survival was 15 months [10] (versus 7.9 months in patients with CC 2 score), with an overall mortality rate of 4.8%.

Yonemura et al. [8] in an RCT of 139 patients with T2-4 GC randomized into 3 groups (HIPEC and surgery, intraperitoneal normothermic chemotherapy plus surgery, and surgery alone) show that in the first group the survival rate was significantly higher (61% versus 43% and 42% of the other two groups), particularly in patients with serosal infiltration and lymph node positive metastases. Similar results were published by Fujimoto et al. [21] in stage II-III GC patients, and by Kim and Bae [7] in patients affected by stage III and IV GC treated with HIPEC + CRS versus surgery alone.

Kim and Bae [7] analysed 103 patients with GC stage III-IV: 51 underwent surgical resection alone and 52 received surgery plus HIPEC. Mitomycin-C at 44°C was used in the HIPEC group as intraperitoneal chemotherapy. The 5 years overall survival rate in the 103 patients was 29.97%. It was higher but not statistically significant in the HIPEC + CRS group (32.7% versus 27.1% control group). The difference, considering exclusively the survival rate of the 65 patients with stage III GC, was statistically significant (58.6% versus 44.4% control group).

In a retrospective multicentric French study undertaken between February 1989 and August 2007, Glehen et al. [10] evaluated 159 patients that underwent cytoreductive surgery and perioperative intraperitoneal chemotherapy (HIPEC and EPIC or both) and showed 1-, 3-, and 5-year survival rates of 43%, 18%, and 13%, respectively, that increase up to 61%, 30%, and 23%, respectively, in patients with a complete cytoreduction. Thanks to multivariate analysis, the authors reported the completeness of cytoreduction as being the principal independent prognostic factor. In order to correctly execute cytoreduction, the staging system should be corroborated by PCI assessment. The study showed that if cytoreductive surgery does not allow a sufficient downstaging, particularly in HIPEC, the survival rates are poor (median survival of 6–8 months).

Three recent meta-analysis [11–13] of RCTs, assessing patients with GC (with or without PC), demonstrates the survival benefit offered by HIPEC. Already in 2007, Yan et al. [11] conducted 13 studies on 1648 patients and demonstrated the positive effects in terms of overall survival rates, when adding HIPEC or HIPEC with EPIC to surgery. These studies also showed how these procedures can be complementary to

TABLE 1: Comparing main studies in terms of median survival, 5-year survival rates, and morbidity.

Authors	Year published	Type of study	Stage of GC	Number of patients	Type of protocol	Median survival (months)	5-year survival rates	Morbidity
Fujimoto et al. [21]	1999	RCT	Stage II-III	141	HIPEC + surgery versus surgery alone	N/A	76% versus 57%	N/A
Kim and Bae [7]	2001	PCS	Stage III-IV	103	HIPEC + CRS versus surgery alone	36 versus 22.9	32.7% versus 27.1%	33.2% versus 36.5%
Yonemura et al. [8]	2001	RCT	Stage II-III	139	HIPEC + surgery versus NIC + surgery versus surgery alone	N/A	61% versus 43% versus 42%	4% versus 0% versus 4%
Yonemura et al. [9]	2009	PCS	Stage III-IV	79	NIPS versus NIPS + surgery	N/A	20.4% versus 40%*	11.4%
Glehen et al. [10]	2010	RCS	Stage III-IV	159	HIPEC + EPIC versus EPIC HIPEC	9.2 (overall)	13% (overall)	27.8% (overall)

HIPEC: hyperthermic intraperitoneal chemotherapy; EPIC: early postoperative intraperitoneal chemotherapy; PIC: perioperative intraperitoneal chemotherapy; NIC: normothermic intraperitoneal chemotherapy; NIPS: neoadjuvant intraperitoneal and systemic chemotherapy; NIIC: normothermic Intraoperative Intraperitoneal Chemotherapy; DPIC: Delayed Postoperative Intraperitoneal Chemotherapy; RCS: Retrospective Case Series; PCS: Prospective cohort study; PCS: prospective case series; N/A: not available.
*2-year survival rates.

TABLE 2: Comparing main meta-analysis in terms of overall survival and morbidity.

Authors	Year published	Type of study	Stage of GC	Number of patients	Type of protocol	Overall survival	Peritoneal recurrence	Mortality and morbidity
Yan et al. [11]	2007	Meta-analysis (13 RCTs)	Stage I-IV	1648	Surgery + HIPEC/HIPEC + EPIC/NIIC versus surgery alone ± systemic chemotherapy	HR = 0.60[1] HR = 0.45[2] HR = 0.67[3]	RR = 0.84$ RR = 0.51 RR = 1.00$	RR = 1.43 RR = 1.01/1.81/0.76/2.37/4.33#
Jin-Yu et al. [12]	2012	Meta-analysis (15 RCTs)	N/A	1713	HIPEC versus HIPEC + PIC versus NIIC	HR = 0.60 HR = 0.47 HR = 0.70	OR = 0.69	OR = 2.29 OR = 1.04/2.60/1.61/0.39/5.74/3.67/3.57$
Sun et al. [13]	2012	Meta-analysis (10 RCTs)	Stage II-III	1062	HIPEC* versus surgery	MMC RR = 0.75 5-FU RR = 0.69	RR = 0.45	N/A for Mortality RR = 1.68/0.52/1.38/0.79/1.47£

HR: hazard ratio; RR: risk ratio; OR: odds ratio; MMC: mitomycin C; 5-FU: 5-fluorouracil; HIPEC: hyperthermic intraperitoneal chemotherapy; EPIC: early postoperative intraperitoneal chemotherapy; PIC: perioperative intraperitoneal chemotherapy; NIC: NIIC: normothermic intraoperative intraperitoneal chemotherapy; RCS: retrospective case series; PCS: prospective case series; N/A: not available; PC: peritoneal carcinomatosis.
[1,2,3]HIPEC, HIPEC + EPIC, and NIIC, respectively.
$No differences in morbidity between HIPEC and NIIC groups and the respective control arms.
#Morbidity of anastomotic leak, bowel fistula, pancreatic fistula, intra-abdominal abscess, and neutropenia, respectively.
*Data calculated with risk ratio (RR) and divided in two subgroups for analysis: mitomycin C subgroup RR = 0.75, 5-Fluorouracil RR = 0.69 versus control group RR = 0.45.
£Morbidity of bone marrow suppression, anastomotic leak, bowel fistula, adhesive ileus, and liver disfunction, respectively.
$Morbidity of anastomotic leak, ileus, bowel perforation, pancreatic fistula, marrow depression, fever, and intra-abdominal abscess, respectively.

adjuvant systemic treatment. The efficacy of normothermic intraperitoneal chemotherapy (NIIC) is marginal. Jin-Yu et al. [12] analyzed 15 RCTs and demonstrated that HIPEC and NIIC should be recommended in treating patients with GC, as they significantly improve the overall survival rates. HIPEC results are better, but NIIC's are still statistically significant [8]. This meta-analysis demonstrated that adding postoperative intraperitoneal chemotherapy (PIC) to HIPEC has no additional effect on overall survival rates but it improves costs and toxicity. This study also showed that intraperitoneal chemotherapy (IPC) has no effect on prevention of lymph metastasis, but could decrease by 73% the rate of hepatic metastasis. Authors demonstrated that IPC does not increase perioperative mortality and postoperative anastomotic leaks, ileus, or bowel perforation rates, but it increases the risk of marrow depression, intra-abdominal abscess, and fever. The same results are also confirmed by Sun et al. [13].

In the last decade an interesting new drug, called Catumaxomab, has been developed in Germany [31]. The Catumaxomab is a rat-mouse hybrid monoclonal antibody that is now used for patients with malignant ascites in phase II/III randomized trial. Two studies [32, 33] demonstrate that this drug seems to improve progression-free survival in patients with GC (median 71 versus 44 days; $P = 0.03$) and that it seems to improve the survival in gastrointestinal EpCAM+ tumours (EpCAM: antiepithelial cell adhesion molecule) in intraperitoneal use. However, final results of both studies have yet to be published.

CRS and HIPEC are associated with significant morbidity and mortality, also in high volume centers, and reported rates are included between 0.9–5.8% and 12–52%, respectively [34]. The main postoperative complications after CRS and HIPEC are intra-abdominal abscess, gastric or small intestinal perforation, postoperative ileus, anastomotic leakage, postoperative bleeding, fistula, sepsis, respiratory distress, hematologic toxicity, and urinary disturbance [6, 19]. In the same group of patients, the main causes of death include anastomotic leakage, sepsis, postoperative bleeding, intestinal fistula, and disseminated intravascular coagulation (DIC) [35].

The aggressiveness of GC disease is the main cause of this unfavourable prognosis. Recently, Yonemura et al. [9, 14] proposed a multimodal strategy that associates neoadjuvant intraperitoneal and systemic chemotherapy (NIPS), CRS + HIPEC and EPIC. The rationale of this method is to reduce tumour burden before surgery with NIPS, a bidirectional chemotherapy that attacks PC from both sides of peritoneum (from the peritoneal cavity and from subperitoneal blood vessels), together with CRS and HIPEC, in order to reduce macroscopic and microscopic PC. The aim of EPIC is then to eradicate residual intraperitoneal cancer cells before the development of adhesions.

The NIPS technique is characterized by a first phase in which patients are treated with $60 \, mg/m^2$ of oral S-1 for 21 days, followed by one week of rest. A port system has been previously placed into the abdominal cavity under local anesthesia, with the tip in the Douglas pouch. On the 1st, 8th, and 15th postoperative days, $30 \, mg/m^2$ of Taxotere and $30 \, mg/m^2$ of Cisplatinum with $500 \, mL$ of saline are infused into the peritoneal cavity. Authors recommend two cycles of treatment to achieve a negative cytology status. Complications after NIPS have been reported in 4 out of 79 patients (1 with grade 4 of bone marrow toxicity, 3 with a renal dysfunction). In 3 patients, infections around the periportal space, that led to the port remotion, were reported. This study shows a washing cytology negativization in 41 out of 79 patients (63%) [4].

Also Glehen et al. [10], in a retrospective multicentre study, recommend the routine use of neoadjuvant chemotherapy to improve surgical results and to exclude patients who do not respond to the therapy form HIPEC treatment.

7. Conclusions

The aforementioned procedures should be exclusively performed in highly experienced centres because of the special surgical expertise needed to achieve high rates of complete cytoreduction [14, 19, 23, 32-34].

Patient selection is very crucial and should be carried out by a multidisciplinary group of specialists (anaesthetists, surgeons, clinicians, and oncologists) in order to achieve better results and to reduce the high costs related to these procedures and relevant complications.

An interdisciplinary approach should be developed further: the association of NIPS, CRS, HIPEC, and EPIC could increase the rate of CC-0 procedures and consequently survival rates, particularly for PCI ≤6 [5, 11, 21, 32]. Neoadjuvant chemotherapy, routinely recommended for management of GC without PC, may improve survival also in PC from GC [10, 34–37] and adjuvant chemotherapy could prevent recurrence from GC [10]. Finally, the study of molecular and serum tumour markers could provide valuable prognostic information and would allow for a better selection of subsequent treatment combinations [14, 38].

Acknowledgment

Thanks are due to Ramona Ruggeri for proofreading.

References

[1] P. Bertuccio, L. Chatenoud, F. Levi et al., "Recent patterns in gastric cancer: a global overview," *International Journal of Cancer*, vol. 125, no. 3, pp. 666–673, 2009.

[2] D. M. Parkin, F. Bray, J. Ferlay, and P. Pisani, "Global cancer statistics, 2002," *CA Cancer Journal for Clinicians*, vol. 55, no. 2, pp. 74–108, 2005.

[3] A. Okines, M. Verheij, W. Allum, D. Cunningham, and A. Cervantes, "Gastric cancer: ESMO clinical practice guidelines for diagnosis, treatment and follow-up," *Annals of Oncology*, vol. 21, no. 5, pp. v50–v54, 2010.

[4] A. Nissan, A. Garofalo, and J. Esquivel, "Cytoreductive surgery and hyperthermic intra-peritoneal chemotherapy (HIPEC) for gastric adenocarcinoma: why haven't we reached the promised land?" *Journal of Surgical Oncology*, vol. 102, no. 5, pp. 359–360, 2010.

[5] O. Glehen, F. Mohamed, and F. N. Gilly, "Peritoneal carcinomatosis from digestive tract cancer: new management by cytoreductive surgery and intraperitoneal chemohyperthermia," *The Lancet Oncology*, vol. 5, no. 4, pp. 219–228, 2004.

[6] R. S. Gill, D. P. Al-Adra, J. Nagendran et al., "Treatment of gastric cancer with peritoneal carcinomatosis by cytoreductive surgery and HIPEC: a systematic review of survival, mortality, and morbidity," *Journal of Surgical Oncology*, vol. 104, no. 6, pp. 692–698, 2011.

[7] J.-Y. Kim and H.-S. Bae, "A controlled clinical study of serosa-invasive gastric carcinoma patients who underwent surgery plus intraperitoneal hyperthermo-chemo-perfusion (IHCP)," *Gastric Cancer*, vol. 4, no. 1, pp. 27–33, 2001.

[8] Y. Yonemura, X. de Aretxabala, T. Fujimura et al., "Intraoperative chemohyperthermic peritoneal perfusion as an adjuvant to

gastric cancer: final results of a randomized controlled study," *Hepato-Gastroenterology*, vol. 48, no. 42, pp. 1776–1782, 2001.

[9] Y. Yonemura, Y. Endou, M. Shinbo et al., "Safety and efficacy of bidirectional chemotherapy for treatment of patients with peritoneal dissemination from gastric cancer: selection for cytoreductive surgery," *Journal of Surgical Oncology*, vol. 100, no. 4, pp. 311–316, 2009.

[10] O. Glehen, F. N. Gilly, C. Arvieux et al., "Peritoneal carcinomatosis from gastric cancer: a multi-institutional study of 159 patients treated by cytoreductive surgery combined with perioperative intraperitoneal chemotherapy," *Annals of Surgical Oncology*, vol. 17, no. 9, pp. 2370–2377, 2010.

[11] T. D. Yan, D. Black, P. H. Sugarbaker et al., "A systematic review and meta-analysis of the randomized controlled trials on adjuvant intraperitoneal chemotherapy for resectable gastric cancer," *Annals of Surgical Oncology*, vol. 14, no. 10, pp. 2702–2713, 2007.

[12] H. Jin-Yu, Y.-Y. Xu, Z. Sun et al., "Comparison different methods of intraoperative and intraperitoneal chemotherapy for patients with gastric cancer: a meta-analysis," *Asian Pacific Journal of Cancer Prevention*, vol. 13, no. 9, pp. 4379–4385, 2012.

[13] J. Sun, Y. Song, Z. Wang et al., "Benefit of hyperthermic intraperitoneal chemotherapy for patients with serosal invasion in gastric cancer: a meta-analysis of the randomized controlled trials," *BMC Cancer*, vol. 12, article 526, 2012.

[14] Y. Yonemura, A. Elnemr, Y. Endou et al., "Multidisciplinary therapy for treatment of patients with peritoneal carcinomatosis from gastric cancer," *World Journal of Gastrointestinal Oncology*, vol. 2, no. 2, pp. 85–97, 2010.

[15] F. Carboni, A. di Giorgio, L. di Lauro et al., "Criteri di appropriatezza clinica ed organizzativa nella diagnosi, terapia e follow-up delle carcinosi peritoneali," SICO, 2012, http://www.sicoonline.org/00_allegati_news/15_CarcinosiPeritoneali.pdf.

[16] S. Pyrhonen, T. Kuitunen, P. Nyandoto, and M. Kouri, "Randomised comparison of fluorouracil, epidoxorubicin and methotrexate (FEMTX) plus supportive care with supportive care alone in patients with non-resectable gastric cancer," *British Journal of Cancer*, vol. 71, no. 3, pp. 587–591, 1995.

[17] K. Hanazaki, Y. Mochizuki, T. Machida et al., "Post-operative chemotherapy in non-curative gastrectomy for advanced gastric cancer," *Hepato-Gastroenterology*, vol. 46, no. 26, pp. 1238–1243, 1999.

[18] Y. Kodera, Y. Yamamura, Y. Shimizu et al., "Peritoneal washing cytology: prognostic value of positive findings in patients with gastric carcinoma undergoing a potentially curative resection," *Journal of Surgical Oncology*, vol. 72, no. 2, pp. 60–64, 1999.

[19] F. Roviello, S. Caruso, D. Marrelli et al., "Treatment of peritoneal carcinomatosis with cytoreductive surgery and hyperthermic intraperitoneal chemotherapy: state of the art and future developments," *Surgical Oncology*, vol. 20, no. 1, pp. e38–e54, 2011.

[20] F. Roviello, D. Marrelli, A. Neri et al., "Treatment of peritoneal carcinomatosis by cytoreductive surgery and intraperitoneal hyperthermic chemoperfusion (IHCP): postoperative outcome and risk factors for morbidity," *World Journal of Surgery*, vol. 30, no. 11, pp. 2033–2040, 2006.

[21] S. Fujimoto, M. Takahashi, T. Mutou et al., "Successful intraperitoneal hyperthermic chemoperfusion for the prevention of post-operative peritoneal recurrence in patiens with advanced gastric carcinoma," *Cancer*, vol. 85, no. 3, pp. 529–534, 1999.

[22] P. H. Sugarbaker, "Peritonectomy procedures," *Annals of Surgery*, vol. 221, no. 1, pp. 29–42, 1995.

[23] P. H. Sugarbaker, "Intraperitoneal chemotherapy and cytoreductive surgery for the prevention and treatment of peritoneal carcinomatosis and sarcomatosis," *Seminars in Surgical Oncology*, vol. 14, no. 3, pp. 254–261, 1998.

[24] P. H. Sugarbaker, "Observations concerning cancer spread within the peritoneal cavity and concepts supporting an ordered pathophysiology," in *Peritoneal Carcinomatosis: Principles and Management*, pp. 79–100, Kluwer Academic, Boston, Mass, USA, 1996.

[25] Y. Yonemura, N. Nojima, T. Kawamura et al., "Mechanisms of formation of peritoneal dissemination," in *Peritoneal Dissemination: Molecular Mechanisms and the Latest Therapy*, pp. 1–46, Maeda Shoten, Kanazawa, Japan, 1998.

[26] J. H. Stewart IV, P. Shen, A. Edward et al., "Intraperitoneal hyperthermic chemotherapy for peritoneal surface malignancy: current status and future directions," *Annals of Surgical Oncology*, vol. 12, no. 10, pp. 765–777, 2005.

[27] R. S. Gill, D. Al-Adra, J. Nagendran et al., "Tretement of gastric cancer with peritoneal carcinomatosis by cytoredctive surgery and HIPEC: a systematic review of survival, mortality, and morbidity," *Journal of Surgical Oncology*, vol. 104, no. 6, pp. 692–698, 2011.

[28] Q.-M. Yang, T. Kawamura, H. Itoh et al., "Is PET-CT suitable for predicting lymph node status for gastric cancer?" *Hepato-Gastroenterology*, vol. 55, no. 82-83, pp. 782–785, 2008.

[29] Japanese Research Society for Gastric Cancer, *The General Rules for Gastric Cancer Study*, Kanahara Shuppan, Tokyo, Japan, 1st edition, 1995.

[30] P. Jacquet and P. H. Sugarbaker, "Clinical research methodologies in diagnosis and staging of patients with peritoneal carcinomatosis," in *Peritoneal Carcinomatosis: Principles of Management*, P. H. Sugarbaker, Ed., pp. 359–374, Kluwer Academic, Boston, Mass, USA, 1996.

[31] L. Ansaloni, M. Lotti, and L. Campanati, "The prevention and treatement of peritoneal carcinomatosis from gastric cancer: a 2013 update," *Journal of Cancer Research & Therapy*, vol. 1, no. 1, pp. 54–59, 2013.

[32] M. M. Heiss, P. Murawa, P. Koralewski et al., "The trifunctional antibody catumaxomab for the treatment of malignant ascites due to epithelial cancer: results of a prospective randomized phase II/III trial," *International Journal of Cancer*, vol. 127, no. 9, pp. 2209–2221, 2010.

[33] M. A. Ströhlein, F. Lordick, D. Rüttinger et al., "Immunotherapy of peritoneal carcinomatosis with the antibody catumaxomab in colon, gastric, or pancreatic cancer: an open-label, multicenter, phase I/II trial," *Onkologie*, vol. 34, no. 3, pp. 101–108, 2011.

[34] I. T. Konstantinidis, C. Young, V. L. Tsikitis et al., "Cytoreductive surgery and hyperthermic intraperitoneal chemoperfusione: the University of Arizona early experience," *World Journal of Gastrointestinal Surgery*, vol. 4, no. 6, pp. 135–140, 2012.

[35] A. Mizumoto, E. Canabay, M. Hiranoand et al., "Morbidity and mortality outcomes of cytoreductive surgery and hyperthermic intraperitoneal chemotherapy at a single institution in Japan," *Gastroenterology Research and Practice*, vol. 2012, Article ID 836425, 5 pages, 2012.

[36] S. Fujimoto, M. Takahashi, T. Mutou et al., "Improved mortality rate of gastric carcinoma patients with peritoneal carcinomatosis treated with intraperitoneal hyperthermic chemoperfusion combined with surgery," *Cancer*, vol. 79, no. 5, pp. 884–891, 1997.

20

Prognostic Relevance of the Peritoneal Surface Disease Severity Score Compared to the Peritoneal Cancer Index for Colorectal Peritoneal Carcinomatosis

Jia Lin Ng,[1] Whee Sze Ong,[2] Claramae Shulyn Chia,[1] Grace Hwei Ching Tan,[1] Khee-Chee Soo,[1] and Melissa Ching Ching Teo[1]

[1]*Department of Surgical Oncology, National Cancer Centre Singapore, 11 Hospital Drive, Singapore 169610*
[2]*Division of Clinical Trials & Epidemiological Sciences, National Cancer Centre Singapore, 11 Hospital Drive, Singapore 169610*

Correspondence should be addressed to Melissa Ching Ching Teo; melissa.teo.c.c@nccs.com.sg

Academic Editor: Perry Shen

Background. Peritoneal Carcinomatosis Index (PCI) is a widely established scoring system that describes disease burden in isolated colorectal peritoneal carcinomatosis (CPC). Its significance may be diminished with complete cytoreduction. We explore the utility of the recently described Peritoneal Surface Disease Severity Score (PSDSS) and compare its prognostic value against PCI. *Methods.* The endpoints were overall survival (OS), progression-free survival (PFS), and survival less than 18 months (18 MS). *Results.* Fifty patients underwent cytoreductive surgery and hyperthermic intraperitoneal chemotherapy (CRS/HIPEC) for CPC from 2003 to 2014, with 98% achieving complete cytoreduction. Median OS was 28.8 months (95% CI, 18.0–39.1); median PFS was 9.4 months (95% CI, 7.7–13.9). Univariate analysis showed that higher PCI was significantly associated with poorer OS (HR 1.11; 95% CI, 1.03–1.20) and PFS (HR 1.09; 95% CI, 1.03–1.14). Conversely, PSDSS was not associated with either endpoint. Multivariate analysis showed that PCI, but not PSDSS, was predictive of OS and PFS. PCI was also able to discriminate survival outcomes better than PSDSS for both OS and PFS. There was no association between 18 MS and either score. *Conclusion.* PCI is superior to PSDSS in predicting OS and PFS and remains the prognostic score of choice in CPC patients undergoing CRS/HIPEC.

1. Introduction

Cytoreductive surgery and hyperthermic intraperitoneal chemotherapy (CRS/HIPEC) have resulted in improved survival outcomes for patients with isolated colorectal peritoneal carcinomatosis (CPC) [1–4]. Improved operative morbidity and mortality, that is, on a par with liver resections for isolated colorectal liver metastases, have also contributed to the increasing acceptance of this treatment modality [5]. The Peritoneal Cancer Index (PCI) and Completeness of Cytoreduction (CC) scores, as described by Jacquet and Sugarbaker [6], aid in predicting postoperative survival outcomes. However, in the presence of optimal cytoreduction regardless of PCI score, one wonders if the prognostic significance of PCI may be rendered irrelevant.

First described by Sugarbaker in 1998 [7], the Peritoneal Surface Disease Severity Score (PSDSS) incorporates clinical symptoms and primary tumour histology with the PCI. There is a growing interest in PSDSS after studies showed its utility in prognostication. However, there is a paucity of data directly comparing it to the more established PCI used in many institutions, including ours. Therefore, the aim of this study was to compare the predictive value of PCI versus PSDSS in our study population where complete cytoreduction was almost always achieved.

2. Materials and Methods

2.1. Patient Selection. In this Singapore Health Services Ethics Board approved study, a retrospective review of a prospectively maintained database was performed for patients who had undergone CRS/HIPEC for peritoneal carcinomatosis from colorectal cancer. As the only tertiary centre offering

CRS/HIPEC in South East Asia, these surgeries performed between February 2003 and April 2014 were carried out by two surgeons with special interest in advanced surgical oncology and CRS/HIPEC, with the second surgeon beginning midway into the period of analysis. CRS/HIPEC performed for appendiceal malignancies and other noncolorectal malignancies were excluded. Cases in which complete cytoreduction was deemed not feasible during exploratory laparotomy, and in which CRS/HIPEC was eventually not performed, were also excluded from analysis. Patients were routinely followed up closely with clinical examination and tumour markers every 3 months, and radiological imaging at least every 6 months, at the discretion of the treating surgeon.

2.2. Prognostic Scores. Peritoneal Cancer Index (PCI) and the Peritoneal Surface Disease Severity Score (PSDSS) were calculated and compared. PCI was calculated according to lesion size and its distribution in 9 abdominopelvic regions and 4 small bowel segments noted intraoperatively [6]. During exploratory laparotomy, patients in whom optimal cytoreduction was not deemed possible had their planned CRS/HIPEC procedure abandoned. Optimal cytoreduction in invasive cancers like CRC is defined as achieving a CC score of 0 to 1, with CC-0 indicating no macroscopic residual disease and CC-1 indicating no residual nodules greater than 2.5 mm. The prognosis for suboptimal or incomplete cytoreduction is universally dismal, with the risks of undertaking further morbid surgery far greater than any potential therapeutic gains [7]. PSDSS consists of 3 prognostic categories: clinical symptoms, primary tumour pathology, and PCI score [8], each of which is subcategorized according to severity. The endpoints used were overall survival (OS), progression-free survival (PFS), and survival less than 18 months (18 MS), as most patients survived beyond that. Demographic data and surgical outcomes were also obtained.

2.3. Statistical Analysis. A total of 61 laparotomy procedures were performed, but 7 did not complete CRS/HIPEC as the volume of disease determined intraoperatively was not found to be amenable for optimal CRS. In total, 54 CRS/HIPEC operations were completed on 51 patients. Three patients had redone CRS/HIPEC, and only their first operative records were selected for analysis. In addition, one patient with a PCI score of zero was excluded from the study. A total of 50 patients were analysed for OS and PFS. For the 18 MS analysis, 24 patients who were still alive or who were lost to follow-up before 18 months were further excluded.

PCI was analysed both as a continuous variable and as a categorical variable with 3 levels (<10, 10–20, and >10). PSDSS was also analysed as a continuous variable and as a categorical variable with 4 levels (<3, 4–7, 8–10, and >10). Categorical cutoffs for analysis were based on evidence from similar recently published prognostication studies [9–12].

OS was calculated from the date of surgery to the date of demise from any cause. PFS was calculated from the date of surgery to the date of disease relapse or demise, whichever occurred first. All survival distributions were estimated using Kaplan-Meier curves, and the log-rank test was used to test differences between curves. Cox proportional hazard regression models were fitted to estimate hazard ratios. For multivariate analysis, only PCI and PSDSS were fitted in the Cox model after considering the relatively small number of events for OS and PFS and that the primary objective of the study was to compare the prognostic value of PCI against PSDSS. Proportional hazards assumption was verified for each fitted model using Schoenfeld residuals. The discriminative ability of each prognostic score for OS/PFS was evaluated based on Harrell's concordance index for censored data (c-index) [13] and the D-statistics (D-stats) of Royston and Sauerbrei [14]. The c-index represents the probability of concordance between predicted and observed survival, taking value from 0.5 (random prediction) to 1 (perfect ability to discriminate). The D-stats measure a prognostic score's ability to separate the risk of death and/or relapse. The larger the D-stats, the greater the degree of separation for a prognostic score.

Logistic regression models were fitted to estimate the odds ratios to assess the association of various variables with 18 MS. The ability of the prognostic score to correctly classify patients who were dead or not within 18 months after CRS/HIPEC was evaluated based on the area under the receiver operating characteristics curve (AUC). The AUC takes value from 0.5 (random prediction) to 1 (perfect discrimination ability).

Statistical significance was set at $p < 0.05$. Analyses were performed using SAS version 9.4 (SAS Institute Inc., Cary, NC) with the D-stats generated using STATA 12.0 (Stata Corp, College Station, TX).

3. Results

Demographic data and surgical outcomes of the 50 patients were summarised in Table 1. The median age was 50 years (range, 14–71), and Eastern Cooperative Oncology Group performance status was 0 (82.0%) or 1 (18.0%). CC-0 score was achieved in 98% of cases, with only one case of moderately differentiated adenocarcinoma achieving CC-1 score. The median operative time was 457.5 minutes (range, 120–960). All patients underwent HIPEC (intraperitoneal mitomycin C or oxaliplatin, leucovorin and 5-fluorouracil combination, at a temperature of 39 to 43 degrees Celsius for 60 to 90 minutes). Twenty-four patients underwent early postoperative intraperitoneal chemotherapy, which was within the treatment protocol before October 2012. The median hospitalisation duration was 13.5 days (range, 9–43), and 22% of patients received adjuvant therapy after surgery at the discretion of the treating physician.

The median PCI was 10 (range, 1–27), and the median PSDSS was 6 (range, 2–22). In terms of cancer grade, 54.0% of patients had moderately differentiated carcinoma, 26.0% had poorly differentiated or mucinous carcinoma, and 2.0% had signet ring cell carcinoma.

The median follow-up duration was 13.3 months (range, 0.8–87.1 months) (Table 2). The median OS was 28.8 months (range, 18.3–39.1) with 87.6% surviving at 1 year. The median

TABLE 1: Baseline demographics and operative findings.

	Number	%
Total	50	100.0
Age at CRS/HIPEC, years		
Median (range)	50 (14–71)	
Gender		
Female	32	64.0
Male	18	36.0
ECOG performance status		
0	41	82.0
1	9	18.0
Presence of comorbidities		
No	19	38.0
Yes	31	62.0
Primary tumour site		
Colon	49	98.0
Rectum	1	2.0
Histology		
Well differentiated	6	12.0
Moderately differentiated	27	54.0
Poorly differentiated or mucinous	13	26
Signet ring cell	1	2.0
Missing data	3	6.0
Preoperation CEA, μg/L		
Median (range)	5.1 (0.2–501.0)	
Type of CRS procedure		
Subdiaphragmatic stripping	30	60.0
Gastrectomy	4	8.0
Colectomy	24	48.0
Small bowel resection	21	42.0
Splenectomy	6	12.0
THBSO	15	30.0
Cholecystectomy	8	16.0
Bladder resection	5	10.0
Others	17	34.0
Number of CRS procedures performed		
0	1[a]	2.0
1	14	28.0
2	18	36.0
3 and over	17	34.0
Median (range)	2 (0–5)	
Duration of operation, mins		
Median (range)	457.5 (120–960)	
Completion of Cytoreduction score		
0	49	98.0
1	1	2.0
≥ 2	0	0
Hospitalization duration, days		
Median (range)	13.5 (9–43)	
Post-CRS/HIPEC adjuvant therapy		
No	26	52.0
Yes	11	22.0
Missing data	13	26.0

CRS, cytoreductive surgery; HIPEC, hyperthermic intraperitoneal chemotherapy; ECOG, Eastern Cooperative Oncology Group; CEA, carcinoembryonic antigen; THBSO, Total Abdominal Hysterectomy Bilateral Salpingo Oophorectomy.

[a]The patient had omentectomy.

TABLE 2: Survival outcomes and relapses.

	Number	%
Follow-up duration, months		
Median (range)	13.3 (0.8–87.1)	
Overall survival (OS)		
Events/patients	18/50	
Median OS, months (95% CI)	28.8 (18.3–39.1)	
1-year OS, % (95% CI)	87.6 (72.7–94.7)	
Progression-free survival (PFS)		
Events/patients	33/50	
Median PFS, months (95% CI)	9.4 (7.7–13.9)	
1-year PFS, % (95% CI)	37.6 (22.7–52.5)	
Among relapsed patients	*32*	*100.0*
Site of relapse		
Peritoneum	28	87.5
Lymph nodes	11	34.4
Lung	15	46.9
Liver	8	25.0
Bones	5	15.6
Others	8	25.0

CI, confidence interval.

PFS was 9.4 months (range, 7.7–13.9), and 1-year PFS was 37.6%.

The results of univariate Cox-regression analysis, D-stats, and c-index for both PCI and PSDSS as continuous variables are summarised in Table 3. Higher PCI values were significantly associated with poorer OS (hazard ratio (HR) = 1.11; 95% CI, 1.03–1.20; and p = 0.005). PSDSS was not associated with OS (HR = 1.06; 95% CI, 0.97–1.14; and p = 0.191). Based on D-stats and c-index, PCI had higher discrimination ability than PSDSS for OS. On multivariate Cox analysis by PCI and PSDSS, only PCI was shown to be an independent significant predictor for OS (HR = 1.16; 95% CI 1.04–1.30; and p = 0.008) (Table 4).

As for PFS, higher PCI values were significantly associated with poorer PFS (HR = 1.09; 95% CI, 1.03–1.14; and p = 0.001). There was no significant association between PFS and PSDSS (HR = 1.05; 95% CI 0.99–1.11; and p = 0.096). PCI had a higher discrimination ability than PSDSS for PFS, with higher D-stats and c-index scores. On multivariate analysis, PCI was again shown to be an independent significant predictor for PFS (HR = 1.11; 95% CI 1.03–1.20; and p = 0.005).

Neither PCI nor PSDSS had any significant association with 18 MS (PCI: odds ratio (OR) = 1.14; 95% CI, 0.99–1.31 versus PSDSS: OR = 1.03; 95% CI, 0.89–1.19). While PCI had higher AUC than PSDSS (0.742 versus 0.585), there was no significant difference between both AUCs (difference = 0.157; 95% CI, −0.03–0.34; and p = 0.091).

4. Discussion

Prognostication scores have gained interest in the field of colorectal cancer with isolated peritoneal carcinomatosis in recent years [8–12]. The ideal score is easy to apply in clinical practice and backed by robust evidence in predicting overall survival and disease progression. Some studies have begun formulating and evaluating scores to predict resectability prior to surgery [9–12].

One such score is the PSDSS. This study explored the utility of using PSDSS in lieu of intraoperative PCI as a prognostic score. Nonetheless, we have found the PCI to be superior to PSDSS in prognosticating overall survival and disease progression. The inclusion of tumour biology and patient symptomology did not aid in discriminating outcome among our patients. This may be due to all but 1 patient achieving macroscopic complete cytoreduction (CC-0), regardless of disease burden. Our commitment to eradicate all disease in the peritoneal cavity, no matter how minute, may have rendered this additional information in the scoring system superfluous.

Furthermore, histopathology of the primary tumour plays a less definitive role in CPC. A French multicentre study [15] showed that positive independent prognostic factors include PCI, completeness of surgery, lymph node status, experience of the centre, and the use of adjuvant chemotherapy. Tumour grade did not appear to be significantly related to overall survival or progress-free survival.

Most of the patients developed progressive disease with interval development of CPC after the initial colorectal surgery. With many on regular postoperative surveillance and early referrals from other practitioners, not many develop symptoms before their early diagnosis of peritoneal carcinomatosis. With 32 of 50 patients asymptomatic on presentation, the inclusion of patient symptomology in PSDSS may not have helped in discriminating for outcome.

Neither PCI nor PSDSS was able to predict 18-month survival. The results may be limited by the relatively small number of patients available for analysis and those who survived less than 18 months, resulting in few measured events.

Surgical treatment of peritoneal metastases has gained momentum from oncologic communities around the world in the past decade. Initially viewed as an advanced disease doomed for palliative chemotherapy, referrals to the surgeons were scanty in the early 2000s and only began to pick up from 2010 onwards. The indications for CRS/HIPEC for colorectal peritoneal carcinomatosis have also broadened in recent years, compared to the initial years when the program initially started. We are in the midst of performing a learning curve analysis for all cases, but it is not inconceivable that our results are typical of any institution with the introduction of a complex procedure.

A potential drawback to the current study is the small sample size, contributed by the factors mentioned above, with a heterogeneous population, as typical of a retrospective analysis of our experience. The cut-offs for categorical analysis of PCI and PSDSS were based on evidence from recently published prognostication studies. While the precision of these analyses was affected by the small sample in some of the categories, it is essential to allow for meaningful comparisons across other similar publications comparing the two prognostic scores [9–12]. We performed sensitivity

TABLE 3: Univariate Cox-regression analysis, D-stats, and c-index of PCI and PSDSS for OS and PFS.

| | | Overall survival (OS) | | | | | | Progression-free survival (PFS) | | | | |
	E/N	Median OS, month	HR (95% CI)	$p^{\wedge}$	D-stats	c-index	E/N	Median PFS, month	HR (95% CI)	$p^{\wedge}$	D-stats	c-index
PCI												
Per unit increase	18/50	28.8	1.11 (1.03–1.20)	**0.005**[#]	—	0.737	33/50	9.4	1.09 (1.03–1.14)	**0.001**[#]	—	0.680
0 ≤ PCI ≤ 9	4/25	NR	1	0.059	1.033	0.693	10/25	17.6	1	**0.004**	0.870	0.668
10 ≤ PCI ≤ 20	11/20	27.1	3.23 (1.03–10.19)				19/20	7.2	3.45 (1.59–7.49)			
PCI > 20	3/5	19.9	4.55 (0.99–20.98)				4/5	7.8	2.85 (0.88–9.27)			
PSDSS												
Per unit increase	18/50	28.8	1.06 (0.97–1.14)	0.191[#]	—	0.613	33/50	9.4	1.05 (0.99–1.11)	0.096[#]	—	0.599
2 ≤ PSDSS ≤ 3	0/5	NR	1	0.139	0.686	0.603	0/5	NR	1	0.077	0.652	0.561
4 ≤ PSDSS ≤ 7	10/26	28.8	a				18/26	9.4	a			
8 ≤ PSDSS ≤ 10	2/5	18.5	a				3/5	8.4	a			
PSDSS > 10	6/14	34.5	a				12/14	9.4	a			

E, events; N, patients; HR, hazard ratio; CI, confidence interval; NR, not reached; PCI, Peritoneal Cancer Index; PSDSS, Peritoneal Surface Disease Severity Score.
a Not estimable as there were no events in the reference group.
^ Based on log-rank test, unless otherwise specified.
# Based on Wald's test.

TABLE 4: Multivariate Cox-regression analysis of OS and PFS by PCI and PSDSS.

	Overall survival (OS)		Progression-free survival (PFS)	
	HR (95% CI)	$p^{\#}$	HR (95% CI)	$p^{\#}$
PCI	1.16 (1.04–1.30)	**0.008**	1.11 (1.03–1.20)	**0.005**
PSDSS	0.93 (0.82–1.06)	0.271	0.97 (0.89–1.05)	0.403

HR, hazard ratio; CI, confidence interval; PCI, Peritoneal Cancer Index; PSDSS, Peritoneal Surface Disease Severity Score.
$^{\#}$Based on Wald's test.

analyses to evaluate the effect of small PCI and PSDSS categories. The conclusion remained similar when the small categories with less than 10 patients were combined with larger categories (results not shown).

Moving forward, we will continue to use intraoperative PCI as a tool for prognostication for overall survival and progression-free survival. With an increasing acceptance of CRS/HIPEC in treating colorectal peritoneal carcinomatosis, improving chemotherapy options and enhanced learning curves, one can look forward to a larger sample size with enhanced outcomes.

With that, we will continue to compare the utility of prognostic scores like PSDSS, and even the COREP score [9], which includes tumour markers to attempt to prognosticate outcomes and predict feasibility of achieving CC-0 resections prior to surgery.

We have also embarked on comparing preoperative PCI and PSDSS based on interpretation of radiological findings and are exploring the utility of radiologically calculated PCI and PSDSS for all patients considered for CRS and HIPEC. CT-PCI has been shown to have a sensitivity of 0.55 and a specificity of 0.86, compared to MRI-PCI with a sensitivity of 0.95 and specificity of 0.70 in a recently published paper comparing these scores amongst patients with appendiceal and ovarian cancer [16]. These adjunct imaging modalities may allow discrimination between those who would go on to have successful CRS and HIPEC and those in whom complete cytoreduction is not possible.

5. Conclusion

PCI remains the prognostic score of choice for patients with CPC undergoing CRS/HIPEC, as it is superior to PSDSS in prognosticating OS and PFS.

References

[1] D. Elias, J. H. Lefevre, J. Chevalier et al., "Complete cytoreductive surgery plus intraperitoneal chemohyperthermia with oxaliplatin for peritoneal carcinomatosis of colorectal origin," *Journal of Clinical Oncology*, vol. 27, no. 5, pp. 681–685, 2009.

[2] J. Franko, Z. Ibrahim, N. J. Gusani, M. P. Holtzman, D. L. Bartlett, and H. J. Zeh III, "Cytoreductive surgery and hyperthermic intraperitoneal chemoperfusion versus systemic chemotherapy alone for colorectal peritoneal carcinomatosis," *Cancer*, vol. 116, no. 16, pp. 3756–3762, 2010.

[3] V. J. Verwaal, S. van Ruth, E. de Bree et al., "Randomized trial of cytoreduction and hyperthermic intraperitoneal chemotherapy versus systemic chemotherapy and palliative surgery in patients with peritoneal carcinomatosis of colorectal cancer," *Journal of Clinical Oncology*, vol. 21, no. 20, pp. 3737–3743, 2003.

[4] P. H. Cashin, W. Graf, P. Nygren, and H. Mahteme, "Cytoreductive surgery and intraperitoneal chemotherapy for colorectal peritoneal carcinomatosis: prognosis and treatment of recurrences in a cohort study," *European Journal of Surgical Oncology*, vol. 38, no. 6, pp. 509–515, 2012.

[5] A. U. Blackham, G. B. Russell, J. H. Stewart IV, K. Votanopoulos, E. A. Levine, and P. Shen, "Metastatic colorectal cancer: survival comparison of hepatic resection versus cytoreductive surgery and hyperthermic intraperitoneal chemotherapy," *Annals of Surgical Oncology*, vol. 21, no. 8, pp. 2667–2674, 2014.

[6] P. Jacquet and P. H. Sugarbaker, "Clinical research methodologies in diagnosis and staging of patients with peritoneal carcinomatosis," *Cancer Treatment and Research*, vol. 82, pp. 359–374, 1996.

[7] P. H. Sugarbaker, *Management of Peritoneal Surface Malignancy Using Intraperitoneal Chemotherapy and Cytoredutive Surgery—A Manual for Physicians and Nurses*, The Ludann Company, Grand Rapids, Mich, USA, 3rd edition, 1998.

[8] J. O. Pelz, A. Stojadinovic, A. Nissan, W. Hohenberger, and J. Esquivel, "Evaluation of a peritoneal surface disease severity score in patients with colon cancer with peritoneal carcinomatosis," *Journal of Surgical Oncology*, vol. 99, no. 1, pp. 9–15, 2009.

[9] P. H. Cashin, W. Graf, P. Nygren, and H. Mahteme, "Comparison of prognostic scores for patients with colorectal cancer peritoneal metastases treated with cytoreductive surgery and hyperthermic intraperitoneal chemotherapy," *Annals of Surgical Oncology*, vol. 20, no. 13, pp. 4183–4189, 2013.

[10] T. C. Chua, D. L. Morris, and J. Esquivel, "Impact of the peritoneal surface disease severity score on survival in patients with colorectal cancer peritoneal carcinomatosis undergoing complete cytoreduction and hyperthermic intraperitoneal chemotherapy," *Annals of Surgical Oncology*, vol. 17, no. 5, pp. 1330–1336, 2010.

[11] W. Yoon, A. Alame, and R. Berri, "Peritoneal surface disease severity score as a predictor of resectability in the treatment of peritoneal surface malignancies," *The American Journal of Surgery*, vol. 207, no. 3, pp. 403–407, 2014.

[12] J. O. W. Pelz, T. C. Chua, J. Esquivel et al., "Evaluation of best supportive care and systemic chemotherapy as treatment stratified according to the retrospective Peritoneal Surface Disease Severity Score (PSDSS) for peritoneal carcinomatosis of colorectal origin," *BMC Cancer*, vol. 10, article 689, 2010.

[13] F. E. Harrell Jr., K. L. Lee, and D. B. Mark, "Multivariable prognostic models: issues in developing models, evaluating assumptions and adequacy, and measuring and reducing errors," *Statistics in Medicine*, vol. 15, no. 4, pp. 361–387, 1996.

[14] P. Royston and W. Sauerbrei, "A new measure of prognostic separation in survival data," *Statistics in Medicine*, vol. 23, no. 5, pp. 723–748, 2004.

21

A Review of the Literature on Extrarenal Retroperitoneal Angiomyolipoma

Anthony Kodzo-Grey Venyo

North Manchester General Hospital Department of Urology, Delaunay's Road, Manchester, UK

Correspondence should be addressed to Anthony Kodzo-Grey Venyo; akodzogrey@yahoo.co.uk

Academic Editor: S. Curley

Background. Extrarenal retroperitoneal angiomyolipomas are rare. *Aim.* To review the literature. *Results.* Angiomyolipomas, previously classified as hamartomas, are now classified as benign tumours. Thirty cases of primary retroperitoneal angiomyolipomas have been reported. Diagnosis of the disease upon is based radiological and pathological findings of triphasic features of (a) fat and (b) blood vessels and myoid tissue. Immunohistochemistry tends to be positive for HMB45, MART1, HHF35, calponin, NKI-C3, and CD117. The lesion is common in women. Treatment options have included the following: (a) radical surgical excision of the lesion with renal sparing surgery or radical nephrectomy in cases where malignant tumours could not be excluded and (b) selective embolization of the lesion alone or prior to surgical excision. One case of retroperitoneal angiomyolipoma was reported in a patient 15 years after undergoing radical nephrectomy for angiomyolipoma of kidney and two cases of distant metastases of angiomyolipoma have been reported following radical resection of the tumour. *Conclusions.* With the report of two cases of metastases ensuing surgical resection of the primary lesions there is need for academic pathologists to debate and review angiomyolipomas to decide whether to reclassify angiomyolipomas as slow-growing malignant tumours or whether the reported cases of metastases were de novo tumours or metastatic lesions.

1. Introduction

Extrarenal retroperitoneal angiomyolipomas (ERAMLs) also referred to as retroperitoneal angiomyolipomas (RAMLs) by some authors are rare lesions which may mimic other retroperitoneal tumours and thus pose a diagnostic problem to the clinician. There are on the whole three tissue components that constitute angiomyolipomas (AMLs) including mature adipose tissue, thick-walled blood vessels, and smooth muscle cells [1, 2]. AMLs were previously classified as hamartomas; however, AMLs are now regarded as belonging to the family of perivascular epithelioid cell tumours (PEComas) [1, 2]. Rare cases of ERAMLs have been reported. It has been documented that ultrasound scan and CT scan can diagnose correctly AMLs of the kidney in 86% of cases [3]. Nevertheless, ERAMLs are more difficult to diagnose on imaging in view of the fact that they tend to lack fat densities [4]. The ensuing review of the literature on extrarenal retroperitoneal angiomyolipoma (ERAMLs) is divided into two parts: (A) overview and (B) miscellaneous narrations and discussions from reported cases of extrarenal retroperitoneal angiomyolipoma and an article related to treatment of angiomyolipoma.

2. Methods

Various internet data bases were searched for the literature on extrarenal retroperitoneal angiomyolipoma (retroperitoneal angiomyolipoma) including Google, Google Scholar, PubMed, and Educus. The search words that were used included extrarenal retroperitoneal angiomyolipoma, retroperitoneal angiomyolipoma, and angiomyolipoma. Information obtained from 69 references mainly related to retroperitoneal angiomyolipoma and one on treatment of angiomyolipoma using mTor inhibitor rapamycin was used to write the literature review.

3. Literature Review

3.1. Overview (A)

3.1.1. General Comments about Angiomyolipomas (AMLs). The following has been stated [33]:

(i) AMLs tend to be benign neoplasms which comprise thick-walled vessels, smooth muscles, and fat (adipose) tissue with spindle and epithelioid cells but the amount of each of the aforementioned components is variable in different AMLs [33].

(ii) AMLs may occur in the kidney and at times AMLs may be found in extrarenal sites. In 2012 Minja et al. [18] summarized the extrarenal sites of AMLs they had encountered in their literature review as follows: uterus (7 cases) [34], hard palate (1 case) [35], head (2 cases) [36], abdominal wall (1 case) [37], penis (1 case) [38], fallopian tube (1 case) [39], liver (18 cases) [40], nasal cavity (1 case) [41], vagina (2 cases) [42, 43], spermatic cord (1 case) [44], and colon (1 case) [45], and the retroperitoneum (16 cases) [18]. A total of 52 cases of extrarenal angiomyolipomas had been reported according to Minja et al. [18] at the time of publication of their paper in 2012.

(iii) The occurrence of AML could be sporadic; nevertheless, AML has been associated with epiloia (tuberous sclerosis) and also with TSC/PKD1 contiguous gene syndrome [33].

3.1.2. Epidemiology

(i) It has been stated that AML tends to be diagnosed in adults and that AMLs of the kidney constitute less than one percent of kidney tumours [33].

(ii) The ages of the patients who have been reported to have been diagnosed with extrarenal retroperitoneal angiomyolipoma (ERAML), also called retroperitoneal angiomyolipoma (RAML) by other authors, have ranged between 22 years and 80 years (see Table 1).

(iii) The occurrence of AML in the retroperitoneum is rare and to the knowledge of the author 30 cases have been reported in the literature and the retroperitoneum constitutes the second most common site of extrarenal angiomyolipoma [18].

(iv) Extrarenal retroperitoneal angiomyolipoma (ERAML), also called retroperitoneal angiomyolipoma (RAML) by other authors, has been reported more commonly in females in comparison with males. Out of the 30 cases of extrarenal retroperitoneal angiomyolipomas (ERAMLs) reported the sex of the patients was available in 25 cases of which 24 (84%) were reported in women and 4 (16%) were reported in men (see Table 1).

3.1.3. Pathophysiology

(i) Stone et al. [46] stated that angiomyolipoma (AML) is a member of the epithelioid cell (PEC) AML which includes pulmonary lymphangioleiomyomatosis; clear cell sugar tumours of the pancreas, lung, and uterus; and also rhabdomyomas of the heart [33].

(ii) It has also been stated that angiomyolipomas (AMLs) are neoplasms and not hamartomas and that a number of cases of angiomyolipomas (AMLs) have loss of heterozygosity of TSC2 gene [33].

3.1.4. Molecular Genetic Studies

(i) Cheng et al. [47] iterated that smooth muscle cells and adipose tissue tend to be monoclonal but they may arise independently. Cheng et al. [47] reported that they had undertaken a study in which smooth muscle, adipose tissue, blood vessels, and adjacent normal tissue of the kidney were separately microdissected from formalin-fixed, paraffin-embedded, processed tissues of angiomyolipomas of 18 women. They studied the clonal origin of each component of angiomyolipoma by means of X chromosome inactivation analysis by using the methylation pattern of exon 1 of the human androgen receptor gene on chromosome Xq11-12. Cheng et al. [47] reported that they found nonrandom inactivation of X chromosomes in six out of the 15 informative tumours; the smooth muscle and adipose tissue did show differing patterns of nonrandom inactivation of X chromosomes in 5 angiomyolipomas and the same pattern of nonrandom inactivation of one; samples taken from blood vessels did show random inactivation of X chromosomes in all of the informative cases. Cheng et al. [47] concluded that their data had illustrated that the adipose tissue and smooth muscle cells of angiomyolipoma of the kidney are both monoclonal but they may arise independently; the coexistence of tumour subclones with morphologic heterogeneity could lead to the formation of a clinically detected tumour.

3.1.5. Clinical Characteristics

(i) Angiomyolipomas (AMLs) occur in the kidney but sporadic cases occur in other sites above with the liver being the commonest site where the tumour tends to have dominant epithelioid smooth muscle component [33].

(ii) It has been stated that angiomyolipomas (AMLs) may be found contemporaneously in association with renal cell carcinoma in cases of nonepiloia (nontuberous sclerosis) patients, especially clear cell carcinoma of the kidney which tends to stain negatively on immunohistochemistry studies [33, 48].

(iii) Angiomyolipomas (AMLs) tend to be benign; nevertheless, they may be associated with haemorrhage,

TABLE 1: A table of reported cases of extrarenal retroperitoneal angiomyolipoma.

Case	Reference	Presentation	Age (years)/ sex	Size	Imaging	Location	Treatment	Outcome/follow-up
1	Friis and Hjorttrup 1982 [5]	Pain and weight gain	22/ female	11 kilograms	Intravenous urography	Peripancreatic space	Radical nephrectomy	Asymptomatic/36 months
2	Randazzo et al. 1987 [6]	Pain and bleeding	64/ female	6 cubic cms	IVU and CT scan	Right perinephric space	Renal sparing surgery	Asymptomatic/2 months
3	Ditonno et al. 1992 [7]	Pain and bleeding	37/ male	5 cm	IVU and CT scan and angiography	Right perinephric space	Radical nephrectomy	Details not available
4	Peh et al. 1994 [8]	Abdominal mass and weight loss	32/ female	3.7 kilograms (7980 cubic cms)	Ultrasound scan and CT scan	Left perinephric space	Radical nephrectomy	Asymptomatic/8 months
5	Angulo et al. 1994 [9]	Abdominal pain and flank pain	53/ female	336 cubic cms	Ultrasound scan, CT scan, and angiography	Left perinephric space	Radical nephrectomy	Details not available
6	Gupta and Guleria 2011 [10]	Abdominal pain	42/ Male	220 cubic cms.	Ultrasound scan and CT scan	Right adrenal space	Renal sparing resection	Details not available
7	Liwnicz et al. 1994 [11]	Abdominal pain	39/ female	1.1 kilograms (216 cubic cm)	CT scan	Right perinephric space	Radical nephrectomy	Asymptomatic/18 months
8	Law et al. 1994 [12]	Incidental finding	59/ female	22.5 cubic cm	CT scan and MRI scan	Left perinephric space	Radical nephrectomy	Details not available
9	Law et al. 1994 [12]	Pain	56/ female	11 cm	IVU, CT Scan, ultrasound and fine needle aspiration	Left perinephric space	Radical nephrectomy	Asymptomatic/8 months
10	Mogi et al. 1998 [13]	Abdominal fullness and pain	41/ female	648 cubic cm	CT scan and MRI scan	Right perinephric space and perihepatic space	Renal sparing resection of mass	Details not available
11	Murphy et al. 2000 [14]	Abdominal pain and bleeding	51/ female	Details not described	CT scan and angiography	Left perinephric space	Selective angiography embolization	Asymptomatic/12 months
12	Tsutsumi et al. 2001 [15]	Abdominal pain and fatigue (lethargy)	60/ female	3.5 kilograms (4840 cubic cm)	CT scan and angiography	Right perinephric space	Radical nephrectomy	Asymptomatic/60 months
13	Tseng et al. 2004 [16]	Fullness of abdomen	35/ female	2.8 kilograms (3726 cubic cm)	Ultrasound scan, CT scan and angiography	Right perinephric space	Renal sparing resection	Details not available
14	Obara et al. 2005 [17]	Visible haematuria	31/ male	Details not documented	CT scan and angiography	Right perinephric space	Radical nephrectomy	Details not available
15	Gupta et al. 2007 [4]	Abdominal pain	80/ female	16 cm	CT scan and MRI scan	Left perinephric space	Radical nephrectomy	Distant metastases in bone and liver/12 months
16	Minja et al. 2012 [18]	Asymptomatic	39/ female	1.7 kilograms (2898 cubic cm)	Ultrasound scan/CT scan	Left perinephric space	Radical nephrectomy	Asymptomatic/16 months

TABLE 1: Continued.

Case	Reference	Presentation	Age (years)/ sex	Size	Imaging	Location	Treatment	Outcome/follow-up
17	Lee et al. 2003 [19]	Increasing abdominal circumference and urinary frequency	35/ female	24 cm × 21 cm × 16 cm	CT scan	Right retroperitoneal region displacing right kidney to left	Wide excision with preservation of kidney (kidney sparing resection of mass)	Asymptomatic/4 months
18	Soni et al. 2013 [20]	Left sided abdominal pain	33/ female	9.3 cm × 6.1 cm × 7.7 cm	CT scan	Left pararenal retroperitoneal space	Kidney preservation excision of mass	Follow-up information was not available
19	Ivanova et al. 2014 [21]	Right sided lumbar ache	33/ female	10 cm × 6 cm	Radiological imaging type not available	Right retroperitoneal space	Kidney preserving resection	Follow-up information was not available
20	Welling et al. 2012 [22]	Incidental finding of staging FDG PET/CT scan for melanoma of right flank	38/ male	Hypermetabolic extrarenal mass size not available	FDG PET/CT scan done as staging CT for melanoma	Left retroperitoneal space	Details of surgery not available	Follow-up information not available
21	Fegan et al. 1997 [23]	Details not available	Details not available	Details not available	Details not available	Extrarenal retroperitoneal details not available	Details not available	Metastases reported in the abstract to the liver and mediastinum (the questions needed to be asked: are the lesions true metastases? Or are they de novo primaries in the liver and mediastinum? If they are metastases then should angiomyolipoma not be classified as malignant tumours?)
22	Lau et al. 2003 [24]	Details not available	Details not available	Details not available	Details not available	Extrarenal retroperitoneal details not available	Details not available	
23	Wen et al. 2014 [25]	History of tuberous sclerosis and left renal AML had preoperative embolization plus left nephrectomy 15 years earlier. Presented with loss of appetite, vomiting, abdominal pain, constipation, and palpable mass in abdomen	45/ female	Large right extrarenal retroperitoneal mass and lesions in other sites	CT scan	Right retroperitoneal AML and lesions elsewhere	Radical excision of mass sparing the kidney	Asymptomatic at 1-year follow-up (in view of the fact that patients with tuberous sclerosis have a tendency to develop lesions in multiple sites, it would be argued that the ERAML that developed 15 years later was a de novo lesion rather than metastatic lesion. On the contrary other people could argue that perhaps the lesion was a late metastatic lesion).
24	Wang et al. 1997 [26]	Abdominal pain and weight loss plus spontaneous bleeding in the tumour	48/ female	Size not available	CT scan	Left retroperitoneal space	Left nephrectomy together with excision of the mass	Follow-up information not available

TABLE 1: Continued.

Case	Reference	Presentation	Age (years)/ sex	Size	Imaging	Location	Treatment	Outcome/follow-up
25	Daniel et al. 2010 [27]	Details not available	34/ female	Large	No available information on imaging	Left retroperitoneal space		Follow-up details not available
26	Vilcea et al. 2015 [28]	Irreducible right inguinofemoral mass considered to be irreducible hernia	65/ male	Large; 15 cm × 25 cm	CT scan and intravenous urography	Large right retroperitoneal mass down to inguinal femoral canal and pushing away nearby organs	Wide excision	Asymptomatic/7 years
27	Mansi et al. 2002 [29]	Details not available	Details not available	Details not available but large	Details not available	Retroperitoneal but details not available		Details not available
28	Ahmad et al. 2006 [30]	Right back pain	44/ female	14 cm × 10 cm × 6 cm	MRI scan; CT guided biopsy of mass	Right retroperitoneal	Excision of the mass	Follow-up details not available
29	Molina et al. 2001 [31]	Spontaneous abortion in first pregnancy associated with complications; diagnosis was incidentally made during imaging investigations	28/ female	Size not available	Ultrasound scan and CT scan	Left retroperitoneum	Excision of mass	Follow-up information not available
30	Medina et al. 2002 [32]	Abdominal distension	25/ sex of patient not available	Large extending from pelvis to umbilical region	Ultrasound scan and CT scan and radiological imaging biopsy	Retroperitoneal space extending from pelvis to umbilical region	Details of treatment not available	Follow-up details not available

invasion of nearby organs, or involvement of organs that are not contiguous [33].

(iv) Angiomyolipomas (AMLs) tend to have characteristic features on radiological imaging which helps in the establishment of the diagnosis [33].

3.1.6. Tuberous Sclerosis

(i) Tuberous sclerosis is an autosomal dominant neurocutaneous disorder which occurs in 1 out of 6 thousand to 11 thousand individuals and it is characterized by the developments of hamartomas/tumours in the brain (subependymal giant cell tumour), retina, skin (angiofibromas of skin), bone, lung (lymphangioleiomyomas, multifocal micronodular pneumocyte hyperplasia), and renal (angiomyolipoma in 40% to 80%, cysts, and renal cell carcinoma; nevertheless, some epithelioid tumours may be unclassified) as well as mental retardation and infantile/childhood convulsions [33].

(ii) Tuberous sclerosis tends to be caused by alterations of TSC1 gene (9q34, which encodes hamartin) as well as TSC2 gene (16p13.3 which encodes tuberin that interacts with hamartin) [33].

(iii) It has been stated that, in TSC/PKD1 contiguous gene syndrome, both the left and the right kidneys tend to be enlarged and cystic and they tend to be associated with classic angiomyosarcomas and rare intraglomerular microlesions [33, 49].

3.1.7. Presentation.
Extrarenal retroperitoneal angiomyolipoma (ERAML) may manifest in a variety of ways including the following (see Table 1):

(i) as an incidental finding, following radiological imaging investigation for various symptoms,

(ii) pain in the abdomen, loin, or back,

(iii) history of gain in weight,

(iv) fullness in epigastrium and tiredness,

(v) feeling of fullness in the abdomen or abdominal distension and pain,

(vi) pain and bleeding,

(vii) haematuria,

(viii) vomiting or constipation,

(ix) abdominal mass and weight loss,

(x) there may or may not be a history or clinical features of tuberous sclerosis.

3.1.8. Laboratory Investigations

(1) Hematological Investigations. Full blood count and coagulation screen are basic investigations that are undertaken in the assessment of a patient who has extrarenal retroperitoneal angiomyolipoma (ERAML); however, there is nothing specific in the tests that would be diagnostic of angiomyolipoma (AML).

(2) Serum Biochemistry Investigations. Serum urea and electrolytes/renal function tests, liver function tests, bone profile, and serum glucose are basic tests that are undertaken in the assessment of a patient with angiomyolipoma (AML) but none of the test results are specific for the diagnosis of extrarenal retroperitoneal angiomyolipoma (ERAML) which has also been referred to by other authors as retroperitoneal angiomyolipoma (RAML).

(3) Urinalysis, Urine Microscopy, and Culture. These tests are basic tests undertaken in the assessment of the patient but they are not investigations that would diagnose angiomyolipoma (AML).

3.1.9. Radiological Investigations

(1) Ultrasound Scan

(i) Ultrasound scan of the abdomen and pelvis can be undertaken which would tend to show the mass in the retroperitoneum; it would also reveal the size and extent of the tumour and show whether or not the tumour mass has displaced any nearby organ.

(ii) If there is hydronephrosis due to obstruction of the ureter by the angiomyolipoma (AML) tumour mass, the ultrasound scan would demonstrate it.

(iii) In cases of hydronephrosis plus or minus impaired renal function, ultrasound guided insertion of percutaneous nephrostomy can be undertaken to help improve renal function or avoid deterioration in renal function.

(iv) Ultrasound of abdomen and pelvis may also demonstrate on rare occasions a metastatic lesion in the liver. Gupta et al. [4] stated that ultrasound scan is useful for the detection of angiomyolipoma (AML).

(v) Antegrade ureteric stenting can be undertaken following insertion of nephrostomy to help the surgeon identify the ureter during surgical excision/resection of the angiomyolipoma (AML) that has encased the ureter to avoid ureteric injury during the surgical procedure.

(vi) Ultrasound guided biopsy of the angiomyolipoma (AML) can also be undertaken.

(2) Computed Tomography (CT) Scan. Minja et al. [18] stated the following:

(i) CT scan and CT angiography (CTA) are the commonest used imaging techniques in the investigation of angiomyolipomas (AMLs) [18].

(ii) Wang et al. [50] undertook an analysis of the radiological characteristics of CT scans of the abdomen in cases of extrarenal retroperitoneal angiomyolipomas (ERAMLs) and observed that extrarenal retroperitoneal angiomyolipomas (ERAMLs) typically tend to show aneurysmal dilatation of the intramural vessels, intramural linear vascularity, bridging veins beak sign, hematomas, and discrete intrarenal/extrarenal fatty tumours, but none of these are pathogenic.

(iii) CT scans of the brain have been recommended in relation to patients who have angiomyolipomas (AMLs) of the kidney, considering the fact that 30% to 40% of such patients may also have CT brain scan features of epiloia (tuberous sclerosis) and likewise 80% of such patients would end up developing angiomyolipoma (AML) of the kidney [51–53]. The CT scan of the brain in such patients typically tends to reveal characteristic periventricular subependymal nodules with calcifications [15].

(iv) CT-guided biopsy of the retroperitoneal mass can be undertaken for pathological examination

(3) Magnetic Resonance Imaging (MRI) Scan

(i) Minja et al. [18] stated that MRI scan could be utilized in addition to CT and that MRI scan is particularly useful for the delineation of the anatomical relationship between extrarenal retroperitoneal angiomyolipomas (ERAMLs), the kidney, as well as its vasculature, particularly in cases of perinephric and retroperitoneal angiomyolipomas.

(ii) MRI-guided biopsy of the retroperitoneal mass can be undertaken to obtain specimen for histological examination.

(4) PET/CT Scan

(i) In extrarenal retroperitoneal angiomyolipoma (ERAML), PET/CT scan would demonstrate a hypermetabolic extrarenal mass in an extrarenal location which on further investigation by means of pathological examination of the specimens obtained from the excised specimen or radiological imaging guidance biopsies would confirm the diagnosis of angiomyolipoma (AML) [22].

(ii) PET/CT scan done as part of an investigation of a different condition could lead to the incidental finding of a retroperitoneal mass [22].

3.1.10. Macroscopic Features. It has been stated that gross examination of angiomyolipomas (AMLs) tends to show red areas in the vascular component, gray-white areas in the smooth muscle component, and yellow areas in the adipose component of the tumour which mimic clear cell carcinoma [33].

It has also been iterated that gross inspection of angiomyolipoma (AML) may reveal evidence of invasion of local lymph nodes and renal vein by the tumour even though the tumour is benign, and invasion of the capsule of the tumour may be observed in 25% of cases [33, 54].

Angiomyolipomas (AMLs) on gross examination tend to be found in unilateral positions and they also tend to be unifocal [33].

In angiomyolipomas (AMLs), gross inspection tends to reveal multiple tumours in one-third of the cases or bilateral in 15% of the tumours which would be suggestive of epiloia (tuberous sclerosis) [33].

On rare occasions of angiomyolipoma (AML) there may be evidence of gross or microscopic cysts [33, 55].

3.1.11. Microscopic Features

(i) Microscopic examinations of angiomyolipomas (AMLs) classically trend to reveal triphasic features which include myoid spindle cells, islands of mature adipose tissue (fat), and dysmorphic blood vessels that are thick-walled and which do not have elastic lamina [33].

(ii) The smooth muscle component of angiomyolipomas (AMLs) on microscopic examination tend to appear to have originated from walls of vessels and they may appear to be hypercellular, atypical, pleomorphic, or epithelioid [33].

(iii) On microscopic examination, angiomyolipoma (AML) may mimic a high grade sarcoma if it metastasizes [33].

(iv) With regard to epithelioid variant of angiomyolipoma (AML), microscopic examination of the lesion tends to show pure or predominant population of large, epithelioid cells that have clear or eosinophilic cytoplasm, large hyperchromatic bizarre-looking nucleus, and possibly multinucleation which include an intimate relationship with vessel wall [33].

(v) Microscopic examination of angiomyolipomas (AMLs) show common areas of haemorrhage and necrosis [33].

(vi) Microscopic examination of angiomyolipoma (AML) may reveal adipose tissue which could be scanty or dominant and this may mimic well-differentiated liposarcoma [33].

(vii) Microscopic examination may show small mesenchymal nodules that are less than 2 cm which are precursors of angiomyolipoma (AML) [56].

(viii) Microscopic examination of angiomyolipoma (AML) may show epithelial cysts [55, 57] and prominent sclerosis [58].

3.1.12. Cytology Features

(i) Cytological examination of specimens of angiomyolipoma (AML) tends to reveal oval to spindled cells and cohesive stromal fragments, adipose tissue, and branching blood vessels within a haemorrhagic background [33].

(ii) Cytological examination of angiomyolipomas (AMLs) also tend to show mitotic figures [59].

3.1.13. Immunohistochemistry of Angiomyolipomas (AMLs)

(1) Positive Staining. In angiomyolipoma (AML) immunohistochemical studies of adipose tissue, myoid, and epithelioid cells tend to show positive staining with regard to various markers as follows:

(i) They are HMB45 (100%) [60], MART1/Melan-A, muscle specific actin (HHF35, 100%), calponin (100%), and NKI-C3 (70–100%) [33].

(ii) CD117 tends to be positive [61], desmin tends to be positive in 20% of cases [62], HMB50 in 100% of cases, microphthalmia transcription factor in 50% of cases [63], and progesterone receptor in 28% of cases and these tend to occur in women who are aged less than 50 years and associated with tuberous sclerosis, smooth muscle actin, and tyrosinase in 20% to 50% of cases, and in vimentin [33].

(iii) Immunohistochemistry tends to show evidence of lymphatic differentiation podoplanin and D2-40 [64] and S100 (fat component) [33].

(iv) HMB45 and Melan-A tend to be positive in descending order of percentage positivity in fat, followed by in smooth muscle and then followed by blood vessels [65].

(2) Negative Staining. Immunohistochemical staining of angiomyolipoma (AML) tends to be negative for Keratin and renin [33].

3.1.14. Molecular Characteristics

5q-Changes. Kattar et al. [66] stated that angiomyolipoma had previously been stated to be a hamartomatous polyclonal proliferation. Nevertheless, recent molecular analysis studies had indicated that angiomyolipomas (AMLs) may be clonal neoplasms rather than polyclonal proliferations. Kattar et al. [66] investigated the chromosomal imbalances in angiomyolipoma (AML) by comparative genomic hybridization. They extracted DNA from paraffin-embedded and frozen tissues of 12 angiomyolipomas (10 usual variants and 2 epithelioid variants). The 10 angiomyolipomas (AMLs) of the usual variant included bilateral tumours from one tuberous sclerosis patient. Fluorescence ratio distributions from tumour hybridizations were compared with those from control hybridizations to detect changes in DNA copy number with sensitivity and specificity. Kattar et al. [66] identified 20 chromosomal imbalances in 7 sporadic angiomyolipomas (AMLs) which included both tumours of the epithelioid variant. The remaining 6 tumours including the two angiomyolipomas (AMLs) from a tuberous sclerosis patient lacked chromosomal imbalances. Seventy percent of the imbalances were partial or whole chromosomal deletions involving disparate genomic regions, some of which had earlier been reported to be associated with tumours of adipose tissue and smooth muscle tumours. Four angiomyolipomas (AMLs) of the usual variant had shown 5q deletions with a common region

of deletion spanning 5q33 to q34. In two of the tumours, deletion on 5q was the sole abnormality. One epithelioid angiomyolipoma showed 5q gain encompassing the same region in addition to other alterations. Kattar et al. [66] concluded that (I) chromosomal imbalances are common in angiomyolipomas (AMLs) of the kidney; (II) presence of clonal genomic alterations would additionally be supportive of the neoplastic pathogenesis of these tumours; (III) the 5q33-q34 region may contain a tumour suppressor gene significant in the histogenesis of some kidney angiomyolipomas.

3.1.15. Monoclonal Proliferation of an Uncommitted Cell.

Paradis et al. [67] stated that angiomyolipomas (AMLs) of kidney had been considered as hamartomas but little data had been available concerning their pathogenesis. It had not been known for sure if angiomyolipoma (AML) is a congenital malformation or a neoplastic process. In order to answer the aforementioned question, Paradis et al. [67] assessed the clonality of sporadic angiomyolipoma (AML) using molecular analysis. Seven women with a mean age of 59 years with angiomyolipoma (AML) of the kidney were included in the study. DNA of the tumour and the normal adjacent kidney was extracted from paraffin-embedded tissue. Paradis et al. [67] studied the DNA methylation pattern at a polymorphic site on the HUMARA gene by polymerase chain reaction (PCR) amplification after methylation-sensitive enzyme digestion. This procedure does enable the differentiation between polyclonal and monoclonal lesions according to the X chromosome inactivation pattern. Five of the 7 women included in the study were informative for the HUMARA gene. The mean size of the AMLs was 53 mm (this had ranged from 18 mm to 110 mm). In one of the cases, a tumour thrombus was found in the inferior vena cava. Clonal analysis had shown that all the angiomyolipomas (AMLs) and the tumour thrombus studied were monoclonal lesions consistent with neoplastic disorders. Paradis et al. [67] concluded that the results strongly support the postulate that angiomyolipomas (AMLs) arise from the clonal proliferation of an uncommitted cell, which will further evolve towards different cell types.

3.1.16. Electron Microscopic Feature.

Electron microscopic examination of angiomyolipoma (AML) tends to show premelanosomes [33].

3.1.17. Differential Diagnoses.

Some of the lesions that may mimic angiomyolipoma (AML) include the following:

(i) oncocytoma in which microscopic examination of the lesion tends to show prominent oncocytes, no evidence of prominent adipose component, and immunohistochemistry study which is negative for melanocyte markers [33],

(ii) leiomyoma in which microscopic examination of the lesion tends to show no evidence of prominent vascular or adipose component and the immunohistochemistry study of the lesion tends to be negative for melanocytic markers [33],

(iii) leiomyosarcoma in which microscopic examination of the lesion tends to show infiltrative lesion, evidence of prominent atypia, and quite commonly no prominent vascular or adipose component and immunohistochemistry studies of the lesion tend to be negative for melanocytic markers [33],

(iv) melanoma in which microscopic examination of the lesion tends to show marked atypia, no evidence of prominent adipose, or vascular component in the lesion [33],

(v) pleomorphic rhabdomyosarcoma in which microscopic examination of the lesion tends to show smooth muscle component which is often an infiltrative tumour that is markedly atypical, no evidence of prominent adipose, or vascular component and immunohistochemical staining of the tumour tends to show negative staining for melanocytic markers [33],

(vi) renal cell carcinoma in which microscopic examination of the lesion tends to show marked atypia and infiltrative margins and no evidence of being triphasic, and immunohistochemistry study of the lesion tends to be negative for melanocytic markers [33].

3.1.18. Treatment. Minja et al. [18] stated the following:

(i) The primary treatments for extrarenal retroperitoneal angiomyolipomas (ERAMLs) have commonly involved surgery (surgical excisions but less often embolization of the tumour have been undertaken).

(ii) Surgical excision is indicated in cases of symptomatic, complex appearing, radiologically enlarging, or large extrarenal retroperitoneal angiomyolipomas (ERAMLs), which tend to be associated with a higher potential to bleed spontaneously.

(iii) With regard to the patients who present in emergency situations symptomatically as a result of spontaneous retroperitoneal bleeding, selective arterial angiography and embolization have been undertaken effectively to control bleeding from haemorrhagic lesions in patients who are hemodynamically unstable which tend to result in involution of the tumour and which tend to allow for subsequent elective surgical excision or clinical observation (see [12, 14, 16]).

(iv) Surgical excision has always been recommended in order to allow for histological examination to differentiate suspected extrarenal retroperitoneal angiomyolipomas (ERAMLs) from the differential diagnoses of lesions involving the retroperitoneum. The establishment of definitive diagnosis by means of pathological examination of surgically resected specimens of extrarenal retroperitoneal angiomyolipomas (ERAMLs) would dictate the length and type of appropriate follow-up considering that extrarenal retroperitoneal angiomyolipomas (ERAMLs), unlike malignant retroperitoneal sarcomas or renal/adrenal

carcinomas which may require long-term surveillance.

3.1.19. Follow-Up of Patients. Angiomyolipomas (AMLs) and extrarenal angiomyolipomas (ERAMLs) used to be defined as hamartomas but these lesions have subsequently been classified as benign tumours. Considering the fact that angiomyolipomas have been documented to have metastasized to lymph node and to the liver it is the opinion of the author that angiomyolipomas should be regarded as tumours that often exhibit benign biological behaviour but a subset of such tumours would metastasize; therefore, perhaps angiomyolipomas should be regarded as slow-growing malignant tumours with the potential to metastasize. In view of the fact that angiomyolipomas could metastasize it would be recommended that whether or not patients with extrarenal retroperitoneal angiomyolipomas (ERAMLs) have been treated by selective angiography and superselective embolization or surgical excision the patients should be followed up over a long period of time by means of appropriate radiological imaging that would minimize extensive cumulative radiation and perhaps a 5-year follow-up may be sufficient.

3.1.20. Outcome. With regard to the outcome of ERAMLs following treatment, Minja et al. [18] stated the following:

(i) Out of the cases they had reviewed, 56% of the patients had been followed up over a period of time which had ranged between 2 months and 60 months after they had undergone surgical excision of their tumours.

(ii) Outside the context of epiloia (tuberous sclerosis), they had encountered only one reported case of tumour recurrence up to the time of publication of their paper which occurred pursuant to a radical en bloc nephrectomy with the development of distant metastasis to the liver and bone 12 months after the surgical operation [4]. The rest of the patients had remained asymptomatic and free of disease at their last follow-up, and there had not been any documentation of recurrence of disease following a renal sparing nephrectomy or embolization.

(iii) Considering the fact that the only recurrence they found in their review of the literature had occurred 12 months after an en bloc radical nephrectomy, they were of the opinion that extrarenal retroperitoneal angiomyolipomas (ERAMLs) should be followed closely with CT scans during the first year after surgical excision of the lesions, with continued yearly follow-up for 5 years or the duration of follow-up should be dictated by the symptoms of the patient.

3.2. Miscellaneous Narrations and Discussions from Some Reported Cases of Retroperitoneal Angiomyolipoma (B). Friis and Hjortrup [5] in 1982 reported a 22-year-old woman who presented with pain and weight gain. She had intravenous urography which revealed an extrarenal retroperitoneal mass.

For which she underwent exploratory laparotomy with radical nephrectomy including excision of the mass in the peripancreatic space and histological examination of the specimen which weighed 11 kilograms revealed features consistent with angiomyolipoma (AML). She was asymptomatic at her 30 months' follow-up. They stated that angiomyolipoma (AML) is a benign tumour and its treatment should always be surgical in view of the fact that it is difficult to establish the differential diagnosis preoperatively. Nevertheless, angiomyolipoma (AML) has a tendency toward recurrence if the entire tumour is not removed [5].

Randazoo et al. [6] in 1987 reported a 64-year-old woman with epiloia (tuberous sclerosis) who presented with abdominal pain due to spontaneous rupture of a 6 cubic centimetres retroperitoneal angiomyolipoma situated in the right perinephric space which was diagnosed by means of intravenous urography and CT scan of abdomen. She underwent right renal sparing excision of the mass. Pathological examination of the tumour mass showed features consistent with angiomyolipoma (AML). The patient was well at her 2 months' follow-up. Randazoo et al. [6] stated that their case was the first case of extrarenal angiomyolipoma associated with tuberous sclerosis.

Ditonno et al. [7] in 1992 reported two cases of extrarenal angiomyolipoma. One of the two cases involved a 37-year-old man who presented with abdominal pain. He had intravenous urography, CT scan of abdomen, and angiography which revealed 5 cm bleeding right extrarenal mass in the perinephric space. He underwent radical nephrectomy. Pathological examination finding of the specimen was consistent with a diagnosis of angiomyolipoma (AML). His follow-up data was not available.

Peh et al. [8] in 1994 reported a 32-year-old woman who presented with weight loss and abdominal mass. She had ultrasound scan and CT scan of the abdomen which revealed a mass in her left perinephric space. She underwent left radical nephrectomy which included the mass lesion which weighed 3.7 kilograms. Pathological examination of the specimen revealed features that were adjudged to be consistent with a diagnosis of angiomyolipoma (AML). She was asymptomatic at her 8-month follow-up.

Angulo et al. [9] in 1994 reported a 53-year-old female who presented with abdominal and left loin pain. She has ultrasound scan, CT scan, and angiography which showed a mass in the left perinephric space 336 cubic centimetres. She underwent left radical nephrectomy and pathological examination finding of the specimen was consistent with a diagnosis of angiomyolipoma (AML). There was no follow-up data available on the patient.

Liwnicz et al. [11] in 1994 reported a 39-year-old woman who presented with abdominal pain. She had a CT scan which showed a mass in her right perinephric space. She underwent a right radical nephrectomy with removal of a 1.1 kilogram mass. Histological examination of the specimen revealed features that had been adjudged to be consistent with angiomyolipoma (AML). Pathological examination of the tumour revealed tumour fat on the whole which was inconspicuous and manifested largely as hibernoma-like

microvesicular lipid. The tumour cells also did on Immunohistological staining showed that the tumour cells were positively stained for HMB-45 and S-100 protein. The cells on electron microscopy studies showed occasional cytoplasmic striated granules which were indistinguishable from stage II premelanosomes. Nevertheless, electron microscopy and immunohistochemistry studies of the tumour also did confirm the presence of a substantial myogenous component of the tumour which established the diagnosis of AML. She was asymptomatic at her 18 months' follow-up.

Law et al. [12] reported two cases as follows.

Case 1. Law et al. [12] in 1994 reported a 59-year-old woman who was found incidentally to have a mass in her left perinephric space when she had CT scan and MRI scan of the abdomen and pelvis. She underwent a left radical nephrectomy with excision of a 22.5 cubic centimetres mass. Pathological examination of the specimen revealed features that were adjudged to be consistent with the diagnosis of angiomyolipoma (AML). Her follow-up outcome data was not available.

Case 2. Law et al. [12] in 1994 reported a 56-year-old woman who presented with abdominal pain. She had a number of investigations including intravenous urography, ultrasound scan of abdomen and pelvis, and CT scan of abdomen and as well as fine needle aspiration of a mass which was found in her left perinephric space. She underwent left radical nephrectomy and histological examination of the excised 11 cm mass revealed features that were consistent with a diagnosis of angiomyolipoma (AML). She was asymptomatic at her 8-month follow-up.

Mogi et al. [13] in 1998 reported a 41-year-old woman who 2 years earlier undergone surgery for type IIc early gastric cancer and who presented with back pain and fullness of her abdomen. She had CT scan and MRI scan of her abdomen and pelvis which revealed a massive fat tumour mass that had extended from the hepatic hilus to the retroperitoneum (in her right perinephric space as well as her perihepatic space). She underwent renal sparing excision of a 648 cubic centimetres mass located in her right perinephric and perihepatic space and the pathological examination of the specimen revealed features consistent with angiomyolipoma (AML) which did not involve the kidney. Her follow-up outcome data was not available.

Murphy et al. [14] in 2000 reported a 51-year-old woman who presented with abdominal pain due to bleeding from her angiomyolipoma (AML). She had a CT scan of her abdomen and angiography which revealed a bleeding from a mass in her left perinephric space. She underwent selective angiography and superselective embolization of the mass which had radiological imaging characteristics of angiomyolipoma (AML). She was asymptomatic at her 12-month follow-up.

Tsutsumi et al. [15] in 2001 reported a 60-year-old man who presented with fullness in the epigastrium and tiredness. A smooth, round soft painless mass was palpable on his abdominal examination. He had CT scan of her abdomen and pelvis which revealed a 22 cm × 22 cm × 10 cm lobulated fatty mass around the right kidney and a small fatty mass in the left kidney. The tumour was well delineated from the surrounding organs. She had abdominal angiography which demonstrated that the mass which had scattered aneurysmal lesions was fed by the right renal, adrenal, and lumbar arteries. He had a CT scan of the brain which did show multiple small calcified subependymal nodules which had extended from the lateral margins into both ventricles that was suggestive of tuberous sclerosis. He underwent en bloc resection of the mass together with the right kidney via a thoracoabdominal incision with radical nephrectomy with excision of 3.5 kilogram mass. The tumour was noted to be well encapsulated and was easily dissected from the surrounding tissues as well as it was noted that the regional lymph nodes had not been involved. Pathological examination of the specimen revealed features consistent with angiomyolipoma (AML) in that microscopic examination of the tumour revealed that the tumour comprised of mature fat cells which contained smooth muscle and thick-walled blood vessels, all of which characteristically typify angiomyolipoma (AML). He was alive and asymptomatic at her 60-month follow-up. Tsutsumi et al. [15] stated that the diagnostic dilemma of the tumour could be solved by performing renal arteriography and CT scan of the brain and in their case the two studies had been helpful in that the renal arteriogram had revealed the aneurysmal dilatation of the intratumoural vessels, which typifies angiomyolipoma (AML), and the CT scan of the brain did show periventricular subependymal nodules with calcification which had be indicative of tuberous sclerosis.

Tseng et al. [16] in 2004 reported a 35-year-old woman who presented with symptom of fullness in her abdomen. She had ultrasound scan and CT scan of her abdomen and pelvis as well as angiography which revealed a mass in her right perinephric space (retroperitoneum). She underwent arterial embolization and renal sparing excision of the lesion which weighed 2.8 kilograms. Pathological examination of the specimen revealed features consistent with angiomyolipoma (AML). Her follow-up outcome data was not available.

Obara et al. [17] in 2005 reported a 31-year-old man who presented with painless visible haematuria. He had a CT scan of abdomen which revealed a large perinephric mass in his right kidney without any evidence of contrast enhancement. The mass was separated from the kidney and appeared to have surrounded the kidney. There was no evidence of intrarenal mass on the CT scan. He had abdominal aortography and right renal angiography which revealed no evidence of hypervascular tumour. He underwent right radical nephrectomy and macroscopic examination of the specimen revealed that the tumour had originated from the perinephric fat and was separated from the kidney. The tumour had compressed the ureter causing hydronephrosis. The pathological examination of the specimen revealed features that were considered to be consistent with a diagnosis of angiomyolipoma (AML) of the perinephric space and this showed mature fat, blood vessels, and smooth muscle. His follow-up outcome data was not available.

Gupta et al. [4] in 2007 reported an 80-year-old woman who presented with abdominal pain. She had CT scan and MRI scan of abdomen and pelvis which showed a mass in her left perinephric space. She underwent left radical nephrectomy with excision of a 16 cm mass. Macroscopic examination of the specimen revealed a perinephric mass with cystic areas that contained dilated vascular spaces intermingled with necrotic tissue which had alternated with more solid, better preserved areas which contained spindled cells with elongated and hyperchromatic nuclei. Immunohistochemistry of the tumour showed positive staining for HMB-45 and focally for smooth muscle actin but negative staining was shown for chromogranin, synaptophysin, epithelial membrane antigen, vimentin, carcinoembryonic antigen, S100, desmin, CD45, CD20, and cytokeratin. The features of the pathological examination of the specimen were adjudged to be consistent with angiomyolipoma (AML) with atypical features in the retroperitoneum. At her 1-year follow-up she was found to have distant metastases in the bone and liver.

Gupta and Guleira [10] in 2011 reported a 42-year-old man who presented with abdominal pain. He had ultrasound scan and CT scan of the abdomen and pelvis which revealed a 220 cubic centimetres mass in his right adrenal space. He underwent renal sparing excision of the lesion and pathological examination finding of the tumour was consistent with angiomyolipoma (AML). His follow-up outcome data was not available.

Minja et al. [18] in 2012 reported the case of a 39-year-old woman who in 2011 had initially presented with dysfunctional uterine bleeding and who had transvaginal ultrasound scan which was normal. She developed protracted respiratory tract infection for which she had been on antibiotics and because of the unexpected duration of her symptoms she had CT scan of the thorax which revealed unremarkable findings in the chest. However, the lower Ct images of the chest did reveal a large retroperitoneal mass which had abutted the left kidney. She subsequently had contrast enhanced CT scan of the abdomen which showed an encapsulated mass that measured 19.3 cm × 13.5 cm × 10.7 cm with associated prominent vascularity which arose from the left renal vasculature. Additionally, there was evidence of a 2 cm homogeneous fatty renal lesion in the inferior midpole which was adjudged to be consistent with angiomyolipoma of the kidney (see Figures 1(a) and 1(b)). She also had MRI scan of abdomen and pelvis which showed a well-encapsulated fatty tumour that had displaced the left hemicolon laterally and this measured 19 cm × 14.4 cm × 13.8 cm. The mass was seen to have abutted tightly to the upper pole of the left kidney as well as a small 2 cm lesion was shown inferiorly which was considered to be most likely representing an angiomyolipoma of the kidney (see Figures 2(a) and 2(b)). Minja et al. [18] considered a number of differential diagnoses which included a retroperitoneal liposarcoma, leiomyosarcoma, lipoma, angiomyolipoma, adrenal adenocarcinoma, renal cell carcinoma, or leiomyoma with fatty change. She was asymptomatic with regard to the mass. Minja et al. [18] stated that the patient underwent en bloc resection of the mass with the left kidney via midline incision as well as total abdominal hysterectomy to treat her dysfunctional uterine bleeding contemporaneously. The kidney measured 11.5 cm × 4.5 cm × 3 cm and the mass which was situated near the upper pole of the kidney measured

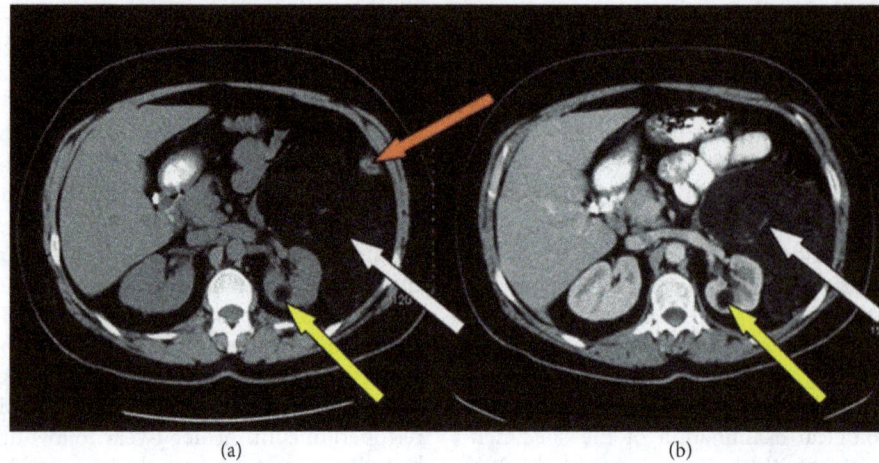

(a)   (b)

FIGURE 1: (a) Oral contrast and (b) IV and oral contrast: abdominal computerized tomography demonstrating an encapsulated fatty vascular mass (white arrows) lateral to the left kidney measuring 19.3 cm × 13.5 cm × 10.7 cm with prominent vascular dependence on the left renal vein and artery as well as a 2 cm posterior midpole homogeneous fatty density (yellow arrow). Left colon is laterally displaced (orange arrow). Reproduced from [18].

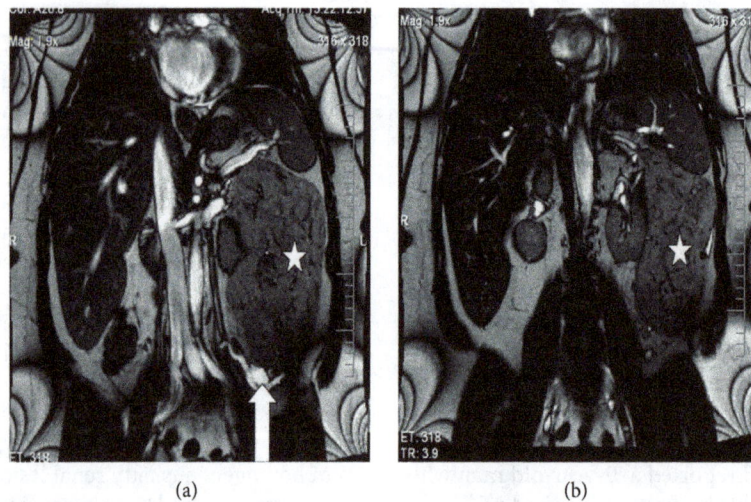

(a)   (b)

FIGURE 2: Abdominal magnetic resonance imaging demonstrating a large fatty encapsulated mass (white asterisk) measuring 19.3 cm × 13.5 cm × 10.7 cm with prominent vascularity (white arrows). The anatomic relationship between the mass and the left kidney can be well seen in Figure 2(b). Reproduced from [18].

23 cm × 14 cm × 9 cm (see Figure 3). Serial sections of the mass and kidney did reveal the lesion to be well and fully circumscribed and separate from the parenchyma of the kidney. Gross examination revealed the mass to be homogeneously yellow without any stigmata of necrosis or haemorrhage. Another well-circumscribed, intrarenal mass, which measured 2 cm × 1.8 cm × 1 cm, was also found within the lower midportion of the renal cortex. Macroscopic and microscopic examinations of the two lesions revealed similar features in that they had predominance of adipose tissue and smaller areas of smooth muscle with epithelioid features and characteristically abnormal vessels. The larger lesion was separate and distinct from the parenchyma of the kidney.

Immunohistochemistry study of the larger lesion showed positive staining for HMB-45 which is characteristic for an angiomyolipoma (see Figure 4). Microscopic examinations of the uterus and cervix were normal. At her 16-month follow-up she was alive and asymptomatic. Minja et al. [18] stated that presence of perivascular epithelioid cells (PEC) tends often to be used to characterize angiomyolipomas in view of the fact that these cells exhibit immunoreactivity for muscle markers (epithelial membrane antigen, keratin, vimentin, desmin, and actin) and HMB-45 [68]. It has been stated that positive immunoreactivity for HM-45, a monoclonal antibody which has been raised against melanoma-associated antigen, is characteristic of angiomyolipomas (AMLs) and it

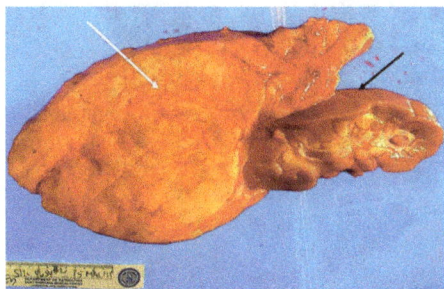

FIGURE 3: Gross image of the en bloc resected mass including the left kidney (black arrow), demonstrating a well-encapsulated fatty mass attached to the upper pole of the kidney (white arrow), with a smooth outer surface measuring 23 cm × 14 cm × 9 cm. Reproduced from [18].

can be used to differentiate angiomyolipomas (AMLs) from other similar appearing lesions, for example, liposarcomas, lipomas, leiomyosarcomas, or leiomyomas [11, 17].

Lee et al. [19] reported a 35-year-old woman who presented with symptoms of increased abdominal circumference and urinary frequency. She had a CT scan of abdomen which showed a 24 cm × 21 cm × 16 cm retroperitoneal fatty tumour which had displaced the right kidney to the left upper quadrant of the abdomen. She underwent laparotomy and wide excision of the tumour and preservation of the right kidney. Pathological examination of the excised tumour revealed features consistent with the diagnosis of angiomyolipoma (AML). At her 4-month follow-up, she was well with no evidence of tumour recurrence and her right kidney was functioning well.

Soni et al. [20] reported a 33-year-old woman who presented with left sided flank pain. She had CT scan of abdomen which showed a large angiomyolipoma that measured 9.3 cm × 6.1 cm × 7.7 cm located in the lower pole of the kidney. During her surgical operation the tumour was found to be located in a pararenal retroperitoneal position without involving the kidney. Surgical excision of the mass was undertaken with preservation of the kidney. Pathological examination of the excised tumour revealed predominantly adipose tissue with multiple thick-walled vascular channels that were lined by flattened endothelial cells. Perivascular epithelioid cells were proliferating and emanated from blood vessel wall and had extended into the surrounding adipose tissue. Immunohistochemical staining of the tumour showed strong positivity for HMB-45 and smooth muscle actin. The pathological examination findings were consistent with a diagnosis of pararenal angiomyolipoma. She was evaluated for evidence of tuberous sclerosis and this was negative. There was no long-term follow-up data on the patient.

Ivanova et al. [21] reported a 33-year-old woman who presented with dull pain in the right lumbar region. She had radiological imaging studies which showed a tumour mass in the right retroperitoneal space without any clear evidence of the kidney. During her surgical operation an ill-defined tumour mass was found to have encased the right kidney and hence an en bloc resection of the mass was undertaken.

Macroscopic examination of the excised specimen showed an intact kidney which measured 10 cm × 6 cm and which was surrounded by multinodular, yellowish soft tumour which added about 6 cm to each side of the kidney. Microscopic examination of the specimen showed mature fat, an unevenly dispersed abnormal blood vessel of variable thickness, and spindle cell component which appeared to irradiate from vessel walls, which occasionally fused into solid areas with hyperchromatic nuclei. Neoplastic nests with similar appearance were observed within the superficial part of the renal cortex. Multiple small foci appeared to contain larger polygonal cells which had abundant clear cytoplasm which had epithelioid appearance. Few of the cells had exhibited increased nuclear atypia, and almost no evidence of mitotic figures was observed. A provisional diagnosis of liposarcoma was made based upon the high fat content, presence of spindle, and epithelioid cells which had mildly atypical nuclei and rare whirling pattern of spindle cell growth. Nevertheless, second opinion evaluation led to immunohistochemistry studies of the tumour which showed negative staining for cytokeratin AE1-AE3 and S100 protein but positive staining in scattered majority of the cells for HMB-45 and furthermore synchronous strong positive expression of smooth muscle actin was observed. A final diagnosis of angiomyolipoma (AML) was established. There was no follow-up data on the long-term outcome of the patient.

Welling et al. [22] reported a 38-year-old man who had melanoma of the right flank region. He had a staging 18F-fluoro-2-doxyglucose (FDG) PET/CT scan which showed a hypermetabolic extrarenal mass in the left retroperitoneal space which was reported to be concerning for metastatic melanoma. Nevertheless, pathological examination of the mass revealed features, that were adjudged to be consistent with angiomyolipoma (AML). Welling et al. [22] stated that angiomyolipomas (AMLs) tend to have a variety of radiological imaging appearances on multiple imaging modalities, including FDG PET, and can confound accurate diagnosis when the mass is in an extrarenal location. They also stated that their case had demonstrated the only known description of an extrarenal retroperitoneal angiomyolipoma (ERAML) and this would highlight the challenge of accurate diagnosis based upon FDG PET findings.

Fegan et al. [23] in 1997 reported a case of extrarenal retroperitoneal AML. The details of the case are not available but Fegan et al. [23] stated that their case was the 5th case of extrarenal retroperitoneal angiomyolipoma (ERAML) to be reported and in their case as well as in the other four previously reported cases, the correct diagnosis was made only after laparotomy, despite a number of prospective imaging studies. They suggested that careful exploration should in the future result in more renal sparing approaches to the management of extrarenal retroperitoneal angiomyolipoma (ERAML).

Lau et al. [24] in 2003 reported a patient who had primary retroperitoneal monotypic epithelioid angiomyolipoma which was composed exclusively of atypical epithelioid cells which had subsequently metastasized to the liver and the mediastinum. Lau et al. [24] stated that monotypic epithelioid angiomyolipoma has generally been considered to be

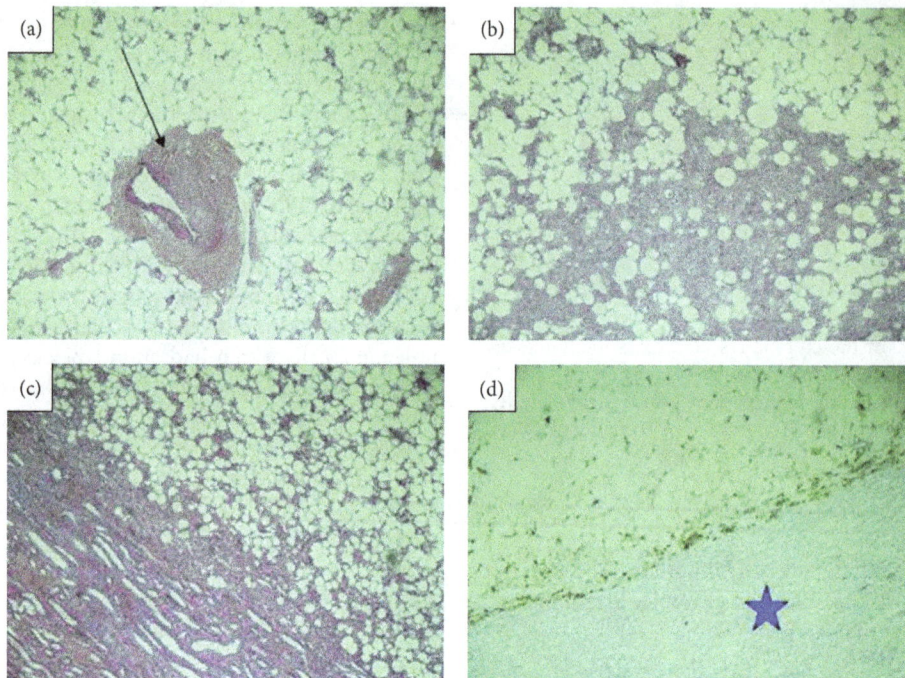

FIGURE 4: Extrarenal mass (haematoxylin and eosin). Photomicrograph of the mass demonstrate mature adipose tissue with a tortuous thick blood vessel (black arrow) ((a); ×20) and bundles of smooth muscles lacking elastic tissue lamina ((b); ×40), adipose tissue with small areas of smooth muscle with epithelioid features ((c); ×40). Focal staining with HMB45 antibody was positive (blue star) ((d); ×40), consistent with angiomyolipoma. Reproduced from [18].

a benign neoplasm even though rare cases of such lesions exhibiting malignant behaviour had been reported. They also stated that to their knowledge their case was the first report of metastatic disease which had occurred in an extrarenal retroperitoneal angiomyolipoma (ERAML).

Wen et al. [25] reported a 45-year-old woman with a history of tuberous sclerosis and left renal angiomyolipoma and had 15 years earlier undergone left radical nephrectomy and preoperative embolization of left kidney due to a huge AML which had compressed the descending colon to the right side and caused loss of appetite and constipation. Pathological examination of the specimen confirmed angiomyolipoma (AML) of left kidney without invasion of the renal vessel. She presented 15 years after her left nephrectomy with loss of appetite, vomiting, abdominal pain, and constipation. She was found on examination to have a palpable, huge, painless mass which had elastic to firm consistency and adenoma sebaceum skin lesions in the malar regions of her face. Her urinalysis and blood biochemistry tests were normal. She had CT scan which showed an adhesion ileus, a giant retroperitoneal tumour in the left side that had extended over the right retroperitoneum, and multifocal lipomatosis that had involved the posterior mediastinum, right kidney, and liver. The CT scan also revealed multiple pulmonary nodules in the right, middle, and the lower lobes of the lung and a focal right pneumothorax at the area of the pericardium. She underwent laparotomy during which a brown to yellowish tumour that had a fibrotic capsule and tortuous vessels was found in the entire left retroperitoneum. The tumour mass was excised and the right kidney was left

intact. Pathological examination of the specimen did show that the tumour comprised of mature adipose tissue, large blood vessels which had thick muscular walls, and a number of foci that showed epithelioid cells surrounding the vessels. All the pathological features were adjudged to be consistent with the diagnosis of angiomyolipoma (AML). She did not have any gastrointestinal symptoms for one year.

Wang et al. [26] reported a 48-year-old woman who presented with abdominal pain and weight loss. On examination she was found to have a palpable mass in the left side of her abdomen. She was referred from her initial hospital after she had had a CT scan which was provisionally reported as showing features suggestive of a retroperitoneal liposarcoma. She had another CT scan of abdomen in the second hospital on her admission which revealed a huge left sided retroperitoneal fatty tumour which had encompassed the left kidney. The CT scans also showed that the tumour had extended caudally into the pelvis, anterior to the uterus, and many intrarenal fatty nodules that were clearly separated from huge tumour and all these radiological findings were adjudged to be consistent with the diagnosis of retroperitoneal angiomyolipoma (RAML). Four days after her admission she developed sudden onset of severe abdominal pain which was ensued by her development of shock for which she was resuscitated and for which she underwent an emergency laparotomy which revealed that she had developed spontaneous haemorrhage of her large retroperitoneal angiomyolipoma (RAML). Excision of the mass as well as left nephrectomy was undertaken. The pathological examination of the specimen did confirm the radiological diagnosis of retroperitoneal angiomyolipoma. Microscopic examination of the specimen also showed scattered small angiomyolipomas of the left kidney. The case was reported without any long-term follow-up information which would indicate that the case was published not long after the patient was discharged.

Daniel et al. [27] reported a 34-year-old woman who underwent excision of a large left retroperitoneal mass which had extended between the diaphragm and the bifurcation of the iliac vessels. They stated that the pathological features of the lesion were consistent with the diagnosis of retroperitoneal angiomyolipoma (RAML) and their reported case was the 19th case of extrarenal retroperitoneal angiomyolipoma (ERAML) to be reported.

Vîlcea et al. [28] reported a 65-year-old man who presented with an irreducible tumour in the right inguino-femoral region which he had had for four years with no subjective symptoms. A provisional preoperative diagnosis of irreducible right inguinal hernia was made. During the surgical procedure upon the inguinal canal a lipomatous mass was found which was in continuity with the scrotum and which was continuous through the deep inguinal canal (internal ring) with a retroperitoneal tumour. Two ureters in the right inguinal canal as well as absence of a peritoneal sac were observed. The lipomatous mass was excised en bloc with the right testis; nevertheless, the section of the tumour was limited to the deep inguinal (internal) ring. Both ureters were reduced into the retroperitoneal space. Postoperatively, he had a CT scan of abdomen and pelvis which showed a 15 cm × 25 cm inhomogeneous retroperitoneal tumour, the location of which had extended from the lower pole of the kidney to the inguinal arch. The CT scan also showed that the tumour contained fat tissue densities, areas of haemorrhage in the tumour, calcifications, and sclerosis; the tumour had pushed the right kidney superiorly and laterally and included two ureteric ducts. Furthermore, the CT scan did show thickening of the pararenal fascia, cleavage plane with the inferior vena cava, and abdominal wall, and it showed right sided hydronephrosis. He had an intravenous urography which showed grade 2 right sided hydronephrosis and a single right sided ureter which was amputated at the level of the iliac crest. He underwent another laparotomy three weeks later which revealed the following: a 15 cm × 25 cm lipomatous tumour extending caudally from the lower pole of the right kidney; the tumour had encased two ureteric ducts (one of the ureters had originated from the right renal pelvis and the second ureter had developed from the upper pole of the right kidney without any relationship to the renal pelvis). At laparotomy the tumour was found to have smooth, elastic areas, which were adjudged to be specific to a lipoma, but the distal part of the tumour was found to be hardened and at that level (the distal part) the surgeon found dissection of the ureter impossible. The tumour was excised en bloc with both ureters and the kidney. Macroscopic examination of the excised specimen showed a 15 cm × 25 cm mass which had lipomatous appearance and areas of haemorrhage that had alternated with areas of necrosis as well as hardened areas with sclerosis and calcifications; the two right ureters were stuck tightly in the fibrosclerosis process. Pathological

examination of the specimen showed a mature adipose tissue admixed with smooth muscle tissue proliferation, occasional giant cells that surrounded medium calibre blood vessels. The microscopic features of the tumour were adjudged to be conclusive with a diagnosis of angiomyolipoma (AML). At his 7-year follow-up, the patient was alive and well with no evidence of recurrence of his disease.

Mansi et al. [29] in 2002 reported a case of a large extrarenal angiomyolipoma which had mimicked a large locally advanced renal parenchymal tumour. They stated that the diagnosis by means of histopathology examination of the specimen after radical nephrectomy had been performed and that even though angiomyolipoma (AML) is rare, angiomyolipoma (AML) of the perinephric fat may present in various ways and should be considered in the differential diagnosis of large renal tumours especially in view of the possibility of kidney sparing management.

Ahmad et al. [30] reported a 44-year-old woman who presented with right sided back pain. She had MRI scan and CT scan which showed a 10 cm retroperitoneal mass lying posterior to the right kidney and pushing the kidney anteriorly, and the mass was not connected to the kidney, adrenal gland, vascular, or other structures. She had CT scan guided biopsy but the histological features of the specimen were nondiagnostic. She underwent excision of the mass which was well-encapsulated, firm, and ovoid and measured 14 cm × 10 cm × 6 cm with fibrofatty tissue. Macroscopic examination of the specimen revealed a lobulated grey homogeneous tumour with a cystic area in a peripheral location. Microscopic examination of the specimen showed myoid spindle proliferation which was arranged in irregular sheets and nests that had been separated by prominent stromal hyalinization. The tumour cells exhibited vacuolated to eosinophilic cytoplasm with pink globules. In some areas there was evidence of dense hypercellularity and fascicular arrangement. Radial and concentric arrangement of the tumour cells was seen around thick-walled medium sized malformed blood vessels. There was evidence of mild nuclear pleomorphism and mitosis was rare. There was no tumour necrosis, vascular invasion, or infiltrative growth pattern. Immunohistochemistry revealed diffuse positive staining for desmin and smooth muscle actin, and scattered positivity for HMB-45 as well as S-100 protein. CD34 highlighted the vascular endothelial lining but the tumour cells were negatively stained. Immunohistochemistry of the tumour was negative for Melan-A, CD99, Cd10, inhibin, calretinin, and pancytokeratin (CK AE1/AE3). The pathological features of the tumour were diagnostic of angiomyolipoma (AML).

Molina et al. [31] reported a 28-year-old woman in her first pregnancy who presented with loin pain during the 17th week of her pregnancy which eventually resulted in spontaneous abortion and retained placenta. She was managed for the complications of her spontaneous abortion and her radiological imaging studies including ultrasound scan and CT scan showed a large mass in the left side of her retroperitoneum abutting the Gerota fascia of the left kidney displacing the left kidney. The mass was located between the splenic flexure and the iliac region. She underwent excision of the mass and pathological examination of the excised specimen showed features consistent with extrarenal retroperitoneal angiomyolipoma.

Medina et al. [32] reported a 25-year-old patient who presented with abdominal distension and whose ultrasound scan of abdomen had shown a large solid hypoechogenic mass which had occupied the whole pelvis and extended to the umbilical region displacing the adjacent organs. A CT scan which was subsequently done confirmed presence of the mass. An imaging guided per-cutaneous biopsy of the mass was undertaken and pathological examination of the specimen confirmed extrarenal retroperitoneal angiomyolipoma (ERAML).

Peces et al. [69] reported a 40-year-old man with a history of sporadic tuberous sclerosis and with a history of spontaneous bleeding from his left kidney angiomyolipoma. He received a low-dose mTor inhibitor and rapamycin for 12 months and this was noted to be associated with a reduction in the volume of his bilateral angiomyolipomas (AMLs) and it was noted to have resulted in stabilization as well as improvement of his renal function. Furthermore, there was additionally a reduction of his facial angiofibromas, improvement in the control of his blood pressure, and absence of angiomyolipoma (AML) bleeding over the 12-month period. His tuberous sclerosis brain lesion images did remain stable, and there was no significant rapamycin associated side-effects. Peces et al. [69] stated that to the best of their knowledge, their reported case was the first reported case of reduction in the volume of angiomyolipoma (AML) together with preservation of renal function in a patient with tuberous sclerosis who had received low-dose rapamycin. They also iterated that these data would suggest that it could be the result of the antiangiogenic, antifibrotic, and antiproliferative effects of rapamycin.

It is known that in tuberous sclerosis a number of tumours develop in various parts of the patient's body. A case of retroperitoneal angiomyolipoma has been reported in a patient 15 years after the patient had undergone radical nephrectomy. It could be argued that the new reported angiomyolipoma was a de novo benign angiomyolipoma due to the fact that the patient had tuberous sclerosis. On the contrary some people could argue that perhaps the newly reported angiomyolipoma could have been a metastatic angiomyolipoma that developed very late. Furthermore, two cases of distant metastases have been reported in two patients following radical resection of their retroperitoneal angiomyolipomas. Some people would argue that if angiomyolipomas are benign tumours then the subsequent development of angiomyolipomas in the liver, bone, and mediastinum could be considered as the subsequent development of de novo benign angiomyolipomas in other sites. However, it could be argued that the development of distant metastases occurring in a nontuberous sclerosis patient is the development of true metastases rather than de novo primary tumours. If that is the case, it would further be argued that there is the need for academic pathologists and oncologists globally to have a consensus opinion meeting discussion on angiomyolipomas to decide whether angiomyolipomas should still be regarded

as benign tumours or they should be regarded as slow-growing malignant tumours. There is also the need to discuss further if in event of reclassification of angiomyolipomas as potentially slow-growing malignant tumours should patients undergoing selective embolization or surgical resection of angiomyolipomas be given adjuvant rapamycin.

There is no consensus opinion on what angiomyolipomas occurring in the retroperitoneum. Some authors have referred to the lesions as retroperitoneal angiomyolipomas but other authors have referred to the lesions as extrarenal retroperitoneal angiomyolipomas. Some people would argue that the kidney lies in the retroperitoneum and thus angiomyolipomas of the kidney are also retroperitoneal angiomyolipomas and that by using the terminology extrarenal retroperitoneal angiomyolipoma every one would understand that the angiomyolipoma does not involve the kidney. Those who use the terminology retroperitoneal angiomyolipoma use the terminology knowing that angiomyolipomas of the kidney are strictly confined to the kidney and should not be regarded as retroperitoneal angiomyolipomas. With regard to the two different terminologies used in the literature, the author has observed from a review of the literature that all angiomyolipomas of the kidney have always been referred to as angiomyolipomas of the kidney or renal angiomyolipomas and these lesions had not been regarded as retroperitoneal angiomyolipomas even though the kidney could be said to be located in the retroperitoneum.

4. Conclusions and Recommendations

Extrarenal retroperitoneal angiomyolipoma (ERAML) is a rare tumour which could be confused with other tumours; ERAML was previously regarded as a hamartoma but is now classified as a benign tumour. Considering the fact that there are reports of the occurrence of distant metastases following complete excision of ERAML it would be recommended that academic pathologists and oncologists globally should convene a consensus opinion meeting to discuss the pathology and biological behaviour of the lesion in order to classify ERAML as a malignant neoplasm which tends usually to exhibit benign biological behaviour but has the potential to metastasize. Pathologists globally should also review the pathological features of ERAML that would indicate the possibility of malignant biological behaviour of the lesion. In view of the fact that there is evidence to show that mTor inhibitor rapamycin has been reported to be associated with reduction of the volume of angiomyolipoma (AML), perhaps it would be a good idea to give all patients who have undergone embolization of resection of angiomyolipoma (AML) as adjuvant treatment. Perhaps patients with extrarenal retroperitoneal angiomyolipoma (ERAML) who are not fit to undergo surgical procedures should be considered for rapamycin treatment.

Acknowledgment

Thanks are due to Dr. Siddick Dullo, a nephrologist of North Manchester General Hospital, Manchester United Kingdom, for translating one of the articles written in Spanish for the author.

References

[1] A. Strahan, J. King, and S. McClintock, "Retroperitoneal angiomyolipoma: a case report and review of the literature," *Case Reports in Radiology*, vol. 2013, Article ID 457383, 2 pages, 2013.

[2] A. R. Lienert and D. Nicol, "Renal angiomyolipoma," *BJU International*, vol. 110, supplement 4, pp. 25–27, 2012.

[3] C. P. Nelson and M. G. Sanda, "Contemporary diagnosis and management of renal angiomyolipoma," *The Journal of Urology*, vol. 168, no. 4, part 1, pp. 1315–1325, 2002.

[4] C. Gupta, A. K. Malani, V. Gupta, J. Singh, and H. Ammar, "Metastatic retroperitoneal epithelioid angiomyolipoma," *Journal of Clinical Pathology*, vol. 60, no. 4, pp. 428–431, 2007.

[5] J. Friis and A. Hjortrup, "Extrarenal angiomyolipoma: diagnosis and management," *The Journal of Urology*, vol. 127, no. 3, pp. 528–529, 1982.

[6] R. F. Randazzo, P. Neustein, and M. A. Koyle, "Spontaneous perinephric hemorrhage from extrarenal angiomyolipoma," *Urology*, vol. 29, no. 4, pp. 428–431, 1987.

[7] P. Ditonno, R. B. Smith, M. A. Koyle, J. Hannah, and A. Belldegrun, "Extrarenal angiomyolipomas of the perinephric space," *The Journal of Urology*, vol. 147, no. 2, pp. 447–450, 1992.

[8] W. C. G. Peh, B. H. Lim, and P. C. Tam, "Case report: perinephric angiomyolipomas in tuberous sclerosis," *British Journal of Radiology*, vol. 67, no. 802, pp. 1026–1029, 1994.

[9] J. C. Angulo, J. I. Lopez, J. A. Carnicero, and N. Flores, "Extrarenal retroperitoneal angiomyolipoma," *Urologia Internationalis*, vol. 52, no. 1, pp. 58–60, 1994.

[10] P. Gupta and S. Guleria, "Adrenal angiomyolipoma: a case report and review of literature," *Research Journal of Medical Sciences*, vol. 5, no. 5, pp. 243–246, 2011.

[11] B. H. Liwnicz, D. A. Weeks, and C. W. Zuppan, "Extrarenal angiomyolipoma with melanocytic and hibernoma-like features," *Ultrastructural Pathology*, vol. 18, no. 4, pp. 443–448, 1994.

[12] S. Y. K. Law, M. Fok, W. H. Shek, L. T. Ma, and J. Wong, "Retroperitoneal extrarenal angiomyolipoma," *Australian and New Zealand Journal of Surgery*, vol. 64, no. 6, pp. 449–451, 1994.

[13] Y. Mogi, R. Takimoto, T. Kura, M. Tamakawa, S. Sakamaki, and Y. Niitsu, "Retroperitoneal extrarenal angiomyolipoma with early gastric carcinoma," *Journal of Gastroenterology*, vol. 33, no. 1, pp. 86–90, 1998.

[14] D. P. Murphy, D. B. Glazier, E. S. Chenven, R. Principato, and S. M. Diamond, "Extrarenal retroperitoneal angiomyolipoma: nonoperative management," *The Journal of Urology*, vol. 163, no. 1, pp. 234–235, 2000.

[15] M. Tsutsumi, A. Yamauchi, S. Tsukamoto, and S. Ishikawa, "A case of angiomyolipoma presenting as a huge retroperitoneal mass," *International Journal of Urology*, vol. 8, no. 8, pp. 470–471, 2001.

[16] C.-A. Tseng, Y.-S. Pan, Y.-C. Su, D.-C. Wu, C.-M. Jan, and W.-M. Wang, "Extrarenal retroperitoneal angiomyolipoma: case report and review of the literature," *Abdominal Imaging*, vol. 29, no. 6, pp. 721–723, 2004.

[17] W. Obara, K. Sato, Y. Owari et al., "Perinephric angiomyolipoma: a unique development pattern surrounding the kidney," *International Journal of Urology*, vol. 12, no. 3, pp. 305–307, 2005.

[18] E. J. Minja, M. Pellerin, N. Saviano, and R. S. Chamberlain, "Retroperitoneal extrarenal angiomyolipomas: an evidence-based approach to a rare clinical entity," *Case Reports in Nephrology*, vol. 2012, Article ID 374107, 7 pages, 2012.

[19] Y.-C. Lee, S.-P. Huang, C.-C. Liu, W.-J. Wu, Y.-H. Chou, and C.-H. Huang, "Giant extrarenal retroperitoneal angiomyolipoma: a case report and literature review," *Kaohsiung Journal of Medical Sciences*, vol. 19, no. 11, pp. 579–582, 2003.

[20] S. Soni, A. Singhvi, and R. C. Purohit, "Pararenal retroperitoneal angiomyolipoma: a rare case report," *International Journal of Science Research*, vol. 4, no. 9, pp. 1225–1226, 2013.

[21] V. Ivanova, T. Dikov, G. Derimachkovski et al., "Retroperitoneal tumor: differential diagnosis beyond 'the usually suspected,'" *Science & Technologies Medicine*, vol. 4, no. 1, pp. 437–440, 2014.

[22] R. D. Welling, M. P. Lungren, and R. E. Coleman, "Extrarenal retroperitoneal angiomyolipoma mimicking metastatic melanoma: CT and FDG PET correlation," *Clinical Nuclear Medicine*, vol. 37, no. 7, pp. 705–706, 2012.

[23] J. E. Fegan, H. R. Shah, P. Mukunyadzi, and M. J. Schutz, "Extrarenal retroperitoneal angiomyolipoma," *Southern Medical Journal*, vol. 90, no. 1, pp. 59–62, 1997.

[24] S. K. Lau, A. M. Marchevsky, and D. J. Luthringer, "Malignant monotypic epithelioid epithelioid angiomolipoma of the retroperitoneum," *International Journal of Surgical Pathology*, vol. 11, no. 3, pp. 223–228, 2003.

[25] C. S.-C. Wen, Y.-S. Juan, Y.-C. Lee et al., "Concomitant mediastinal and extrarenal retroperitoneal angiomyolipomas in a patient who previously underwent ipsilateral radical nephrectomy," *Urological Science*, vol. 25, no. 4, pp. 115–118, 2014.

[26] L. J. Wang, K. E. Lim, Y. C. Wong, and C. J. Chen, "Giant retroperitoneal angiomyolipoma mimicking liposarcoma," *British Journal of Urology*, vol. 79, no. 6, pp. 1001–1002, 1997.

[27] L. R. Daniel, L. G. Sabela, R. R. Jorge, and O. C. Antonio, "Angiomiolipoma retroperitoneal: revisión de la literatura y reporte de un nuevo caso," *Actas Urológicas Españolas*, vol. 34, no. 9, pp. 815–826, 2010.

[28] I. D. Vilcea, R. Victor, C. S. Mirea et al., "Extrarenal retroperitoneal angiomyolipoma with unusual evolution," *Romanian Journal of Morphology and Embryology*, vol. 56, no. 1, pp. 263–266, 2015.

[29] M. K. Mansi, W. K. Al-Khudair, N. M. Al-Bqami et al., "Extrarenal angiomyolipa," *Saudi Medical Journal*, vol. 23, no. 9, pp. 1124–1126, 2002.

[30] M. Ahmad, S. Shuja, and R. A. Makary, "44 Year old woman with retroperitoneal mass: a pathology quiz," *Internet Journal of Anesthesiology*, vol. 14, no. 2, 2006.

[31] M. Molina, J. Ruiperez, N. Ortega et al., "Angiomiolipoma retroperitoneal en una embarazada," *Medicina Clínica*, vol. 117, no. 5, 2001, http://www.elsevier.es/en-revista-medicina-clinica-2-articulo-angiomiolipoma-retroperitoneal-una-embarasa-13017329.

[32] M. Medina, J. Ruiperez, N. Ortega et al., "Angiomiolipoma retroperitoneal/extrarenal retroperitoneal angiomyolipoma," *Revista Argentina de Radiología*, vol. 66, no. 2, pp. 129–133, 2002.

[33] M. Ziadie, "Kidney tumor—cysts, children, adult benign Benign (usually) adult tumors Angiomyolipoma," PathologyOutlines.com, 2015, http://www.pathologyoutlines.com/topic/kidneytumorangiomyolipoma.html.

[34] R. I. Demopoulos, F. Denarvaez, and V. Kaji, "Benign mixed mesodermal tumors of the uterus: a histogenetic study," American Journal of Clinical Pathology, vol. 60, no. 3, pp. 377–383, 1973.

[35] J. Gutmann, C. Cifuentes, R. Vicuña, V. Sobarzo, and M. A. Balzarini, "Intraoral angiomyolipoma," Oral Surgery, Oral Medicine, Oral Pathology, vol. 39, no. 6, pp. 945–948, 1975.

[36] C. Bures and L. Barnes, "Benign mesenchymomas of the head and neck," Archives of Pathology and Laboratory Medicine, vol. 102, no. 5, pp. 237–241, 1978.

[37] K. T. K. Chen and V. Bauer, "Extrarenal angiomyolipoma," Journal of Surgical Oncology, vol. 25, no. 2, pp. 89–91, 1984.

[38] B. A. Chaitin, R. L. Goldman, and D. G. Linker, "Angiomyolipoma of penis," Urology, vol. 23, no. 3, pp. 305–306, 1984.

[39] D. A. Katz, D. Thom, P. Bogard, and M. S. Dermer, "Angiomyolipoma of the fallopian tube," American Journal of Obstetrics and Gynecology, vol. 148, no. 3, pp. 341–343, 1984.

[40] M. Miyahara, M. Kobayashi, I. Tada et al., "Giant hepatic angiomyolipoma simulating focal nodular hyperplasia," The Japanese Journal of Surgery, vol. 18, no. 3, pp. 346–350, 1988.

[41] E. E. Dawlatly, J. T. Anim, and A. Y. El-Hassan, "Angiomyolipoma of the nasal cavity," Journal of Laryngology and Otology, vol. 102, no. 12, pp. 1156–1158, 1988.

[42] S. C. Peh and V. Sivanesaratnam, "Angiomyolipoma of the vagina—an uncommon tumour. Case report," British Journal of Obstetrics and Gynaecology, vol. 95, no. 8, pp. 820–823, 1988.

[43] K. T. K. Chen, "Angiomyolipoma of the vagina," Gynecologic Oncology, vol. 37, no. 2, pp. 302–304, 1990.

[44] T. A. Castillenti and A. P. Bertin, "Angiomyolipoma of the spermatic cord: case report and literature review," The Journal of Urology, vol. 142, no. 5, pp. 1308–1309, 1989.

[45] Y. Hikasa, T. Narabayashi, M. Yamamura et al., "Angiomyolipoma of the colon: a new entity in colonic polypoid lesions," Gastroenterologia Japonica, vol. 24, no. 4, pp. 407–409, 1989.

[46] C. H. Stone, M. W. Lee, M. B. Amin et al., "Renal angiomyolipoma: further immunophenotypic characterization of an expanding morphologic spectrum," Archives of Pathology and Laboratory Medicine, vol. 125, no. 6, pp. 751–758, 2001.

[47] L. Cheng, J. Gu, J. N. Eble et al., "Molecular genetic evidence for different clonal origin of components of human renal angiomyolipomas," The American Journal of Surgical Pathology, vol. 25, no. 10, pp. 1231–1236, 2001.

[48] R. E. Jimenez, J. N. Eble, V. E. Reuter et al., "Concurrent angiomyolipoma and renal cell neoplasia: a study of 36 cases," Modern Pathology, vol. 14, no. 3, pp. 157–163, 2001.

[49] G. Martignoni, F. Bonetti, M. Pea, R. Tardanico, M. Brunelli, and J. N. Eble, "Renal disease in adults with TSC2/PKD1 contiguous gene syndrome," The American Journal of Surgical Pathology, vol. 26, no. 2, pp. 198–205, 2002.

[50] L.-J. Wang, Y.-C. Wong, C.-J. Chen, and L.-C. See, "Computerized tomography characteristics that differentiate angiomyolipomas from liposarcomas in the perinephric space," The Journal of Urology, vol. 167, no. 2, part 1, pp. 490–493, 2002.

[51] J. E. Osterling, E. K. Fishman, S. M. Goldman, and F. F. Marshall, "The management of renal angiomyolipoma," The Journal of Urology, vol. 135, no. 6, pp. 1121–1124, 1986.

[52] M. S. Steiner, S. M. Goldman, E. K. Fishman, and F. F. Marshall, "The natural history of renal angiomyolipoma," The Journal of Urology, vol. 150, no. 6, pp. 1782–1786, 1993.

[53] S. I. Hajdu and F. W. Foote Jr., "Angiomyolipoma of the kidney: report of 27 cases and review of the literature," The Journal of Urology, vol. 102, no. 4, pp. 396–401, 1969.

[54] J. Y. Ro, A. G. Ayala, A. El-Naggar, D. J. Grignon, S. F. Hogan, and D. R. Howard, "Angiomyolipoma of kidney with lymph node involvement. DNA flow cytometric analysis," Archives of Pathology and Laboratory Medicine, vol. 114, no. 1, pp. 65–67, 1990.

[55] C. J. Davis, J. H. Barton, and I. A. Sesterhenn, "Cystic angiomyolipoma of the kidney: a clinicopathologic description of 11 cases," Modern Pathology, vol. 19, no. 5, pp. 669–674, 2006.

[56] P. R. Chowdhury, N. Tsuda, M. Anami et al., "A histopathologic and immunohistochemical study of small nodules of renal angiomyolipoma: a comparison of small nodules with angiomyolipoma," Modern Pathology, vol. 9, no. 11, pp. 1081–1088, 1996.

[57] S. W. Fine, V. E. Reuter, J. I. Epstein, and P. Argani, "Angiomyolipoma with epithelial cysts (AMLEC): a distinct cystic variant of angiomyolipoma," The American Journal of Surgical Pathology, vol. 30, no. 5, pp. 593–599, 2006.

[58] A. Matsuyama, M. Hissaoka, K. Ichikawa et al., "Sclerosing variant of epithelioid angiomyolipoma," Pathology International, vol. 58, no. 5, pp. 306–310, 2008.

[59] U. Handa, A. Nanda, and H. Mohan, "Fine-needle aspiration of renal angiomyolipoma: a report of four cases," Cytopathology, vol. 18, no. 4, pp. 250–254, 2007.

[60] H. R. Makhlouf, K. G. Ishak, R. Shekar, I. A. Sesterhenn, D. Y. Young, and J. C. Fanburg-Smith, "Melanoma markers in angiomyolipoma of the liver and kidney: a comparative study," Archives of Pathology and Laboratory Medicine, vol. 126, no. 1, pp. 49–55, 2002.

[61] H. R. Makhlouf, H. E. Remotti, and K. G. Ishak, "Expression of KIT (CD117) in angiomyolipoma," The American Journal of Surgical Pathology, vol. 26, no. 4, pp. 493–497, 2002.

[62] H. L'Hostis, C. Deminiere, J.-M. Ferriere, and J.-M. Coindre, "Renal angiomyolipoma: a clinicopathologic, immunohistochemical, and follow-up study of 46 cases," The American Journal of Surgical Pathology, vol. 23, no. 9, pp. 1011–1020, 1999.

[63] A. Zavala-Pompa, A. L. Folpe, R. E. Jimenez et al., "Immunohistochemical study of microphthalmia transcription factor and tyrosinase in angiomyolipoma of the kidney, renal cell carcinoma, and renal and retroperitoneal sarcomas: comparative evaluation with traditional diagnostic markers," The American Journal of Surgical Pathology, vol. 25, no. 1, pp. 65–70, 2001.

[64] S. M. Bonsib, M. Moghadamfalahi, and A. Bhalodia, "Lymphatic differentiation in renal angiomyolipomas," Human Pathology, vol. 40, no. 3, pp. 374–380, 2009.

[65] A. A. Roma, C. Magi-Galluzzi, and M. Zhou, "Differential expression of melanocytic markers in myoid, lipomatous, and vascular components of renal angiomyolipomas," Archives of Pathology and Laboratory Medicine, vol. 131, no. 1, pp. 122–125, 2007.

[66] M. M. Kattar, D. J. Grignon, J. N. Eble et al., "Chromosomal analysis of renal angiomyolipoma by comparative genomic hybridization: evidence for clonal origin," Human Pathology, vol. 30, no. 3, pp. 295–299, 1999.

[67] V. Paradis, I. Leurendesu, A. Viellefond et al., "Clonal analysis of renal sporadic angiomyolipomas," Human Pathology, vol. 29, no. 10, pp. 1063–1067, 1998.

[68] N. Takahashi, R. Kitahara, Y. Hishimoto, A. Ohguro, Y. Hashimoto, and T. Suzuki, "Malignant transformation of renal angiomyolipoma," *International Journal of Urology*, vol. 10, no. 5, pp. 271–273, 2003.

[69] R. Peces, C. Peces, E. Cuesta-López et al., "Low-dose rapamycin reduces kidney volume angiomyolipomas and prevents the loss of renal function in a patient with tuberous sclerosis complex," *Nephrology Dialysis Transplantation*, vol. 25, no. 11, pp. 3787–3791, 2010.

22

Contralateral Risk-Reducing Mastectomy: Review of Risk Factors and Risk-Reducing Strategies

N. N. Basu,[1,2] **L. Barr,**[1] **G. L. Ross,**[3] **and D. G. Evans**[1,4]

[1]*Nightingale and Genesis Prevention Centre, University Hospital South Manchester, Southmoor Road, Manchester M23 9LT, UK*
[2]*Department of Breast Surgery, Queen Elizabeth Hospital, Birmingham B15 2TH, UK*
[3]*The Institute of Cancer Sciences, The University of Manchester, Oxford Road, Manchester M13 9PL, UK*
[4]*University of Manchester Department of Genomic Medicine, Institute of Human Development, St. Mary's Hospital, Oxford Road, Manchester M13 9WL, UK*

Correspondence should be addressed to N. N. Basu; naren_basu@hotmail.com

Academic Editor: Kazuhiro Yoshida

Rates of contralateral risk-reducing mastectomy have increased substantially over the last decade. Surgical oncologists are often in the frontline, dealing with requests for this procedure. This paper reviews the current evidence base regarding contralateral breast cancer, assesses the various risk-reducing strategies, and evaluates the cost-effectiveness of contralateral risk-reducing mastectomy.

1. Introduction

Breast cancer is the most common cancer in women worldwide, with 1.7 million new cases diagnosed in 2012 [1, 2]. It accounts for 25% of all cancers in women and in the UK; it is estimated that 1 in 8–10 women will develop breast cancer [3] during their lifetime.

Breast cancer survivorship has improved as a result of early detection and advancing treatment modalities [3]. As such, management of this group of women requires healthcare professionals to be familiar with additional risks factors so that timely recommendations may be made on surveillance or risk-reducting strategies.

Once diagnosed with breast cancer, these women will have an increased risk of developing a contralateral, metachronous breast cancer [4]. The level of this risk is multifactorial, dependent on tumour biology, adjuvant treatment, and oncogenetics.

There is ongoing interest in contralateral breast cancer (CBC). Surveillance, Epidemiology, and End Results Program (SEER) data from the US [5] has confirmed a 150% increase in rates of contralateral risk-reducing mastectomy (CRRM) over the last decade, although this may not be the case in Europe [6]. This rise is somewhat surprising, given that rates of CBC are decreasing (due to endocrine

therapy especially with aromatase inhibitors) and may be a reflection of a heightened perceived risk in this vulnerable group of women. Clinicians are at the frontline of many of these complex decisions and need to make evidence-based recommendations.

We examine the multiple risk factors known to contribute to developing CBC. Survival data are analysed and the contribution of the following risk factors is discussed: gene mutation and family history, histology, ER status, and HER2 status. We evaluate the different risk-reducing strategies (surgery and chemoprevention) and their efficacy and cost and finally consider the patient's perspective. We have included chemoprevention using antiendocrine treatment in the section of ER status as this is relevant to this section.

This review aims to serve as an aide-memoire for clinicians to refer to when counselling women on CBC.

2. Incidence of CBC

High-risk patients include breast cancer sufferers with known genetic mutations (*BRCA1/2, TP53*) and a significant family history. *BRCA1/2* mutation carriers have a CBC risk of 2-3% per annum [8]. This is likely to be higher in *TP53* patients, though there is limited data on this group of patients [9]. This heightened risk, particularly in women diagnosed with their primary cancer before 40 years, lasts for at least 20 years. Risk-reducing bilateral salpingo-oophorectomy (RRBSO) and menopause before the age of 40 [8, 10, 11] are protective factors.

The remainder of patients without a known genetic mutation or significant family history represent the majority of breast cancer sufferers. SEER historical data (1973–1996) quote actuarial incidence rates of CBC in this group of women at 5, 10, 15, and 20 years were 3%, 6.1%, 9.1%, and 12%, respectively, amounting to 0.6% per annum [4]. This level of risk is likely to be outdated with several studies supporting a global decrease in CBC, with almost a 30% reduction in parts of Europe over the last 10-year period [4]. This trend is likely to be a reflection of successful adjuvant treatment, in particular antiendocrine treatment.

2.1. Risk Factors

2.1.1. Gene Mutation. The two most commonly studied breast cancer susceptibility genes are BRCA1 and BRCA2. Mutations in these tumour suppressor genes confer an up to 80–90% lifetime risk of developing breast cancer [12–14].

These women have a significant CBC risk once diagnosed with breast cancer.

The risk, up to age 70 years, of a CBC in BRCA1 mutation carriers has been estimated to be above 60% [15] and in BRCA2 mutation carriers slightly lower at around 50% [12]. However, a recent prospective study [16] has shown that these risks may be even higher at 83% and 63%, respectively, representing higher risks in the modern era particularly for BRCA1 where the majority of tumours would not receive endocrine therapy.

Several studies have evaluated further CBC risk factors within BRCA1/2 mutation carriers [8, 10, 11]. Early age of first breast cancer diagnosis (<50 years) with increasing numbers of first-degree relatives with breast cancer at a young age heightens that risk. Protective factors that reduce CBC risk include the use of tamoxifen (HR 0.59; 95% CI 0.31–1.01) [8, 17] and oophorectomy (HR 0.44; 95% CI 0.21–0.91), with additional benefit of oophorectomy prior to the age of 49 years (HR 0.24; 95% CI 0.07–0.77).

Breast cancer remains the most common malignancy in women harbouring a TP53 mutation in Li-Fraumeni syndrome. These mutation carriers will have a nearly 100% lifetime risk of developing cancer with the vast majority developing breast cancer by the age of 46 [18].

Given the rarity of this condition, there is very limited data on CBC risk. Evans et al. [9] studied women under the age of 30 years with breast cancer and found that rates of CBC were approximately 2-3% annually in all mutations carriers (TP53 and BRCA1/2), although only 11 TP53 mutation carriers were included in their extended analysis. It is possible that adjuvant endocrine and anti-HER2 treatment will influence CBC risk in TP53 mutation carriers as the majority of these patients are ER and HER2 positive [19]. Efforts are underway to assess this risk further.

2.1.2. Family History. A positive family history of breast cancer increases the risk of CBC although this risk pattern is

complex. Vichapat et al. [7] studied 8478 women with breast cancer over a 31-year period (1975–2006) and found that there was a 2.8-fold increase in relative risk with a positive family history of breast cancer. Subgroup analysis revealed that the highest risks were those with a first- and second-degree relative (RR 2.33) followed by first-degree alone (RR 1.38) and second- or third-degree (RR 1.13). Numerous first-degree relatives will confer an even higher risk.

The WECARE study (Women's Environment Cancer and Radiation Epidemiology Study) conducted a population-based case control study comparing asynchronous bilateral breast cancer patients (case) against unilateral breast cancer (control) patients [20]. They confirmed that the risk of CBC in noncarriers of BRCA1/2 mutation with a family history was highest in women diagnosed at an earlier age with their index breast cancer (<45 years), those with a young first-degree relative, particularly with bilateral disease. The 10-year cumulative CBC risk stratified by age was 6.7% (50–54 years), 9.0% (40–44 years), and 14.7% (30–34 years).

A study from the Mayo Clinic [21] followed up 745 women with breast cancer and a positive family history who underwent a CRRM between 1960 and 1993. They had predicted (without CRRM) 106 CBCs in the premenopausal group and 50 CBCs in the postmenopausal group. CRRM had resulted in an approximate 95% reduction in relative risk as only 6 and 2 actual CBCs occurred in pre- and postmenopausal women, respectively.

2.1.3. Histology of Index Breast Cancer. The Vichapat et al. study [7] assessed histological type and found no significant increase in CBC in those with lobular breast cancer. This is an interesting finding given that lobular breast cancer has been shown previously to be an independent predictor of increased CRRM rates [22] and possibly arises from previous studies that have shown an association of lobular cancer and CBC [23].

High grade of primary tumours (RR 1.3 for Grade 3 cancer compared to Grade 1), increasing size (<2 cm RR 1.0, 2–5 cm RR 1.51, and >5 cm RR 1.89), and number of positive lymph nodes (non-RR 1.0, 4–9 RR 1.12, and >10 RR 1.62) were all shown to be important risk factors [7]. Table 1 summarises the known risk factors for developing contralateral breast cancer while Table 2 shows the risk reduction strategies of CBC.

2.1.4. HER2 Status and Anti-HER2 Treatment. Up to 30% of breast cancers [24] express HER2 receptor tyrosine-protein kinase. Use of the monoclonal antibody trastuzumab (Herceptin) has been shown to improve disease-free survival [25]. The HERA study (Herceptin Adjuvant Trial) recently reported outcomes after a 4-year follow-up [26]. In the observation group there were 19/320 (1.1%) CBCs compared to 14/251 (0.8%) in the trastuzumab group. Although this represents a small reduction in CBC in women treated with trastuzumab, its clinical application for risk reduction of CBC remains debatable.

Saltzman et al. [27] performed a case-control study of 29,126 women using the Cancer Surveillance System (CSS) cancer registry. They were able to show that women with

TABLE 1: Risk factors for developing CBC (estimated annual risk) [4, 7].

	Estimated annual risk (%) [4]	Relative risk—multivariate (95% CI) [7]
Patient factors		
Age at first diagnosis		
<30 yrs	0.5–1.3	
40–50 yrs		
ER +ve	0.2-0.3	
ER −ve	0.4-0.5	
Gene mutation		
BRCA1	2.0–3.0	
BRCA2	2.0–3.0	
Family history		
None		1 (reference)
First- and second-degree	0.4–1.3	2.8 (1.4–5.5)
First-degree	0.2–0.8	1.4 (0.9–2.1)
Second- or third-degree	Baseline	1.1 (0.7–1.9)
Tumour factors		
Size		
<2 cm (T1)		1 (reference)
2–5 cm (T2)		1.5 (1.1–2.0)
>5 cm (T3)		1.9 (1.1–3.3)
LN status		
None		1 (reference)
1–3		0.9 (0.6–1.2)
4–9		1.1 (0.7–1.9)
>10		1.6 (0.8–3.1)
Histology		
Ductal		1 (reference)
Lobular		1.2 (0.6–2.1)
ER status		
ER positive		1.0 (reference)
ER negative		1.3 (0.9–1.9)
HER2 status		
HER2 positive		1.0 (reference)
HER2 negative		1.02 (0.6–1.8)

TABLE 2: Risk reduction of CBC associated with chemoprevention and surgery.

	Risk reduction (95% CI)
Chemoprevention	
Antiendocrine	
Tamoxifen in *BRCA1/2* mutation carriers	OR 0.5 (0.3–0.9)
Tamoxifen in noncarriers	50% risk reduction
Aromatase inhibitors in noncarriers	70% risk reduction
Chemotherapy	
Chemo versus no chemo	RR 0.6 (0.4–0.8)
Surgery	20-year survival benefit
CRRM	
CRRM in *BRCA1/2* mutation carriers	14.9%
CRRM in nonmutation carriers	<1%

HER2 overexpression (ER negative/HER2 positive) and those with triple negative cancer (ER negative, PR negative, and HER2 negative) had a 2.0-fold and 1.4-fold increased risk of developing CBC, respectively. Therefore, in addition to having a higher risk of recurrent disease and death, this subgroup of patients will have an elevated risk of CBC and surveillance strategies need to be considered in monitoring this cohort.

2.1.5. ER Status and Chemoprevention. Several studies (ATAC, IBIS I, IBIS II, and STAR) have confirmed that antihormonal agents (SERM and aromatase inhibitors) given to high-risk women for up to 10 years can reduce the incidence of CBC and primary breast cancer [28]. Women with hormone sensitive index breast cancers are routinely offered antihormonal agents as part of their adjuvant treatment and can expect an up to 50% reduction in their risk of developing a CBC with recent studies showing favouring aromatase inhibitors over tamoxifen (ATAC) in the postmenopausal setting [29]. Women considering antihormonal agents need to be appraised of significant adverse effects including thromboembolic phenomenon, osteoporosis, and uterine carcinoma.

Recently, Gronwald et al. [17] were able to confirm previous studies showing an approximately 50% reduction in CBC risk in *BRCA1/2* mutation carriers who took Tamoxifen following their index breast cancer. Of interest was the similar risk-reduction of a short period of Tamoxifen (<1 year) compared to longer use (>4 years). This has implications on women who have concerns over the side effect profile of long term Tamoxifen use and may rationalise the short-term use of this drug.

2.1.6. Chemotherapy. Cytotoxic chemotherapy agent recommended as adjuvant or neoadjuvant treatment of primary breast cancer has been shown to reduce the risk of CBC. The Early Breast Cancer Trialists Group (EBCTG) showed a marginal reduction in the incidence of CBC over a 15-year follow-up period [30], which was more definite in women under the age of 50 years.

The WECARE group carried out a case-control study [31] and found that chemotherapy use was associated with a 35–40% reduction in risk of CBC in women under the age of 55 and that this protective effect lasted up to 10 years. In addition, those who became postmenopausal within 1 year of diagnosis had the greatest risk reduction.

PARP inhibitors and their effect on triple negative and *BRCA1/2* mutation related breast cancers are the subject of much interest [32]. Initial reports from proof-of-concept trials [33] have confirmed their safety and efficacy, and phase III studies with an extended follow-up may determine whether these targeted therapy modalities affect contralateral breast cancer risk.

2.2. Contralateral Risk-Reducing Mastectomy

2.2.1. Survival. The aftermath of Angelina Jolie's announcement of her bilateral risk-reducing mastectomy (BRRM) has raised public awareness of risk-reducing surgery [34, 35]. Several studies have confirmed a survival benefit in high-risk patients (BRCA1/2 and FH) undergoing BRRM and CRRM [36–39]. Our own experience [39] compared 105 female BRCA1/2 mutation carriers with unilateral breast cancer to matched mutation carriers who did not undergo CRRM. The overall 10-year survival was 89% in the CRRM group compared to 71% in the non-CRRM group ($P < 0.001$), which was independent of RRBSO. This is in contrast to van Sprundel et al. [40] who found that, after adjusting for RRBSO, there was no overall survival benefit from CRRM. Metcalfe et al. [38] followed a similar group of 390 BRCA1/2 mutation carriers and found that at 20 years the survival rate of those who underwent CRRM was 88% (CI 83–93%) compared to 65% (CI 59–73%) who did not undergo CRRM.

The survival benefit in non-BRCA mutation patients is less clear. Younger women under the age of 49 [41, 42] with ER −ve disease are likely to have an improved disease-specific survival, which is thought to be due to a higher baseline risk of CBC. A clear survival benefit on the remainder of patients seems less likely [37]. Portschy et al. [43] used a Markov model to compare survival outcomes between CRRM and non-CRRM in non-BRCA patients. They estimated a less than 1% absolute 20-year survival benefit from CRRM amongst all age groups, ER status, and cancer stage groups.

2.2.2. Breast Reconstruction. Several studies have shown that access to immediate breast reconstruction positively affects the decision for CRRM [44, 45]. Recently, Ashfaq et al. [45] identified 102,674 patients (2004–2008) with a diagnosis of DCIS (15%) or invasive breast cancer (85%) from SEER registry data. Those undergoing mastectomy were 3 times more likely to request CRRM if offered immediate reconstruction. Overall, 16% of all patients underwent CRRM with a significant proportion undergoing reconstruction (46%, $P < 0.001$). Similar proportions of patients underwent implant-based reconstruction (36%) and tissue-based reconstruction (37%). There was a trend of increasing numbers of reconstructions during this time period, and Caucasian women, under the age of 45 years with a diagnosis of a node-negative lobular carcinoma or DCIS, were more likely to choose reconstruction.

Women undergoing reconstruction following CRRM are 1.5 times more likely to have a major complication requiring hospitalisation or reoperation [46] compared to unilateral mastectomy. Limited data is available comparing CRRM and reconstruction with unilateral mastectomy and reconstruction. Crosby et al. [47] assessed 497 patients undergoing CRRM with reconstruction and concluded that a third of patients experiencing at least one complication may not have developed a complication if they had only had a mastectomy and reconstruction of their index side.

2.2.3. Sentinel Lymph Node Biopsy (SLNB). SLNB at the time of risk-reducing surgery remains controversial. A recent meta-analysis of 1251 patients [48] showed that 1.7% ($n = 21$) of women undergoing RRM harboured occult invasive cancer in the mastectomy specimen. Of these 21 patients, the SLN was positive in only 4/21 patients and negative in the remainder (17/21). This was higher in women with advanced cancer in the contralateral breast. Overall, 2.8% ($n = 36$) of women benefited from SLNB that included 19 cases of a positive SLNB result requiring completion axillary surgery and 17 women who had invasive disease in the mastectomy specimen but a negative SLNB, thus avoiding further axillary surgery. This is offset against the 5% lymphoedema rate associated with SLNB [49]. Kuwajerwala et al. [50] retrospectively assessed 170 patients undergoing CRRM and found that of the 21.8% who had a SLNB at the surgeon's discretion, none had positive SLNB.

2.2.4. Cost. Health care economics contribute to the decision making process. Cost-effectiveness with life expectancy gains is well established in the setting of bilateral RRM in women harbouring BRCA1/2 mutations [51, 52]. Few studies have looked at this in the setting of CRRM [53–55]. Deshmukh et al. [54] analysed matched groups (CRRM and non-CRRM) and showed that CRRM significantly increases short-term healthcare cost by $7,749. In addition, women who had a reconstruction and in particular a delayed type had significantly higher cost associated as well as those who had HER2 positive disease and received radiotherapy.

In contrast, Roberts et al. [55] found that CRRM was cost-effective in the prevention of CBC in women under the age of 50 years. From their decision tree-model, they concluded that 68,000 women under the age of 50 years would have been diagnosed with early breast cancer in 2010. If all women had undergone CRRM, savings of $19 million would have been made to avoid 3,900 contralateral breast cancers that would have developed over the next 10 years. Their CRRM group had 0.2 quality-adjusted life years (QUALYs) less than the non-CRRM that may have been accounted for by complications of reconstruction. They highlighted a potential greater benefit of CRRM in ER −ve disease compared to ER +ve disease, given that the latter would receive adjuvant endocrine treatment, shown to reduce CBC.

Zendejas et al. [53] used a Markov model to compare cost-effectiveness in women undergoing CRRM compared to routine surveillance (including annual mammography). They found that CRRM prior to the age of 70 years was cost-effective and in particular in those who were BRCA-positive.

Currently in the UK, there are no funding restrictions within the National Health Service on CRRM. Breast cancer patients can choose between delayed and immediate (performed at the same time as the therapeutic mastectomy) without financial scrutiny provided that there is backing from the relevant clinicians.

2.2.5. Patient's Perspective. One of the main driving forces for CRRM is patients' worry and anxiety about developing another breast cancer and having to undergo further treatment including chemotherapy. This is often the most difficult component to assess, as the psychology behind it is multifactorial. A recent US study reported that 68.9% of patients undergoing CRRM did not have genetic or familial risk factors for CBC [56] and that the main driving force for this was worry about recurrence. Patients overestimate their risk of contralateral breast cancer [57] and in doing so can compound their anxiety.

A recent study [58] assessed the perspective from 60 consecutive patients choosing CRRM. In almost all cases, requests for CRRM were instigated by the patient and every patient unambiguously wanted CRRM. Patients responded to risk in an "all or nothing" manner and the majority did not objectively quantify this risk. The risk assessment in those that did quantify risk had little role in their decision for surgery. The authors concluded that "patients' subjective sense of vulnerability overwhelmed their appreciation of risk so that, so that regardless of level of risk of CBC, they found this risk intolerable and felt that only CRRM could reduce it." This showed that a rate limiting factor will be the availability of immediate reconstruction and if this is not made possible for patients as part of their primary surgical treatment rates of CRRM are likely to be lower.

3. Discussion

Rates of CRRM have increased in the US, a trend that in the future other countries may follow. This is of concern given that the actual incidence on CBC is on the decrease as a result of successful adjuvant treatments.

CBC risk assessment is multifactorial and may be assessed in a multidisciplinary setting. The most significant risk factors are gene mutation status and significant family history, which can result in at least a fourfold increase in CBC risk. Patients harbouring a *BRCA1/2* mutation have an approximate 2-3% annual incidence on developing CBC. In nonmutation carriers with a family history, young age at first diagnosis and first-degree relative are particularly strong risk factors.

Tumour biology is important. The ER status is of particular importance given that approximately 70% of all breast cancers are hormone sensitive. Risk reduction with antiendocrine treatment is approximately 50% with tamoxifen and 70% with aromatase inhibitors. As predicted, women with ER negative breast cancer have an increased risk of CBC. The use of cytotoxic agents and targeted treatments (e.g., Herceptin) marginally reduces CBC, with the greatest benefit for young women having chemotherapy.

CRRM offers the greatest risk reduction of CBC, up to 95% in women with a family history. Survival benefits are conferred on those high-risk patients with a *BRCA1/2* mutation. There is no survival benefit in the non-high-risk group.

Access to immediate breast reconstruction positively affects a woman's decision to opt for CRRM, with a significant number experiencing operative complications. Occult disease in the CRRM specimen occurs in less than 2% of women with no clear evidence to support sentinel lymph node biopsy.

Survival benefits and cost-effectiveness are seen in those at the highest risk of CBC (gene mutation carriers) and these patients are likely to benefit most from CRRM.

The assessment of CBC risk is multifactorial and may be assessed in a multidisciplinary setting. Arrington et al. [22] showed that surgeon and patient characteristics determine CRRM and include independent factors like young patient age (<40 years), large tumour size (>5 cm), lobular histology, positive family history, multicentric disease, and female surgeon. In addition, patients' anxiety about developing another breast cancer and going through subsequent treatment is a real entity, albeit difficult to quantify.

All clinicians treating breast cancer patients should be familiar with CBC risk and have the opportunity to discuss the various options including CRRM, chemoprevention, and routine surveillance. The multidisciplinary team is invaluable in guiding women based on objective assessment of genetic and family history, tumour biology, and psychological support.

It is becoming apparent that women seeking CRRM are categorised into different risk groups [59] and that clinicians are faced with differing challenges when managing these different groups. This review has focused on the different risk factors and risk-reducing strategies to give clinicians a comprehensive overview of the current literature.

References

[1] D. M. Parkin, P. Pisani, and J. Ferlay, "Estimates of the worldwide mortality from 25 cancers in 1990," *International Journal of Cancer*, vol. 83, no. 1, pp. 18–29, 1999.

[2] World Cancer Research Fund International, Breast Cancer Statistics, 2012, http://www.wcrf.org/int/cancer-facts-figures/data-specific-cancers/breast-cancer-statistics.

[3] Cancer Research UK, 2014, http://cancerresearchuk.org/cancer.

[4] I. M. Lizarraga, S. L. Sugg, R. J. Weigel, and C. E. H. Scott-Conner, "Review of risk factors for the development of contralateral breast cancer," *The American Journal of Surgery*, vol. 206, no. 5, pp. 704–708, 2013.

[5] T. M. Tuttle, E. B. Habermann, E. H. Grund, T. J. Morris, and B. A. Virnig, "Increasing use of contralateral prophylactic mastectomy for breast cancer patients: a trend toward more aggressive surgical treatment," *Journal of Clinical Oncology*, vol. 25, no. 33, pp. 5203–5209, 2007.

[6] U. Güth, M. E. Myrick, C. T. Viehl, W. P. Weber, A. M. Lardi, and S. M. Schmid, "Increasing rates of contralateral prophylactic mastectomy—a trend made in USA?" *European Journal of Surgical Oncology*, vol. 38, no. 4, pp. 296–301, 2012.

[7] V. Vichapat, C. Gillett, I. S. Fentiman, A. Tutt, L. Holmberg, and M. Lüchtenborg, "Risk factors for metachronous contralateral breast cancer suggest two aetiological pathways," *European Journal of Cancer*, vol. 47, no. 13, pp. 1919–1927, 2011.

[8] K. Metcalfe, H. T. Lynch, P. Ghadirian et al., "Contralateral breast cancer in BRCA1 and BRCA2 mutation carriers," *Journal of Clinical Oncology*, vol. 22, no. 12, pp. 2328–2335, 2004.

[9] D. G. R. Evans, A. Moran, R. Hartley et al., "Long-term outcomes of breast cancer in women aged 30 years or younger, based on family history, pathology and *BRCA1/BRCA2/TP53*

status," *British Journal of Cancer*, vol. 102, no. 7, pp. 1091–1098, 2010.

[10] K. Metcalfe, S. Gershman, H. T. Lynch et al., "Predictors of contralateral breast cancer in BRCA1 and BRCA2 mutation carriers," *British Journal of Cancer*, vol. 104, no. 9, pp. 1384–1392, 2011.

[11] M. K. Graeser, C. Engel, K. Rhiem et al., "Contralateral breast cancer risk in BRCA1 and BRCA2 mutation carriers," *Journal of Clinical Oncology*, vol. 27, no. 35, pp. 5887–5892, 2009.

[12] D. Ford, D. F. Easton, M. Stratton et al., "Genetic heterogeneity and penetrance analysis of the BRCA1 and BRCA2 genes in breast cancer families," *The American Journal of Human Genetics*, vol. 62, no. 3, pp. 676–689, 1998.

[13] D. G. Evans, A. Shenton, E. Woodward, F. Lalloo, A. Howell, and E. R. Maher, "Penetrance estimates for BRCA1 and BRCA2 based on genetic testing in a Clinical Cancer Genetics service setting: risks of breast/ovarian cancer quoted should reflect the cancer burden in the family," *BMC cancer*, vol. 8, article 155, 2008.

[14] F. Lalloo and D. G. Evans, "Familial breast cancer," *Clinical Genetics*, vol. 82, no. 2, pp. 105–114, 2012.

[15] D. Thompson and D. F. Easton, "Breast Cancer Linkage Consortium. Cancer incidence in BRCA1 mutation carriers," *Journal of the National Cancer Institute*, vol. 94, no. 18, pp. 1358–1365, 2002.

[16] N. Mavaddat, S. Peock, D. Frost et al., "Cancer risks for *BRCA1* and *BRCA2* mutation carriers: results from prospective analysis of EMBRACE," *Journal of the National Cancer Institute*, vol. 105, no. 11, pp. 812–822, 2013.

[17] J. Gronwald, A. Robidoux, C. Kim-Sing et al., "Duration of tamoxifen use and the risk of contralateral breast cancer in BRCA1 and BRCA2 mutation carriers," *Breast Cancer Research and Treatment*, vol. 146, no. 2, pp. 421–427, 2014.

[18] A. Chompret, L. Brugières, M. Ronsin et al., "P53 germline mutations in childhood cancers and cancer risk for carrier individuals," *British Journal of Cancer*, vol. 82, no. 12, pp. 1932–1937, 2000.

[19] S. Masciari, D. A. Dillon, M. Rath et al., "Breast cancer phenotype in women with TP53 germline mutations: a Li-Fraumeni syndrome consortium effort," *Breast Cancer Research and Treatment*, vol. 133, no. 3, pp. 1125–1130, 2012.

[20] A. S. Reiner, E. M. John, J. D. Brooks et al., "Risk of asynchronous contralateral breast cancer in noncarriers of *BRCA1* and *BRCA2* mutations with a family history of breast cancer: a report from the women's environmental cancer and radiation epidemiology study," *Journal of Clinical Oncology*, vol. 31, no. 4, pp. 433–439, 2013.

[21] S. K. McDonnell, D. J. Schaid, J. L. Myers et al., "Efficacy of contralateral prophylactic mastectomy in women with a personal and family history of breast cancer," *Journal of Clinical Oncology*, vol. 19, no. 19, pp. 3938–3943, 2001.

[22] A. K. Arrington, S. L. Jarosek, B. A. Virnig, E. B. Habermann, and T. M. Tuttle, "Patient and surgeon characteristics associated with increased use of contralateral prophylactic mastectomy in patients with breast cancer," *Annals of Surgical Oncology*, vol. 16, no. 10, pp. 2697–2704, 2009.

[23] J. L. Bernstein, R. H. Lapinski, S. S. Thakore, J. T. Doucette, and W. D. Thompson, "The descriptive epidemiology of second primary breast cancer," *Epidemiology*, vol. 14, no. 5, pp. 552–558, 2003.

[24] Z. Mitri, T. Constantine, and R. O'Regan, "The HER2 receptor in breast cancer: pathophysiology, clinical use, and new advances in therapy," *Chemotherapy Research and Practice*, vol. 2012, Article ID 743193, 7 pages, 2012.

[25] M. J. Piccart-Gebhart, M. Procter, B. Leyland-Jones et al., "Trastuzumab after adjuvant chemotherapy in HER2-positive breast cancer," *New England Journal of Medicine*, vol. 353, no. 16, pp. 1659–1672, 2005.

[26] L. Gianni, U. Dafni, R. D. Gelber et al., "Treatment with trastuzumab for 1 year after adjuvant chemotherapy in patients with HER2-positive early breast cancer: a 4-year follow-up of a randomised controlled trial," *The Lancet Oncology*, vol. 12, no. 3, pp. 236–244, 2011.

[27] B. S. Saltzman, K. E. Malone, J. A. McDougall, J. R. Daling, and C. I. Li, "Estrogen receptor, progesterone receptor, and HER2-neu expression in first primary breast cancers and risk of second primary contralateral breast cancer," *Breast Cancer Research and Treatment*, vol. 135, no. 3, pp. 849–855, 2012.

[28] J. Cuzick, I. Sestak, J. F. Forbes et al., "Anastrozole for prevention of breast cancer in high-risk postmenopausal women (IBIS-II): an international, double-blind, randomised placebo-controlled trial," *The Lancet*, vol. 383, no. 9922, pp. 1041–1048, 2014.

[29] J. Cuzick, I. Sestak, M. Baum et al., "Effect of anastrozole and tamoxifen as adjuvant treatment for early-stage breast cancer: 10-year analysis of the ATAC trial," *The Lancet Oncology*, vol. 11, no. 12, pp. 1135–1141, 2010.

[30] Early Breast Cancer Trialists' Collaborative Group (EBCTCG), "Effects of chemotherapy and hormonal therapy for early breast cancer on recurrence and 15-year survival: an overview of the randomised trials," *The Lancet*, vol. 365, no. 9472, pp. 1687–1717, 2005.

[31] J. L. Bernstein, D. C. Thomas, R. E. Shore et al., "Contralateral breast cancer after radiotherapy among *BRCA1* and *BRCA2* mutation carriers: a WECARE Study Report," *European Journal of Cancer*, vol. 49, no. 14, pp. 2979–2985, 2013.

[32] R. Plummer, "Poly(ADP-ribose) polymerase inhibition: a new direction for BRCA and triple-negative breast cancer?" *Breast Cancer Research*, vol. 13, no. 4, article 218, 2011.

[33] A. Tutt, M. Robson, J. E. Garber et al., "Oral poly(ADP-ribose) polymerase inhibitor olaparib in patients with BRCA1 or BRCA2 mutations and advanced breast cancer: a proof-of-concept trial," *The Lancet*, vol. 376, no. 9737, pp. 235–244, 2010.

[34] N. N. Basu, L. Barr, D. G. Evans, and G. L. Ross, "Threshold for genetic testing in women with breast cancer needs to be determined," *British Medical Journal*, vol. 348, Article ID g1863, 2014.

[35] D. G. Evans, J. Barwell, D. M. Eccles et al., "The Angelina Jolie effect: how high celebrity profile can have a major effect on provision of cancer related services," *Breast Cancer Research*, vol. 16, no. 5, article 442, 2014.

[36] S. M. Domchek, T. M. Friebel, C. F. Singer et al., "Association of risk-reducing surgery in BRCA1 or BRCA2 mutation carriers with cancer risk and mortality," *JAMA—Journal of the American Medical Association*, vol. 304, no. 9, pp. 967–975, 2010.

[37] L. Lostumbo, N. E. Carbine, and J. Wallace, "Prophylactic mastectomy for the prevention of breast cancer," *Cochrane Database of Systematic Reviews*, vol. 11, Article ID CD002748, 2010.

[38] K. Metcalfe, S. Gershman, P. Ghadirian et al., "Contralateral mastectomy and survival after breast cancer in carriers of BRCA1 and BRCA2 mutations: retrospective analysis," *British Medical Journal*, vol. 348, article g226, 2014.

[39] D. G. R. Evans, S. L. Ingham, A. Baildam et al., "Contralateral mastectomy improves survival in women with *BRCA1/2*-associated breast cancer," *Breast Cancer Research and Treatment*, vol. 140, no. 1, pp. 135–142, 2013.

[40] T. C. van Sprundel, M. K. Schmidt, M. A. Rookus et al., "Risk reduction of contralateral breast cancer and survival after contralateral prophylactic mastectomy in *BRCA1* or *BRCA2* mutation carriers," *British Journal of Cancer*, vol. 93, no. 3, pp. 287–292, 2005.

[41] S. B. Zeichner, A. L. Ruiz, N. J. Markward, and E. Rodriguez, "Improved long-term survival with contralateral prophylactic mastectomy among young women," *Asian Pacific Journal of Cancer Prevention*, vol. 15, no. 3, pp. 1155–1162, 2014.

[42] I. Bedrosian, C. Y. Hu, and G. J. Chang, "Population-based study of mastectomy and survival outcomes of breast cancer patients," *Journal of the National Cancer Institute*, vol. 102, no. 6, pp. 401–409, 2010.

[43] P. R. Portschy, K. M. Kuntz, and T. M. Tuttle, "Survival outcomes after contralateral prophylactic mastectomy: a decision analysis," *Journal of the National Cancer Institute*, vol. 106, no. 8, Article ID dju160, 2014.

[44] T. A. King, R. Sakr, S. Patil et al., "Clinical management factors contribute to the decision for contralateral prophylactic mastectomy," *Journal of Clinical Oncology*, vol. 29, no. 16, pp. 2158–2164, 2011.

[45] A. Ashfaq, L. J. McGhan, B. A. Pockaj et al., "Impact of breast reconstruction on the decision to undergo contralateral prophylactic mastectomy," *Annals of Surgical Oncology*, vol. 21, no. 9, pp. 2934–2940, 2014.

[46] M. E. Miller, T. Czechura, B. Martz et al., "Operative risks associated with contralateral prophylactic mastectomy: a single institution experience," *Annals of Surgical Oncology*, vol. 20, no. 13, pp. 4113–4120, 2013.

[47] M. A. Crosby, P. B. Garvey, J. C. Selber et al., "Reconstructive outcomes in patients undergoing contralateral prophylactic mastectomy," *Plastic and Reconstructive Surgery*, vol. 128, no. 5, pp. 1025–1033, 2011.

[48] W.-B. Zhou, X.-A. Liu, J.-C. Dai, and S. Wang, "Meta-analysis of sentinel lymph node biopsy at the time of prophylactic mastectomy of the breast," *Canadian Journal of Surgery*, vol. 54, no. 5, pp. 300–306, 2011.

[49] R. E. Mansel, L. Fallowfield, M. Kissin et al., "Randomized multicenter trial of sentinel node biopsy versus standard axillary treatment in operable breast cancer: the ALMANAC trial," *Journal of the National Cancer Institute*, vol. 98, no. 9, pp. 599–609, 2006.

[50] N. K. Kuwajerwala, N. S. Dekhne, P. A. Pentiak et al., "Sentinel lymph node biopsy in contralateral prophylactic mastectomy: are we overtreating? Experience at a tertiary care hospital," *Clinical Breast Cancer*, vol. 13, no. 4, pp. 287–291, 2013.

[51] V. R. Grann, P. R. Patel, J. S. Jacobson et al., "Comparative effectiveness of screening and prevention strategies among BRCA1/2-affected mutation carriers," *Breast Cancer Research and Treatment*, vol. 125, no. 3, pp. 837–847, 2011.

[52] D. Schrag, K. M. Kuntz, J. E. Garber, and J. C. Weeks, "Life expectancy gains from cancer prevention strategies for women with breast cancer and BRCA1 or BRCA2 mutations," *Journal of the American Medical Association*, vol. 283, no. 5, pp. 617–624, 2000.

[53] B. Zendejas, J. P. Moriarty, J. O'Byrne, A. C. Degnim, D. R. Farley, and J. C. Boughey, "Cost-effectiveness of contralateral prophylactic mastectomy versus routine surveillance in patients with unilateral breast cancer," *Journal of Clinical Oncology*, vol. 29, no. 22, pp. 2993–3000, 2011.

[54] A. A. Deshmukh, S. B. Cantor, M. A. Crosby et al., "Cost of contralateral prophylactic mastectomy," *Annals of Surgical Oncology*, vol. 21, no. 9, pp. 2823–2830, 2014.

[55] A. Roberts, M. Habibi, and K. D. Frick, "Cost-effectiveness of contralateral prophylactic mastectomy for prevention of contralateral breast cancer," *Annals of Surgical Oncology*, vol. 21, no. 7, pp. 2209–2217, 2014.

[56] S. T. Hawley, R. Jagsi, M. Morrow et al., "Social and clinical determinants of contralateral prophylactic mastectomy," *JAMA Surgery*, vol. 149, no. 6, pp. 582–589, 2014.

[57] A. Abbott, N. Rueth, S. Pappas-Varco, K. Kuntz, E. Kerr, and T. Tuttle, "Perceptions of contralateral breast cancer: an overestimation of risk," *Annals of Surgical Oncology*, vol. 18, no. 11, pp. 3129–3136, 2011.

[58] H. Beesley, C. Holcombe, S. L. Brown, and P. Salmon, "Risk, worry and cosmesis in decision-making for contralateral risk-reducing mastectomy: analysis of 60 consecutive cases in a specialist breast unit," *The Breast*, vol. 22, no. 2, pp. 179–184, 2013.

[59] J. A. Murphy, T. D. Milner, and J. M. O'Donoghue, "Contralateral risk-reducing mastectomy in sporadic breast cancer," *The Lancet Oncology*, vol. 14, no. 7, pp. e262–e269, 2013.

23

Myxoid Liposarcoma: Prognostic Factors and Metastatic Pattern in a Series of 148 Patients Treated at a Single Institution

Francesco Muratori ⑩,[1] Leonardo Bettini,[1] Filippo Frenos,[1] Nicola Mondanelli,[1] Daniela Greto,[2] Lorenzo Livi,[2] Alessandro Franchi,[3] Giuliana Roselli,[4] Maurizio Scorianz,[1] Rodolfo Capanna,[3] and Domenico Campanacci[1]

[1]Divisione di Ortopedia Oncologica e Ricostruttiva Ospedale, Azienda Universitaria Ospedaliera Careggi Firenze, Firenze, Italy
[2]Dipartimento di Radioterapia Azienda Ospedaliera Universitaria Careggi, Firenze, Italy
[3]Dipartimento di Ricerca Traslazionale e delle Nuove Tecnologie in Medicina e Chirurgia, Università di Pisa, Pisa, Italy
[4]Divisione di Radiologia Ospedale, Azienda Universitaria Ospedaliera Careggi Firenze, Firenze, Italy

Correspondence should be addressed to Francesco Muratori; fmuratori@inwind.it

Academic Editor: C. H. Yip

Objectives. The authors reported a retrospective study on myxoid liposarcomas (MLs), evaluating factors that may influence overall survival (OS), local recurrence-free survival (LRFS), metastasis-free survival (MFS), and analyzing the metastatic pattern. *Methods.* 148 MLs were analyzed. The sites of metastases were investigated. *Results.* Margins ($p = 0.002$), grading ($p = 0,0479$), and metastasis ($p < 0,0001$) were significant risk factors affecting overall survival (OS). Type of presentation ($p = 0.0243$), grading ($p = 0,0055$), margin ($p = 0.0001$), and local recurrence (0.0437) were risk factors on metastasis-free survival (MFS). Authors did not observe statistically significant risk factors for local recurrence-free survival (LRFS) and reported 55% extrapulmonary metastases and 45% pulmonary metastases. *Conclusion.* Margins, grading, presentation, local recurrence, and metastasis were prognostic factors. Extrapulmonary metastases were more frequent in myxoid liposarcoma.

1. Introduction

Liposarcoma is one of the most common sarcomas found in adults [1, 2] and it can be defined as a mesenchymal malignancy characterized by adipocyte differentiation. Different forms of liposarcoma are described: atypical lipomatous tumor/well differentiated (ALT/WD), dedifferentiated liposarcoma (DDLs), myxoid liposarcoma (MLs), and pleomorphic liposarcoma (PLs) [2–5].

Myxoid liposarcoma is the second most common subtype (MLs). It accounts for 15–20% of liposarcomas and represents about 5% of all soft tissue sarcomas in adults. Histologically MLs show a continuous spectrum of lesions with low grade forms and others poorly differentiated round cells forms [2].

MLs presents the recurrent translocation $t(12;16)(q13;p11)$ that results in *FUS-DDIT3* gene fusion, present in >95% of cases. In the remaining cases, a variant $t(12;22)(q13;q12)$ is present in which *DDIT3* (also known as *CHOP*) fuses instead with *EWSR1*, a gene that is highly related to *FUS*. They have a peak incidence in the fourth and fifth decade of life, in particular on the lower extremities and buttock [2, 6, 7].

Another feature that distinguishes the MLs than other liposarcomas is the tendency to metastasize in unusual regions correlated to worst prognosis and more precisely where fat tissue is present as the trunk, extremities, bone, retroperitoneal site, the chest wall, the pleura, and pericardium [8–11].

Factors affecting the prognosis in MLs include age at diagnosis, tumor size, tumor grade, depth of tumor, and surgical margins [12–16]. Differentiation, necrosis, mitotic rate, proliferation index (MIB-1, Ki-67 immunostain), and overexpression of P53 represent morphological prognostic factors in MLs [12, 13, 16]. Surgical excision with or without radiation therapy is the treatment of choice in the localized MLs. Chemotherapy is generally reserved for patients with high risk disease such as high grade, deep sited tumor, tumor size > 5 cm, and positive surgical margins.

The aim of our retrospective study was to evaluate factors that may influence overall survival (OS), local recurrence-free survival (LRFS), and metastasis-free survival (MFS) in a series of 148 patients with MLs treated in a single center. We analyzed the metastatic pattern of MLs and the propensity to give extrapulmonary metastases to define a proper clinic and imaging pathway.

2. Materials and Methods

We retrospectively reviewed histological and clinical records of 148 patients treated between 1994 and 2015. The mean age was 49 years (16–82), 142 (96%) liposarcomas localized in the limbs and 6 (4%) in the trunk.

All data collected included patient characteristics (age, gender), tumor characteristics (site, size, clinical symptoms, stage, and histology), the diagnostic and therapeutic procedures (type of biopsy, type of surgery, margins, neoadjuvant, and adjuvant therapy), and clinical outcome.

The data were obtained from the patient's medical records. Local recurrence and distant metastasis after treatment were recorded. Each patient underwent anamnestic collection of his medical history, physical examination, and routine blood tests; electrocardiogram and chest X-ray were obtained. Considering that X-ray or CT were not useful to identify the features and the edges of the primary tumor, MRI was performed in most patients. MRI was particularly useful in defining certain characteristics such as homogeneity, necrosis, hemorrhagic areas, the local spread of the disease (size), and tumor stages. Chest CT scan, bone scan, or PET (from 2009) was performed preoperatively.

At diagnosis, all patients had a localized soft tissue sarcoma in absence of metastases.

Histological diagnosis was confirmed by open incisional biopsy, ultrasound needle biopsy, or previous inadvertent excision performed at other centers. All available histologic slides were reviewed and tumors were graded according to WHO 2013 classification of soft tissue sarcomas [2]. High grade ("round cell") areas were characterized by solid sheets of back-to-back primitive round cells with a high nuclear to cytoplasmic ratio, with no intervening myxoid stroma [2]. If these areas represented more than 5% of the tumor, this was considered as high grade. FISH for *DDIT3* was performed in dubious forms of high grade MLs for the differential diagnosis with other soft tissue sarcomas.

Following the initial work-up the surgical approach was the main treatment that attempts to get wide margins. When the tumor was adjacent to critical structures such as nerves, blood vessels, or bones, a planned marginal surgery has been accepted.

Radiotherapy (RT) in preoperative or postoperative setting was performed in patients with high grade disease or tumor size > 5 cm and deep sited tumors or in case of close/positive margins.

External beam radiotherapy was delivered with 6–10 MeV photons; Gtv (Gross Tumor Volume) was obtained contouring the surgical bed or the gross tumor in case of preoperative RT on T1 weighted MRI images, CTV (clinical target Volume) derived from an expansion of 1.5 cm radially, and 4 cm longitudinally from the GTV, and finally 0.5 cm were added to the CTV to obtain the PTV (planning target volume). There was a total dose of 50 Gy and 60 Gy in preoperative and postoperative setting, respectively.

A standard fraction schedule was used: 2 Gy per fraction, 5 days a week.

Chemotherapy was performed in patients with more than two of these unfavourable prognostic factors: high grade disease, tumor size > 5 cm, deep sited tumors, and positive surgical margins. Chemotherapy consisted of three or five cycles of epirubicin (60 mg/m2, Days 1-2) and ifosfamide (3 g/m2, Days 1–3) administered every 21 days.

The patients were followed every 3 months for the first 2 years, every 4 months during 3rd year, every 6 months for 4th-5th years, and annually from 6th to 10th year.

The statistical analysis was performed with MedCalc software version 16.8.4. Values of $p \leq 0,05$ were considered statistically significant. All variables were analyzed for their impact on overall survival, local recurrence-free survival, and metastasis-free survival with a follow-up of 5 and 10 years. In univariate analysis of the overall survival estimates, local recurrence-free survival and metastasis-free survival were calculated according to the method of Kaplan-Meier.

The comparison of survival curves calculated was performed by the log-rank test media. The hazard ratios and confidence intervals (95%) were calculated using the Cox hazard test.

3. Results

Our data included 103 (70%) primitive liposarcomas, 26 (17%) local recurrences of primitive liposarcoma, and 19 (13%) radicalizations of liposarcoma treated elsewhere. The locations were the lower extremities in 129 (87%) cases, the upper limb in 13 (9%) cases, and trunk in 6 (4%) cases. Specifically 5 (3%) liposarcomas were localized at the muscles of the shoulder, 3 at the arm, 5 at the elbow and distal to the elbow, 10 in pelvic muscles, 76 in the thigh, and 43 in the knee and distal to the knee. Six liposarcomas were localized in the muscle of the trunk. The preoperative MRI showed size > to 10 cm in 47 (32%) patients, between 5 and 10 cm in 67 (45%) patients, and <5 cm in 34 (23%) patients (Table 1).

100 (68%) tumors were classified low grade (<5% round cells) and 48 (32%) high grade (>5% round cells).

At the final histology 105 (71%) MLs were treated with radical or wide surgery, 41 (28%) with marginal surgery, and 2 (1%) with intralesional excision. The preoperative radiotherapy was performed in 41 MLs (14 cases with size > 10 cm, 18 cases between 5 and 10 cm, and 9 cases with dimensions < 5); the postoperative radiotherapy was performed in 63 patients (14 < 5 cm, 32 between 5 and 10 cm, and 17 > 10 cm) of which 17 patients had marginal or compromised margins at histological examination and in 30 patients with high grade MLs (Table 2).

Chemotherapy was administered in 45 MLs patients with aggressive histological type, 25 neoadjuvant chemotherapy, and 29 postoperative chemotherapy (Table 2).

TABLE 1: Main features.

Characteristics	N°	%
Patients	148	100
Presentation:		
Primary	103	70
Local recurrence	26	17
Radicalization	19	13
Grading:		
Low grade (<5% round cell)	100	68
High grade (>5% round cell)	48	32
Site:		
Lower limb	129	87
Upper limb	13	9
Trunk	6	4
Size:		
>10 cm	47	32
5–10 cm	67	45
<5 cm	34	23

TABLE 2: Surgical margins, radiotherapy, chemotherapy, local recurrence, and metastasis.

	Wide/radical	Marginal	Intralesional
Margin	105	41	2
	Preoperative		Postoperative
Radiotherapy	41		63
Chemotherapy	Neoadjuvant		Adjuvant
	25		29
Local recurrence	15 (10%)	8 (wide/radical surgery),	7 (marginal surgery)
Metastasis	20 (14%)	7 (wide/radical surgery),	15 (marginal surgery)
Site metastasis	55% extrapulmonary, 45% pulmonary (9 lung, 2 liver, 5 spine, 1 peritoneum, 1 kidney, 1 dorsal soft tissue, and 1 chest wall)		

The average follow-up was 73 months (range 6–257); 76 patients had a greater than 5-year follow-up.

4. Local Recurrence

We observed 15 (10%) local recurrences with mean free interval of 29 months (range 1–81 months).

Eight MLs treated with radical or wide excision developed local recurrence, 3 with size > 10 cm, 3 with size > 5 cm, and only 2 with sizes < 5 cm. A patient with local recurrence underwent amputation for involvement of neurovascular bundle, six patients were treated with excision, and one patient was lost.

Seven MLs treated with marginal excision developed local recurrence, 4 with size > 10 cm, 2 with size > 5 cm, and 1 with size < 5 cm. Five local recurrences were treated with excision and 2 with amputation for involvement of neurovascular bundle.

No patients treated with intralesional surgery developed local recurrence.

We did not observe statistically significant risk factors for the local recurrence-free survival (LRFS) (Table 4).

LRFS was 89% at 5 years and 86% at 10 years.

5. Metastasis

Twenty MLs (14%), 7 MLs treated with wide resection and 13 with marginal surgery, developed metastases. The sites of metastases were 9 lung, 2 liver, 5 spine, 1 chest wall, 1 peritoneum, 1 kidney, and 1 dorsal soft tissue

One patient treated with intralesional excision died after 3 months, while one patient with MLs (size > 5 cm) treated with intralesional excision and postoperative radiation therapy has not developed local recurrence and metastases after 142 months of follow-up.

Margins ($p = 0.0001$), grading ($p = 0,0055$) (Figure 4), type of presentation ($p = 0,0243$) (Figure 6), and local recurrence ($p = 0,0437$) (Figure 5) are risk factors on metastasis-free survival (MFS) (Table 5).

Five MLs with local recurrences developed distant metastases.

MFS was 85% at 5 years and 82% 10 years.

6. Overall Survival

Statistical analysis indicates margins ($p = 0.002$) (Figure 1) and grading ($p = 0.0479$) (Figure 2) are a risk factor on overall survival (OS) and the appearance of metastases is a highly significant Factor ($p < 0.0001$) (Figure 3) (Table 3).

OS was 90% at 5 years and 85%, respectively, at 10 years.

7. Multivariate Analysis

In multivariate analysis for MFS only the margins ($p = 0.0004$) was statistically significant, unlike the type of presentation ($p = 0.0906$) and the event local recurrence ($p = 0.0821$). In the multivariate analysis for OS only metastasis was statistically significant ($p < 0,0001$), unlike margins ($p = 0,1039$).

8. Discussion

The study reports the outcome in terms of recurrence-free survival, metastasis-free survival, and overall survival, in a series of 148 patients with MLs diagnosed and treated in a single center over the last 21 years.

Limb salvage with wide margin is the main treatment in soft tissue sarcomas surgery. Amputation is reserved only when neurovascular bundle is involved, in cases of severe tissue impairment caused by radiotherapy and finally in unsolvable postsurgical infectious complications. Our results showed that surgical margins had an impact on metastasis-free survival (MFS) and overall survival (OS) while local recurrence-free survival (LRFS) was not correlated with margins. Inadequate surgical margins increased the risk to develop metastasis ($p = 0,0001$) affecting negatively OS ($p = 0.002$), according to other reported series [12, 13, 17, 18].

TABLE 3: Statistical analysis indicates that margins ($p = 0.002$), grading ($p = 0,0479$), and the metastasis ($p < 0,001$) are risk factors on overall survival (OS).

Variables	Survival at 5 years (%)	Survival at 10 years (%)	p value (LR test)
Overall survival			
Site			
Upper limb	92	73	
Lower limb	89	86	0,6215
Trunk	100	100	
Size			
<5 cm	81	81	
5–10 cm	95	88	0,4268
>10 cm	89	89	
Grading, round cell (RC)			
Low (RC < 5%)	95	87	0,0479
High (RC > 5%)	80	80	
Margin			
Wide/radical	96	92	
Marginal	76	66	0,002
Intralesional	50	50	
Presentation			
Primitive	91	91	
Local Recurrence	78	72	0,0755
Radicalization	100	80	
LR			
No	92	86	0,2821
Yes	76	76	
RT			
No	90	90	0,7921
Yes	90	85	
CHT			
No	94	87	0,1766
Yes	83	83	
Metastases			
No	98	98	<0,0001
Yes	42	22	

TABLE 4: Statistical analysis shows no significant risk factors for the local recurrence-free survival (LRFS).

Variables	Survival at 5 years (%)	Survival at 10 years (%)	p value (LR test)
Local recurrence-free survival			
Site			
Upper limb	91	91	
Lower limb	89	85	0,5852
Trunk	67	67	
Size			
<5 cm	97	82	
5–10 cm	91	91	0,2883
>10 cm	77	77	
Grading, round cell (RC)			
Low (RC < 5%)	89	87	0,4824
High (RC > 5%)	87	83	
Margin			
Wide/radical	92	88	
Marginal	78	78	0,1085
Intralesional	100	100	
Presentation			
Primitive	87	85	
Local recurrence	86	78	0,2061
Radicalization	100	100	
RT			
No	94	81	0,9303
Yes	88	86	
CHT			
No	90	88	0,2035
Yes	85	81	

Surgical excision should be carefully planned by experienced surgeons considering the areas in proximity of vascular structures, nerves, and bone [19, 20]. The treatment of MLs in facilities not specialized in cancer care is an important risk factor for local recurrence. Lemeur reported 23% of local recurrence in a series with six patients treated initially in nonspecialized centers, including 4 managed with intralesional excision; only one had a preoperative MRI and no patient underwent preoperative biopsy [14], stressing the importance of surgical planning in agreement with other authors [12, 13, 17, 18]. Engström et al. reported a 47% recurrence for tumors operated in nonspecialized setting [20]. Chandrasekhar et al. reported 59% of local recurrences on 363 cases treated inadequately [21]. This finding is also confirmed by our data: local recurrence of tumors treated in nonspecialized center in cancer care had a higher risk to develop distant metastases ($p = 0.0243$) (Table 5). In our series we observed 15 recurrences (10.1%) in 8 MLs treated with wide and in 7 with marginal surgery. Local recurrence rate was lower compared to 14% observed by Mayo Clinic group [22] and 21.7% at 5 years observed by Fiore et al. [13]. The low rate of local recurrence in our series can be explained by the fact that 70.2% of patients received prior postoperative radiotherapy. Accordingly Guadagnolo et al. observed 3% of local recurrences in 127 MLs treated with preoperative or postoperative radiation therapy [23]. It was postulated that the effectiveness of radiation therapy in myxoid liposarcomas is related to radiosensitivity of the delicate blood supply, characteristic of this tumor [24]. Hannibal et al. observed a very low rate of local recurrence (4%) in patients with purely myxoid liposarcoma (low grade) treated with wide margins. For these patients, the role of radiation therapy appears more questionable [17].

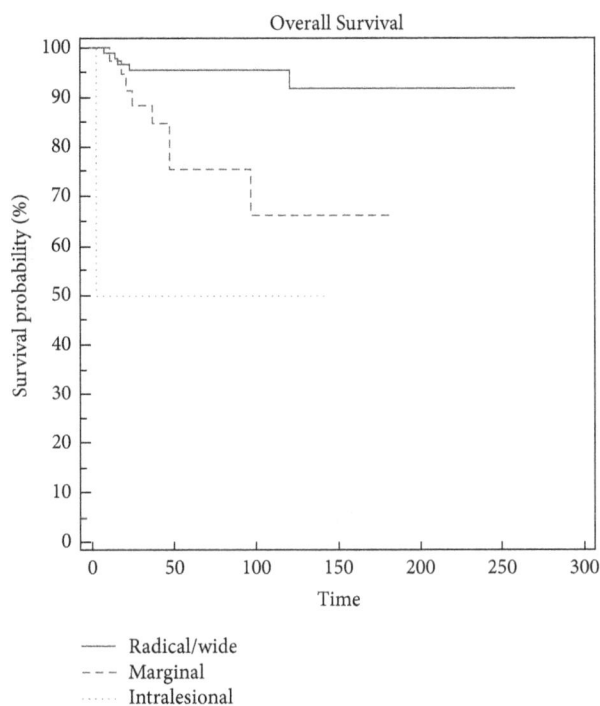

FIGURE 1: Margins represent a significant risk factor ($p = 0,002$) in overall survival (OS).

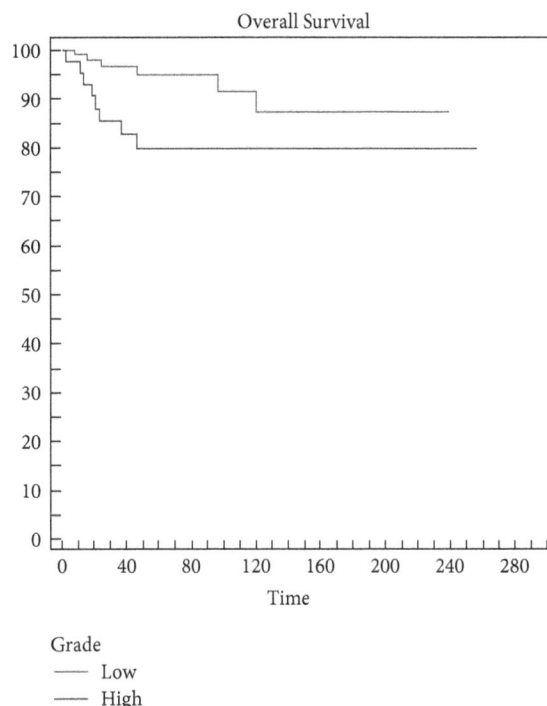

FIGURE 2: Grading is a significant risk factor ($p = 0,0479$) in overall survival (OS).

In several series, the proportion of round cell and the histologic grade represent a prognostic factor influencing the overall survival. This was confirmed by our data: overall survival was 95% at 5 years and 87% at 10 years for MLs with round cells < 5% and 80% at 5 years and 80% at 10 years for MLs with round cells > 5%. Fiore et al. reported 93% overall survival for patients with MLs including round cell forms [13]. Haniball et al. reported a dramatically worse 5-year survival of 58% [17] highlighting that round cell > 5% increases the risk of local recurrence by more than 3 times and concluding that this subgroup of patients should primarily be treated by radiotherapy and chemotherapy. Dalal found an overall survival rate of 92% at 5 years for patients with round cells < 5% compared to 74% of patients with round cells > 5% [25].

The role of chemotherapy in patients with soft tissue sarcomas has been extensively investigated [26] and several studies highlighted the potential sensitivity of liposarcoma to chemotherapy [23, 26–28]. Given the high risk of developing metastases, high grade MLs are suitable to chemotherapy and to new experimental protocols.

Tumoral site (upper limb, lower limb, and trunk) did not result in a significant risk factor, even though the few number of patients with trunk localization could have hampered statistical significance.

Tumor size is generally considered a prognostic factor for soft tissue sarcomas. Several studies have reported that larger tumors > 10 cm are associated with a poor prognosis [19, 20, 22, 29]. Size did not represent a significant prognostic factors in our series.

Local recurrence in our series was associated with an increased risk to develop metastases ($p = 0.0437$) and death

due to cancer. Five patients who developed early local recurrence, simultaneously or subsequently developed metastases and all died. Early local recurrence is generally considered a poor prognostic indicator [19].

According to other authors, we observed a high rate of extrapulmonary metastases in MLs. Metastatic spread involved the lungs in 45% of cases and extrapulmonary sites in 55% of cases. Estourgie reported extrapulmonary metastases in 55% of patients with metastatic disease and recommended to follow up the patients with regular CT scan of the abdomen and pelvis [11]. Guadagnolo et al. reported 78% of metastasis localized in extrapulmonary sites, of which 48% in retroperitoneal space [23]. Several other authors found a high rate of extrapulmonary metastases in MLs, ranging from 41% to 77% [10, 12, 13, 18]. From these reports, common sites of metastases were the retroperitoneum, the abdominal and thoracic wall, and the abdominal cavity. Schwab et al. reported the skeleton as the most frequent site of metastasis, identifying 8 patients with skeletal lesions in a population of 184 MLs (4.3%). In this series, more than half of metastases (56%) were skeletal lesions, in particular localized to the spine, 70% in the absence of pulmonary localizations [8].

The reason of the tendency of MLs to metastatic spread in extrapulmonary sites is not clear. Ogose et al. speculated that the abundance of fat tissue in metastatic sites, such as the subcutaneous tissue, retroperitoneum, bone marrow, and the epidural space might favour the metastatic seeding [30].

An important issue is to assess whether extrapulmonary lesions are metastatic lesions or different sites of metachronous disease. Smith et al., analyzing the genomic rearrangement of TLS, CHOP, or EWS in six patients, confirmed the

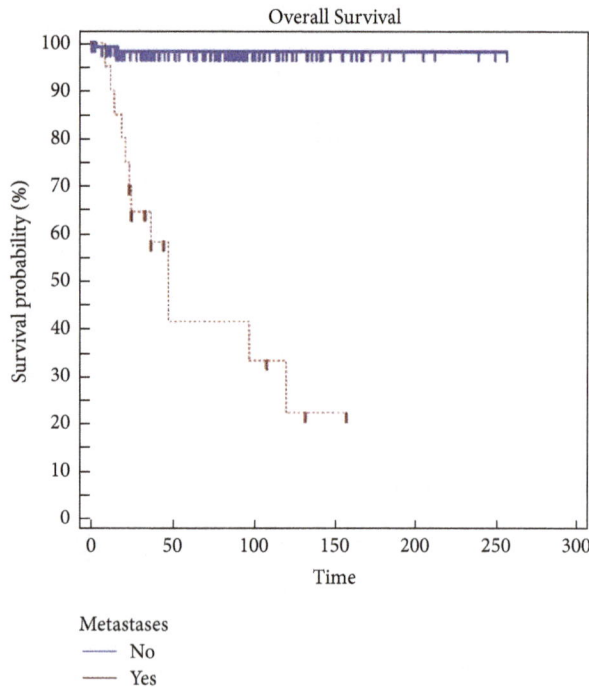

FIGURE 3: Metastasis is a high significant risk factor ($p < 0,0001$) in overall survival (OS).

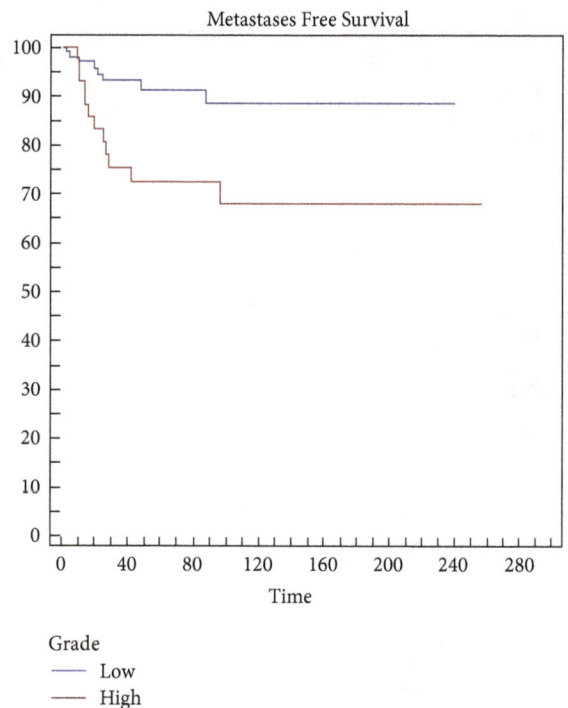

FIGURE 4: Grading is a significant risk factor ($p = 0,0055$) in metastasis-free survival (MFS).

monoclonal origin of myxoid multifocal liposarcoma. They concluded that this unusual clinical phenomenon may represent a pattern of hematogenous metastatic spreading to other soft tissue sites, with cells unable to colonize the lungs [31].

Some authors highlighted an influence in the prognosis of some factors such as adipophilin, a well-known adipogenesis marker that appears early in the differentiation process [32], perhaps suggesting that MLs differentiate beyond the initial stage before the interruption of complete adipocyte maturation. Hoffmann et al. observed a significantly higher level of adipophilin in high grade than in low grade MLs, suggesting a role in the progression of the disease [33]. Other factors which are particularly expressed in MLs are the adipogenesis regulator PPARγ [34] and CXCR4 (chemokine receptor), overexpressed in high grade tumors [35]. Overexpression of p53 in MLs [12] correlated with a poor chemotherapeutic response. The PDGFR-βexpression in the MLs was found most frequently in metastatic forms (especially to bone) than in localized lesions [36].

An issue is what kind of imaging to use during follow-up of MLs for an early detection of extrapulmonary metastases. Some authors reported the failure of both PET scan and bone scan to detect metastases of myxoid liposarcoma [8]. Other options are total body CT and MRI who remain the most reliable screening tools. In particular, total body MRI may reveal the presence of extrapulmonary metastases at an early stage, when they are still not symptomatic, without radiation exposure.

9. Conclusion

Our study confirmed that inadequate surgical margins in MLs represent a significant risk factor to develop metastases ($p = 0.001$) with consequent negative influence on overall survival ($p = 0.002$). Surgical excision of MLs should be performed in specialized centers by experienced sarcoma surgeons. Inadequate primary treatment more frequently leads to local recurrence and metastasis ($p = 0.0243$). Local recurrences increase the risk to develop metastases ($p = 0.0437$) and metastatic event has a highly significant impact on overall survival ($p < 0.001$). Grading affects OS ($p = 0,0479$) and MFS ($p = 0,0055$). A multidisciplinary approach to MLs is recommended, considering combining surgery to radiation therapy and/or chemotherapy in selected cases. The awareness of the high incidence of extrapulmonary metastases, especially in fat-rich areas, should lead to clinical and imaging investigation such as total body MRI, aiming to an early diagnosis.

Authors' Contributions

Francesco Muratori designed, wrote, and revised the study. Domenico Campanacci, Nicola Mondanelli, Giuliana Roselli, and Rodolfo Capanna contributed to review of the study. Lorenzo Livi and Daniela Greto revised medical oncological results. Alessandro Franchi revised histological and pathological results. Statistical analyses were run by Leonardo Bettini and Filippo Frenos. Maurizio Scorianz revised graphic format of figures. All the authors interpreted the results,

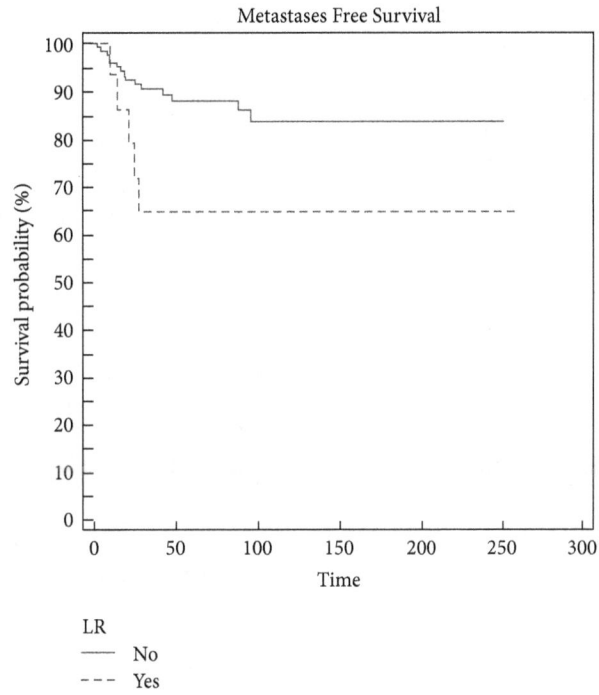

FIGURE 5: Local recurrence is a significant risk factor ($p = 0{,}0437$) in metastasis-free survival (MFS).

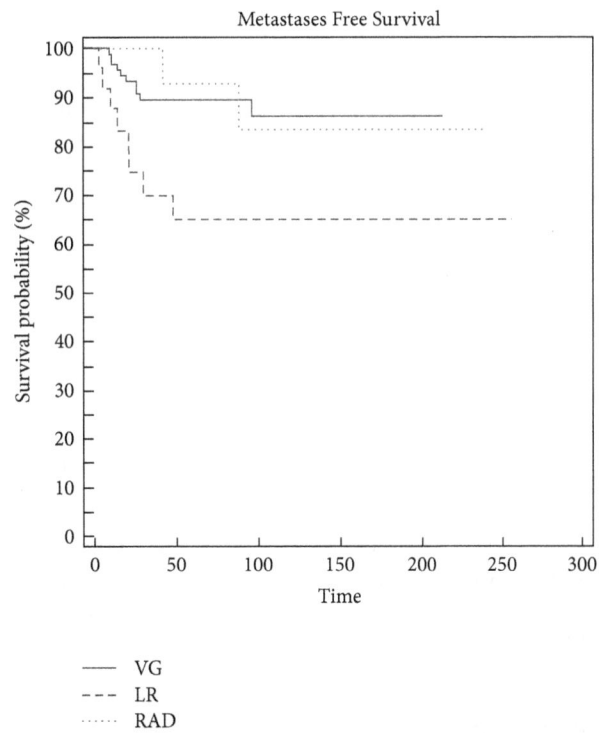

FIGURE 6: Presentation is a significant risk factor ($p = 0{,}0243$) in metastasis-free survival (MFS).

TABLE 5: Statistical analysis indicates margins ($p = 0.0001$), grading (0,0055), type of presentation ($p = 0.0243$), and local recurrence (0.0437) as risk factors on metastasis-free survival (MFS).

Variables	Metastases-free survival		
	Survival at 5 years (%)	Survival at 10 years (%)	p value (LR test)
Site			
Upper limb	72	72	
Lower limb	86	82	0,4542
Trunk	100	100	
Size			
<5 cm	86	86	
5–10 cm	88	86	0,2716
>10 cm	80	70	
Grading, round cell (RC)			
Low (RC < 5%)	91	88	0,0055
High (RC > 5%)	72	68	
Margin			
Wide/radical	94	88	
Marginal	62	62	0,0001
Intralesional	100	100	
Presentation			
Primitive	90	86	
Local recurrence	65	65	0,0243
Radicalization	93	84	
LR			
No	88	84	0,0437
Yes	65	65	
RT			
No	82	82	0,9645
Yes	86	82	
CHT			
No	87	84	0,2363
Yes	81	76	

critically revised the manuscript, and approved the final version.

References

[1] K. J. Fritchie, J. R. Goldblum, R. R. Tubbs et al., "The expanded histologic spectrum of myxoid liposarcoma with an emphasis on newly described patterns: Implications for diagnosis on small biopsy specimens," *American Journal of Clinical Pathology*, vol. 137, no. 2, pp. 229–239, 2012.

[2] C. D. Fletcher, P. Hogendoorn, and F. Mertens, *WHO Classification of Tumours of Soft Tissue and Bone*, IARC Press, Lyon, France, 4th edition, 2013.

[3] J. J. Lewis, D. Leung, J. M. Woodruff, and M. F. Brennan, "Retroperitoneal soft-tissue sarcoma: Analysis of 500 patients treated and followed at a single institution," *Annals of Surgery*, vol. 228, no. 3, pp. 355–365, 1998.

[4] D. C. Linehan, J. J. Lewis, D. Leung, and M. F. Brennan, "Influence of Biologic Factors and Anatomic Site in Completely Resected Liposarcoma," *Journal of Clinical Oncology*, vol. 18, no. 8, pp. 1637–1643, 2000.

[5] D. McCormick, T. Mentzel, A. Beham, and C. D. M. Fletcher, "Dedifferentiated liposarcoma: clinicopathologic analysis of 32 cases suggesting a better prognostic subgroup among pleomorphic sarcomas," *The American Journal of Surgical Pathology*, vol. 18, no. 12, pp. 1213–1223, 1994.

[6] L. Panagopoulos, N. Mandahl, F. Mitelman, and P. Aman, "Two distinct FUS breakpoint clusters in myxoid liposarcoma and acute myeloid leukemia with the translocations t(12;16) and t(16;21)," *Oncogene*, vol. 11, no. 6, pp. 1133–1137, 1995.

[7] J. Pérez-Losada, M. Sánchez-Martín, M. A. Rodríguez-García et al., "Liposarcoma initiated by FUS/TLS-CHOP: The FUS/TLS domain plays a critical role in the pathogenesis of liposarcoma," *Oncogene*, vol. 19, no. 52, pp. 6015–6022, 2000.

[8] J. H. Schwab, P. Boland, T. Guo et al., "Skeletal metastases in myxoid liposarcoma: An unusual pattern of distant spread," *Annals of Surgical Oncology*, vol. 14, no. 4, pp. 1507–1514, 2007.

[9] C. D. M. Fletcher, K. K. Unni, and F. Mertens, "Atypical lipomatous tumour/Well differentiated liposarcoma, Dedifferentiated liposarcoma, Myxoidliposarcoma, Pleomorphic liposarcoma," in *Pathology & Genetics, Tumours of Soft Tissue and Bone*, P. Kleihues, Ed., pp. 35–46, IARC Press, Lyon, France, 2002.

[10] E. Y. Cheng, D. S. Springfield, and H. J. Mankin, "Frequent incidence of extrapulmonary sites of initial metastasis in patients with liposarcoma," *Cancer*, vol. 75, no. 5, pp. 1120–1127, 1995.

[11] S. H. Estourgie, G. P. Nielsen, and M. J. Ott, "Metastatic patterns of extremity myxoid liposarcoma and their outcome," *Journal of Surgical Oncology*, vol. 80, no. 2, pp. 89–93, 2002.

[12] C. R. Antonescu, S. J. Tschernyavsky, R. Decuseara et al., "Prognostic impact of P53 status, TLS-CHOP fusion transcript structure, and histological grade in myxoid liposarcoma: a molecular and clinicopathologic study of 82 cases," *Clinical Cancer Research*, vol. 7, no. 12, pp. 3977–3987, 2001.

[13] M. Fiore, F. Grosso, S. Lo Vullo et al., "Myxoid/round cell and pleomorphic liposarcomas: prognostic factors and survival in a series of patients treated at a single institution," *Cancer*, vol. 109, no. 12, pp. 2522–2531, 2007.

[14] M. Lemeur, J.-C. Mattei, P. Souteyrand, C. Chagnaud, G. Curvale, and A. Rochwerger, "Prognostic factors for the recurrence of myxoid liposarcoma: 20 cases with up to 8 years follow-up," *Orthopaedics & Traumatology: Surgery & Research*, vol. 101, no. 1, pp. 103–107, 2015.

[15] Y. Nishida, S. Tsukushi, H. Nakashima, and N. Ishiguro, "Clinicopathologic prognostic factors of pure myxoid liposarcoma of the extremities and trunk wall," *Clinical Orthopaedics and Related Research*, vol. 468, no. 11, pp. 3041–3046, 2010.

[16] L.-C. Moreau, R. Turcotte, P. Ferguson et al., "Myxoid\round cell liposarcoma (MRCLS) revisited: An analysis of 418 primarily managed cases," *Annals of Surgical Oncology*, vol. 19, no. 4, pp. 1081–1088, 2012.

[17] J. Haniball, V. P. Sumathi, L.-G. Kindblom et al., "Prognostic factors and metastatic patterns in primary myxoid/round-cell liposarcoma," *Sarcoma*, vol. 2011, Article ID 538085, 2011.

[18] S. E. Ten Heuvel, H. J. Hoekstra, R. J. Van Ginkel, E. Bastiaannet, and A. J. H. Suurmeijer, "Clinicopathologic prognostic factors in myxoid liposarcoma: A retrospective study of 49 patients with long-term follow-up," *Annals of Surgical Oncology*, vol. 14, no. 1, pp. 222–229, 2007.

[19] G. K. Zagars, M. T. Ballo, P. W. T. Pisters et al., "Prognostic factors for patients with localized soft-tissue sarcoma treated with conservation surgery and radiation therapy: an analysis of 1225 patients," *Cancer*, vol. 97, no. 10, pp. 2530–2543, 2003.

[20] K. Engström, P. Bergh, P. Gustafson et al., "Liposarcoma: outcome based on the Scandinavian Sarcoma Group register," *Cancer*, vol. 113, no. 7, pp. 1649–1656, 2008.

[21] C. R. Chandrasekar, H. Wafa, R. J. Grimer, S. R. Carter, R. M. Tillman, and A. Abudu, "The effect of an unplanned excision of a soft-tissue sarcoma on prognosis," *The Journal of Bone and Joint Surgery—British Volume*, vol. 90, no. 2, pp. 203–208, 2008.

[22] S. E. Kilpatrick, J. Doyon, P. F. M. Choong, F. H. Sim, and A. G. Nascimento, "The clinicopathologic spectrum of myxoid and round cell liposarcoma: A study of 95 cases," *Cancer*, vol. 77, no. 8, pp. 1450–1458, 1996.

[23] B. A. Guadagnolo, G. K. Zagars, M. T. Ballo et al., "Excellent Local Control Rates and Distinctive Patterns of Failure in Myxoid Liposarcoma Treated With Conservation Surgery and Radiotherapy," *International Journal of Radiation Oncology Biology Physics*, vol. 70, no. 3, pp. 760–765, 2008.

[24] R. S. A. de Vreeze, D. de Jong, R. L. Haas, F. Stewart, and F. van Coevorden, "Effectiveness of Radiotherapy in Myxoid Sarcomas Is Associated With a Dense Vascular Pattern," *International Journal of Radiation Oncology • Biology • Physics*, vol. 72, no. 5, pp. 1480–1487, 2008.

[25] K. M. Dalal, M. W. Kattan, C. R. Antonescu, M. F. Brennan, and S. Singer, "Subtype specific prognostic nomogram for patients with primary liposarcoma of the retroperitoneum, extremity, or trunk," *Annals of Surgery*, vol. 244, no. 3, pp. 381–389, 2006.

[26] S. R. Patel, M. Andrew Burgess, C. Plager, N. E. Papadopoulos, K. A. Linke, and R. S. Benjamin, "Myxoid liposarcoma. Experience with chemotherapy," *Cancer*, vol. 74, no. 4, pp. 1265–1269, 1994.

[27] R. L. Jones, C. Fisher, O. Al-Muderis, and I. R. Judson, "Differential sensitivity of liposarcoma subtypes to chemotherapy," *European Journal of Cancer*, vol. 41, no. 18, pp. 2853–2860, 2005.

[28] F. Grosso, R. L. Jones, G. D. Demetri et al., "Efficacy of trabectedin (ecteinascidin-743) in advanced pretreated myxoid liposarcomas: a retrospective study," *The Lancet Oncology*, vol. 8, no. 7, pp. 595–602, 2007.

[29] G. Pitson, P. Robinson, D. Wilke et al., "Radiation response: an additional unique signature of myxoid liposarcoma," *International Journal of Radiation Oncology • Biology • Physics*, vol. 60, no. 2, pp. 522–526, 2004.

[30] A. Ogose, T. Hotta, Y. Inoue, S. Sakata, R. Takano, and S. Yamamura, "Myxoid liposarcoma metastatic to the thoracic epidural space without bone involvement: report of two cases," *Japanese Journal of Clinical Oncology*, vol. 31, no. 9, pp. 447–449, 2001.

[31] T. A. Smith, K. A. Easley, and J. R. Goldblum, "Myxoid/round cell liposarcoma of the extremities: A clinicopathologic study of 29 cases with particular attention to extent of round cell liposarcoma," *The American Journal of Surgical Pathology*, vol. 20, no. 2, pp. 171–180, 1996.

[32] H. W. Heid, R. Moll, I. Schewetlick, and etal., "Adipophilin is a specific marker of lipid accumation in diverse cell types and diseases," *Cell Tissue Res*, p. 2, 2012.

[33] A. Hoffman, M. P. Ghadimi, E. G. Demicco et al., "Localized and metastatic myxoid/round cell liposarcoma," *Cancer*, vol. 119, no. 10, pp. 1868–1877, 2013.

[34] H. Cheng, J. Dodge, E. Mehl et al., Validation of immature adiogenic status and identification of prognostic biomarkers in myxidliposarcoma using tissue microarray. Hum Pathol. 2009; 40:1244-1251.

[35] R. H. Kim, B. D. Li, and Q. D. Chu, "The Role of Chemokine Receptor CXCR4 in the Biologic Behavior of Human Soft Tissue Sarcoma," *Sarcoma*, vol. 2011, pp. 1–4, 2011.

[36] A. Olofsson, H. Willén, M. Göransson et al., "Abnormal expression of cell cycle regulators in FUS-CHOP carrying liposarcomas," *International Journal of Oncology*, 2004.

24

Invasive *Candida* Infection after Upper Gastrointestinal Tract Surgery for Gastric Cancer

Evgeni Brotfain,[1] **Gilbert Sebbag,**[2] **Michael Friger,**[3] **Boris Kirshtein,**[4] **Abraham Borer,**[5] **Leonid Koyfman,**[1] **Dmitry Frank,**[1] **Yoav Bichovsky,**[1] **Jochanan G. Peiser,**[6] **and Moti Klein**[1]

[1]*Department of Anesthesiology and Critical Care, General Intensive Care Unit, Soroka Medical Center, Ben-Gurion University of the Negev, Beer Sheva, Israel*
[2]*Department of General Surgery B, Soroka Medical Center, Ben-Gurion University of the Negev, Beer Sheva, Israel*
[3]*Department of Public Health, Faculty of Health Sciences, Ben-Gurion University of the Negev, Beer Sheva, Israel*
[4]*Department of General Surgery A, Soroka Medical Center, Ben-Gurion University of the Negev, Beer Sheva, Israel*
[5]*Department of Infectious Disease, Soroka Medical Center, Ben-Gurion University of the Negev, Beer Sheva, Israel*
[6]*Department of Medical Management, Soroka Medical Center, Ben-Gurion University of the Negev, Beer Sheva, Israel*

Correspondence should be addressed to Evgeni Brotfain; bem1975@gmail.com

Evgeni Brotfain and Gilbert Sebbag contributed equally to this work.

Academic Editor: S. Curley

Upper gastrointestinal tract (GIT) surgical procedures are more likely to cause nosocomial *Candida peritonitis* than lower GIT procedures and they thus constitute an independent risk factor for mortality. Because of the severity of postsurgical fungal infections complications, intensivists and surgeons need to be extremely aware of their clinical importance in critically ill postsurgical intensive care unit (ICU) patients. We analyzed the clinical and microbiological data of 149 oncologic patients who were hospitalized in the ICU at Soroka Medical Center between January 2010 and January 2015 after undergoing upper GIT surgery for gastric cancer. Invasive fungal infections related to secondary peritonitis following oncologic upper GIT surgery had a higher mortality rate than patients with nonfungal postoperative infectious complications. The presence of gastroesophageal junction leakage and advanced age were found to be independent risk factors for invasive fungal infection after oncologic upper GIT surgery.

1. Introduction

Gastrointestinal tract (GIT) surgery is a major risk factor for secondary peritonitis [1]. Surgical intervention causes this complication by altering the physiologic flora of the GIT and by directly damaging the natural barriers of infection [2]. In the wake of surgical intervention, the GIT is most often colonized by Gram-negative invasive microorganisms. However, under certain postsurgical conditions *Candida* fungi are liable to colonize the peritoneal cavity and cause infection [3]. It is known that upper GIT surgical procedures are more likely to cause nosocomial *Candida peritonitis* than lower GIT procedures [1, 4–6] and consequently upper GIT surgery constitutes an independent risk factor for mortality [4]. Underlying comorbidities, such as immunosuppression,

cancer, the frequently malnourished state of critical care patients, administration of total parenteral nutrition (TPN), and use of intravenous catheters, are additional factors that tend to increase the frequency of *Candida* colonization and peritonitis in oncologic surgical patients undergoing upper GIT surgery [7, 8]. All the above factors when present in oncologic surgical patients undergoing upper GIT surgery significantly increase their risk for developing intra-abdominal *Candida* infections. Importantly, the overall mortality rate is much higher in surgical critically ill patients with intra-abdominal *Candida* infections than in those with purely bacterial infections [9, 10]. Furthermore, postsurgical patients who are critically ill with fungal or nonfungal secondary generalized peritonitis often require repeated laparotomies, which in turn are associated with a high incidence of yeast superinfection in the peritoneal fluid [4, 11]. Because of its severity, intensivists and surgeons need to be extremely aware of the clinical importance of fungal superinfection in critically ill postsurgical intensive care unit (ICU) patients and to pay scrupulous attention to the factors that predispose to these infections.

In the present study, we reviewed and analyzed the clinical and microbiological data of oncologic patients who were hospitalized in the General Intensive Care Unit (GICU) at Soroka Medical Center between January 2010 and January 2015 after having undergone upper GIT surgery for gastric cancer.

2. Patients and Methods

Soroka Medical Center is a 1000-bed tertiary care university teaching hospital located in the city of Beer Sheva in Israel's southern Negev region. We retrospectively collected the clinical and laboratory data on all patients who underwent oncologic upper GI surgery for gastric cancer and who were hospitalized postoperatively in the GICU at the Soroka Medical Center between January 2010 and June 2015. All the clinical data were extracted from the OFEK™ Registry Information System, the Operating Room Registry System, and the Metavision ICU Registry Information System. The study was reviewed and approved by the Human Research and Ethics Committee at Soroka Medical Center (RN 0334-15-SOR).

2.1. Inclusion Criteria. All patients aged ≥ 18 who underwent any type of oncologic upper GIT surgery for gastric cancer between January 2010 and January 2015 and who were hospitalized postoperatively in the GICU at Soroka Medical Center were eligible for inclusion in the study.

2.2. Exclusion Criteria. The following patients were excluded from the study: patients who were immunosuppressed (including those who had undergone preoperative chemo- and/or radiotherapy); patients with chronic and/or recurrent skin or mucosal fungal infections, such as intertrigo/oral candidosis, who were treated with antifungal therapy one month prior to hospital admission or who were known carriers of a fungal infection; and patients who had been hospitalized for more than one month prior to the upper GIT surgical procedure.

2.3. Variables and Measures. We recorded the following parameters: demographic data; the presence or absence of comorbid conditions; the patients' chronic medications; the type of primary surgery undergone by the patients as well as information regarding any reoperations; data on interventional procedures performed postoperatively; and the results of relevant imaging studies. Information regarding laboratory and microbiological studies was also recorded. Clinical data recorded included the patients' diagnoses on admission, the Acute Physiology and Chronic Health Evaluation-II (APACHE II) score, and the Therapeutic Intervention Scoring System (TISS) score. Other recorded parameters included the rate of success in weaning the patients from mechanical ventilation (the number of ventilator-free days);

the therapeutic management of the patients; their nutritional state during their ICU stay; the development of infectious complications; and the intra-ICU and intrahospital mortality rates among the study patients.

2.4. Microbiology. The microbiological data included the results of blood, peritoneal fluid, and pleural fluid cultures sampled during the patients' hospital and ICU admissions. Intra-abdominal infection (peritonitis), bacteremia (non-central line-associated blood stream infection {BSI}), and empyema were diagnosed according to the criteria specified in the international surveillance guidelines of the Centers for Disease Control [12]. An *invasive fungal infection* was defined as a new event of fungemia, fungal peritonitis, or fungal empyema after oncologic upper GIT surgery.

2.5. Definitions. The severity of illness and the presence or absence of multiorgan failure were evaluated using the patients' APACHE II and TISS scores as recorded within 24 hours of ICU admission.

2.6. Study Groups. The patients were divided into two groups. Group 1 comprised oncologic surgical patients who underwent elective upper GIT surgery for gastric cancer and had an uneventful postoperative course. Group 2 comprised oncologic surgical patients who underwent elective upper GIT surgery for gastric cancer and developed new postoperative intra-abdominal infectious complications.

2.7. Statistical Analysis. Data analysis was performed with SPSS (version 18.0 or higher). Data collected in this study was summarized using frequency tables, summary statistics, confidence intervals, and p values as appropriate. Continuous variables were compared by t-tests or analyses of variance. For continuous variables with nonnormal distribution, comparisons were evaluated for significance using the Wilcoxon rank-sum test. For categorical variables, the 95% confidence interval was analyzed using binomial distribution. For continuous variables, the 95% confidence interval was calculated using means and standard errors derived from Student's t-test statistical method.

3. Results

The clinical and laboratory data of 149 patients who underwent oncologic upper GIT surgery for gastric cancer were analyzed. Forty-nine (33%) of the patients developed secondary peritonitis and were hospitalized in our GICU during the study period (Group 2). The remaining one hundred patients (67%) had an uneventful postoperative course (Group 1). The patients' demographic data, their past medical history, and their clinical and nutritional parameters are presented in Table 1. The patients in Group 2 were significantly older than those in Group 1 (p value 0.002, Table 1). The two groups were similar for gender, weight, and type of upper GIT surgery. Underlying diabetes (type II) was more frequent among the Group 2 patients. In contrast, Group 1 included more patients with arterial hypertensive disease (Table 1). There was a significant difference in the

TABLE 1: Patient demographics, underlying conditions, nutritional data, length of ICU, and hospital stay (Group 1: no infectious complications; Group 2: patients who developed documented intra-abdominal infection).

	Group 1 (n = 100)	Group 2 (n = 49)	p value*
Age, years (mean ± SD)	62.67 ± 9.1	72.38 ± 14.2*	0.002
Weight, Kg (mean ± SD)	72.78 ± 12.75	72.85 ± 13.7	0.7
Gender (male)	48/100 (48%)	24/49 (49%)	0.5
Type of upper GIT[a] surgery			
Total gastrectomy	56/100 (56%)	26/49 (53.1%)	0.8
Partial gastrectomy	44/100 (44%)	23/49 (46.9%)	0.9
Underlying condition (%)			
Without chronic disease	36/100 (36%)	15/49 (30.6%)	0.6
Diabetes mellitus	10/100 (10%)	18/49 (36.7%)*	0.04
CIHD[b]	31/100 (31%)	14/49 (35.8%)	0.5
Hypertension	23/100 (23%)	1/49 (2.04%)*	<0.001
Chronic therapy (%)			
Without chronic therapy	36/100 (36%)	15/49 (30.6%)	0.46
Statins	20/100 (20%)	16/49 (32.6%)	0.04
ACE[c]	44/100 (44%)	18/49 (36.7%)	0.29
TPN (n, %)[d]	27/100 (27%)	36/49 (73.5%)	<0.001
Length of stay (day ± SD)			
ICU length of stay[e] (day, mean ± SD)	1.25 ± 0.67	12.04 ± 1.49	<0.001
Hospital length of stay (day, mean ± SD)	10.84 ± 4.8	32.2 ± 2.4	<0.001

*$p < 0.05$ is considered to be significant; [a]GIT: gastrointestinal tract; [b]CIHD: chronic ischemic heart disease; [c]ACE: angiotensin-converting enzyme. [d]Percent total parenteral nutrition after oncologic upper GIT surgery. [e]Some of the patients from Group 1 were also hospitalized in the GICU for a postoperative observation period.

frequency of chronic statin therapy between the two groups (Table 1). TPN after upper GIT surgery was initiated more often in Group 2 patients than in Group 1 patients (73.5% versus 27%, $p < 0.001$, Table 1). The duration of the patients' admissions, both in the ICU and in the hospital, was significantly longer in the Group 2 patients compared to the Group 1 patients ($p < 0.001$, Table 1).

Table 2 shows demographic data, postoperative infectious complications, and clinical outcome data of Group 2 patients only. All 49 patients in Group 2 had documented intra-abdominal infections (peritonitis). Ten of the 49 patients (20.4%) also had invasive fungal (Candida albicans) infection (Candida peritonitis, n = 5; candidemia, n = 3; Candida empyema, n = 2) on admission to the ICU (Table 2). Importantly, all three cases of candidemia were noncentral line-associated blood stream infection. There was no difference in the demographic data, type of surgery, and past medical history between the patients with and without fungal infections. A large proportion of the patients with nonfungal infections were receiving chronic therapy with ACE inhibitors (Table 2).

Patients with nonfungal and invasive fungal infectious complications had similar APACHE and TISS scores within 24 hours of ICU admission and similar lengths of ICU and hospital admissions (Table 2). Patients with invasive

fungal infection had a higher incidence of intraperitoneal leak documented during surgery compared to patients with nonfungal infections (90% versus 69%, p value 0.01) (Table 2).

In the patients with invasive fungal infection, leakage was more frequently found at the gastroesophageal junction area compared to the patients with nonfungal infections (80% versus 34%, $p < 0.02$, Table 2). In contrast, the patients in the nonfungal subgroup had a higher frequency of leak at the gastrointestinal anastomosis and in the small bowel area (30–34% versus 10%, p 0.01 and 0.02, resp., Table 2). Also, there was a higher frequency of intra-abdominal abscesses and pleural effusions in the patients with invasive fungal complications as compared to those with nonfungal infections (p value 0.006 and 0.04, resp., Table 2).

The ICU mortality rate was much higher in patients with invasive fungal infectious complications compared to those without fungal infection (50% versus 15%, p value 0.03, Table 2).

Microbiological data of the Group 2 patients (Table 3) showed similar culture growth of Streptococcus constellatus and coagulase negative Staphylococcus spp. in the abdominal fluid, the pleural fluid, and the blood in both the nonfungal and the fungal subgroups. In contrast, there was a higher frequency of positive cultures of Gram-negative flora (Escherichia coli, Pseudomonas spp., and Klebsiella spp.)

TABLE 2: Demographic data, postoperative infectious complications, and clinical outcomes endpoints of Group 2 patients divided into nonfungal and invasive fungal subgroups (n, %, mean ± SD).

	Nonfungal (n = 39)	Invasive fungal[a] (n = 10)	p value*
Age, years (mean ± SD)	72.25 ± 14.29	72.9 ± 14.9	0.15
Weight, Kg (mean ± SD)	72.9 ± 12.9	72.6 ± 13.57	0.9
Gender (male)	21/39 (53.8%)	3/10 (30%)	0.4
Type of upper GIT[b] surgery			
Total gastrectomy	22/39 (56.4)	4/10 (40%)	0.61
Partial gastrectomy	17/39 (43.6%)	6/10 (60%)	0.5
Underlying condition (%)			
Without chronic disease	10/39 (25.6%)	5/10 (50%)	0.08
Diabetes mellitus	16/39 (41%)	3/10 (30%)	0.08
CIHD[c]	12/39 (30.7%)	2/10 (20%)	0.16
Hypertension	1/39 (2.5%)	0	NA
Chronic therapy (%)			
Without chronic therapy	10/39 (25.6%)	5/10 (50%)	0.04
Statins	13/39 (33.3%)	3/10 (30%)	0.48
ACE[d]	16/39 (41%)	2/10 (20%)	0.03
Postoperative complications			
Intraperitoneal leak (n, %) (documented)	27/39 (69.2%)	9/10 (90%)	0.01
Leak location (n, %)			
Gastroesophageal junction	8/39 (34.8%)	8/10 (80%)	0.02
Gastrointestinal anastomosis	7/39 (30.4%)	1/10 (10%)	0.01
Duodenum/small bowel	8/39 (34.8%)	1/10 (10%)	0.02
Intra-abdominal abscesses (n, %)	16/39 (41%)	9/10 (90%)	0.006
Presence of pleural effusion (n, %)	4/39 (10.3%)	4/10 (40%)	0.04
Clinical outcome endpoints			
APACHE 24[e] (units, mean ± SD)	24.51 ± 6.06	24.2 ± 5.37	0.67
TISS score 24[e] (units, mean ± SD)	22.48 ± 6.03	22.2 ± 5.37	0.72
ICU length of stay (day, mean ± SD)	11.6 ± 1.5	13.9 ± 1.4	0.65
Hospital length of stay (day, mean ± SD)	34.84 ± 2.6	25.2 ± 1.5	0.11
ICU mortality (%)	6/39 (15.4%)	5/10 (50%)	0.03

*p < 0.05 was found to be statistically significant. [a]Invasive fungal (Candida) complications: Candida peritonitis, candidemia, and Candida empyema. [b]Gastrointestinal tract; [c]CIHD: chronic ischemic heart disease; [d]ACE: angiotensin-converting enzyme. [e]Within 24 hours of ICU admission.

in the abdominal fluid, the pleural fluid, and the blood in patients with nonfungal infectious complications (see Table 3) compared to those with fungal infections.

Patients with invasive fungal infections had a higher creatinine level on admission to the ICU than those with nonfungal infections (1.6 ± 0.2 versus 0.94 ± 0.58, p value 0.01). Other laboratory data did not differ between the fungal and the nonfungal subgroups (Table 3).

No difference was found between the fungal and the nonfungal subgroups in regard to the following therapeutic measures that were implemented while the patients were in the ICU: CT-guided drainage of pleural effusions and abdominal abscesses; nutritional care; administration of steroids; vasopressor therapy; and additional surgical interventions (Table 4).

Table 4 shows the results of multivariate logistic regression analysis of postoperative peritonitis after oncologic

upper GIT surgery. Advanced age, underlying diabetes mellitus, and postoperative TPN treatment were found to be independent risk factors for postoperative secondary peritonitis in patients who underwent oncologic upper GIT surgery (Table 4).

Further multivariate analysis of postoperative invasive fungal infections in the wake of oncologic upper GIT surgery is shown in Table 5. Gastroesophageal junction leak and advanced age were found to be independent predictors for invasive fungal infections after oncologic upper GIT surgery (Table 5).

4. Discussion

Postoperative infectious complications following oncologic gastric surgery are known to be associated with a significant decrease in 5-year overall and relapse-free survival (66% and

TABLE 3: Microbiological data (from intraabdominal fluid, blood, and pleural effusions) and other laboratory parameters of the Group 2 patients during their ICU stay.

	Nonfungal (n = 39)	Invasive fungal[a] (n = 10)	p value[*]
Intraabdominal positive cultures (%):			
No organisms	22/39 (56.4%)	5/10 (50%)	0.59
E. coli	10/39 (25.6%)	2/10 (20%)	0.61
Klebsiella spp.	1/39 (2.6%)	0	NA
Enterococcus spp.	1/39 (2.6%)	0	NA
Staph. aureus	1/39 (2.6%)	0	NA
Staph. coagulase negative	1/39 (2.6%)	0	NA
Streptococcusconstellatus[b]	1/39 (2.6%)	1/10 (10%)	0.17
Pseudomonas spp.	1/39 (2.6%)	0	NA
Pleural effusion positive cultures (%)			
No organisms	35/39 (89.7%)	9/10 (90%)	0.8
Streptococcusconstellatus[b]	2/39 (5.1%)	1/10 (10%)	0.75
Staph. coagulase negative	1/39 (2.6%)	0	NA
Pseudomonas spp.	1/39 (2.6%)	0	NA
Blood cultures (%):			
No organisms	21/39 (53.8%)	5/10 (50%)	0.35
E. coli	1/39 (2.6%)	0	NA
Klebsiella spp.	8/39 (20.5%)	0	NA
Staph. coagulase negative	4/39 (10.3%)	4/10 (40%)	0.23
Streptococcus constellatus	2/39 (5.1%)	1/10 (10%)	0.3
Pseudomonas spp.	3/39 (7.6%)	0	NA
Laboratory data[b]:			
WBC (cells/mcq, mean ± SD)	16410.7 ± 1421.4	17800 ± 1389.4	0.41
Neutrophil (%)	85.8 ± 8.4	83 ± 11.1	0.27
Creatinine (mg/dl)	0.94 ± 0.58	1.6 ± 0.2	0.01
Phosphorus (mmol/L)	3.78 ± 1.4	4.06 ± 1.44	0.75
pH arterial blood	7.31 ± 0.1	7.32 ± 0.12	0.24
Lactate arterial blood (mmol)	1.96 ± 1.8	2.67 ± 0.7	0.11

[*]$p < 0.05$ was found to be statistically significant. [a]Invasive fungal (*Candida*) complications: *Candida peritonitis*, candidemia, and *Candida empyema*. [b]All laboratory data presented are those recorded on admission to the ICU.

TABLE 4: Multivariate logistic regression analysis of risk factors for postoperative secondary peritonitis after oncologic upper GIT surgery.

	OR	95% CI	p value
Age	1.1	1.07–1.29	0.001
Diabetes mellitus (type II)[a]	4.3	1.56–13.1	0.001
Total parenteral nutrition	1.1	1.0–1.9	0.04

[a]Underlying medical conditions.

TABLE 5: Multivariate logistic regression analysis of risk factors for invasive fungal infection after oncologic upper GIT surgery.

	OR	95% CI	p value
Age	1.2	1.07–1.29	0.04
Gastroesophageal leak[a]	2.66	1.16–5.26	0.02

[a]Documented intraperitoneal leak location during first recurrent surgical procedure.

64%, resp., in patients with infectious complications versus 87% and 85%, resp., in an uncomplicated population group) [13]. Advanced age, male gender, underlying cirrhosis, prolonged operative time, suturing or anastomosis of the small bowel, and total gastrectomy were found to be independent risk factors for postoperative infectious complications in patients undergoing upper GIT oncologic surgery [13, 14].

In our study, we retrospectively analyzed 149 cases of oncologic surgical patients who underwent upper GIT surgery for gastric cancer. The postoperative course of 49 patients (Group 2) was complicated by secondary peritonitis with an overall ICU mortality rate of 22% (11 patients). Advanced age, underlying diabetes mellitus, and postoperative parenteral nutrition were found to be independent risk factors for postoperative secondary peritonitis in these patients. In our study, ten (20%) of the Group 2 patients had the following invasive fungal (*Candida*) infections: candidemia, *Candida peritonitis,* and *Candida empyema.*

Over the last two decades several studies have described fungal complications after upper GIT surgery. Candidemia was reported in 10–20% of patients with nosocomial or complicated secondary and tertiary peritonitis [4]. *Candida peritonitis* is associated with a markedly raised mortality rate which can reach as high as 60–70% [4, 5, 15], reinforcing the contention that *Candida* is an independent risk factor for mortality in peritonitis. Some authors [4, 5, 15, 16] have demonstrated almost a double mortality rate (48% versus 28%) in critically ill surgical patients with nosocomial fungal peritonitis compared to those without fungal superinfection [4].

Surgery itself is a major risk factor for *Candida peritonitis* [17–19]. Other risk factors for fungal infections after abdominal surgery were found to be recurrent gastrointestinal perforation, previous treatment with broad-spectrum antibiotics, parenteral nutrition, and central venous catheter insertions. The frequency of invasive fungal infections in the oncologic population continues to increase due to impaired host defenses resulting from underlying disease and/or immunosuppressive therapy [20]; however, the precise incidence of *Candida* infection after oncologic upper GI surgical procedures remains indeterminate.

In our study, in multivariate analysis, advanced age and the presence of a gastroesophageal junction leak were identified as independent risk factors for invasive fungal infectious complications after oncologic upper GIT surgery. In fact, the frequent occurrence of leakage at a high GIT location in our patients supports a primary source of *Candida* in the oral cavity. In previous studies, *Candida* colonization was isolated in 41% of upper GIT sites [6, 17]. Several studies [1, 4, 21] have demonstrated that the presence of yeast isolates in the oral cavity is about 35% in patients aged 56 to 70 but is much more frequent (up to 74%) in patients aged 71–92 years. It is not surprising, therefore, that up to 30–40% of patients with secondary peritonitis are liable to develop *Candida peritonitis* or intra-abdominal abscesses [4, 11]. Importantly, 90% of our patients with invasive fungal infections had a documented postoperative leak as well as a higher frequency of intra-abdominal abscesses and pleural effusions than those without fungal superinfection.

Of note, Edwards Jr. et al. [7] demonstrated that critical illness, parenteral nutrition, and corticosteroid therapy are also independent risk factors for fungal infection in the ICU. However, in our study, no differences in severity of critical illness, postoperative therapeutic management, and type of nutrition were demonstrated between the nonfungal and the invasive fungal populations.

Several previously published data have demonstrated an increased mortality rate in patients with dual infections with *Candida albicans* and *E. coli* [22, 23]. Furthermore, Sawyer et al., investigating the role of *Candida albicans* in the pathogenesis of mixed fungal and bacterial infections, found a synergistic effect on mortality rates in patients with *E. coli* and *B. fragilis* who suffered from simultaneous fungal superinfections [2]. In the present study, microbiological analysis of the peritoneal fluid, blood, and pleural effusions of the patients with invasive fungal infections showed a high frequency of concomitant *Streptococcus constellatus* and coagulase negative *Staphylococcus* spp. cultures (Table 3). In contrast, the frequency of *E. coli* positive cultures was similar (20–25%) in the peritoneal fluid of patients with nonfungal peritonitis and in that of the patients with concomitant invasive fungal infections and mixed abdominal flora (Table 3).

Our study has several limitations, the most important of which is its retrospective design. Another limitation was our inability to make an appropriate selection of the patients and to take into account the administration of antifungal therapy. The significance of our results for the long-term outcomes of our study patients is unclear because the study did not incorporate follow-up of these patients after discharge from the hospital.

5. Conclusion

In conclusion, secondary peritonitis has emerged as a significant postoperative infectious complication after upper GIT surgery for gastric cancer. In the present study, underlying diabetes mellitus, advanced age, and postoperative parenteral nutrition were independent risk factors for the development of peritonitis after oncologic upper GIT surgery. In addition, our study demonstrated that surgical patients who developed invasive fungal infections related to secondary peritonitis had a higher mortality rate than patients with nonfungal postoperative infectious complications. The presence of gastroesophageal junction leakage and advanced age were found to be independent risk factors for invasive fungal infection after oncologic upper GI surgery.

Authors' Contributions

Drs. Evgeni Brotfain and Gilbert Sebbag contributed equally to the paper.

References

[1] H. A. Carneiro, A. Mavrakis, and E. Mylonakis, "Candida peritonitis: An update on the latest research and treatments," *World Journal of Surgery*, vol. 35, no. 12, pp. 2650–2659, 2011.

[2] R. G. Sawyer, L. K. Rosenlof, R. B. Adams, A. K. May, M. D. Spengler, and T. L. Pruett, "Peritonitis into the 1990s: changing pathogens and changing strategies in the critically ill," *The American Surgeon*, vol. 58, pp. 82–87, 1992.

[3] D. W. Johnson and J. P. Cobb, "Candida infection and colonization in critically ill surgical patients," *Virulence*, vol. 1, no. 5, pp. 355-356, 2010.

[4] P. Montravers, H. Dupont, R. Gauzit et al., "Candida as a risk factor for mortality in peritonitis," *Critical Care Medicine*, vol. 34, no. 3, pp. 646–652, 2006.

[5] H. Dupont, C. Paugam-Burtz, C. Muller-Serieys et al., "Predictive factors of mortality due to polymicrobial peritonitis with

Candida isolation in peritoneal fluid in critically III patients," *JAMA Surgery*, vol. 137, no. 12, pp. 1341–1347, 2002.

[6] S.-C. Lee, C.-P. Fung, H.-Y. Chen et al., "Candida peritonitis due to peptic ulcer perforation: Incidence rate, risk factors, prognosis and susceptibility to fluconazole and amphotericin B," *Diagnostic Microbiology and Infectious Disease*, vol. 44, no. 1, Article ID 10895, pp. 23–27, 2002.

[7] J. E. Edwards Jr., G. P. Bodey, R. A. Bowden et al., "International conference for the development of a consensus on the management and prevention of severe candidal infections," *Clinical Infectious Diseases*, vol. 25, no. 1, pp. 43–62, 1997.

[8] S. I. Blot, K. H. Vandewoude, and J. J. De Waele, "Candida peritonitis," *Current Opinion in Critical Care*, vol. 13, no. 2, pp. 195–199, 2007.

[9] O. D. Rotstein, T. L. Pruett, and R. L. Simmons, "Microbiologic features and treatment of persistent peritonitis in patients in the intensive care unit," *Canadian Journal of Surgery*, vol. 29, pp. 247–250, 1986.

[10] D. Manolakaki, G. C. Velmahos, T. Kourkoumpetis et al., "Candida infection and colonization among trauma patients," *Virulence*, vol. 1, no. 5, pp. 367–375, 2010.

[11] M. Bassetti, M. Marchetti, A. Chakrabarti et al., "A research agenda on the management of intra-abdominal candidiasis: Results from a consensus of multinational experts," *Intensive Care Medicine*, vol. 39, no. 12, pp. 2092–2106, 2013.

[12] "Guidelines of the Centers for Disease Control," 2003, https://www.cdc.gov/oralhealth/infectioncontrol/guidelines/.

[13] H. Onodera, A. Tokunaga, T. Yoshiyuki et al., "Surgical Outcome of 483 Patients with Early Gastric Cancer: Prognosis, Postoperative Morbidity and Mortality, and Gastric Remnant Cancer," *Hepato-Gastroenterology*, vol. 51, no. 55, pp. 82–85, 2004.

[14] J.-J. Tuech, C. Cervi, P. Pessaux et al., "Early gastric cancer: Univariate and multivariate analysis for survival," *Hepato-Gastroenterology*, vol. 46, no. 30, pp. 3276–3280, 1999.

[15] P. Sandven, H. Qvist, E. Skovlund, and K. E. Giercksky, "Significance of Candida recovered from intraoperative specimens in patients with intra-abdominal perforations," *Critical Care Medicine*, vol. 30, no. 3, pp. 541–547, 2002.

[16] P. Montravers, J.-P. Mira, J.-P. Gangneux, O. Leroy, and O. Lortholary, "A multicentre study of antifungal strategies and outcome of Candida spp. peritonitis in intensive-care units," *Clinical Microbiology and Infection*, vol. 17, no. 7, pp. 1061–1067, 2011.

[17] J. De Ruiter, J. Weel, E. Manusama, W. P. Kingma, and P. H. J. Van Der Voort, "The epidemiology of intra-abdominal flora in critically Ill patients with secondary and tertiary abdominal sepsis," *Infection*, vol. 37, no. 6, pp. 522–527, 2009.

[18] Y.-S. Shan, H.-P. Hsu, Y.-H. Hsieh, E. D. Sy, J.-C. Lee, and P.-W. Lin, "Significance of intraoperative peritoneal culture of fungus in perforated peptic ulcer," *British Journal of Surgery*, vol. 90, no. 10, pp. 1215–1219, 2003.

[19] T. Calandra, R. Schneider, J. Bille, F. Mosimann, and P. Francioli, "Clinical significance of candida isolated from peritoneum in surgical patients," *The Lancet*, vol. 334, no. 8677, pp. 1437–1440, 1989.

[20] K. Rolston, "Overview of systemic fungal infections," *Oncology (Williston Park)*, vol. 15, no. 11, article 4, 2001.

[21] M. L. Zaremba, T. Daniluk, D. Rozkiewicz et al., "Incidence rate of Candida species in the oral cavity of middle-aged and elderly subjects.," *Advances in Medical Sciences*, vol. 51, pp. 233–236, 2006.

[22] A. Y. Peleg, D. A. Hogan, and E. Mylonakis, "Medically important bacterialg-fungal interactions," *Nature Reviews Microbiology*, vol. 8, no. 5, pp. 340–349, 2010.

[23] G. Akagawa, S. Abe, and H. Yamaguchi, "Mortality of candida albicans-infected mice is facilitated by superinfection of escherichia coli or administration of its lipopolysaccharide," *The Journal of Infectious Diseases*, vol. 171, no. 6, pp. 1539–1544, 1995.

25

Radical Gastrectomy: Still the Cornerstone of Curative Treatment for Gastric Cancer in the Perioperative Chemotherapy Era—A Single Institute Experience over a Decade

Harsh Kanhere [iD],[1] Raghav Goel,[2] Ben Finlay,[2] Markus Trochsler,[1] and Guy Maddern [iD][1]

[1]University of Adelaide Discipline of Surgery, The Queen Elizabeth Hospital, Woodville, Adelaide, SA, Australia
[2]Division of Surgery, The Queen Elizabeth Hospital, Woodville, Adelaide, SA, Australia

Correspondence should be addressed to Harsh Kanhere; harsh.kanhere@sa.gov.au

Academic Editor: Theodore D. Liakakos

Background and Objectives. Most gastric cancer patients now undergo perioperative chemotherapy (POCT) based on the MAGIC trial results. POCT consists of neoadjuvant chemotherapy (NACT) as well as postoperative adjuvant chemotherapy. This study assessed the applicability of perioperative chemotherapy and the impact of radical gastrectomy encompassing a detailed lymph-node resection on outcomes of gastric cancer. *Methods.* Medical and pathology records of all gastric carcinoma resections were reviewed from 2006 onwards. Pathological details, number of lymph-nodes resected, and proportion of involved nodes, reasons for nonadministration of NACT, complications, recurrence, and survival data were analysed. *Results.* Only twenty-eight (37.8%) out of 74 patients underwent NACT and only nine completed POCT. NACT was declined due to comorbidities/patient refusal $n = 24$, early stage $n = 14$, and emergency presentation $n = 8$. Patients receiving NACT were much younger. Anastomotic leaks, hospital-mortality, lymph-node yield, and proportion of involved lymph-nodes were similar in both groups. Thirty-two patients died due to recurrence with lymph-node involvement heralding higher recurrence risk and much poorer survival (HR 2.66; $p = 0.013$). *Conclusion.* More than 60% patients with resectable gastric carcinoma did not undergo NACT. Radical gastrectomy with lymphadenectomy remained the cornerstone of treatment in this period.

1. Introduction

Gastric carcinoma remains a leading cause of cancer related death [1]. Although there is a trend towards improved survival in the last decades, the survival rates remain low at 5 years [2]. Since the publication of the MAGIC [3] trial which showed a 13% improvement in 5-year survival with perioperative chemotherapy (POCT) (36% versus 23%), most units have adopted this approach in treatment of advanced stage gastric cancers.

Randomised trials provide the highest level of evidence in patient management. Adoption and implementation of the trial protocols in daily practice however are not always easy. It is important to assess the feasibility, adoption, implementation, and benefits achieved from change of practice based on trial results in day to day practice to gauge the true impact on patient management.

This study was undertaken to assess the outcomes of all resectable gastric cancers that presented to a tertiary referral centre in South Australia. The aim was to identify the applicability of the POCT protocol, pattern of treatment, the pathological features, and the clinical outcomes in this cohort over a period of 10 years. The reasons for patients not undergoing neoadjuvant chemotherapy (NACT)/POCT were identified and factors impacting the oncological outcomes were analysed. The use of POCT in all patients with resectable gastric cancers was scrutinised.

2. Materials and Methods

This study was approved by the Human Research Ethics Committee of The Queen Elizabeth Hospital as a part of the audit process of an existing database.

A prospective database for all patients with upper gastrointestinal cancer resections has been maintained at our institute from 2005. POCT protocol for gastric cancers based on the MAGIC trial results [3] was adopted at the hospital in 2006. This study was a retrospective analysis of all gastric cancer resections from then until June 2016. Patient data such as age, gender, presence of significant comorbidities, date of diagnosis, and surgery were recorded. All surgeries were performed with an open approach. The authors believe this is the best approach in their hands with an oncological perspective. Surgeons performing gastrectomy are skilled in minimal invasive and laparoscopic surgery and utilise this approach regularly for benign upper GI pathologies as well as complex bariatric surgeries. All patients with stages T2 or N1 disease were considered for NACT. A standard subtotal/total gastrectomy in conjunction with a lymphadenectomy was performed. Routine lymphadenectomy involved Level 1–12 clearance. Level 10 clearance (splenic hilar nodes) was performed selectively. Lymph-node resections from levels 1–6 were performed based on site of the primary disease. Lymphadenectomy was less radical in some settings such as emergency cases or when the procedure was performed with more of a palliative intent or in patients with borderline fitness. In terms of fitness, the patients were evaluated initially at the surgical review with regard to number of comorbidities and their respective severity. Accordingly they were referred to high-risk preoperative clinic for further evaluation. Patients underwent an echocardiogram and pulmonary function tests as part of the preassessment for NACT. The decision for NACT was ultimately taken by the medical oncology team based on their assessment and MDT evaluation. All patients underwent an endoscopy, staging CT of chest, abdomen, and pelvis as well as a laparoscopy prior to NACT. These investigations were repeated in the interval between NACT and surgery with EUS performed in selected cases. The preoperative staging, site of disease (proximal versus distal), type of surgery, intra- and postoperative complications, and detailed histopathology results were documented. Case records of all patients were retrieved and data regarding neoadjuvant and postoperative treatment was collected. Reasons for not undergoing NACT/POCT were documented in patients who underwent surgical resection only.

Every case was discussed in both an institute based meeting and statewide Multidisciplinary Team Meeting (MDT). Decision to proceed to NACT or directly to surgery was based on the recommendations of the MDTs. A study to look at the concordance between the two meetings is in the pipeline. In the instances of disagreement, the decisions from both meetings were discussed with the patient with precedence given to the statewide MDT decision.

2.1. Statistics. All continuous data was compared using a paired T-test while categorical data was expressed in proportions and compared using Fischer's exact test and Chi2 test where appropriate. Survival was presented as Kaplan-Meier curves and assessed using Cox proportional hazards model. Time to recurrence was presented as cumulative incidence function curves and assessed using Fine and Gray competing risk regression models.

TABLE 1: Sample characteristics.

Sex	
Males	42 (56.7%)
Females	32 (43.2%)
Site	
Proximal	21 (28.8%)
Distal	52 (71.2%)
Neoadjuvant chemotherapy	
No	46 (62.2%)
Yes	28 (37.8%)
Reason for not having NACT ($n = 46$)	
Comorbidities	24 (52.2%)
Early stage	14 (30.4%)
Emergency presentation	8 (17.4%)

NACT: neoadjuvant chemotherapy.

3. Results

3.1. Sample Characteristics. A total of 74 patients underwent surgical resection for gastric carcinoma during the study period. Of these only 28 (37.8%) were deemed eligible as per MDT recommendation and received NACT prior to surgery. Mean age was 67.9 years (32–87 years). Patients undergoing surgery alone were significantly older than those that underwent NACT and surgery (mean age 69.9 versus 64.1 years; $p = 0.04$). Patients deemed ineligible for chemotherapy based on comorbidities were even older with a mean age of 76.6 years (65–86 years; $p = 0.0002$). Comorbidities included cardiac failure or cardiomyopathy precluding platin based chemotherapy. The sample characteristics and reasons for not receiving NACT are summarised in Table 1. Associated comorbidities and age were the most common reasons for declining NACT (24/46 patients). Prevalent comorbidities included cardiac failure/ischaemic heart disease (20%), severe COPD (15%), and multiple medical problems (10%). Fourteen patients were declined because of presumed early stage disease on preoperative staging and eight due to emergency presentation of obstruction or bleeding. There were 53 distal and 21 proximal cancers in the patient cohort. A high proportion of patients with proximal cancers underwent NACT (15/21). All 21 patients with proximal cancers underwent a radical total gastrectomy while a subtotal radical gastrectomy was performed in those with distal cancers. A median of 16 (3–49) lymph-nodes were resected per patient. The number of lymph-nodes resected were similar in patients undergoing NACT and surgery and those undergoing surgery alone (19 versus 15; $p = 0.053$). Of the 74 resections, 45 had a lymph-node yield of more than 15 nodes and 15 of these were more than 25 nodes. The proportion of positive lymph-nodes was also similar in the two groups (2.15 versus 1.9; $p = 0.7$). Of the 28 patients in the NACT group, 17 had positive lymph-nodes on histology. Only 9/28 (32%) patients went on to complete the postoperative arm of the chemotherapy in the POCT group. Of the 23 patients with node positive disease in the no NACT arm, seven (30.4%) went on to receive postoperative

TABLE 2: Pathology and morbidity characteristics.

	NACT $n = 28$	No NACT $n = 46$	p
Age [mean, (range)]	64.1 (47–76 years)	69.9 (32–86)	0.04[*]
Proximal/distal	15/13	6/40	0.0004[*]
Number of lymph-nodes harvested [mean, (range)]	20.6 (7–49)	15.8 (3–36)	0.053
Number of positive lymph-nodes [mean, (range)]	2.15 (0–13)	1.90 (0–10)	0.72
Patients with positive lymph-nodes [n, % total]	17 (60.7%)	23 (50%)	0.47
Patients with anastomotic leak [n, % total]	1 (3.5%)	2 (4.3%)	1.00
Proportion of patients with postoperative complications (%)	28.5%	34.7%	0.23

NACT: neoadjuvant chemotherapy; [*]statistically significant ($p < 0.05$).

chemoradiotherapy. Only two patients deemed early stage showed positive lymph-nodes on final histology. Further details are illustrated in Table 2.

3.2. Morbidity. Significant morbidity due to chemotherapy occurred in 5 (17.8%) patients (4 DVT, 1 febrile neutropenia). Postoperative morbidity (Clavien-Dindo grade 3 and above) and anastomotic leaks were similar in both groups as shown in Table 2. There were 2 (2.7%) postoperative mortalities within 30 days. One patient died on postoperative day 1 with small bowel ischemia, considered to be a vascular event (with no evidence of internal herniation/strangulation at reexploration), and the other had a myocardial infarct. Both occurred in patients not receiving neoadjuvant chemotherapy with significant comorbidities.

3.3. Recurrence and Survival. Thirty-two (43.2%) patients died of disease during the observation period. Amongst the patients who died (10 NACT, 22 no NACT), overall survival ranged from 0 to 65.7 months with a mean of 19.2 months and median of 13.6 months. Median survival was significantly poorer in patients with positive lymph-nodes than those without (17.1 versus 24.3 months, HR 2.66; p = 0.013). Survival was slightly better in patients undergoing neoadjuvant chemotherapy but did not reach statistical significance (20.8 versus 19.0 months p = 0.128). Survival curves and time to recurrence cumulative incidence function curves are depicted in Figures 1 and 2.

4. Discussion

This study details the 10-year experience with perioperative chemotherapy in gastric carcinoma at a tertiary centre in

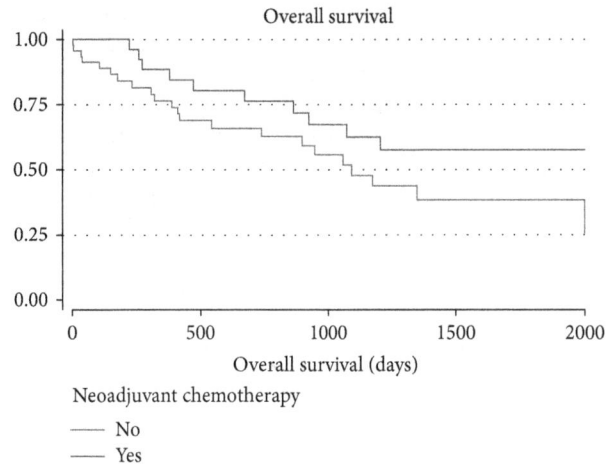

FIGURE 1: NACT versus no NACT HR = 1.00 no NACT; 0.56 NACT; 95% CI 0.26–1.18. p = 0.128.

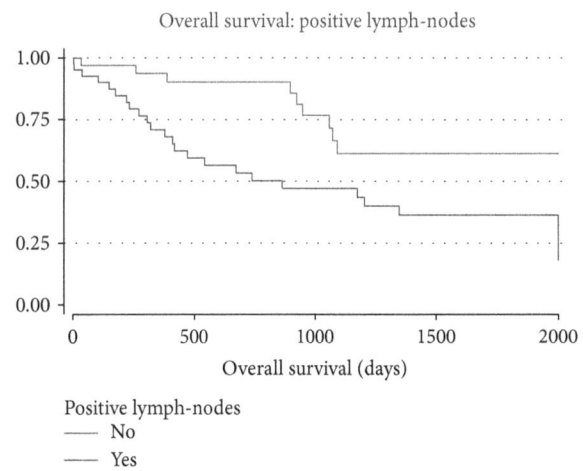

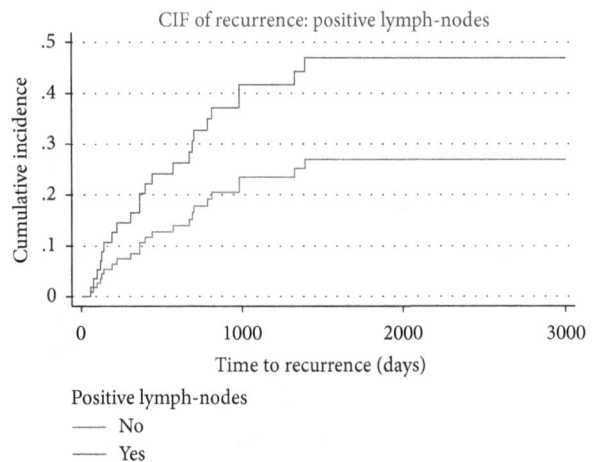

FIGURE 2: (a) Overall survival: positive lymph-node versus negative lymph-node status. (b) Risk of recurrence: positive lymph-node versus negative lymph-node status.

South Australia. The protocol for perioperative chemotherapy was introduced at the hospital after the publication of the results of the MAGIC trial [3]. The improvement in 5-year survival with perioperative chemotherapy was significant in this trial even with a major proportion of patients not completing the postoperative treatment.

Significant advantages seen in the trial setting however may not be evident in wider community based clinical practice for various reasons, especially if the treatment cannot be provided to all patients. According to Post et al. [4] randomised controlled trials (RCTs) are the preferred source of evidence for the effect of treatment but patients participating in RCTs often manifest important differences from patients seen in clinical practice. These differences may be in the form of age, comorbidities, and type of presentation, which will have an important bearing on the outcomes.

4.1. Eligibility and Uptake of POCT.

Just over a third (37%) of all patients presenting with resectable gastric cancers were deemed eligible for perioperative chemotherapy after thorough evaluation by the Surgical and Medical Oncology teams. All cases were discussed in an institute based MDT as well as a statewide MDT and treatment decisions were made on the basis of consensus opinion at both meetings. The most common reason for not receiving chemotherapy preoperatively was comorbidities precluding multimodality treatment (n = 24; 32.4%). Emergency presentations with gastric outlet obstruction and/or bleeding were the other main reasons to proceed directly to surgery. These results are consistent with many studies [5]. A large study based on American College of Surgeons data showed a similar uptake of NACT (36.6%) with large academic centres using NACT more frequently [6]. Shrikhande et al. [7] reported that up to 40% patients did not receive NACT due to emergency presentation or early stage disease. It is the authors' belief that this data reflects the real clinical practice situation in most countries and centres.

Only nine of the 28 patients (32.1%) went on to complete the postoperative chemotherapy arm in this study. Others have shown that more than 60% of patients who undergo NACT are unable to complete the postoperative treatment [5]. The role of the postoperative part of the chemotherapy is thus questionable. The MAGIC trial itself showed survival benefit despite majority of the patients in the chemotherapy arm not completing the postoperative component of the chemotherapy. The authors believe that further trials or meta-analyses are required to test the benefit/risk ration and effectiveness of this part of the regimen.

The patients who did not receive NACT were significantly older than the NACT patients (69.9 versus 64.0 years). The average age of the whole cohort was older than the MAGIC trial (67.7 versus 62 years). Most studies show a similar pattern [7]. A larger proportion of proximal gastric cancers were treated with NACT than upfront surgery (15/21). Similar results are reported by other authors [8]. The perception that proximal gastric cancers present at a later stage and consequently have a poorer prognosis [9] may be responsible for this phenomenon.

4.2. Lymphadenectomy.

The role of lymphadenectomy cannot be understated. A modified D2 gastrectomy is the accepted norm in today's practice [10]. Almost all patients in this study cohort undergoing elective surgery underwent a modified spleen preserving D2 lymphadenectomy. The number of nodes retrieved is particularly relevant in gastric cancer resections. A recent study shows that retrieving more than 25 lymph-nodes during curative-intent gastrectomy substantially improved survival of advanced gastric cancer without compromising patient safety [11]. Previous studies have shown that retrieval of 15 lymph-nodes constitutes an adequate lymphadenectomy [12]. In stage II and III disease, removal of >15 LN appears to contribute to a considerable survival advantage [12, 13]. An extended lymphadenectomy will most reliably allow >15 LN to be removed and adds no operative morbidity and mortality according to Li et al. [8]. They strongly recommend such a lymphadenectomy in curative resections of gastric cancer. A D2 lymphadenectomy thus provides vital information in prognostication of the disease and affords survival benefit as well [11, 13].

It is important to note that the number of lymph-nodes harvested was not affected by NACT (20.6 NACT group versus 15.8 no NACT). Some studies have indicated that NACT reduces the number of lymph-nodes harvested as compared to upfront surgery. Wu et al. [14] found a reduced lymph-node yield (<15 harvested lymph-nodes) following NACT compared to patients who underwent upfront surgery for gastric cancer (7.7% versus 24.1%); however other large series dispute this observation [15].

Seventeen of the 28 patients (60%) had lymph-node metastases on final histology after NACT. Similar data is reported by other authors [7]. This underscores the importance of a good lymph-node clearance even with NACT. It also highlights the fact that NACT may not produce a significant response in lymph-node metastases.

4.3. Morbidity and Mortality.

There was no difference in the postoperative morbidity or mortality in patients undergoing NACT as compared to those undergoing upfront surgery. NACT is regarded safe in relation to postoperative morbidity and mortality based on the MAGIC trial [3] and recently published data [8]. Some authors have reported an increase in wound infection rates and duodenal stump insufficiency in the NACT group [16]. Such issues were not evident in this study. Chemotherapy related DVT/PE was however noted in 4/28 (14.2%) patients in the NACT group. This constituted the significant morbidity from chemotherapy but did not affect the surgical outcomes. Neoadjuvant chemotherapy has been shown to be an independent risk factor for DVT in oesophageal and gastric cancers in a recent publication which recommends pharmacological and mechanical prophylaxis to be commenced in the neoadjuvant period [17, 18]. Targeted and considered use of NACT would be very useful in this regard.

4.4. Survival.

Survival was only slightly better in the NACT group as compared to the no NACT group (20.8 versus 19.0 months). This may be due to the fact that the two groups were not exactly comparable. There were 14 early stage cancers in the no NACT group, but patients in this group were older and had more comorbidity as well. A recent meta-analysis has suggested that neoadjuvant chemotherapy improves survival in patients with gastric and gastro-oesophageal junctional cancers [19]. Given that all patients are not eligible for NACT, these results are not applicable to all patients. Furthermore, a meta-analysis of 6 randomised trials (781 patients) failed to find any benefit in survival specifically in gastric cancer patients with NACT as compared to surgery alone [20]. It appears therefore that evidence for NACT is robust when gastric, gastro-oesophageal junctional, and distal oesophageal cancers are grouped together as was the case in the MAGIC trial as well as a French trial in perioperative chemotherapy [21]. The authors therefore believe that further investigation is warranted for the use of NACT purely in gastric cancers where the benefit may not be as significant. Cost benefit analyses should also be included in such investigative trials and "value for expense" taken into account while treating gastric cancers with NACT [22].

The authors believe that NACT and indeed multimodality therapy need to be tailored and individualised for gastric cancers. Recent advances in biomarkers predicting chemotherapy response (HER2, P53) show promising results and will be useful to tailor NACT for gastric carcinoma based on the profile of each patient [23]. Newer biomarkers like angiopoietin-2 show promising results for targeted therapy in gastric cancers as well [24]. These approaches are perhaps useful in providing low toxicity targeted treatment that can be tolerated by elderly individuals and those with significant comorbidities instead of NACT and improve survival in this group as well.

4.5. Limitations. Being a retrospective analysis, this study has inherent limitations. The final histology of all patients who underwent NACT was not reviewed to assess the tumor response. It is however reported that on the whole only up to 50% gastric carcinomas show tumor response (partial or complete) with NACT [25]. This highlights the fact that 50% of gastric cancers do not show any response to NACT and hence makes a further argument for a targeted approach to NACT. In our cohort, clinical progression was seen in only 2 patients on NACT, but both underwent surgical resections and no metastatic disease was evident. Since it was a retrospective review of patients undergoing surgery till date, 5-year survival is difficult to calculate. The authors acknowledge the fact that most trials of perioperative chemotherapy exclude emergency presentations and early-stage disease. Thus, the denominator of patients eligible for NACT may be 74 − 14 − 8 = 52. It is however our desire to show the real world experience, but even considering the eligibility for most trials based on presentation and stage, close to 50% (24/52), did not receive NACT.

4.6. Conclusion. Only about 40% of patients presenting with resectable locally advanced gastric cancers can undergo NACT. A majority of patients will be treated with surgery alone due to various reasons. Targeted low toxicity therapy should be investigated further to improve survival from gastric cancers in all patients. While a proportion of patients benefit from neoadjuvant chemotherapy, radical gastrectomy remains the cornerstone for treatment of gastric carcinoma and an appropriate lymphadenectomy is advocated for prognostic and treatment purposes.

Additional Points

Synopsis of Table of Contents. This study looked at the eligibility of administering perioperative chemotherapy for all resectable gastric cancer patients in a clinical setting. Reasons for ineligibility and problems with administering NACT to all patients are highlighted. Modified D2 lymphadenectomy is important for prognostication and surgical clearance.

References

[1] D. M. Parkin, F. Bray, J. Ferlay, and P. Pisani, "Global cancer statistics, 2002," *CA: A Cancer Journal for Clinicians*, vol. 55, no. 2, pp. 74–108, 2005.

[2] Australian Institute of Health and Welfare, "Cancer in Australia 2014: Actual incidence data from 1982 to 2011 and mortality data from 1982 to 2012 with projections to 2014," *Asia-Pacific Journal of Clinical Oncology*, vol. 11, no. 3, pp. 208–220, 2015.

[3] D. Cunningham, W. H. Allum, S. P. Stenning et al., "Perioperative chemotherapy versus surgery alone for resectable gastroesophageal cancer," *The New England Journal of Medicine*, vol. 355, pp. 11–20, 2006.

[4] P. N. Post, H. De Beer, and G. H. Guyatt, "How to generalize efficacy results of randomized trials: Recommendations based on a systematic review of possible approaches," *Journal of Evaluation in Clinical Practice*, vol. 19, no. 4, pp. 638–643, 2013.

[5] E. A. Bringeland, H. H. Wasmuth, R. Fougner, P. Mjønes, and J. E. Grønbech, "Impact of perioperative chemotherapy on oncological outcomes after gastric cancer surgery," *British Journal of Surgery*, vol. 101, no. 13, pp. 1712–1720, 2014.

[6] E. K. Greenleaf, C. S. Hollenbeak, and J. Wong, "Trends in the use and impact of neoadjuvant chemotherapy on perioperative outcomes for resected gastric cancer: Evidence from the American College of Surgeons National Cancer," *Surgery*, vol. 159, no. 4, pp. 1099–1112, 2016.

[7] S. V. Shrikhande, S. G. Barreto, S. D. Talole et al., "D2 lymphadenectomy is not only safe but necessary in the era of neoadjuvant chemotherapy," *World Journal of Surgical Oncology*, vol. 11, article no. 31, 2013.

[8] Z.-Y. Li, F. Shan, L.-H. Zhang et al., "Complications after radical gastrectomy following FOLFOX7 neoadjuvant chemotherapy for gastric cancer," *World Journal of Surgical Oncology*, vol. 9, article 110, 2011.

[9] P. Piso, U. Werner, H. Lang, P. Mirena, and J. Klempnauer, "Proximal versus distal gastric carcinoma - What are the differences?" *Annals of Surgical Oncology*, vol. 7, no. 7, pp. 520–525, 2000.

[10] H. J. F. Brenkman, L. Haverkamp, J. P. Ruurda, and R. Van Hillegersberg, "Worldwide practice in gastric cancer surgery," *World Journal of Gastroenterology*, vol. 22, no. 15, pp. 4041–4048, 2016.

[11] Y.-Y. Liu, W.-L. Fang, F. Wang et al., "Does a higher cutoff value of lymph node retrieval substantially improve survival in

patientswith advanced gastric cancer?—Time to embrace a new digit," *The Oncologist*, vol. 22, no. 1, pp. 97–106, 2017.

[12] C. M. Volpe, D. L. Driscoll, and H. O. Douglass Jr., "Outcome of patients with proximal gastric cancer depends on extent of resection and number of resected lymph nodes," *Annals of Surgical Oncology*, vol. 7, no. 2, pp. 139–144, 2000.

[13] K. J. M. Liu, M. Loewen, M. J. Atten et al., "The survival of stage III gastric cancer patients is affected by the number of lymph nodes removed," *Surgery*, vol. 134, no. 4, pp. 639–646, 2003.

[14] Z.-M. Wu, R.-Y. Teng, J.-G. Shen, S.-D. Xie, C.-Y. Xu, and L.-B. Wang, "Reduced lymph node harvest after neoadjuvant chemotherapy in gastric cancer," *Journal of International Medical Research*, vol. 39, no. 6, pp. 2086–2095, 2011.

[15] J. L. Dikken, N. C. T. Van Grieken, P. Krijnen et al., "Preoperative chemotherapy does not influence the number of evaluable lymph nodes in resected gastric cancer," *European Journal of Surgical Oncology*, vol. 38, no. 4, pp. 319–325, 2012.

[16] P. Téoule, J. Trojan, W. Bechstein, and G. Woeste, "Impact of Neoadjuvant Chemotherapy on Postoperative Morbidity after Gastrectomy for Gastric Cancer," *Digestive Surgery*, vol. 32, no. 4, pp. 229–237, 2015.

[17] M. Marshall-Webb, T. Bright, T. Price, S. K. Thompson, and D. I. Watson, "Venous thromboembolism in patients with esophageal or gastric cancer undergoing neoadjuvant chemotherapy," *Diseases of the Esophagus*, vol. 30, no. 2, pp. 1–7, 2017.

[18] K. E. Rollins, C. J. Peters, P. M. Safranek, H. Ford, T. P. Baglin, and R. H. Hardwick, "Venous thromboembolism in oesophago-gastric carcinoma: Incidence of symptomatic and asymptomatic events following chemotherapy and surgery," *European Journal of Surgical Oncology*, vol. 37, no. 12, pp. 1072–1077, 2011.

[19] L. Jiang, K.-H. Yang, Q.-L. Guan, Y. Chen, P. Zhao, and J.-H. Tian, "Survival benefit of neoadjuvant chemotherapy for resectable cancer of the gastric and gastroesophageal junction," *Journal of Clinical Gastroenterology*, vol. 49, no. 5, pp. 387–394, 2015.

[20] Y. Liao, Z.-L. Yang, J.-S. Peng, J. Xiang, and J.-P. Wang, "Neoadjuvant chemotherapy for gastric cancer: A meta-analysis of randomized, controlled trials," *Journal of Gastroenterology and Hepatology*, vol. 28, no. 5, pp. 777–782, 2013.

[21] M. Ychou, V. Boige, J. Pignon et al., "Perioperative chemotherapy compared with surgery alone for resectable gastroesophageal adenocarcinoma: an FNCLCC and FFCD multicenter phase III trial," *Journal of Clinical Oncology*, vol. 29, no. 13, pp. 1715–1721, 2011.

[22] M. C. Russell, "Comparison of neoadjuvant versus a surgery first approach for gastric and esophagogastric cancer," *Journal of Surgical Oncology*, vol. 114, no. 3, pp. 296–303, 2016.

[23] J. Qu and X. Qu, "The predictors of response to neoadjuvant chemotherapy in patients with locally advanced gastric cancer," *Cancer Biomarkers*, vol. 17, no. 1, pp. 49–54, 2016.

[24] U. T. Hacker, L. Escalona-Espinosa, N. Consalvo et al., "Evaluation of Angiopoietin-2 as a biomarker in gastric cancer: Results from the randomised phase III AVAGAST trial," *British Journal of Cancer*, vol. 114, no. 8, pp. 855–862, 2016.

[25] K. Becker, R. Langer, D. Reim et al., "Significance of histopathological tumor regression after neoadjuvant chemotherapy in gastric adenocarcinomas: A summary of 480 cases," *Annals of Surgery*, vol. 253, no. 5, pp. 934–939, 2011.

26

Resection of Nonalcoholic Steatohepatitis-Associated Hepatocellular Carcinoma: A Western Experience

Brian Shrager,[1] Ghalib A. Jibara,[1] Parissa Tabrizian,[1] Sasan Roayaie,[1] and Stephen C. Ward[2]

[1] Division of Surgical Oncology, Department of Surgery, Mount Sinai School of Medicine, One Gustave Levy Place, Box 1259, New York, NY 10029, USA

[2] Department of Pathology, Mount Sinai School of Medicine, 1468 Madison Avenue, Annenberg Building, 15th Floor, Room 92, New York, NY 10029, USA

Correspondence should be addressed to Brian Shrager, shragermd1@yahoo.com

Academic Editor: S. Curley

Introduction. Hepatocellular carcinoma is now known to arise in association with nonalcoholic steatohepatitis. The aim of this study is to examine the clinicopathological features of this entity using liver resection cases at a large Western center. *Methods.* We retrospectively reviewed all cases of partial liver resection for hepatocellular carcinoma over a 10-year period. We included for the purpose of this study patients with histological evidence of nonalcoholic steatohepatitis and excluded patients with other chronic liver diseases such as viral hepatitis and alcoholic liver disease. *Results.* We identified 9 cases in which malignancy developed against a parenchymal background of histologically-active nonalcoholic steatohepatitis. The median age at diagnosis was 58 (52–82) years, and 8 of the patients were male. Median body mass index was 30.2 (22.7–39.4) kg/m². Hypertension was present in 77.8% of the patients and diabetes mellitus, obesity, and hyperlipidemia in 66.7%, respectively. The background liver parenchyma was noncirrhotic in 44% of the cases. Average tumor diameter was 7.0 ± 4.8 cm. Three-fourths of the patients developed recurrence within two years of resection, and 5-year survival was 44%. *Conclusion.* Hepatocellular carcinoma may arise in the context of nonalcoholic steatohepatitis, often before cirrhosis has developed. Locally advanced tumors are typical, and long-term failure rate following resection is high.

1. Introduction

Nonalcoholic fatty liver disease (NAFLD) is the most prevalent form of chronic liver disease in the West today [1]. NAFLD is associated with the diseases of diabetes mellitus (DM) and obesity and has come to be considered a hepatic manifestation of the metabolic syndrome [2–4]. The most severe form of NAFLD is an inflammatory and fibrosing parenchymal lesion known as nonalcoholic steatohepatitis (NASH) [5]. NASH affects roughly 3% of adults in Western countries [1] and approximately 25–30% of the morbidly obese [6]. A subset of NASH patients will ultimately develop frank cirrhosis, with its potential end-points of liver failure and hepatocellular carcinoma (HCC) [7].

DM and obesity have each been shown to increase risk for liver cancer occurrence or liver cancer-related mortality in large-scale prospective cohort studies [8–11]. It is logical to assume that NASH is the connecting link between these metabolic diseases and liver malignancy. Surprisingly, however, few clinical studies have been devoted to investigating NASH-associated HCC [1, 12–14] (Table 1). Similarly, few surgical series have been published [15–19] (Table 2). Of note, all papers describing partial liver resection for NASH-HCC originate from Japan. In this study, we report a Western series of liver resections for HCCs arising in histologically-active NASH. The aims of the study are to (a) examine the clinical and pathological features of NASH-associated HCC using the accuracy of surgical specimens and to

TABLE 1: Series of NASH-associated HCCs (≥5 patients).

	n	Age (years)*	Gender (M : F)	Comorbidities	Cirrhosis (%)
Shimada et al. [12]	6	65.7	3 : 3	Ob 50%, DM 50%, HL 17%	100
Chagas et al. [13]	7	63	4 : 3	Ob 43%, DM 57%, HL 29%	85.7
Hashimoto et al. [14]	34	70 (median)	21 : 13	Ob 62%, DM 74%, HL 29%, HTN 47%	88
Ertle et al. [1]	36	68.6	32 : 4	Ob 95%, DM 64%, HL~50%, HTN > 70%	52.8

Ob: obesity, DM: diabetes mellitus, HL: hyperlipidemia, HTN: hypertension.
*Expressed as a mean unless otherwise indicated.

TABLE 2: Surgical series of NASH-associated HCCs (≥5 patients).

	n	Age (years)	Gender (M : F)	Tumor size (cm)	Primary Tx	Cirrhosis (%)	Recurrence (%)
Hashizume et al. [15]	9	71.5**	6 : 3	3.8*	LR 67%, RFA 22%, TAE 11%	67	11.1
Kawada et al. [16]	6	73**	3 : 3	3.5**	LR 100%	0	N.R.
Malik et al. [17]	17	63.1*	12 : 5	3.4*	LT 100%	100	5.9
Tokushige et al. [18]	16	N.R.	N.R.	N.R.	LR 81%, RFA 18%	N.R.	88
Takuma and Nouso [19]	11	73.8*	6 : 5	3.3*	LR 64%, RFA 27%, MCT 9%	36	60[a]

LR: liver resection, RFA: radiofrequency ablation, TAE: transarterial embolization, LT: liver transplant, MCT: microwave coagulation therapy.
*Mean, **median, [a]recurrence-free survival.

(b) evaluate long-term survival and recurrence outcomes following curative treatment.

2. Materials and Methods

2.1. Inclusion Criteria.
After obtaining consent from an institutional review board, prospectively collected data on all patients receiving partial liver resection for nonfibrolamellar HCC at Mount Sinai Medical Center from January 2000 to December 2009 was reviewed. The purpose of this paper was to identify all patients with tumors arising against a background of histologically-active NASH.

NASH was defined by the following criteria: (a) histological evidence in the nonneoplastic liver parenchyma of steatosis with varying degrees of ballooning hepatocytes, Mallory bodies, lobular inflammatory infiltrate, and fibrosis [5]; (b) an absence of clinically significant alcohol intake (less than 20 gm/day of ethanol consumption) and no personal history of alcoholism; (c) negative serology for Hepatitis B surface antigen; (d) negative serology for anti-Hepatitis C virus antibody and/or no evidence of Hepatitis C viral RNA on polymerase chain reaction (PCR), and (e) no histological, serological, chemical and/or clinical evidence for other parenchymal liver diseases including, but not limited to, autoimmune hepatitis, primary biliary cirrhosis, hereditary hemochromatosis, Wilson's disease and drug-induced liver injury. For a cirrhotic patient to be included into the study, some degree of residual NASH histology was required.

2.2. Definitions.
DM was defined as a fasting blood glucose ≥126 mg/dL on two occasions or current treatment with insulin or oral hypoglycemic agent(s) [20]. Hypertension (HTN) was defined as a resting blood pressure of ≥140/90 mmHg on two separate occasions or current treatment with antihypertensive medication(s). Hyperlipidemia was defined as total serum cholesterol ≥220 mg/dL or serum triglyceride ≥150 mg/dL on two separate occasions or current treatment with lipid-lowering medication(s) [21]. Obesity was classified by a body mass index (BMI) >28.8 kg/m² [22].

2.3. Diagnosis and Treatment of HCC.
Diagnosis was established using contrast-enhanced CT scan of the chest and abdomen ± MRI of the abdomen as per the radiographic criteria laid out by the European Association for the Study of the Liver [23]. A patient was deemed resectable if synthetic and excretory liver functions were preserved (Child-Pugh class A liver function) and radiographic/hematologic stigmata of portal hypertension were absent.

Following resection, patients were followed with clinical, laboratory, and radiographic assessment every 3 months for the first year, every 4 months for the second year, and bi-annually thereafter. Patients with a solitary liver recurrence and Child-Pugh A liver disease and no evidence of portal hypertension underwent a second hepatic resection. Patients with multiple intrahepatic recurrences or compromised hepatic function were treated with radiofrequency ablation (RFA) and/or transarterial chemoembolization (TACE). Patients with recurrence confined to the liver and without significant comorbidities were also referred for liver transplantation. Patients ultimately receiving liver transplant were censored on the date of transplant. After 2007, patients not

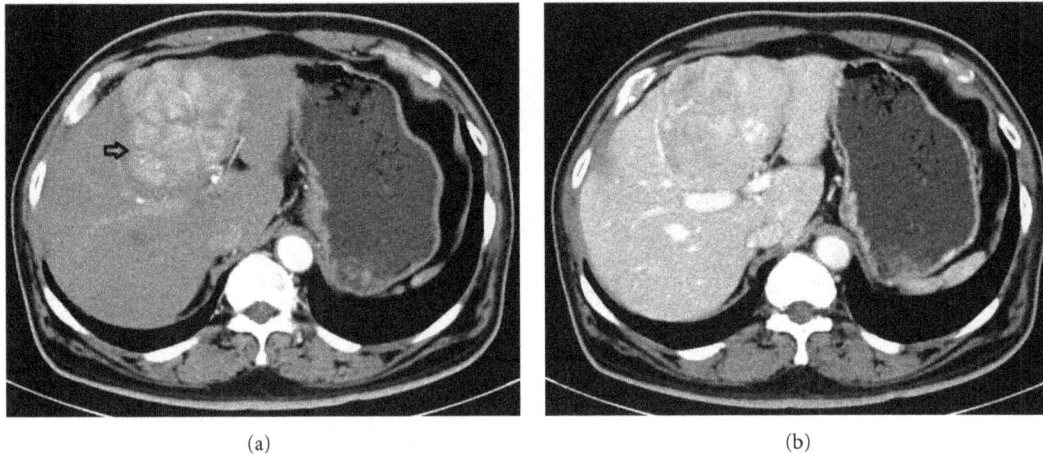

(a)   (b)

FIGURE 1: Contrast-enhanced CT scan of NASH-associated HCC. (a) This arterial-phase image shows an enhancing lesion (arrow) in the left lobe of a steatotic liver. No gross radiographic evidence of cirrhosis is present. (b) The same tumor shows hypoenhancement or "washout" in the delayed portal venous-phase image.

eligible for repeat resection, liver transplantation, or local-regional therapies were treated with sorafenib.

2.4. Pathological Analysis.

Specimens were independently reviewed by two attending pathologists. Specimens were routinely fixed in hemotoxylin and eosin stain, Masson's trichrome stain for collagen fibers, and Prussian blue stain for iron granules. Additional specialized stains were used on a selective basis. Tumor size was measured at the widest diameter of the dominant nodule. Satellite nodules were defined as tumors ≤2 cm in diameter and within 2 cm of the dominant nodule. *"By contrast, additional HCC implants outside of the satellite criteria, that is, >2 cm in diameter or >2 cm away from the index tumor, defined multinodularity."* Tumor grade was reported as well, moderate or poorly differentiated using the Edmonson classification [24]. The Brunt criteria were used to quantify the degree of hepatic steatosis and to grade the level of lobular inflammatory activity [5]. Fibrosis was also staged according to the descriptions of Brunt et al. [5]: F0, no fibrosis; F1, pericellular and/or perivenular fibrosis confined to Zone 3; F2, pericellular fibrosis extending to Zones 2 and 3 with or without portal fibrosis; F3, bridging fibrosis; and F4, cirrhosis. For the purpose of this study, F0 to F2 fibrosis was considered "noncirrhotic."

3. Results

3.1. Patients.

Of the 548 patients undergoing partial liver resection for HCC, 255 (46.5%) showed serological evidence for Hepatitis B viral (HBV) infection, 178 (32.5%) for Hepatitis C viral (HCV) infection, and 5 (0.9%) for coinfection with both viruses. 20 patients (3.6%) displayed alcoholic liver disease. 7 patients (1.3%) had hereditary hemochromatosis. 2 patients had α-1 antitrypsin deficiency, 2 had primary biliary cirrhosis, and one had Gaucher's disease. 18 patients (3.3%) had cryptogenic cirrhosis (CC) and 51 patients (9.3%) had noncirrhotic livers without evidence for underlying parenchymal liver disease despite comprehensive

investigation. The remaining 9 patients (1.6%) developed their tumors in association with histologically-active NASH; these cases form our series.

Of the 9 patients with NASH-associated HCC, 2 presented with tumor-related symptoms, specifically abdominal pain and weight loss; the remaining 7 cases were discovered incidentally. HCC diagnosis was established radiographically in each case (Figure 1), with tissue biopsy acting as a supplement in 6 of the 9 cases.

Median age at diagnosis was 58 (52–82) years, and 8 of the patients were male (Table 3). Median BMI was 30.2 (22.7–39.4) kg/m^2. All of the patients carried a diagnosis of at least one metabolic disease, with HTN displaying the highest prevalence (77.8%). Obesity, DM, and hyperlipidemia each displayed a prevalence of 66.7%, respectively. In only one case was serum α-fetoprotein elevated above 200 ng/mL. All patients demonstrated Child-Pugh class A liver function.

3.2. Pathology.

One resection was noncurative with a positive microscopic surgical margin. Another patient had intraoperative evidence of metastatic disease in the greater omentum that was completely excised. Mean tumor size was 7.0 ± 4.8 cm (Table 4). One patient had a multinodular HCC. Gross vascular invasion was present in 2 cases and microscopic vascular invasion in 4. All tumors except one were well or moderately differentiated, and 4 tumors showed varying degrees of steatosis within neoplastic cells. Of interest, four of the cases (44.4%) showed a noncirrhotic parenchyma (all F1). Figure 2 shows salient histopathological findings from three of these noncirrhotic cases. In accordance with the inclusion criteria of this study, all cases displayed the histological hallmarks of NASH in the background liver.

3.3. Long-Term Outcome.

Median length of followup was 38.3 (1.1–105.2) months. One patient died of sepsis 33 days after surgery. Of the remaining 8 patients, 7 recurred (87.5%). The median time to recurrence was 8.3 (6.2–37.9) months and 6 of the 7 patients that recurred did so within

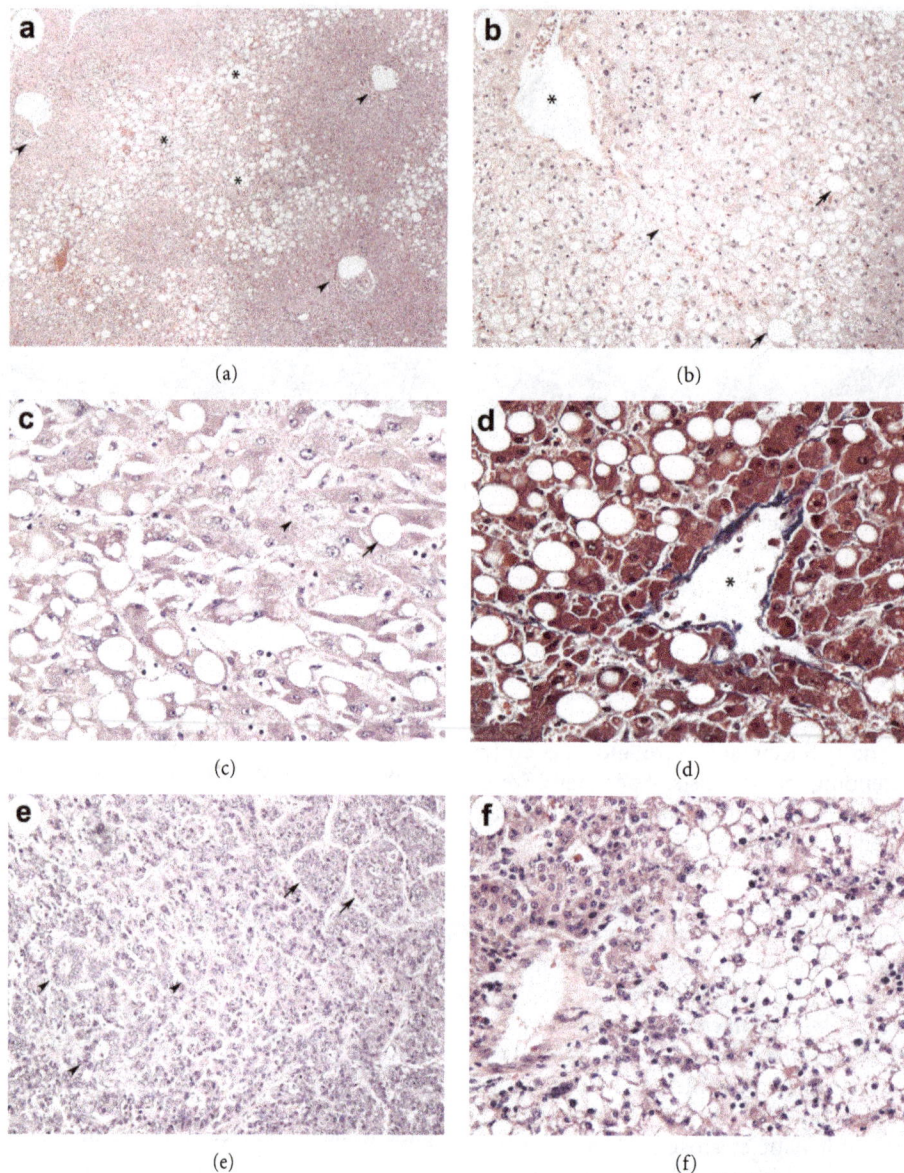

FIGURE 2: Histopathological features of noncirrhotic NASH-associated HCC. (a) The nonneoplastic liver shows macrovesicular steatosis involving the perivenular zone (∗) with sparing of the periportal zones (arrowheads) (patient 8, H&E stain, 40x). (b) and (c) show at greater magnification the steatotic hepatocytes (arrows) and ballooning degeneration of hepatocytes (arrowheads) evident in the perivenular zone of the nonneoplastic parenchyma (patients 4 and 7, H&E stain, 100x and 200x). (d) Specialized collagen staining shows the central venule (∗) to be invested with a band of perivenular fibrosis; bridging fibrosis and cirrhotic nodules are notably absent (patient 7, Masson's trichrome stain, 200x). (e) and (f) show two examples of HCC arising within noncirrhotic NASH showing pseudoglandular (arrowheads) and trabecular (arrows) features and fat within tumor cells (right frame) (patients 7 and 8, H&E stain, 100x).

2 years of the index resection. Initial recurrence was limited to the liver in 6 of 7 cases. One patient received a liver transplant 6.4 months following index resection and is still alive at the time of this report. Median survival was 38.3 (1.1–105.2) months. 5-year survival was 44.4%. Detailed long-term outcome data is provided in Table 4.

4. Discussion

It has become widely accepted that NASH is a hepatic manifestation of the metabolic syndrome. The heavy prevalence of DM, HTN, obesity, and hyperlipidemia in our series gives further clinical support to this concept. Moreover, our study demonstrates the sclerotic spectrum of NASH, with varying degrees of fibrosis seen originating from the centrilobular zone.

Our study consisted of patients with a large mean tumor size of 7.0 cm. The finding of more advanced tumors in our series is related to the modes of presentation; all cases were either discovered incidentally or because of mass-related symptoms. None of the patients had been enrolled in radiographic surveillance programs for HCC. Similarly,

TABLE 3: Demographic and clinical data.

Patient	1	2	3	4	5	6	7	8	9
Age gg	58	57	73	52	78	82	52	57	73
Gender	M	M	F	M	M	M	M	M	M
BMI (kg/m^2)	29.1	30.2	26.4	39.4	32.2	27.4	31.1	34.6	22.7
Metabolic disease	HTN	DM	DM	DM HTN HL	DM HTN HL	HTN HL	HTN HL	DM HTN HL	DM HTN HL
Symptoms	No	No	No	No	No	No	Yes	No	Yes
Biopsy	No	No	Yes	Yes	Yes	Yes	No	Yes	Yes
AFP (ng/mL)	7.1	3.1	100.2	2.1	N.A.	7.4	311,190	9.3	2.5
ALT (IU/L)	60	44	52	N.A.	106	35	49	235	23
Albumin (g/dL)	4.3	3.9	4.2	4.5	3.6	4.3	3.6	3.3	3.7
Bilirubin (mg/dL)	1.1	1.0	0.8	0.3	1.3	1.0	0.8	0.5	0.5
Creatinine (mg/dL)	0.7	1.3	1.?	1.0	0.7	1.1	0.8	0.9	0.9
Platelet ($\times 1000/\mu$L)	133	65	112	362	340	154	590	218	316
INR	1.0	1.3	0.9	1.0	1.1	1.0	1.1	0.9	1.1
CTP class	A	A	A	A	A	A	A	A	A
MELD score	6.6	9.0	7.2	7.3	6.4	6.8	6.9	6.4	6.9

BMI: body mass index, DM: diabetes mellitus, HTN: hypertension, HL: hyperlipidemia, AFP: alpha-fetoprotein, ALT: alanine aminotransferase, INR: international normalization ratio, CTP: Child-Turcotte-Pugh, MELD: model for end stage liver disease, N.A.: data not available.

TABLE 4: Pathological data and longterm outcomes.

Patient	1	2	3	4	5	6	7	8	9
Tumor size (cm)	5.1	1.8	6.2	6.0	4.5	6.3	19.0	6.0	8.4
Number of nodules	1	1	1	1	2	1	1	1	1
Vascular invasion	None	None	Micro	None	Gross	Micro	Gross	Micro	Micro
Satellites	Yes	No	Yes	No	No	No	Yes	No	No
Tumor cell differentiation[a]	Well	Well	Well	Mod	Mod	Mod	Poor	Mod	Mod
Steatotic tumor cells	No	Yes	Yes	No	No	No	No	Yes	Yes
Parenchymal fibrosis[b]	F4	F4	F4	F1	F3	F3	F1	F1	F1
Margin (mm)	3	5	0	20	10	10	10	2	2
Regional lymph nodes (+)	No	No	No	No	No	No	No	No	No
Metastases	No	No	No	No	No	No	Yes	No	No
Recurrence gg	Yes	Yes	Yes	No	Yes	Yes	No	Yes	Yes
Time to recurrence (months)	19.4	6.4	8.3	—	6.2	37.9	—	6.2	16.8
Distribution of 1st recurrence	IH	IH	IH	—	IH	IH	—	IH/EH	IH
Treatment of 1st recurrence	TACE	OLT	TACE	—	RR	RFA	—	RR	RFA
Survival (months)	105.2	32.3	27.8	84.0	62.1	68.0	1.1	34.7	38.3

Micro: microscopic, Mod: moderate, IH: intrahepatic, EH: extrahepatic, TACE: transarterial chemoembolization, OLT: orthotopic liver transplant, RR: repeat resection, RFA: radiofrequency ablation.
[a]Based on Edmonson grading system, [b]based on Brunt criteria.

Giannini et al. found that CC-associated HCCs were more likely to be discovered at an advanced stage and less likely to be amenable to treatment when compared to HCV-associated HCCs; this was also attributed to less surveillance among the former group [25]. It follows that of our 8 patients that survived the postoperative period 6 recurred within two years of resection, a clear sequella of the advanced nature of their initial tumors. Despite this high early recurrence rate, we were able to achieve a 5-year survival of 44%, likely attributable to the aggressive multimodality approach to treating those recurrences.

4.1. Fibrosis: A Necessary Precursor? NASH is felt to progress to cirrhosis in 3–15% of cases [7], and it has been suggested that the development of cirrhosis is a necessary intermediate step in a progression to HCC [6]. This has been a difficult theory to prove, in part due to the disappearance of the histopathological features of NASH once cirrhosis is established [15, 26]. Nevertheless, "cryptogenic cirrhosis" has been shown to likely represent end-stage NASH based on clinical parameters [3, 27], with a risk of HCC development that rivals HCV-associated cirrhosis [7]. In a large case-control study, Hashimoto et al. showed that the strongest independent predictor for HCC development in NASH patients was severe hepatic fibrosis [14].

Despite this evidence, 44% of our patients showed only mild fibrosis in the nonneoplastic liver parenchyma. Similar findings have been echoed in other surgical series. Hashizume et al. found that 3 of 8 patients undergoing curative treatments (6 resections, 2 RFAs) of NASH-associated HCC had noncirrhotic livers [15]. Kawada et al. found that 5 of 8 patients receiving resection of NASH-associated HCC showed only mild fibrosis (F2) in their background livers [16]. Paradis et al. analyzed a group of 31 patients receiving resection of HCC that complicated only metabolic syndrome (81% with some form of NAFLD) and found nonfibrotic or mildly fibrotic livers in 20 (65.5%) of the cases [28].

It is important to point out the natural selection bias for noncirrhotics that exists in a surgical resection series such as ours. Further supporting data, however, exists in nonsurgical studies [1, 29, 30]. Guzman et al. found from a cohort of 50 HCC patients submitted to a wide spectrum of treatments 3 of 5 NAFLD-associated cases that were noncirrhotic [30]. In a larger series, Ertle et al. showed that in a group of 36 NASH-associated HCC patients of which only a minority received resection, the prevalence of noncirrhotic background liver was 47.2% [1].

We chose not to include cases of cryptogenic cirrhosis (CC) in our study group and instead included only patients with histologically-active NASH. Accepting the premise that the 18 CC cases in our entire population represented "burnt-out" NASH, the actual proportion of NASH-associated HCC cases that developed in the absence of cirrhosis becomes 14.8%. This is similar to the rate of noncirrhotic HCV-associated HCCs in our overall cohort (21/178, 11.8%, $P = 0.751$ by Fisher's exact test); it is less but also statistically similar to our rate of noncirrhotic HBV-associated HCCs (68/255, 26.7%, $P = 0.246$ by Fisher's exact test). Indeed, based on our experience and that of other investigators, the relevance of this entity should not be underestimated.

If the carcinogenic milieu of a cirrhotic liver represents only part of the story, the additional mechanisms underlying HCC development in the NASH liver have yet to be fully elucidated. Recent investigation has centered on the oncogenic effects of hyperinsulinemia, a key component of the metabolic syndrome [31–33]. Additional research has focused on the oxidative stress present in the microenvironment of the steatotic liver. Specifically, lipid peroxidation, an important component of disease progression in NASH, has been implicated in the generation of reactive oxygen species that may possess mutagenic qualities sufficient to initiate malignant transformation [6, 34, 35]. An additional effect of this oxidative stress has been shown to include clonal expansion of premalignant oval cells in both mouse and human forms of fatty liver [35–37]. Further proliferation of these neoplastic cells may be driven by disturbances in cytokines and growth factors [6, 38]. Whether HCC development in NASH is an effect of factors directly derived from the underlying metabolic diseases or a result of biochemical derangements in the steatotic liver lesions is a question which remains to be answered.

"While the potential mutagenicity of the noncirrhotic NASH parenchyma is intriguing, we must acknowledge that alternate etiological agents might have been at play in these patients. One possibility is occult HBV infection, as evidenced by the presence of HBV DNA by PCR analysis in the context of a negative serological panel. Unfortunately, only 1 of the 4 noncirrhotic patients in our series received this PCR analysis (negative), and this scenario cannot be ruled out in the other three. Environmental exposure to a hepato-carcinogen such as aflatoxin A, nitrosamine, or benzopyrene serves as an additional plausible, albeit unlikely, etiology. Finally, advanced age (one noncirrhotic over 70) and male gender (all 4 noncirrhotics) placed these patients at slightly increased risk of primary hepatic malignancy."

In conclusion, HCC may arise in a liver affected by NASH, often in association with multiple metabolic comorbidities. Although cirrhosis increases the risk of malignant transformation, it does not appear to be a necessary precursor to such an event. NASH-HCC often presents at a late stage leading to increased local failure following resection; nevertheless, with an aggressive approach to recurrence, long-term survival may still be achieved. With the increasing prevalence of obesity and diabetes mellitus in Western populations, investigation into the utility of HCC surveillance for patients with established NASH seems warranted.

References

[1] J. Ertle, A. Dechêne, J. P. Sowa et al., "Non-alcoholic fatty liver disease progresses to hepatocellular carcinoma in the absence of apparent cirrhosis," *International Journal of Cancer*, vol. 128, no. 10, pp. 2436–2443, 2011.

[2] G. Marchesini, M. Brizi, G. Blanchi et al., "Nonalcoholic fatty liver disease: a feature of the metabolic syndrome," *Diabetes*, vol. 50, no. 8, pp. 1844–1850, 2001.

[3] E. Bugianesi, N. Leone, E. Vanni et al., "Expanding the natural history of nonalcoholic steatohepatitis: from cryptogenic cirrhosis to hepatocellular carcinoma," *Gastroenterology*, vol. 123, no. 1, pp. 134–140, 2002.

[4] G. Marchesini, E. Bugianesi, G. Forlani et al., "Nonalcoholic fatty liver, steatohepatitis, and the metabolic syndrome," *Hepatology*, vol. 37, no. 4, pp. 917–923, 2003.

[5] E. M. Brunt, C. G. Janney, A. M. Di Bisceglie, B. A. Neuschwander-Tetri, and B. R. Bacon, "Nonalcoholic steato-hepatitis: a proposal for grading and staging the histological lesions," *American Journal of Gastroenterology*, vol. 94, no. 9, pp. 2467–2474, 1999.

[6] S. H. Caldwell, D. M. Crespo, H. S. Kang, and A. M. S. Al-Osaimi, "Obesity and hepatocellular carcinoma," *Gastroenterology*, vol. 127, pp. S97–S103, 2004.

[7] M. S. Ascha, I. A. Hanouneh, R. Lopez, T. A. R. Tamimi, A. F. Feldstein, and N. N. Zein, "The incidence and risk factors of hepatocellular carcinoma in patients with nonalcoholic steatohepatitis," *Hepatology*, vol. 51, no. 6, pp. 1972–1978, 2010.

[8] E. E. Calle, C. Rodriguez, K. Walker-Thurmond, and M. J. Thun, "Overweight, obesity, and mortality from cancer in a

prospectively studied cohort of U.S. Adults," *The New England Journal of Medicine*, vol. 348, no. 17, pp. 1625–1638, 2003.

[9] H. O. Adami, W. H. Chow, O. Nyrén et al., "Excess risk of primary liver cancer in patients with diabetes mellitus," *Journal of the National Cancer Institute*, vol. 88, no. 20, pp. 1472–1477, 1996.

[10] L. Wideroff, G. Gridley, L. Mellemkjaer et al., "Cancer incidence in a population-based cohort of patients hospitalized with diabetes mellitus in denmark," *Journal of the National Cancer Institute*, vol. 89, no. 18, pp. 1360–1365, 1997.

[11] H. B. El-Serag, T. Tran, and J. E. Everhart, "Diabetes increases the risk of chronic liver disease and hepatocellular carcinoma," *Gastroenterology*, vol. 126, no. 2, pp. 460–468, 2004.

[12] M. Shimada, E. Hashimoto, M. Taniai et al., "Hepatocellular carcinoma in patients with non-alcoholic steatohepatitis," *Journal of Hepatology*, vol. 37, no. 1, pp. 154–160, 2002.

[13] A. L. Chagas, L. O. O. Kikuchi, C. P. M. S. Oliveira et al., "Does hepatocellular carcinoma in non-alcoholic steatohepatitis exist in cirrhotic and non-cirrhotic patients?" *Brazilian Journal of Medical and Biological Research*, vol. 42, no. 10, pp. 958–962, 2009.

[14] E. Hashimoto, S. Yatsuji, M. Tobari et al., "Hepatocellular carcinoma in patients with nonalcoholic steatohepatitis," *Journal of Gastroenterology*, vol. 44, no. 19, supplement, pp. 89–95, 2009.

[15] H. Hashizume, K. Sato, H. Takagi et al., "Primary liver cancers with nonalcoholic steatohepatitis," *European Journal of Gastroenterology and Hepatology*, vol. 19, no. 10, pp. 827–834, 2007.

[16] N. Kawada, K. Imanaka, T. Kawaguchi et al., "Hepatocellular carcinoma arising from non-cirrhotic nonalcoholic steatohepatitis," *Journal of Gastroenterology*, vol. 44, no. 12, pp. 1190–1194, 2009.

[17] S. M. Malik, P. A. Gupte, M. E. de Vera, and J. Ahmad, "Liver transplantation in patients with nonalcoholic steatohepatitis-related hepatocellular carcinoma," *Clinical Gastroenterology and Hepatology*, vol. 7, no. 7, pp. 800–806, 2009.

[18] K. Tokushige, E. Hashimoto, S. Yatsuji et al., "Prospective study of hepatocellular carcinoma in nonalcoholic steatohepatitis in comparison with hepatocellular carcinoma caused by chronic hepatitis C," *Journal of Gastroenterology*, vol. 45, no. 9, pp. 960–967, 2010.

[19] Y. Takuma and K. Nouso, "Nonalcoholic steatohepatitis-associated hepatocellular carcinoma: our case series and literature review," *World Journal of Gastroenterology*, vol. 16, no. 12, pp. 1436–1441, 2010.

[20] World Health Organization, *Definition, Diagnosis and Classification of Diabetes Mellitus and Its Complications*, World Health Organization, Department of Noncommunicable Disease Surveillance, 1999.

[21] J. I. Cleeman, "Executive summary of the third report of the National Cholesterol Education Program (NCEP) expert panel on detection, evaluation, and treatment of high blood cholesterol in adults (adult treatment panel III)," *Journal of the American Medical Association*, vol. 285, no. 19, pp. 2486–2497, 2001.

[22] N. Sattar, A. Gaw, O. Scherbakova et al., "Metabolic syndrome with and without C-reactive protein as a predictor of coronary heart disease and diabetes in the West of Scotland Coronary Prevention Study," *Circulation*, vol. 108, no. 4, pp. 414–419, 2003.

[23] J. Bruix, M. Sherman, J. M. Llovet et al., "Clinical management of hepatocellular carcinoma. Conclusions of the barcelona-2000 EASL conference," *Journal of Hepatology*, vol. 35, no. 3, pp. 421–430, 2001.

[24] H. A. Edmonson and P. E. Steiner, "Primary carcinoma of the liver: a study of 100 cases among 48,900," *Cancer*, vol. 7, no. 3, pp. 462–503, 1954.

[25] E. G. Giannini, E. Marabotto, V. Savarino et al., "Hepatocellular carcinoma in patients with cryptogenic cirrhosis," *Clinical Gastroenterology and Hepatology*, vol. 7, no. 5, pp. 580–585, 2009.

[26] B. Q. Starley, C. J. Calcagno, and S. A. Harrison, "Nonalcoholic fatty liver disease and hepatocellular carcinoma: a weighty connection," *Hepatology*, vol. 51, no. 5, pp. 1820–1832, 2010.

[27] J. M. Regimbeau, M. Columbat, P. Mognol et al., "Obesity and diabetes as a risk factor for hepatocellular carcinoma," *Liver Transplantation*, vol. 10, no. 2, pp. S69–S73, 2004.

[28] V. Paradis, S. Zalisnski, E. Chelbi et al., "Hepatocellular carcinomas in patients with metabolic syndrome often develop without significant liverfibrosis: a pathological analysis," *Hepatology*, vol. 49, no. 3, pp. 851–859, 2009.

[29] Y. Komorizono, T. Shibatou, K. Saito et al., "Cryptogenic hepatocellular carcinoma and nonalcoholic steatohepatitis: a review of ten Japanese cases [AASLD abstract 1221]," *Hepatology*, vol. 44, no. 4, supplement 1, pp. 644A–645A, 2006.

[30] G. Guzman, E. M. Brunt, L. M. Petrovic, G. Chejfec, T. J. Layden, and S. J. Cotler, "Does nonalcoholic fatty liver disease predispose patients to hepatocellular carcinoma in the absence of cirrhosis?" *Archives of Pathology and Laboratory Medicine*, vol. 132, no. 11, pp. 1761–1766, 2008.

[31] C. Weyer, R. L. Hanson, P. A. Tataranni, C. Bogardus, and R. E. Pratley, "A high fasting plasma insulin concentration predicts type 2 diabetes independent of insulin resistance: evidence for a pathogenic role of relative hyperinsulinemia," *Diabetes*, vol. 49, no. 12, pp. 2094–2101, 2000.

[32] K. Saito, S. Inoue, T. Saito et al., "Augmentation effect of postprandial hyperinsulinaemia on growth of human hepatocellular carcinoma," *Gut*, vol. 51, no. 1, pp. 100–104, 2002.

[33] J. A. Price, S. J. Kovach, T. Johnson et al., "Insulin-like growth factor I is a comitogen for hepatocyte growth factor in a rat model of hepatocellular carcinoma," *Hepatology*, vol. 36, no. 5, pp. 1089–1097, 2002.

[34] L. J. Marnett, "Oxyradicals and DNA damage," *Carcinogenesis*, vol. 21, no. 3, pp. 361–370, 2000.

[35] W. Hu, Z. Feng, J. Eveleigh et al., "The major lipid peroxidation product, trans-4-hydroxy-2-nonenal, preferentially forms DNA adducts at codon 249 of human p53 gene, a unique mutational hotspot in hepatocellular carcinoma," *Carcinogenesis*, vol. 23, no. 11, pp. 1781–1789, 2002.

[36] S. Yang, H. Z. Lin, J. Hwang, V. P. Chacko, and A. M. Diehl, "Hepatic hyperplasia in noncirrhotic fatty livers: is obesity-related hepatic steatosis a premalignant condition?" *Cancer Research*, vol. 61, no. 13, pp. 5016–5023, 2001.

[37] T. Roskams, S. Q. Yang, A. Koteish et al., "Oxidative stress and oval cell accumulation in mice and humans with alcoholic and nonalcoholic fatty liver disease," *American Journal of Pathology*, vol. 163, no. 4, pp. 1301–1311, 2003.

[38] A. Sánchez, V. M. Factor, I. S. Schroeder, P. Nagy, and S. S. Thorgeirsson, "Activation of NF-κB and STAT3 in rat oval cells during 2-acetylaminofluorene/partial hepatectomy-induced liver regeneration," *Hepatology*, vol. 39, no. 2, pp. 376–385, 2004.

27

Genetic Heterogeneity of Breast Cancer Metastasis May Be Related to miR-21 Regulation of TIMP-3 in Translation

Jianyi Li,[1] Yang Zhang,[1] Wenhai Zhang,[1] Shi Jia,[1] Rui Tian,[1] Ye Kang,[1] Yan Ma,[2] and Dan Li[3]

[1] Department of Breast Surgery, Shengjing Hospital of China Medical University, Shenyang, Liaoning 110004, China
[2] Ultrasound Diagnosis Center, Shengjing Hospital of China Medical University, Shenyang, Liaoning 110004, China
[3] Pathological Diagnosis Center, Shengjing Hospital of China Medical University, Shenyang, Liaoning 110004, China

Correspondence should be addressed to Wenhai Zhang; sjbreast@sina.com

Academic Editor: Giuseppe Nigri

Purpose. MicroRNAs are noncoding RNA molecules that posttranscriptionally regulated expression of target gene and implicate the progress of cancer proliferation, differentiation, and apoptosis. The aim of this study is to determine whether microRNA-21 (miR-21), a specific microRNA implicated in multiple aspects of carcinogenesis, promoted breast cancer metastasis by regulating the tissue inhibitor of metalloproteinase 3 (TIMP-3) gene. *Methods.* miR-21 of serum and tissue from 40 patients (30 patients with breast cancer) were detected by real-time quantitative reverse transcriptase polymerase chain reaction (RT-qPCR). TIMP-3 of tissue from the patient was tested by real-time RT-qPCR. Protein expression of TIMP-3 was evaluated by western blotting. Correlation analysis was performed between miR-21 and TIMP-3. *Results.* Of the 40 samples from tissue and serum analyzed, the miR-21 expression was significantly higher in high invasion metastasis group (HIMG) that in low invasion metastasis group (LIMG); the latter was higher than that in normal group (NG). Additionally, the TIMP-3 expression was significantly lower in HIMG than in LIMG; the latter was lower than that in NG. There was significantly inverse correlation between miR-21 and TIMP-3 extracted from tissue. *Conclusion.* Our data suggest that miR-21 could promote metastasis in breast cancer via the regulation of TIMP3 translation, and there was consistency between miR-21 of serum and miR-21 in tissue.

1. Introduction

Metastasis is the main reason which cause the treatment failure and death in patients with breast cancer [1]. In clinical work, even in the same pathological type, histological grade, clinical stages and molecular typing, differences between the metastatic probability in patients are huge [2]. In fact, tumor metastasis is still poorly understood for researchers, and deconstruction of genetic heterogeneity is the right way. According to findings previously, endogenous inhibitors of matrix metalloproteinases (MMPs) play an important role in extracellular matrix (ECM) homeostasis and deregulate ECM remodeling which contributes to cancer metastasis [3, 4]. Tissue inhibitor of metalloproteinase (TIMP) balanced the role of MMPs involved in organizing remodeling, thus having an impact on cancer metastasis [5]. On the other hand, the discovery of microRNA regulation of tumor metastasis

was considered to be the molecular basis of the genetic heterogeneity of mechanism's important part [6]. Specifically, miR-21 is overexpressed in diverse types of malignancy [7]. Further, recent experiments suggest that miR-21 can regulate the expression of tissue inhibitor of metalloproteinase-3 (TIMP-3) to control the invasion of breast cancer [8]. We sought to determine the role of miR-21 in breast cancer metastasis and to identify whether miR-21-mediated metastasis might be regulated via TIMP-3.

2. Methods

2.1. Patients and Groups. Human tissue and serum samples were obtained by surgical resection and blood drawing from patients who have been treated in Shengjing Hospital of China Medical University from 2009 to 2010. Inclusion

TABLE 1

Grouped criteria	High invasion and metastasis group HIMG	Low invasion and metastasis group LIMG
Diameter by ultrasound (cm)	<2 cm	≧3 cm
Lymph nodes metastasis by HE	Yes	No
Micrometastasis by CK-22	Unnecessary	No
Histological grading	III	I
Tumor embolus	Positive	Negative
Her2 receptor status	Positive	Negative
ER & PR	Negative	Positive
P53	Positive	Negative
Ki67	≧14%	<14%

All indicators of immunohistochemical staining need to meet verification of two pathological diagnosis centers.

TABLE 2

Parameters	HIMG	LIMG	Normal group
Age (years)			
Median	42	48	45
Range	(33~60)	(36~64)	(35~62)
Quadrant			
Areolar	3	2	2
Outer upper	5	6	3
Outer lower	4	5	3
Inner lower	1	1	1
Inner upper	2	1	1
Operation			
Mastectomy	12	10	
Tumorectomy	3	5	

criteria included invasive ductal carcinoma, receiving no neoadjuvant therapy, no history of radiotherapy before, and no previous history of cancer, and no vice-breast cancer. In those patients, there are fifteen persons who entirely meet the following requirements entered the HIMG: tumor diameter less than 2 cm; lymph node metastases; historical grade III; Her2 positive; vascular thrombosis positive; estrogen and progesterone receptor negative; P53 positive; Ki67 positive more than or equal to 14%. There are fifteen persons who completely meet the following requirements entered the LIMG: tumor diameter more than 3 cm; no lymph node metastases and micrometastases; historical grade I; Her2 negative; vascular thrombosis negative; estrogen and progesterone receptor positive; P53 negative; Ki67 positive less than 14% (Table 1). And we choose 10 patients with benign tumor as the control group during the same period (Table 2). By the way, all patients on admission signed complete informed consent.

2.2. Serum and Tissue Samples. The preoperative blood was collected and centrifuged, and volume of 2 mL of serum was kept as above. The samples including serum, tumor tissue and normal breast tissue, were preserved temporarily in liquid nitrogen for 30 min following isolated and for long time in deep freezer at −86°C.

2.3. Micrometastasis Detection. If no carcinoma cells were detected in the nodes, immunohistochemistry with cytokeratin antibody CK-22 (Santa Cruz, USA), using a standard immunoperoxidase method (ABC Elite kit, Vector Laboratories, USA), was performed. Micrometastasis was defined as tumor of the size exceeding 0.2 mm and less than or equal to 2 mm in diameter, according to the American Joint Committee of Cancer (AJCC) 7th classification. Hence, isolated tumor cells or tumor cell clusters measuring less than or equal to 0.2 mm in diameter did not meet the definition of micrometastases [9]. Therefore, the patients with such clusters were considered as micro-metastasis negative. All the analysis above was performed by a pathologist from the Breast Group of Pathology Diagnosis Center of our institute.

2.4. Real-Time RT-qPCR. Small RNA of serum was isolated by mirVana PARIS Kit (AM1556, ABI, USA). Small RNA and total RNA of breast tissue were extracted by mirVana miRNA Isolation Kit (AM1560, ABI, USA). Reverse transcription was performed with PrimeScript RT reagent kit (DRR037A, Takara, Japan) in a final volume of 10 μL containing RNA 200 ng and other elements followed instruction of protocol. Small RNA was added poly-A tail by poly-A polymerase (NEB, M0276) before reverse transcription using primers in Table 3 as before (Table 3). Real-time quantitative PCR was performed on Roche LightCycler 2.0 with SYBR Premix Ex Taq (DRR041A, Takara, Japan). For each sample, real time PCR was performed in a final volume of 10 μL containing PCR master mix, 50 ng of genomic DNA or 5 ng of cDNA, and primers (250 nM). For negative control, template was replaced by purified non-reverse-transcribed RNA. Each experiment was done in triplicate. Averaged Ct values of GAPDH were subtracted from each averaged interest Ct to give ΔCt.

2.5. Western Blot. Protein extracts, SDS-PAGE, electrotransfer, and immunoblotting were following the standard procedure. The TIMP3 expression can be detected by sc-6836 (Santa Cruz, USA), which was against the C-terminal of TIMP3. Internal controls were checked by antibody of GAPDH (KC-5G4, Kangchen Biotech, China). Densitometric analysis was performed using Quantity One (version 4.5, Bio-Rad, USA).

TABLE 3: Primers.

Universal reverse transcription primer	GCTGTCAACGATACGCTACGTAACGGCATGACAGTG(TT$\cdots$TT)$_{24}$N(A, G, C)	
U6	F: CTCGCTTCGGCAGCACA	R: AACGCTTCACGAATTTGCGT
miR-21	F: AGCTTATCAGACTGATGTTG	R: GCTGTCAACGATACGCTACGTAACG
TIMP3	F: CTTCCAAGAACGAGTGTCT	R: GGTCTGTGGCATTGATGA
GAPDH	F: GGTGAAGGTCGGAGTCAACG	R: CCATGTAGTTGAGGTCAATGAAG

TABLE 4

Sample	Group	Mean ± SD	F	P
Tissue miR-21	High	9.34 ± 1.87	70.91	0.000
	Low	4.65 ± 1.44		
	Normal	0.00 ± 2.59		
Serum miR-21	High	10.91 ± 1.82	85.38	0.000
	Low	7.25 ± 1.49		
	Normal	0.00 ± 2.94		
TIMP-3 mRNA	High	−6.90 ± 2.09	35.28	0.000
	Low	−3.21 ± 2.25		
	Normal	0.00 ± 1.55		
TIMP-3 protein	High	0.455 ± 0.062	19.43	0.000
	Low	0.517 ± 0.050		
	Normal	0.592 ± 0.046		

Averaged Ct value of normal samples was chosen as reference ($\Delta\Delta$Ct = 0, relative fold increase, RFI = 1). $\Delta\Delta$Ct was calculated by ΔCt subtracted with this reference. Our datum of relative fold index (RFI = 2 −$\Delta\Delta$Ct) obeyed skewed distribution, so we transformed our datum with log2(RFI) to normal distribution. miR-21 expression of tumor tissue and serum samples in the normal group, high and low invasive group has statistical differences and the comparison between each group is statistically significant ($P < 0.01$).
Tumor tissue TIMP-3 mRNA and protein expression levels in each group has statistical differences and the comparison between each group is statistically significant ($P < 0.01$).

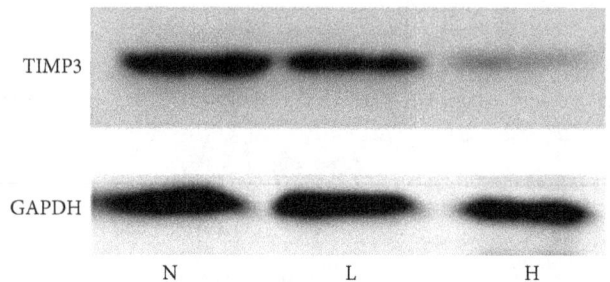

FIGURE 1: Western blot electrophoresis results, N: normal group, L: low invasion and metastasis group, H: high invasion and metastasis group; it can be seen that TIMP3 protein expression was significantly decreased in high invasion and metastasis group.

2.6. Statistical Analysis.

All the data were performed by normality test: the normally distributed data was compared using t-test; other data were log-transforming to meet normally distributed and abnormally distributed using Mann-Whitney U test. Multiple groups were compared using ANOVA analysis, between the two groups using SNK test (Student-Newman-Keuls), and correlation analysis using Pearson test. $P < 0.05$ was defined as being significant. Statistical analysis was performed using the SPSS software (version 17.0, IBM, USA).

3. Result

3.1. miR-21 Is Overexpressed in HIMG (Realtime RT-qPCR).

The relative content of miR-21 extracted from tissue in HIMG was 9.34±1.87, LIMG was 4.65±1.44, and NG was 0.00±2.59. There was significant difference in the three groups ($F = 70.91$, $P < 0.05$) (Table 4). The tissue miR-21 expression was significantly higher in HIMG than in LIMG; the latter was higher than that in NG by SNK test ($P < 0.05$) (Figure 2(a)). The relative content of miR-21 extracted from serum in HIMG was 10.91 ± 1.82, LIMG was 7.25 ± 1.49, and NG was 0.00 ± 2.94. There was marked diffidence in the three groups ($F = 85.38$, $P < 0.05$) (Table 4). The serum miR-21 expression was significantly higher in HIMG than LIMG, the latter was higher than NG by SNK test ($P < 0.05$) (Figure 2(b)). The relative content of miR-21 in tissue positively correlates with that in corresponding serum, and the Pearson coefficient was 0.866 ($P < 0.05$) (Table 5, Figure 3(a)).

3.2. Protein and mRNA of TIMP-3 Was Contradictory-Expressed in HIMG, LIMG, and NG (Western Blot and Real-Time RT-qPCR).

The content of TIMP-3 in HIMG was 0.455 ± 0.062, LIMG was 0.517 ± 0.050, and NG was 0.592 ± 0.046. There was striking difference in the three groups ($F = 19.43$, $P < 0.05$) (Table 4). The TIMP-3 protein expression was apparently lower in HIMG than in LIMG, the latter was lower than that in NG by SNK test ($P < 0.05$) (Figures 1 and 2(c)). The relative content of TIMP-3 mRNA in HIMG was −6.90 ± 2.09, LIMG was −3.21 ± 2.25, and NG was 0.00 ± 1.55. There was remarkable difference in the three groups ($F = 35.28$, $P < 0.05$). The TIMP-3 mRNA expression was apparently lower in HIMG than in LIMG; the latter was lower than that in NG by SNK test ($P < 0.05$) (Figure 2(d)).

3.3. TIMP-3 Expression Inversely Correlates with miR-21 Relative Content in Breast Tissue.

In HIMG with high relative miR-21 expression extracted from tissue, low dose mRNA and protein of TIMP-3 were observed, whereas LIMG with low relative miR-21 expression displayed relatively high amount of TIMP-3 (mRNA and protein), resulting in an apparently inverse correlation between tissue miR-21 expression and TIMP-3 content (Pearson correlation, $r = -0.778$ and −0.692, resp., $P < 0.05$) (Table 5, Figures 3(b) and 3(c)). In HIMG

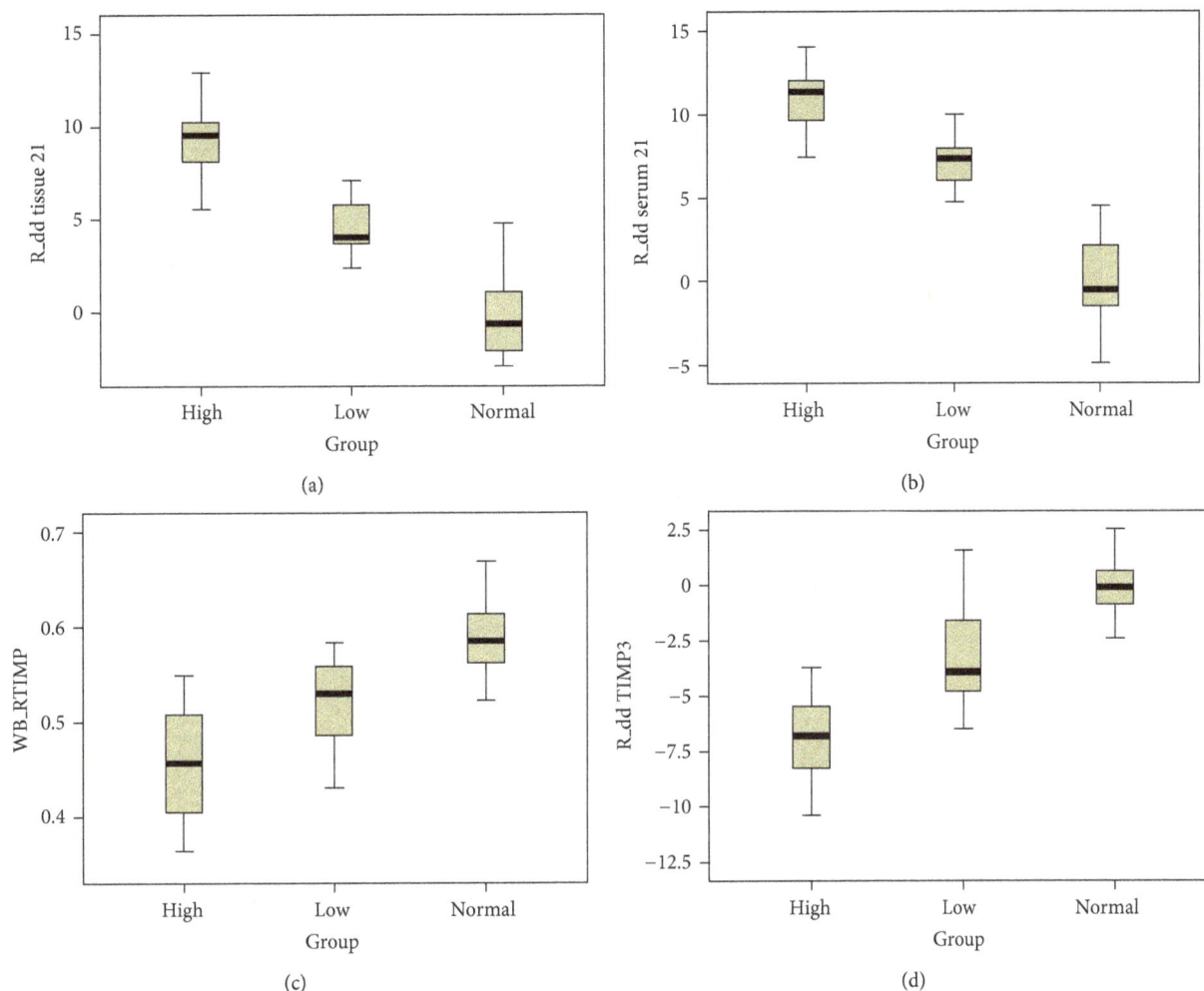

FIGURE 2: (a) miR-21 in various clinical invasions in breast cancer tissue of the different transcripts. Experimental method: realtime RT-PCR; statistical method: ANOVA showed $P < 0.05$; comparison between groups $P < 0.05$, that is, HIMG > LIMG > NG. (b) miR-21 in various clinical invasions in breast cancer patients serum of the different levels. Experimental method: realtime RT-PCR; statistical method: ANOVA showed $P < 0.05$; comparison between groups $P < 0.05$, that is, HIMG > LIMG > NG. (c) TIMP3 in various clinical invasions in breast tissue of different expressions. Experimental methods: western blot; statistical method: ANOVA showed $P < 0.05$; comparison between groups $P < 0.05$, HIMG < LIMG < NG. (d) TIMP3 in various t clinical invasions in breast cancer tissue of the different transcripts. Experimental method: realtime RT-PCR; statistical method: ANOVA showed $P < 0.05$; comparison between groups $P < 0.05$, that is, HIMG < LIMG < NG.

with high relative miR-21 expression extracted from serum, low amounts mRNA and protein of TIMP-3 were observed, whereas LIMG with low relative miR-21 expression displayed relatively high amounts of TIMP-3 (mRNA and protein), resulting in a significantly inverse correlation between serum miR-21 expression and TIMP-3 content (Pearson correlation, $r = -0.762$ and -0.625, resp., $P < 0.05$) (Table 5, Figures 3(d) and 3(e)). There was significant positive correlation between mRNA and protein of TIMP-3 extracted from tissue (Pearson correlation, $r = 0.616$; $P < 0.05$) (Table 5, Figure 3(f)).

4. Discussion

Recent experiments in vitro have suggested that degree of degradation of ECM was determined by the balance between MMPs and TIMP, which affected the epithelial mesenchymal

transformation (EMT) [11]. EMT is considered to be the initial stage of cancer invasion and metastasis of critical process [12]. The same tumor can be significantly different in prognosis caused by different individuals. This is very important in breast cancer patients, because metastasis is the main reason which causes death. The following indicators can predict the metastasis in various degrees, such as historical grading; tumor thrombus; lymph nodes metastasis and micro-metastasis; estrogen receptor and progesterone receptor; human epithelial growth factors receptor-2; P53 and Ki67 [13–16]. Therefore, those generally accepted indicators were grouped criteria through determining the heterogeneity of clinical breast cancer metastasis difference (Table 1). According to Heimann and Hellman's study in 1998, the probability of breast cancer metastasis increased with the tumor diameter [10]. While we can still find that 22% breast cancer patients whose tumor diameter less than 1 cm

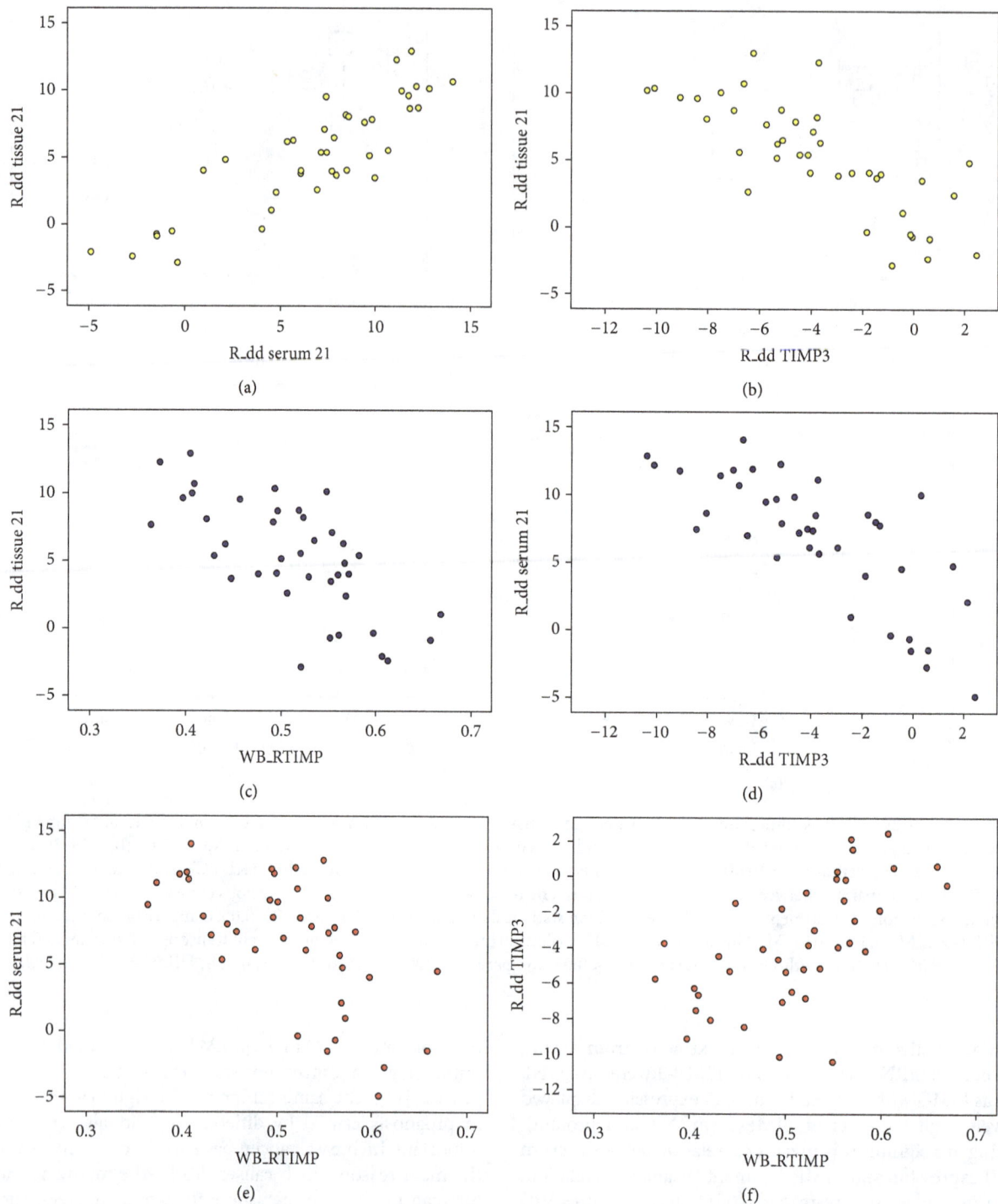

FIGURE 3: (a) miR-21 transcription in volume of breast tissue and corresponding serum levels in patients with significant correlation, Pearson correlation (positive correlation, correlation coefficient = 0.866, $P < 0.05$). (b) Different clinical invasions of breast tissue in the transcription miR-21 and TIMP3 were significantly correlated (negative correlation, correlation coefficient = −0.778, $P < 0.05$). (c) Different clinical invasion of breast tissue in volume of miR-21 transcription and TIMP3 protein expression was significantly correlated (negative correlation, correlation coefficient = −0.692, $P < 0.05$). (d) miR-21 serum levels and breast tissue volume of TIMP transcription were significantly correlated (negative correlation, correlation coefficient = −0.762, $P < 0.05$). (e) miR-21 serum levels and TIMP breast tissue levels of protein expressions were significantly correlated (negative correlation, correlation coefficient = −0.625, $P < 0.05$). (f) Different clinical invasions of breast tissue levels of TIMP3 transcription and protein expression were also correlated (positive correlation, correlation coefficient = 0.616, $P < 0.05$).

TABLE 5

Data A	Data B	Correlation coefficient	Sig.
Tissue miR-21	Serum miR-21	0.866	0.000
Tissue miR-21	TIMP-3 mRNA	−0.778	0.000
Tissue miR-21	TIMP-3 Proteins	−0.692	0.000
Serum miR-21	TIMP-3 mRNA	−0.762	0.000
Serum miR-21	TIMP-3 Proteins	−0.625	0.000
TIMP-3 mRNA	TIMP-3 Proteins	0.616	0.000

Each of the tumor tissue and serum in the miR-21, tumor tissue miR-21 and TIMP-3 of the mRNA, tumor tissue miR-21 and TIMP-3 protein, serum miR-21 and tumor tissue of TIMP-3 mRNA, the miR-21 in serum and tumor tissue TIMP-3 protein, and tumor tissue TIMP-3 mRNA and protein do Pearson correlation analysis; correlation coefficients were 0.866, −0.778, −0.692, −0.762, −0.625, and 0.616, with statistical significance.

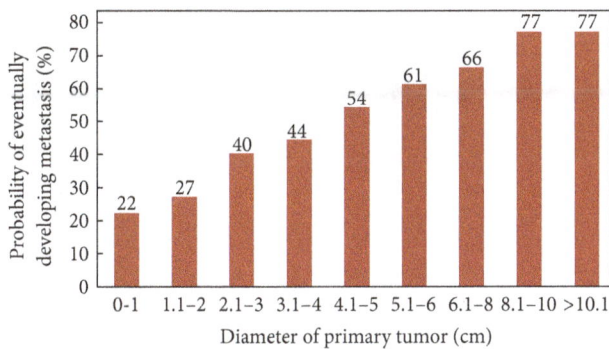

FIGURE 4: From Heimann and Hellman [10].

had metastasis, 23% had no metastasis more than 10 cm (Figure 4). If the increasing rate in tumor volume was certain, it could make larger tumors have no metastasis or the ability of metastasis even worse, and vice versa. In order to compare the ability of metastatic difference better, the aforementioned view was seen as one of grouping criteria in the study (Table 1). It was the aim of grouping criteria to make the genetic heterogeneity become the main reason which cause the metastasis other than the clinical stage. In the present study, we identified increased expression of miR-21, as compared to LIMG (Table 4). These data were consistent with reports indicating that miR-21 expression increased with miR-21 expression was increasing the progression of clinical stage and shortening survival of patients [17]. In fact, the miR-21 gene is located on chromosome 17q23.2, which is located within the common fragile site FRA17B [18]. This region is frequently found amplified in breast, colon, and lung cancer, consistent with the fact that miR-21 overexpression is widespread in many types of cancer, including the breast [19]. Despite the link of miR-21 to carcinogenesis, little was known regarding the specific mechanism of how miR-21 made cancer progression. Several findings suggested that miR-21 could be impacting matrix metalloproteinases inhibitors, such as TIMP3, that played a crucial role in cancer invasion and metastasis including recent studies that identified TIMP3 as a functional target of miR-21 in cell invasion and metastasis in glioma and cholangiocarcinoma [20, 21]. Recently, Song et al. have proved that miR-21 can regulate the expression of TIMP-3 to control the invasion of breast cancer cell [8]. Our finding reported that microRNA-21 negatively regulated

TIMP3 in breast cancer and suggested that TIMP3 might be negatively regulated by miR-21 at the translated level (Table 5). These compelling data supported miR-21 regulation of TIMP3 expression as a novel mechanism impacting genetic heterogeneity of breast cancer invasion and metastasis. But the regulation mechanism needs to be further confirmed by the vitro experiments. Our experiment also demonstrated that the miR-21 in tissue and the miR-21 in serum had a high degree of consistency. Recent study prompted that high circulating miR-21 concentrations correlated significantly with visceral metastasis in patients with breast cancer [22]. This suggested that miR-21 is a predictor of breast cancer metastasis marker with the qualifications.

Authors' Contribution

Li J and Zhang W contributed equally to this work; Li J and Zhang W designed the research; Li J, Zhang Y, Jia S, Tian R, and Kang Y performed the research; Ma Y evaluated axillary lymph nodes by ultrasound before operation; Li D performed the pathological diagnosis; Li J, Zhang Y, and Jia S analyzed the data; and Li J, Zhang Y, and Zhang W wrote the paper.

Acknowledgment

This paper was supported by the Science and Technology Foundation of Shenyang City, no. 1091142-9-02.

References

[1] C. Desantis, R. Siegel, P. Bandi, and A. Jemal, "Breast cancer statistics, 2011," *CA Cancer Journal for Clinicians*, vol. 61, no. 6, pp. 409–418, 2011.

[2] K. Turaga, G. Acs, and C. Laronga, "Gene expression profiling in breast cancer," *Cancer Control*, vol. 17, no. 3, pp. 177–182, 2010.

[3] R. C. S. Figueira, L. R. Gomes, J. S. Neto, F. C. Silva, I. D. C. G. Silva, and M. C. Sogayar, "Correlation between MMPs and their inhibitors in breast cancer tumor tissue specimens and in cell lines with different metastatic potential," *BMC Cancer*, vol. 9, article 20, 2009.

[4] Z.-D. Wang, C. Huang, Z.-F. Li et al., "Chrysanthemum indicum ethanolic extract inhibits invasion of hepatocellular carcinoma via regulation of MMP/TIMP balance as therapeutic target," *Oncology Reports*, vol. 23, no. 2, pp. 413–421, 2010.

[5] D. Bourboulia and W. G. Stetler-Stevenson, "Matrix metalloproteinases (MMPs) and tissue inhibitors of metalloproteinases

(TIMPs): positive and negative regulators in tumor cell adhesion," *Seminars in Cancer Biology*, vol. 20, no. 3, pp. 161–168, 2010.

[6] R. Munker and G. A. Calin, "MicroRNA profiling in cancer," *Clinical Science*, vol. 121, no. 4, pp. 141–158, 2011.

[7] C. H. Yang, J. Yue, S. R. Pfeffer, C. R. Handorf, and L. M. Pfeffer, "MicroRNA miR-21 regulates the metastatic behavior of B16 melanoma cells," *Journal of Biological Chemistry*, vol. 286, no. 45, pp. 39172–39178, 2011.

[8] B. Song, C. Wang, J. Liu et al., "MicroRNA-21 regulates breast cancer invasion partly by targeting tissue inhibitor of metalloproteinase 3 expression," *Journal of Experimental and Clinical Cancer Research*, vol. 29, no. 1, article 29, 2010.

[9] C. Garbe, T. K. Eigentler, J. Bauer et al., "Histopathological diagnostics of malignant melanoma in accordance with the recent AJCC classification 2009: review of the literature and recommendations for general practice," *Journal of the German Society of Dermatology*, vol. 9, no. 9, pp. 690–699, 2011.

[10] R. Heimann and S. Hellman, "Aging, progression, and phenotype in breast cancer," *Journal of Clinical Oncology*, vol. 16, no. 8, pp. 2686–2692, 1998.

[11] L. Aresu, S. Benali, S. Garbisa, E. Gallo, and M. Castagnaro, "Matrix metalloproteinases and their role in the renal epithelial mesenchymal transition," *Histology and Histopathology*, vol. 26, no. 3, pp. 307–313, 2011.

[12] Y. Wang and B. P. Zhou, "Epithelial-mesenchymal transition in breast cancer progression and metastasis," *Chinese Journal of Cancer*, vol. 30, no. 9, pp. 603–611, 2011.

[13] A. Dirier, S. Burhanedtin-Zincircioglu, B. Karadayi, A. Isikdogan, and R. Aksu, "Characteristics and prognosis of breast cancer in younger women," *Journal of B.U.ON*, vol. 14, no. 4, pp. 619–623, 2009.

[14] G.-F. Von Tempelhoff, N. Schönmann, and L. Heilmann, "Thrombosis—a clue of poor prognosis in primary nonmetastatic breast cancer?" *Breast Cancer Research and Treatment*, vol. 73, no. 3, pp. 275–277, 2002.

[15] J. S. Lee, S. I. Kim, S. Y. Choi et al., "Factors influencing the outcome of breast cancer patients with 10 or more metastasized axillary lymph nodes," *International Journal of Clinical Oncology*, vol. 16, no. 5, pp. 473–481, 2011.

[16] E. K. A. Millar, P. H. Graham, C. M. McNeil et al., "Prediction of outcome of early ER+ breast cancer is improved using a biomarker panel, which includes Ki-67 and p53," *British Journal of Cancer*, vol. 105, no. 2, pp. 272–280, 2011.

[17] B. Qian, D. Katsaros, L. Lu et al., "High miR-21 expression in breast cancer associated with poor disease-free survival in early stage disease and high TGF-β1," *Breast Cancer Research and Treatment*, vol. 117, no. 1, pp. 131–140, 2009.

[18] G. A. Calin, C. Sevignani, C. D. Dumitru et al., "Human microRNA genes are frequently located at fragile sites and genomic regions involved in cancers," *Proceedings of the National Academy of Sciences of the United States of America*, vol. 101, no. 9, pp. 2999–3004, 2004.

[19] G. A. Calin and C. M. Croce, "Chromosomal rearrangements and microRNAs: a new cancer link with clinical implications," *Journal of Clinical Investigation*, vol. 117, no. 8, pp. 2059–2066, 2007.

[20] G. Gabriely, T. Wurdinger, S. Kesari et al., "MicroRNA 21 promotes glioma invasion by targeting matrix metalloproteinase regulators," *Molecular and Cellular Biology*, vol. 28, no. 17, pp. 5369–5380, 2008.

[21] F. M. Selaru, A. V. Olaru, T. Kan et al., "MicroRNA-21 is overexpressed in human cholangiocarcinoma and regulates programmed cell death 4 and tissue inhibitor of metalloproteinase 3," *Hepatology*, vol. 49, no. 5, pp. 1595–1601, 2009.

[22] S. Asaga, C. Kuo, T. Nguyen, M. Terpenning, A. E. Giuliano, and D. S. B. Hoon, "Direct serum assay for microRNA-21 concentrations in early and advanced breast cancer," *Clinical Chemistry*, vol. 57, no. 1, pp. 84–91, 2011.

28

Dermal Substitutes Use in Reconstructive Surgery for Skin Tumors: A Single-Center Experience

Mariane Campagnari,[1] **Andrea S. Jafelicci,**[2] **Helio A. Carneiro,**[2] **Eduard R. Brechtbühl,**[1] **Eduardo Bertolli,**[1] **and João P. Duprat Neto**[1]

[1]*Skin Cancer Department, AC Camargo Cancer Center, São Paulo, SP, Brazil*
[2]*Surgical Oncology, AC Camargo Cancer Center, São Paulo, SP, Brazil*

Correspondence should be addressed to Eduardo Bertolli; ebertolli@hotmail.com

Academic Editor: Anil D'cruz

Reconstructive surgery following skin tumor resection can be challenging. Treatment options after removing the tumor are skin grafting, local pedicled and axial flaps, or microsurgery for complex and extensive wounds correction. Recently, the use of dermal substitutes has been extended to reconstructive surgery in cutaneous oncology. *Objectives.* To report both a single-center experience using dermal substitutes in reconstructive surgery for skin malignancies and reconstructive surgery's outcomes. *Methods and Results.* Among thirteen patients, seven (53.8%) were male with mean age of 62.6 years. Regarding diagnosis, there were five cases (38.5%) of basal cell carcinoma (BCC), two (15.4%) of melanoma in situ, two (15.4%) of dermatofibrosarcoma protuberans, one (7.7%) of squamous cell carcinoma (SCC), one (7.7%) of angiosarcoma, and one (7.7%) of eccrine carcinoma (EC). The most common site of injury was scalp (53.8%) and lower limbs (23.1%). Seven (53.8%) patients used NPWT and six (46.2%) patients underwent Brown's dressing. The most frequent complication of the first stage was wound contamination (38.5%). Average time to second-stage skin grafting was 43.9 days. Three (23%) patients developed tumor recurrence and one died. *Conclusions.* Use of dermal substitutes in oncology can be an option for reconstruction after extended resections, providing good aesthetical and functional results.

1. Background

Reconstructive surgery following skin tumor resection can be particularly challenging due to the nature of disease process, including the extent of resection, need for preserving original surgical margin orientation, possibility of tumor recurrence, and requirement for adjuvant radiation therapy. Moreover, following tumor resection, reconstruction must be tailored to clinical prognosis, treatment plan, patient's age, and desired cosmesis [1].

Treatment options after tumor removal are skin grafting, local pedicled and axial flaps, or microsurgery for complex and extensive wounds correction. Each technique has not only its advantages but also its limitations.

Dermal substitutes such as Integra® and Matriderm® were initially used for treating burns and were later extended

for reconstructive surgeries and treatment of chronic wounds [1–5].

Integra (LifeSciences Corporation, NJ, USA) is a bilaminate synthetic construct consisting of an outer silicone layer and an inner collagen-glycosaminoglycan matrix. The first layer is a matrix of bovine collagen and chondroitin-6-sulfate, cross-linked with glutaraldehyde; after grafting, recipient fibroblasts infiltrate the matrix network and synthetize a neodermis, which is histologically very close to normal human dermis. The second layer is a silicone membrane, which acts as a temporary epidermis [6, 7].

Matriderm (Dr. Suwelack Skin & Health Care AG, Billerbeck, Germany) is a single layer composed of bovine collagen and elastin. The collagen promotes rapid cell migration, proliferation, and revascularization and the elastin encourages early neoangiogenesis and elastin synthesis [8, 9].

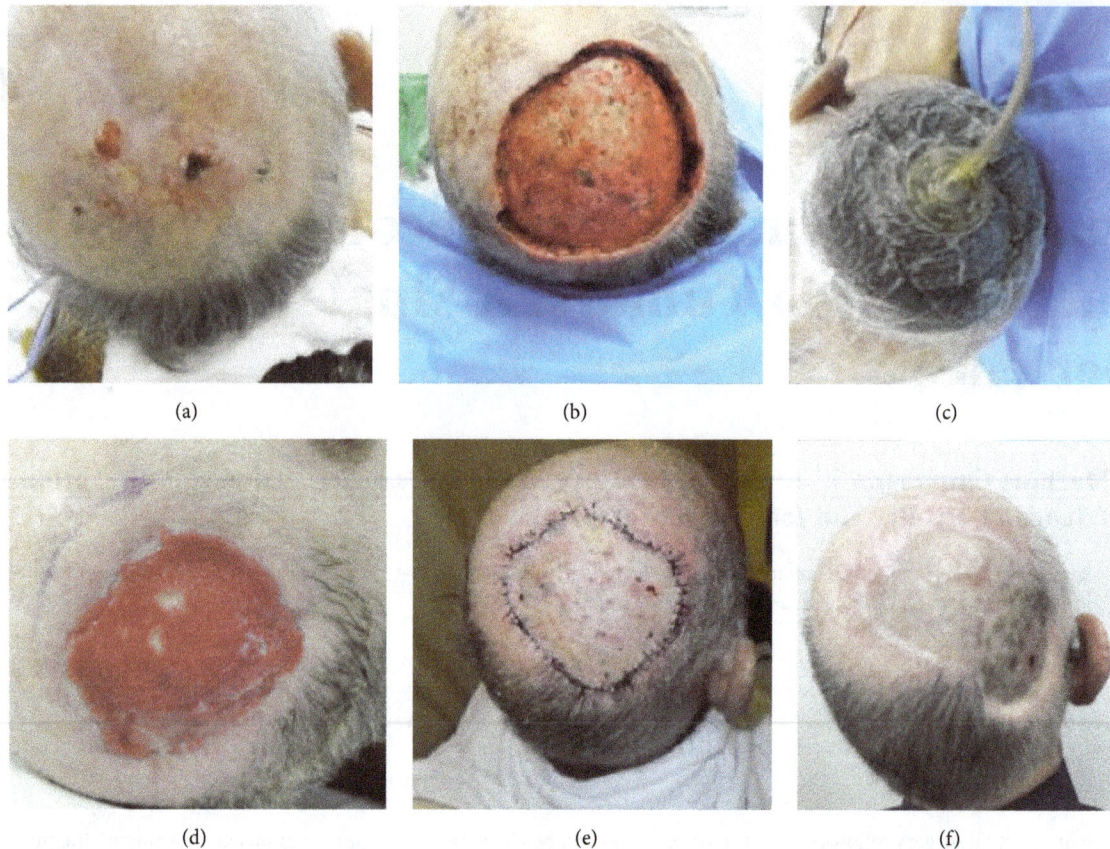

FIGURE 1: (a) Basal cell carcinoma in scalp, clinical aspect before surgery; (b) surgical bed with periosteal removal; (c) negative pressure wound therapy was applied after Matriderm to enhance granulation; (d) granulation tissue; (e) skin graft, early postoperative aspect; (f) late postoperative aspect.

More recently, Matriderm and Integra use in oncology and reconstructive surgery has also been reported [10–12]. These reports show no difference in oncological outcomes and are technically feasible. In addition, good aesthetical results have been achieved.

2. Objectives

We aim to report a single-center experience using dermal substitutes in reconstructive surgery for skin malignancies and the outcomes of those surgeries.

3. Patients and Methods

We present the report of thirteen patients treated in the Skin Cancer Department of AC Camargo Cancer Center, São Paulo/SP, Brazil, who underwent reconstructive surgery with artificial dermis between December 2012 and November 2016. All patients were informed before surgeries, and an informed written consent was provided.

Clinical data was analyzed regarding age, tumor type and location, tumor size in pathology report, comorbidities, postoperative complications, and recurrence. Reconstruction was carried out in a two-stage process and the time interval between them was also analyzed. One patient underwent only

first-stage surgery, due to complete epithelialization. Another patient is still waiting grafting after multiple debridement surgeries of devitalized and necrotic tissue.

First stage involved removal of tumor and application of artificial dermis. Frozen section exam was performed to ensure clear margins, except both in DFSP cases, in which circumferential and deep margin assessment is the standard of care, and in melanoma cases. First stage was followed by Brown's dressing or Negative Pressure Wound Therapy (NPWT) (Figure 1). Our intention was to use NPWT in every patient. However, some of them could not use it due to local pain or in some specific locations such as nail unity. Besides that, some patients had no coverage of their health insurances to this product.

Brown's dressing was removed 5 to 7 days after surgery and new dressings were performed three times a week with Mepilex Ag™ (Mölnlycke Health Care, Göteborg, Sweden) or PolyMem Silver™ (Ferris Mfg. Corp., TX, USA) to help control local contamination. Patients with NPWT were evaluated weekly, following the same procedures as mentioned below. Wound was inspected to assess for contamination or local complications until a well-vascularized neodermis was achieved. Second stage was only performed when the wound showed adequate granulation tissue and subsequently covered with a split-thickness skin graft.

Clinical follow-up of patients was done in outpatient clinics periodically to assess treatment plan, tumor recurrence, and durability of the reconstruction.

4. Results

Clinical data is summarized in Table 1. Mean age was 62.6 years (range 39 to 86 years). Cohort comprised seven (53.8%) male and six (46.2%) female patients. Only two patients had no comorbidities. The most common comorbidities were high blood pressure (46.2%), heart disease (30.8%), former smoking (30.8%), hypothyroidism (23.1%), diabetes mellitus (15.4%), and smoking (7.7%).

Regarding diagnosis, five (38.5%) patients presented with basal cell carcinoma (BCC), all of them with sclerodermiform subtype, two (15.4%) with melanoma in situ, two (15.4%) with dermatofibrosarcoma protuberans, one (7.7%) with eccrine carcinoma, one (7.7%) with squamous cell carcinoma, and one (7.7%) with angiosarcoma. One patient presented with radionecrosis after treatment for malignant fibrohistiocytoma and another used dermal substitutes in the donor area of a frontal skin flap. The most common site of injury was the scalp (53.8%) followed by lower limbs (23.1%) and fingers (15.4%).

Only one patient used Integra. All the others used Matriderm 2 mm. Seven (46.2%) patients used NPWT after first surgery. However, one patient could not tolerate NPWT and had it removed after first week due to local pain. Six (46.2%) patients underwent Brown's dressing.

Average time to second-stage skin grafting was 43.9 days (range 28 to 64 days). The most frequent complication of first stage was wound contamination (38.5%), which was treated with Mepilex Ag or PolyMem Silver and oral antibiotics. Regarding the second stage, partial loss of the graft occurred twice, treated with the same dressing.

Three (23%) patients developed tumor recurrence. And among patients who underwent skin grafting, two (18.2%) experienced partial loss of the graft. One patient did not require a second-stage reconstructive surgery and the other one is still unable to undergo grafting. One patient died due to disease progression. Three patients were lost to follow-up.

Radionecrosis patient's granulation process in surgical bed was slow, which made grafting unfeasible after first surgery. This patient required other surgeries for debridement of devitalized and necrotic tissue. Currently, granulation tissue presents good aspect and skin grafting is being scheduled.

5. Discussion

Reconstructive surgery plays a very important role in cutaneous oncology. Several skin malignancies may lead to complex defects and, therefore, complex reconstructions.

Skin graft may be the simplest option. It is associated with minimal donor-site morbidity and is cost-effective but can be prone to contraction and suboptimal aesthetic appearance [13–15]. In particular skin graft is unreliable on the previously irradiated wound bed and should be avoided whenever there are bones, tendons, and nerves exposed [6].

Locoregional flaps particularly in the scalp and lower limbs can cover exposed bone or tendons but are limited by the size of the defect. Also, the donor site may require grafting. Previous irradiation of tissues can lead to poor take of the flap or delayed healing. Local pedicled and axial flaps are more tolerant to therapeutic radiation. Moreover, the choice of free flap requires the presence of a long vascular pedicle and an adequate surface area of the flap [1].

Free tissue microvascular reconstruction of oncological defects, particularly in larger defects, remains the gold standard for covering large tissue defects, with successful transplant rates ranging from 95 to 99 percent. However, the application of either free or pedicled vascularized tissue transfer is associated with substantial donor-site morbidity, prolonged operative time, and hospital stay [1]. Also, it requires appropriate equipment and enabled professionals.

Artificial dermis is an alternative for the treatment of complex wounds, as it allows their closure with less morbidity and surgical time. Artificial dermis offers lower wound contraction, improved elasticity, and skin thickness in relation to grafts. It is also a simple procedure when compared to microsurgical flap and can be performed in previously irradiated areas, allowing wound cover in complex resection areas, better local control of the disease, and early detection of recurrence. The need for experienced surgeons, weekly returns to dressing change, high product cost, and inability to use artificial dermis on wounds with exposed dura mater [5, 7, 10] can be pointed out as disadvantages.

In summary, the choice of reconstruction is influenced either by patient factors such as age, coexisting medical conditions, length of procedure, and performance for general anaesthesia, as by surgeon's experience and surgical equipment, and/or material availability. Our experience with dermal substitutes is presented since we believe it is a well-tolerated option for the patient, with no prejudice to oncologic principles (Figure 2). We used it in more aggressive tumors such as angiosarcoma and eccrine carcinoma, and both can be easily followed up either by clinical examination or by radiologic exams.

There were three recurrences in our cohort. One of them, the eccrine carcinoma (patient 1), died due to complications of chemotherapy after disease progression. The second case experienced recurrence in scalp and underwent salvage surgery. The third one relapsed in transit disease and parothid and is currently on Vismodegib. They were both diagnosed with sclerodermiform BCC with perineural invasion.

Regarding clinical associated conditions, smoking and diabetes mellitus are known to have higher rate of surgical complications. In this study, the only smoking patient had no wound contamination, progressing with partial loss of the graft after second surgery. Longer dressing care was needed to this patient without prejudice to the aesthetic and functional results. Patients with diabetes mellitus or former smoking showed no surgical complication. No patient had prohibitive risk for anesthetic procedure.

In our data, there were five cases of wound contamination at the first stage. One patient had purulent discharge and necrotic wound, treated with debridement, washing, and dressing with Mepilex Ag or PolyMem Silver and oral

TABLE 1: Clinical features and outcomes summary of the patients who underwent reconstructive surgery with dermal substitutes in AC Camargo Cancer Center, from 2012 to 2016 (M = male, F = female, EC = eccrine carcinoma, DFSP = dermatofibrosarcoma protuberans, BCC = basal cell carcinoma, SCC = squamous cell carcinoma, MMis = malignant melanoma in situ, STSG = split-thickness skin graft, N/A = not available, and * size according to pathology reports, without considering further excisions after frozen section when needed).

Patient	Age	Sex	Abnormality	Tumor location	Size (cm)	Comorbidity	Dressing	Complications after 1st surgery	Application of STSG (days)	Complications after 2nd surgery	Follow-up
1	64	M	EC	Scalp	20,5 × 20	Hypothyroidism Heart disease Rheumatoid arthritis	Brown	Wound secretion/debridement	28	Partial graft loss	Death
2	56	M	DFSP	Scalp	14 × 13	High blood pressure Obesity Former smoking	Vacuum	Wound secretion	50	—	No recurrence
3	84	F	BCC sclerodermiform	Lower limbs	13,8 × 8,6	Heart disease Former smoking Alzheimer's disease	Brown	—	29	—	No recurrence
4	51	M	BCC sclerodermiform	Scalp	N/A	—	Vacuum	Wound secretion	50	—	Parotid metastasis In transit disease
5	56	M	BCC sclerodermiform	Nose	5 × 4,5	High blood pressure Smoking	Brown	Wound secretion	57	Partial graft loss	Lost
6	65	M	MMis	Digital	3,5 × 2,5	Former smoking Chronic obstructive pulmonary diseases	Brown	—	Unnecessary	—	Lost
7	75	M	BCC sclerodermiform	Scalp	8 × 5	High blood pressure Former smoking	Vacuum	—	41	—	Recurrence at 20 months
8	50	F	DFSP	Scalp	7 × 5,5	—	Brown	Wound secretion	35	—	Lost
9	77	F	Radionecrosis	Lower limbs	N/A	High blood pressure Heart disease Hypothyroidism	Vacuum	Slow granulation	Not grafted	—	No recurrence
10	41	F	MMis	Digital	3 × 3	Hypothyroidism	Brown	—	50	—	No recurrence
11	39	F	SCC	Lower limbs	13 × 6	High blood pressure, diabetes mellitus, multiple sclerosis	Vacuum	—	36	—	No recurrence
12	70	M	Angiosarcoma	Scalp	5,2 × 4,5	Parkinson's disease	Vacuum	—	43	—	No recurrence
13	86	F	BCC sclerodermiform	Scalp	12 × 12	High blood pressure Heart disease Diabetes mellitus Renal chronic failure	Vacuum	—	64	—	No recurrence

M = male, F = female, EC = eccrine carcinoma, DFSP = dermatofibrosarcoma protuberans, BCC = basal cell carcinoma, SCC = squamous cell carcinoma, MMis = malignant melanoma in situ, STSG = split-thickness skin graft, and N/A = not available.

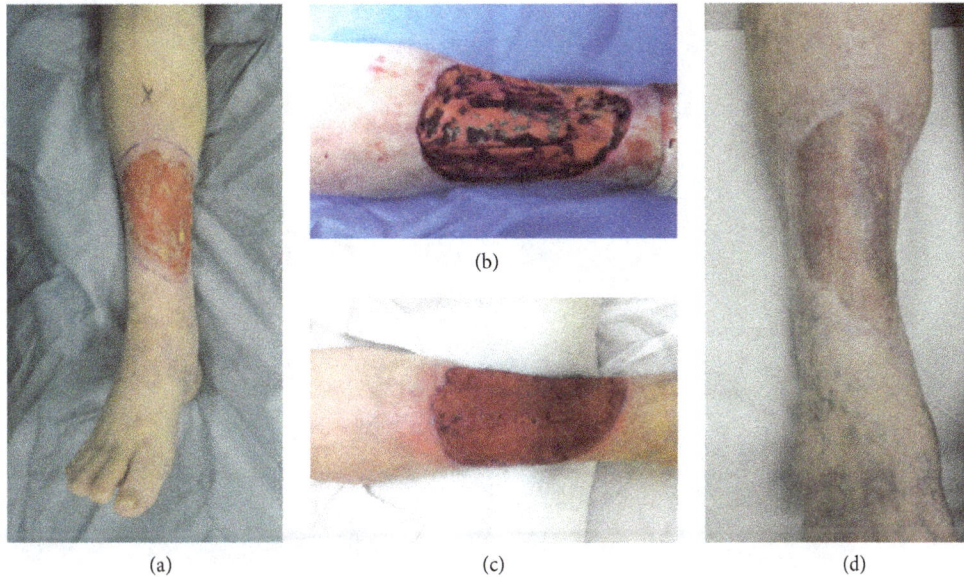

FIGURE 2: (a) Basal cell carcinoma in right leg, clinical aspect before surgery; (b) periosteal removal was necessary to ensure deep margins, which would not allow skin graft; (c) granulation tissue 28 days after Matriderm was placed (no negative pressure wound therapy was used in this case); (d) late postoperative aspect.

antibiotics. Grafting was undergone successfully, but after five months, the patient developed tumor recurrence (eccrine carcinoma) and once again underwent resection of the tumor and reconstruction with regional flap.

The other four patients had only serohematic/serous secretion and underwent only dressing changes before second-stage surgery. Eleven patients underwent grafting in the second stage and only 2 (18.2%) had partial graft loss, but without aesthetic or functional impairment.

In our cohort, the most frequent skin malignancies were sclerodermiform BCC and DFSP, which are frequently associated with wide excisions due to the risk of local recurrence [16]. We also had the scalp as the most prevalent body region, which may also lead to a more challenging reconstruction.

Scalp defects can also be covered using delayed local flaps and tissue expansion. However, in the oncological patient who requires resection, tissue expansion should be used carefully as a reconstructive option since the tumor resection is not delayed because of use of the expansion [6, 17].

As an example, we can mention patients 4 (Figure 3) and 7 (Figure 1) who underwent resection of BCC on the scalp. In both patients, wide excision of the tumor was performed, which was more extensive in patient 4, who needed to have the bone drilled due to involvement of the periosteum.

As reported in other studies, it is known that bone drilling is an important tool used in periosteal involvement of cases to ensure safety margin of tumor resection and even in cases of extensive lesions providing vascularized area to the fixing template. In our data, five (71.4%) patients underwent drilling of scalp injury, due to periosteum involvement by the tumor, to hasten granulation process. The two remaining (28.6%) patients required only periosteum excision.

Two patients had in situ acral melanoma. Digital sparing surgery in this situation can be an option. However, in this scenario, reconstruction after wide local excision can

be associated with functional loss or chronic pain. In such cases, dermal matrix plays an important role as it provides satisfactory aesthetic and functional outcomes [12]. In both cases, amputation could be avoided and the patients report good quality of life after surgery.

Fixing the artificial dermis in the surgical bed can be done either with Brown's dressing or with NPWT. Brown's dressing promotes intimate contact of template with bloody area, providing adequate fixation thereof to wound with tissue neovascularization and granulation tissue. In our routine, we evaluate granulation tissue 3 times a week and Mepilex Ag or Polymem Silver dressings are changed whenever necessary. NPWT can help remove deleterious substances from the wound, relieve edema, and stimulate cell proliferation, thereby promoting granulation and inhibiting chronic inflammation. Furthermore, NPWT also seems to assist in neovascularization of skin grafts and tissue-engineered skin substitutes and can improve the success rate of skin grafting by strengthening bonding between the skin graft and the recipient area. Additionally, NPWT must be evaluated weekly [18].

NPWT was used on 5 patients with lesions of scalp due to extension of the lesion in order to enhance granulation and subsequent grafting. The average time for grafting in these patients was 49.6 days. Also, we used NPWT in 2 patients with lower limbs injury. One patient did not tolerate the pain and the other patient could undergo grafting in 36 days. One patient who underwent resection of a nail melanoma and used Brown's dressing did not require grafting, due to complete epithelialization after 90 days. Average time for grafting in five patients with Brown's dressing was 39.8 days.

There are evidences in literature that the use of vacuum dressing decreases the time required for formation of granulation tissue and subsequent grafting [19–21]. However, in our cohort, patients who used NPWT took on average 47.3 days to

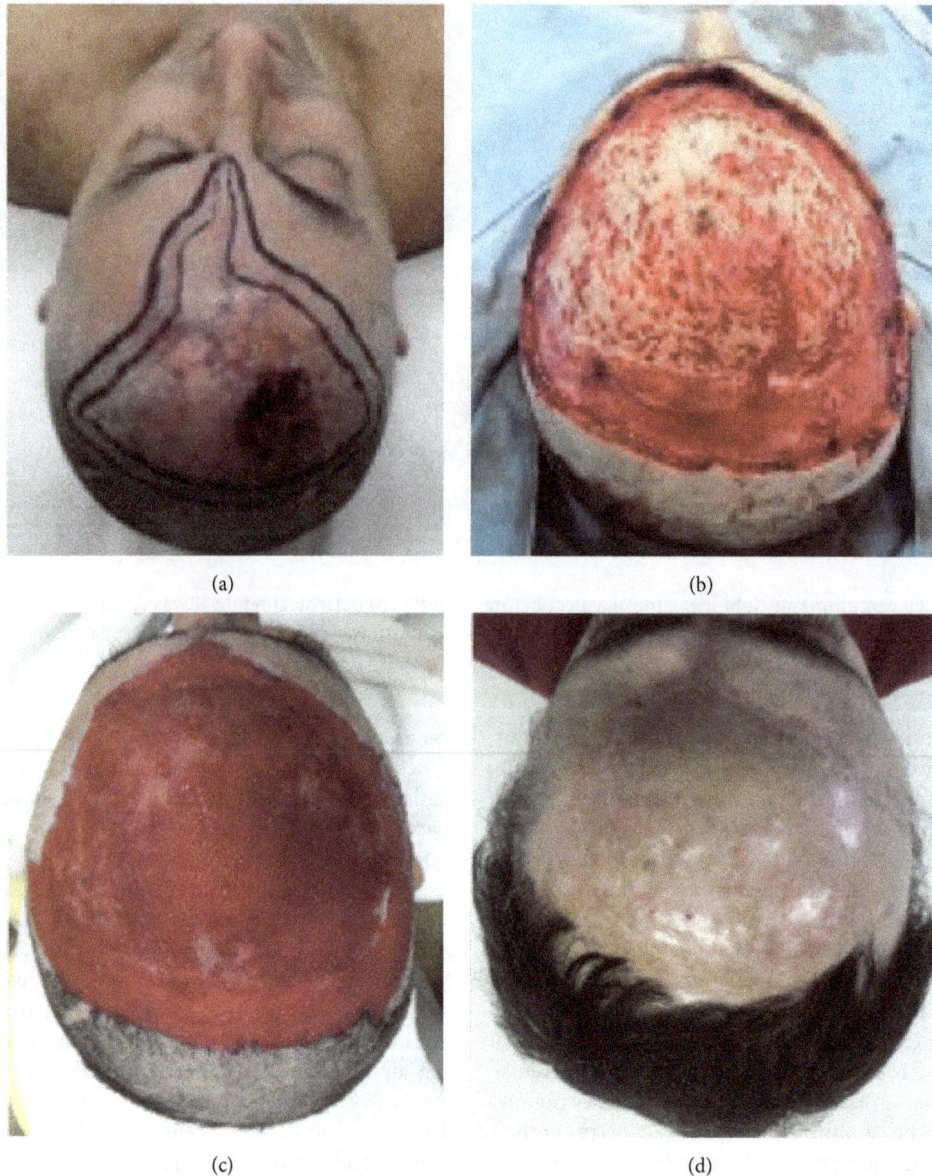

(a)

(b)

(c)

(d)

Figure 3: (a) Basal cell carcinoma, clinical aspect before surgery; (b) once again, periosteal removal was necessary; (c) granulation tissue (negative pressure wound therapy was used); (d) late postoperative aspect.

undergo the second surgery compared to patients who used Brown's dressing with an average of 39.8 days.

We believe that this can be explained by the greater extension of the lesions and the exposed bone. Although our sample is insufficient for statistical validation, we also believe that, even in the absence or inability of NPWT use, Brown's dressing is an acceptable option for the use of dermal substitutes in the reconstructive setting, especially in smaller defects.

Two patients did not achieve second surgery. One patient had complete wound epithelialization with artificial dermis. The other one presented with a complex wound secondary to radionecrosis in her leg after radiotherapy for a malignant fibrohistiocytoma treatment.

She underwent three surgical procedures for debridement of devitalized and necrotic tissue, requiring resection of the

exposed necrotic tendon in the last procedure. Subsequent placement of dermal matrix was performed in all surgical approaches to enhance the formation of feasible tissue to carry out grafting. After her last surgery, the patient has been developing good but still slow formation of granulation tissue (Figure 4). Skin graft is to be scheduled.

There is no report in literature of dermal substitutes use in radionecrosis. However, we believe that, in these complex wounds, dermal matrix could be an ally in its treatment. It could enhance granulation tissue formation for subsequent grafting with an adequate aesthetic and functional result.

We present similar data to what is reported in literature. The use of dermal substitutes in oncology can be an option for reconstruction after extended resections, providing good aesthetical and functional results. Therefore, it can be performed within a shorter period of time, which is useful in

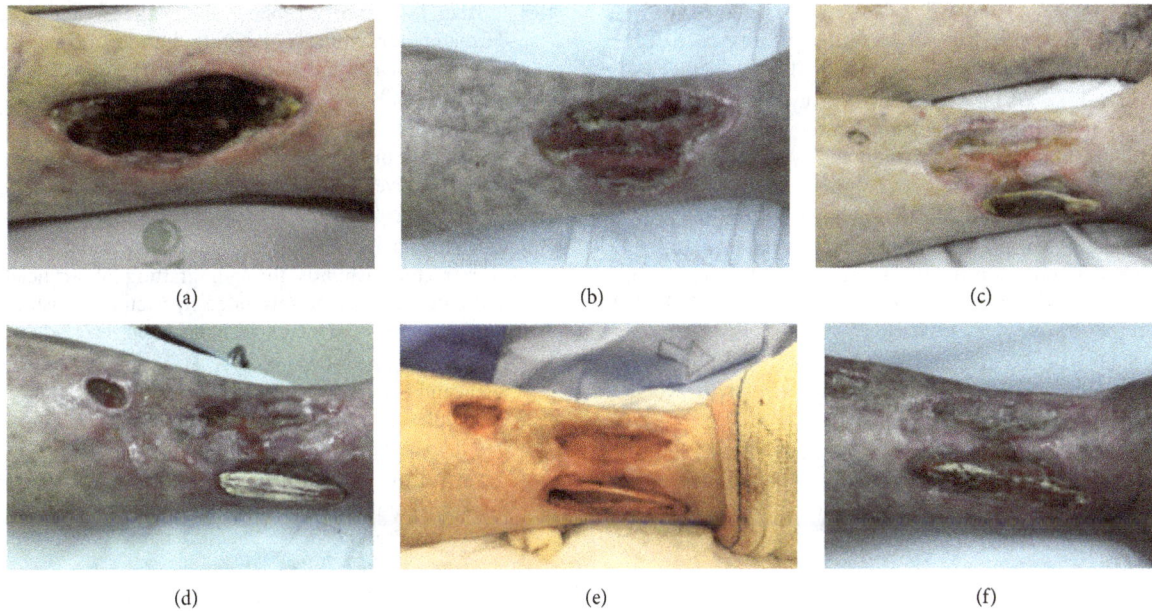

(a)

(b)

(c)

(d)

(e)

(f)

FIGURE 4: (a) Radionecrosis in right leg, clinical aspect before first surgery; ((b) and (c)) there was no granulation in the area of exposed and necrotic tendon, which led to ((d) and (e)) debridement and removal of necrotic tendon. This was the third time that Matriderm was placed; (f) clinical aspect, waiting for skin graft.

patients with clinical comorbidities, such as the ones we had in our patients. Further studies are necessary to validate this procedure.

Disclosure

There was no funding or grants of any kind in the elaboration of this paper.

Authors' Contributions

Mariane Campagnari, Eduardo Bertolli, Eduard R. Brechtbühl, and João P. Duprat Neto were responsible for performing the surgeries mentioned on this paper and for patients' follow-up. Andrea S. Jafelicci and Helio A. Carneiro participated on these procedures and were responsible for collecting the data here presented. All authors were responsible for writing and reviewing this manuscript.

References

[1] E. Komorowska-Timek, A. Gabriel, D. C. Bennett et al., "Artificial dermis as an alternative for coverage of complex scalp defects following excision of malignant tumors," *Plastic and Reconstructive Surgery*, vol. 115, no. 4, pp. 1010–1017, 2005.

[2] J.-Y. Choi, S.-H. Kim, G.-J. Oh, S.-G. Roh, N.-H. Lee, and K.-M. Yang, "Management of defects on lower extremities with the use of Matriderm and skin graft," *Archives of Plastic Surgery*, vol. 41, no. 4, pp. 337–343, 2014.

[3] L. J. M. T. Parren, P. Ferdinandus, V. D. Hulst, J. Frank, and S. Tuinder, "A novel therapeutic strategy for turban tumor : scalp excision and combined reconstruction with artificial dermis and split skin graft," *Dermatologic Surgery*, pp. 246–249, 2013.

[4] S. A. Rehim, M. Singhal, and K. C. Chung, "Dermal skin substitutes for upper limb reconstruction: Current status, indications, and contraindications," *Hand Clinics*, vol. 30, no. 2, pp. 239–252, 2014.

[5] F. Unglaub, D. Ulrich, and N. Pallua, "Reconstructive surgery using an artificial dermis (Integra): results with 19 grafts," *Zentralblatt für Chirurgie*, vol. 130, pp. 157-61, 2005.

[6] R. L. Chalmers, E. Smock, and J. L. C. Geh, "Experience of Integra® in cancer reconstructive surgery," *Journal of Plastic, Reconstructive and Aesthetic Surgery*, vol. 63, pp. 2081–2090, 2010.

[7] E. Dantzer and F. M. Braye, "Reconstructive surgery using an artificial dermis (Integra): results with 39 grafts," *British Journal of Plastic Surgery*, vol. 54, pp. 659–664, 2001.

[8] H. J. C. De Vries, J. E. Zeegelaar, E. Middelkoop et al., "Reduced wound contraction and scar formation in punch biopsy wounds. Native collagen dermal substitutes. A clinical study," *British Journal of Dermatology*, vol. 132, no. 5, pp. 690–697, 1995.

[9] S. Böttcher-Haberzeth, T. Biedermann, C. Schiestl et al., "Matriderm® 1 mm versus Integra® Single Layer 1.3 mm for one-step closure of full thickness skin defects: A comparative experimental study in rats," *Pediatric Surgery International*, vol. 28, no. 2, pp. 171–177, 2012.

[10] E. Bertolli, M. Campagnari, A. S. Molina et al., "Artificial dermis (Matriderm®) followed by skin graft as an option in dermatofibrosarcoma protuberans with complete circumferential and peripheral deep margin assessment," *International Wound Journal*, vol. 12, no. 5, pp. 545–547, 2015.

[11] A. P. Tufaro, D. W. Buck, and A. C. Fischer, "The use of artificial dermis in the reconstruction of oncologic surgical defects," *Plast. Reconstr. Surg*, vol. 120, pp. 638-46, 2007.

[12] K. Hayashi, H. Uhara, H. Koga, R. Okuyama, and T. Saida, "Surgical treatment of nail apparatus melanoma in situ: the use of artificial dermis in reconstruction," *Dermatologic Surgery*, vol. 38, pp. 692–694, 2012.

[13] M. C. T. Bloemen, M. C. E. Van Leeuwen, N. E. Van Vucht, P. P. M. Van Zuijlen, and E. Middelkoop, "Dermal substitution in acute burns and reconstructive surgery: A 12-year follow-up," *Plastic and Reconstructive Surgery*, vol. 125, no. 5, pp. 1450–1459, 2010.

[14] J. T. Shores, A. Gabriel, and S. Gupta, "Skin substitutes and alternatives: a review.," *Advances in skin & wound care*, vol. 20, no. 9, pp. 493–510, 2007.

[15] C. M. Stekelenburg, R. E. Marck, W. E. Tuinebreijer, H. C. W. De Vet, R. Ogawa, and P. P. M. Van Zuijlen, "A Systematic Review on Burn Scar Contracture Treatment: Searching for Evidence," *Journal of Burn Care and Research*, vol. 36, no. 3, pp. e153–e161, 2015.

[16] P. Saiag, J.-J. Grob, C. Lebbe et al., "Diagnosis and treatment of dermatofibrosarcoma protuberans. European consensus-based interdisciplinary guideline," *European Journal of Cancer*, vol. 51, no. 17, pp. 2604–2608, 2015.

[17] E. Bertolli, E. R. Bretchbuhl, W. R. Camarço et al., "Dermatofibrosarcoma protuberans of the vulva: Margins assessment and reconstructive options - A report of two cases," *World Journal of Surgical Oncology*, vol. 12, no. 1, article no. 399, 2014.

[18] C. Zhang, D. Liu, Z. Liang, F. Liu, H. Lin, and Z. Guo, "Repair of refractory wounds through grafting of artificial dermis and autologous epidermis aided by vacuum-assisted closure," *Aesthetic Plastic Surgery*, vol. 38, no. 4, pp. 727–732, 2014.

[19] J. A. Molnar, A. J. DeFranzo, A. Hadaegh, M. J. Morykwas, P. Shen, and L. C. Argenta, "Acceleration of integra incorporation in complex tissue defects with subatmospheric pressure," *Plastic and Reconstructive Surgery*, vol. 113, no. 5, pp. 1339–1346, 2004.

[20] S. Eo, Y. Kim, and S. Cho, "Vacuum-assisted closure improves the incorporation of artificial dermis in soft tissue defects: Terudermis® and Pelnac®," *International Wound Journal*, vol. 8, no. 3, pp. 261–267, 2011.

[21] R. Sinna et al., "Role of the association artificial dermis and negative pressure therapy: about two cases," *Annales de Chirurgie Plastique et Esthétique*, vol. 54, pp. 582–587, 2009.

29

Value of MR and CT Imaging for Assessment of Internal Carotid Artery Encasement in Head and Neck Squamous Cell Carcinoma

W. L. Lodder,[1,2] **C. A. H. Lange,**[3] **H. J. Teertstra,**[3] **F. A. Pameijer,**[4]
M. W. M. van den Brekel,[1,5,6] **and A. J. M. Balm**[1,5]

[1] *Department of Head & Neck Oncology and Surgery, The Netherlands Cancer Institute-Antoni van Leeuwenhoek Hospital, Amsterdam, The Netherlands*
[2] *Department of Otorhinolaryngology/Head and Neck Surgery, The University Medical Center Groningen, University of Groningen, 9700 RB Groningen, The Netherlands*
[3] *Department of Radiology, The Netherlands Cancer Institute-Antoni van Leeuwenhoek Hospital, Amsterdam, The Netherlands*
[4] *Department of Radiology, University Medical Centre Utrecht, Utrecht, The Netherlands*
[5] *Department of Otorhinolaryngology, Academic Medical Centre, University of Amsterdam, Amsterdam, The Netherlands*
[6] *Institute of Phonetic Sciences, ACLC, University of Amsterdam, Amsterdam, The Netherlands*

Correspondence should be addressed to W. L. Lodder; w.l.lodder@gmail.com

Academic Editor: Masaki Mori

Objective. This study was conducted to assess the value of CT and MR imaging in the preoperative evaluation of ICA encasement. *Methods.* Based upon three patient groups this study was performed. Retrospective analysis of 260 neck dissection reports from 2001 to 2010 was performed to determine unexpected peroperative-diagnosed encasement. Two experienced head and neck radiologists reviewed 12 scans for encasement. *Results.* In four out of 260 (1.5%) patients undergoing neck dissection, preoperative imaging was false negative as there was peroperative encasement of the ICA. Of 380 patients undergoing preoperative imaging, the radiologist reported encasement of the ICA in 25 cases. In 342 cases no encasement was described, 125 of these underwent neck dissection, and 2 had encasement peroperatively. The interobserver variation kappa varied from 0.273 to 1 for the different characteristics studied. *Conclusion.* These retrospectively studied cohorts demonstrate that preoperative assessment of encasement of the ICA using MRI and/or CT was of value in evaluation of ICA encasement and therefore contributively in selecting operable patients (without ICA encasement), since in only 1.5% encasement was missed. However, observer variation affects the reliability of this feature.

1. Introduction

Preoperative diagnosis of internal carotid artery (ICA) involvement changes the primary treatment of head and neck tumors. Literature data on carotid encasement in head and neck cancer are scarce. One series reported on a 5% to 10% incidence of cervical lymph node metastases invading the ICA not diagnosed on preoperative imaging using 5 different imaging signs [1]. Encasement of the ICA is both a poor prognostic indicator and often a contraindication to surgical treatment [2]. Removal of lymph node metastases from the ICA may lead to stroke and carotid rupture in 3.3% and 5.5%, respectively [3]. The risk for cerebral damage after removal of the ICA is 3.3% to 30% [1]. Although grafting of the carotid

artery, as generally performed in vascular disease and glomus tumors, is possible, it is generally not advocated because the outcome in oncologic patients is dismal [4].

Many attempts have been undertaken to classify carotid invasion on preoperative imaging including ultrasound, followed by magnetic resonance imaging (MRI) and computed tomography (CT) scan [1, 2, 5–13].

In 1995 Yousem et al. [2] demonstrated in a series of 49 patients undergoing neck dissection for head and neck tumors clinically suspicious for encasement that more than 270 degrees of circumferential involvement of the ICA on MRI predicted unresectable disease. They reached sensitivity and specificity of 100% and 88%. Assessment of carotid invasion by ultrasonography had sensitivity up to 100%

[10–13]. However, in this study we focused on the value of MR and CT imaging.

Until now, no consensus has been reached on standardization of imaging criteria for defining encasement of the carotid artery. MRI seems to be the most sensitive imaging modality to visualize contrasts between soft tissues structures and therefore should be optimal for the assessment of carotid encasement. Apart from the publications of Pons et al. [1] and Yousem et al. [2], no other studies were performed for classifying carotid encasement on MR imaging. Carotid encasement has a low incidence, but a high impact on treatment planning. This study was conducted to assess the value of CT and MR imaging in the preoperative evaluation of ICA encasement. Therefore we studied 3 patient groups/cohorts retrospectively to review the number of cases with peroperative encasement of the ICA in our institution (group 1) and to assess the prevalence of preoperatively diagnosed encasement of the ICA on CT and MR scans (group 2) and interobserver variation (group 3).

2. Materials and Methods

2.1. Ethical Considerations. Institutional approval for the study was received. As patient anonymity was preserved patient consent was not required for the retrospective review of records and images.

The results of this study will be presented based upon following three different patient groups.

(1) Peroperative Assessment of Encasement of the ICA. Between 2001 and 2011 a total of 551 patients (608 neck dissections) who had undergone neck dissection in our institution for head and neck squamous cell carcinoma following a presurgical MRI or CT workup were selected from our operation database. In our center, patients with a tumor located above the level of the hyoid bone or with an unknown primary tumor are preferentially studied with MR imaging. After a first evaluation of the 608 operation reports, 348 patients were excluded (incomplete data, pathological N0-stage, or pathological N1-stage). Two hundred and sixty operation reports were evaluated for the presence of peroperative carotid encasement (Figure 1). All patients received a (modified) radical neck dissection or salvage selective neck dissection or superselective lymph node dissection after chemoradiation therapy and underwent preoperative evaluation with CT or MR imaging.

(2) Preoperative Assessment of Encasement of the ICA. CT- and MR image reports from 2009 to 2010 ($n = 1486$) were reviewed retrospectively for encasement of the ICA to estimate the prevalence of preoperatively diagnosed carotid encasement. After a first evaluation of the reports, 1106 out of the 1486 imaging reports were excluded (cases with no aberrations on imaging or with benign lesions were excluded; see Figure 2). Three hundred and eighty reports were evaluated for the presence of preoperative carotid encasement. These reports were from different radiologists using nonspecified criteria. Most of the radiologists used the criterion of >270 degrees circumferential involvement of the carotid artery

as positive sign for encasement. However, it was unclear whether all radiologists used standardized criteria.

(3) Evaluation of Radiologically Determined Criteria. Twelve patients with peroperative encasement or preoperative encasement or possible encasement of the ICA were selected from the previously claimed cohorts. Their pretreatment MRIs ($n = 6$) and CTs ($n = 6$) were reviewed among 42 other scans (with no ICA encasement) by two experienced head and neck radiologists (JT and CL) using criteria selected from the literature [1, 2]. The observers were unaware of the peroperative findings, of all 54 scans. The results of only the 12 with ICA involvement were used for assessment of the interobserver variation.

2.2. MR Technique. For this study both MRI examinations were performed at 1,5 T. (Magnetom; Siemens Medical Systems, Erlangen, Germany) and 3.0 T. (Philips Achieva release 3.2.1, Philips Medical Systems, Best, The Netherlands) using a dedicated 16-channel SENSE neurovascular coil. The following series were acquired: STIR TSE COR, TR (repetition time), IR (inversion time), TE (echo time) 3,880/180/20 ms, ETL: 12, FOV 300/228/40 mm, matrix: 320/320, 2 nex, slice thickness 4 mm; STIR TSE TRA, TR/IR/TE 4,228/180/20, ETL: 12, FOV: 180/200/80 mm, matrix 300/312, 2 nex, SW 3.5 mm, T1 TSE TRA, TR/TE: 780/10, ETL: 5, FOV 180/180/80, matrix 384/384, 2 nex, slice thickness: 3.5 mm; T1 3D Thrive (performed after intravenous injection of 15 cc gadoterate meglumine (Dotarem)), TR/TE: 5/2,22, ETL: 90, TA: 10, FOV 230/272/220, matrix 288/288, 2 nex, slice thickness: 0.8 mm; T1 TSE COR (postcontrast): TR/TE: 812/10, ETL: 6, FOV: 180/150/96 mm, matrix: 320/320, 3 nex, slice thickness 3.5 mm.

The mean time between imaging and neck dissection was 12 days (range 1–48; SD 19).

2.3. CT Technique. CT studies were performed with one of two multidetector scanners (Philips Gemini TF or Siemens Sensation). Standard CT of the neck was performed, after the injection of nonionic contrast material (Omnipaque 300 mg/mL, GE Health Care, quantity in mL equal to body weight in kilograms) with an injection rate of 4 mL/sec. Acquisition of 1,5 or 2 mm slices started after 55 seconds, and the images were reformatted into 3-mm-thick sections in transverse and coronal directions.

2.4. Studied Radiological Criteria for ICA Encasement. Encasement of the ICA was assessed using the following radiological criteria selected from the literature [1, 2]:

(1) encasement of the artery: none, 180–270, >270 degrees,

(2) obliteration of the fat between the lymph node/primary tumor and the carotid artery,

(3) deformation of the carotid artery,

(4) length of contact between the carotid artery and tumor mass.

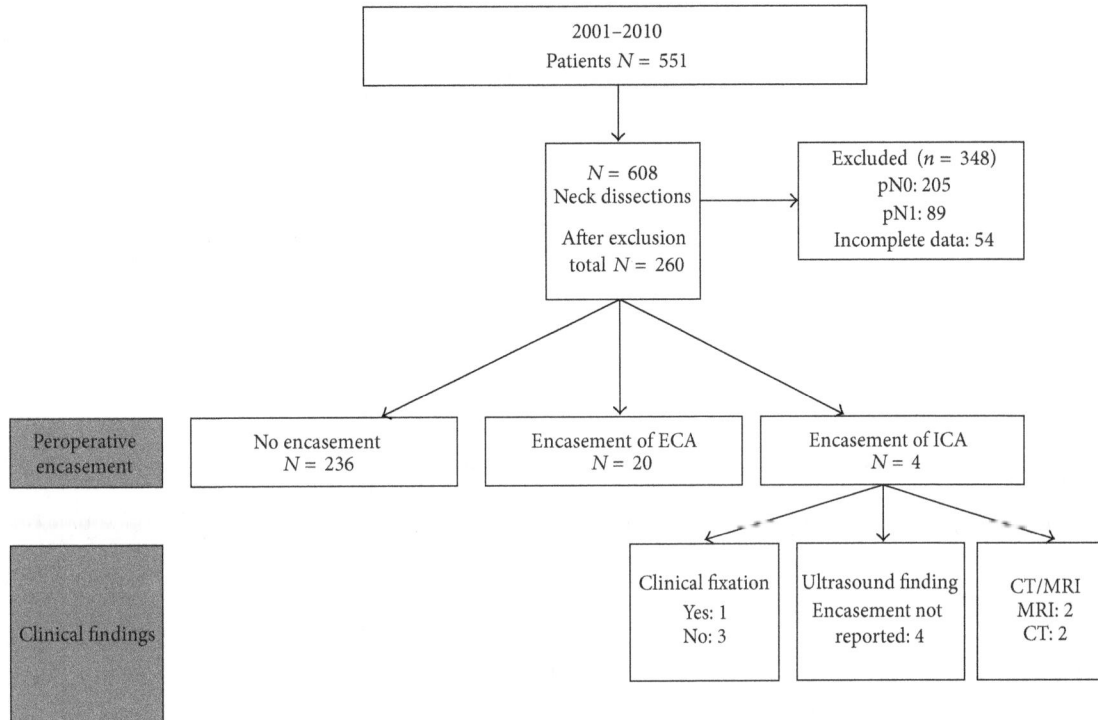

FIGURE 1: Neck dissections performed between 2001 and 2010. ECA: external carotid artery. ICA: internal carotid artery. This figure shows 551 patients in which 608 neck dissections were performed. In total 260 cases were studied after exclusion. In 236 cases no encasement was found during operation. In 20 cases (7.7%) encasement of the external carotid artery was seen. In four cases encasement of the internal carotid artery was present (4/260 = 1.5%). Two cases had MRI and 2 had CT preoperatively.

2.5. Statistics. Logistic regression was used to determine all significant characteristics for carotid encasement on MRI. To measure the interobserver agreement, the kappa coefficient was used. This coefficient can vary between −1 (complete disagreement) and +1 (complete agreement). If this measure takes on the value zero (0), the observer agreement can be interpreted as being the result of mere chance. A value of more than 0.75 can be interpreted as good agreement among observers. The overall kappa coefficient can be interpreted as a measure of agreement between the groups of observers.

3. Results

3.1. Peroperative Assessment of Encasement of the ICA. In 24 of 260 cases (9.2%) peroperative encasement of both the internal or external carotid artery was found: in total 1.5% (4/260) of the cases undergoing a neck dissection had encasement of the ICA (see Figure 1). In one case of encasement of the ICA, clinical fixation of the tumor on physical examination was mentioned.

3.2. Preoperative Assessment of Encasement of the ICA. A total of 380 image reports were studied for the presence of preoperatively reported ICA encasement. In twenty-five cases (6.6%) the radiologist reported encasement. None of these patients were operated. In thirteen cases (3.4%) the radiologist reported possible encasement. Of these 13 patients, five underwent surgery and none had peroperative

encasement. In 342 cases (90%) the radiologist reported no encasement. One hundred and twenty-five of these patients were operated; in two patients peroperative encasement of the ICA was present (2/125 = 1.6%), which was not reported during preoperative imaging (see Figure 2).

3.3. Evaluation of Radiologically Determined Criteria. Two radiologists reviewed 12 preoperative images of patients with known peroperative ICA encasement using the above-mentioned criteria (see Figure 3). Table 1 shows the percentages of the radiologically determined criteria per observer and the interobserver variation. Interobserver kappa values were low with values from 0.273 (deformation of the carotid artery) to high with value of 1 (obliteration of fat planes) for the different parameters.

4. Discussion

4.1. Synopsis of Key/New Findings. These retrospectively studied cohorts demonstrate that preoperative assessment of encasement of the ICA using MRI and/or CT was missed in only 1.5%. However the criteria used in the literature show a high interobserver variation.

4.2. Comparisons with Other Studies. In 2010 Pons et al. [1] studied the relevance of five different imaging parameters for evaluating carotid artery invasion in 22 patients with peroperatively proven encasement of the ICA. Of these

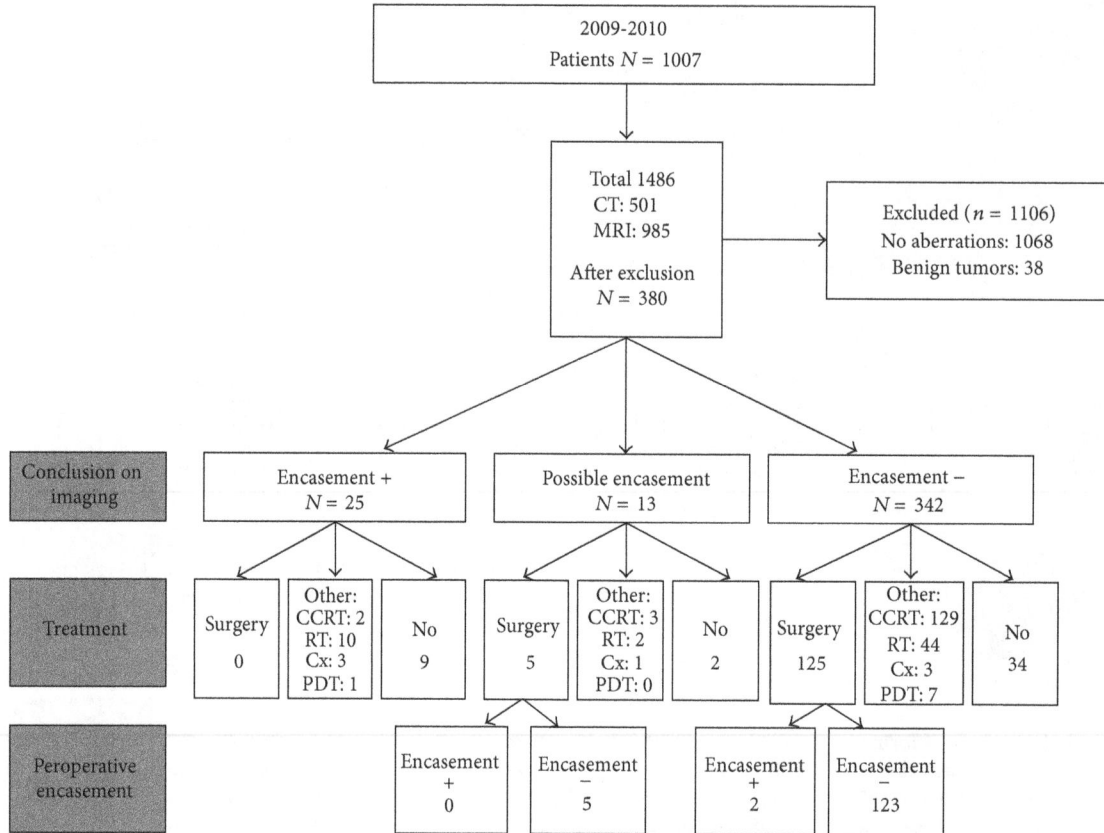

FIGURE 2: Retrospective analysis of all MR and CT images from 2009 to 2010. CCRT: concomitant chemoradiation therapy, RT: radiotherapy, Cx: chemotherapy, and PDT: photodynamic therapy. This figure shows 1486 MR and CT studies performed in 1007 patients between 2009 and 2010. In 1068 cases no aberrations were found, and in 38 cases there were only benign tumors. In 25 cases encasement (>270 degrees encasement) was present at preoperative assessment. In 13 cases the report was not conclusive, and in 342 cases no encasement was seen. During operation in 2/125 = 1.6% cases, encasement of the internal carotid artery was found.

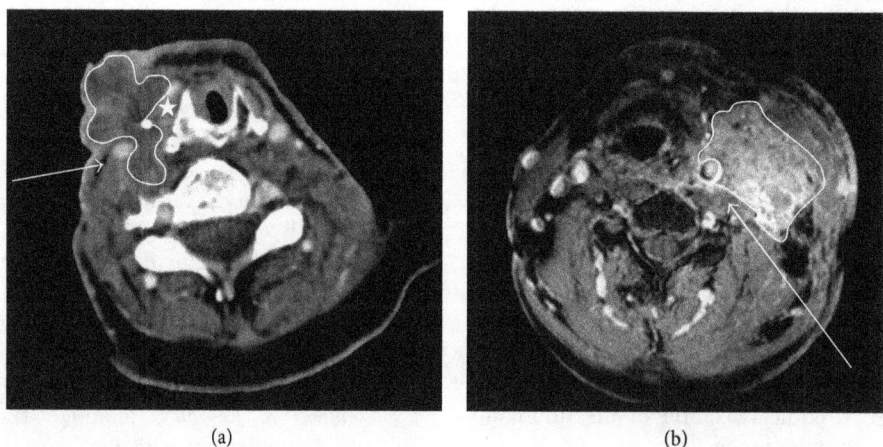

(a)   (b)

FIGURE 3: Examples of CT and MR images showing carotid encasement. (a) Axial CT image of a lymph node metastases (the mass is encircled by a white line) at the right side showing at least 270 degrees of encasement. The confluent lymph node mass is invading into the skin. The right carotid artery (arrow) is covered by the lymph node mass. Note: the right internal jugular vein is not visible, possibly due to compression. Suggestive the high-density structure (white star) lateral to the right lamina of the cricoid is surgical clip from earlier operation. (b) Fat-suppressed T1 contrast-enhanced MR section showing lymph node metastases in the left neck. The left internal carotid artery (arrow) is covered anteriorly and laterally by nodal disease (the mass is encircled by a white line). The circumferential involvement is (just) over 180 degrees.

TABLE 1: Radiologically determined criteria and interobserver kappa.

Radiologically determined criteria	Observer 1 $N = 12$	Observer 2 $N = 12$	Interobserver kappa
Encasement			0.584
<180 degrees	2 (17%)	0 (0%)	
180–270 degrees	0 (0%)	4 (33%)	
>270 degrees	10 (83%)	8 (67%)	
Obliteration of fat planes			1
No	0	0	
Yes	12 (100%)	12 (100%)	
Deformation of the carotid artery			0.273
No	4 (33%)	2 (17%)	
Yes	8 (67%)	10 (83%)	
Length of contact carotid artery			0.488
Mean in cm	3.5 (range: 1.0–5.0; SD 1.3)	3.6 (range: 1.6–6.1; SD 1.6)	

patients, preoperative CT and MR images were analyzed. Size of the adenopathy and intensity of the contact showed no correlation with peroperative findings. However, imaging characteristics such as carotid artery deformation, encasement of >180 degrees, and segmental obliteration of the fat were significantly associated ($P < 0.05$) with massive invasion of the carotid artery. In 1995 Yousem et al. [2] studied MR images of 53 carotid arteries in 49 patients. Twenty-two MR images had a tumor surrounding the carotid artery less than 180 degrees and none of these had carotid artery invasion at surgery. Seventeen arteries had more than 270 degrees of tumor encasement and twelve of these had invasion during surgery (12/17 = 71%). Fourteen arteries had tumor with 180–270 degrees of encasement on the preoperative imaging, with none having invasion at surgery. When the criterion of >270 degrees encasement was used, sensitivity of MRI was 100% and specificity 88%. In our series however, the criterion of 270 degrees resulted in an interobserver kappa value of 0.584.

Five articles reported on the value of preoperative CT imaging. Sarvanan et al. [5] studied 26 patients and compared palpation, ultrasound, and CT imaging. On CT, they studied encasement of >270 degrees and loss of fat planes. Sensitivity reached 75% and specificity 100%. Solano et al. [6] studied loss of a fat interface between the carotid and the neck mass. There were 11 false positive findings and one true positive finding. Rapoport et al. [7] studied in 2008 interobserver agreement based on a simplified two-item classification (0–50% and 51–100% involvement). The general kappa was 0.53. In our specific and selected series interobserver variation for categorical encasement (<180 versus 180–270 versus >270 degrees) was 0.584. Rothstein et al. [8] also studied loss of

fat interface in 17 patients. All CT scans demonstrated this feature; however 16/17 = 94% was false positive.

Yu et al. [9] studied in 2003 the diagnostic value of CT imaging for the detection of carotid encasement. In 27 patients, involvement of the common carotid artery or internal carotid artery (11 tumors) or the jugular vein (25 tumors) was studied. In 17 cases the tumors did not involve the cervical vessels. The compression and deformation, more than 180 degrees circumference, undefined carotid artery wall, and fat or fascial plane deletion between tumor and carotid wall were studied. With specificity ranging from 47.4% to 100% and sensitivity ranging from 18.5% to 90.9% they emphasized that a combination of criteria should be used.

Our results seem to confirm the results from the above-mentioned studies. Overall, it can be questioned whether preoperative imaging assessment of carotid encasement for treatment selection should be used at all with no specific criteria available.

The false negative rate of preoperative assessment of encasement of the ICA was 1.5% in our retrospective cohorts, using the intraoperative findings as "gold standard" for carotid encasement. If the radiologist reported >270 degrees of carotid encasement according to our current protocol, patients were not operated. For the calculation of observer variation we used a small selection of twelve patients. The interobserver kappa varied from 0.273 to 1.00 for the different radiologically determined characteristics.

Various studies showed survival with carotid resection was less than 15 months [14, 15]. In a meta-analysis of Snyderman and D'Amico [16], 2-year disease-free survival was 22% after carotid resection. With these low survival figures in mind, one may seriously doubt whether carotid resection should be part of a standard surgical approach.

4.3. Clinical Applicability of the Study. The importance of carotid artery encasement as a separate prognostic indicator justifying an aggressive surgical approach with a high risk of neurological complications can only be determined by a prospective multivariate analysis using standardized imaging techniques and agreement on radiological criteria. In daily practice we still have to rely on the limitations of preoperative imaging. Most probably the combination of head and neck surgical and radiological expertise remains of crucial importance to assess the resectability of neck node metastases in an individual patient.

Future research efforts should be directed at more detailed depiction of the carotid artery wall. Increased resolution may give more insight in the amount of invasion of malignant neck disease in the various layers of the wall of the carotid artery. Use of high-field strength (3T) and application of surface coils may achieve this goal.

5. Conclusion

These retrospectively studied cohorts demonstrate that preoperative assessment of encasement of the ICA using MRI and/or CT was of value in evaluation of ICA encasement and therefore contributively in selecting operable patients (without ICA encasement), since in only 1.5% encasement was missed. However, observer variation affects the reliability of this feature.

Most probably the combination of head and neck surgical and radiological expertise remains of crucial importance to assess the resectability of neck node metastases in an individual patient. The importance of carotid artery encasement as a separate prognostic indicator justifying an aggressive surgical approach with a high risk of neurological complications can only be determined by a prospective multivariate analysis using standardized imaging techniques and agreement on radiological criteria.

References

[1] Y. Pons, E. Ukkola-Pons, P. Clément, J. Gauthier, and C. Conessa, "Relevance of 5 different imaging signs in the evaluation of carotid artery invasion by cervical lymphadenopathy in head and neck squamous cell carcinoma," *Oral Surgery, Oral Medicine, Oral Pathology, Oral Radiology and Endodontology*, vol. 109, no. 5, pp. 775–778, 2010.

[2] D. M. Yousem, H. Hatabu, R. W. Hurst et al., "Carotid artery invasion by head and neck masses: prediction with MR imaging," *Radiology*, vol. 195, no. 3, pp. 715–720, 1995.

[3] E. Ozer, A. Agrawal, H. G. Ozer, and D. E. Schuller, "The impact of surgery in the management of the head and neck carcinoma involving the carotid artery," *Laryngoscope*, vol. 118, no. 10, pp. 1771–1774, 2008.

[4] Z. S. Nemeth, G. Y. Domotor, M. Talos, J. Barabas, M. Ujpal, and G. Y. Szabo, "Resection and replacement of the carotid artery in metastatic head and neck cancer: literature review and case report," *International Journal of Oral and Maxillofacial Surgery*, pp. 645–650, 2003.

[5] K. Sarvanan, J. Rajiv Bapuraj, S. C. Sharma, B. D. Radotra, N. Khandelwal, and S. Suri, "Computed tomography and ultrasonographic evaluation of metastatic cervical lymph nodes with surgicoclinicopathologic correlation," *Journal of Laryngology and Otology*, vol. 116, no. 3, pp. 194–199, 2002.

[6] J. Solano, V. Garrido, and M. Martínez-Morillo, "Ultrasonography is more effective than computed tomography in excluding invasion of the carotid wall by cervical lymphadenopathies," *European Journal of Radiology*, vol. 17, no. 3, pp. 191–194, 1993.

[7] A. Rapoport, O. D. S. Tornin, I. M. Beserra, P. B. C. De Neto, and R. P. De Souza, "Assessment of carotid artery invasion by lymph node metastasis from squamous cell carcinoma of aerodigestive tract," *Brazilian Journal of Otorhinolaryngology*, vol. 74, no. 1, pp. 79–84, 2008.

[8] S. G. Rothstein, M. S. Persky, and S. Horii, "Evaluation of malignant invasion of the carotid artery by CT scan and ultrasound," *Laryngoscope*, vol. 98, no. 3, pp. 321–324, 1988.

[9] Q. Yu, P. Wang, H. Shi, and J. Luo, "Carotid artery and jugular vein invasion of oral-maxillofacial and neck malignant tumors: diagnostic value of computed tomography," *Oral Surgery, Oral Medicine, Oral Pathology, Oral Radiology, and Endodontics*, vol. 96, no. 3, pp. 368–372, 2003.

[10] G. A. W. Gooding, A. W. Langman, W. P. Dillon, and M. J. Kaplan, "Malignant carotid artery invasion: sonographic detection," *Radiology*, vol. 171, no. 2, pp. 435–438, 1989.

[11] N. Gritzmann, M. C. Grasl, M. Helmer, and E. Steiner, "Invasion of the carotid artery and jugular vein by lymph node metastases: detection with sonography," *American Journal of Roentgenology*, vol. 154, no. 2, pp. 411–414, 1990.

[12] A. W. Langman, M. J. Kaplan, W. P. Dillon, and G. A. W. Gooding, "Radiologic assessment of tumor and the carotid artery: correlation of magnetic resonance imaging, ultrasound, and computed tomography with surgical findings," *Head and Neck*, vol. 11, no. 5, pp. 443–449, 1989.

[13] G. A. W. Gooding, "Malignant carotid invasion: sonographic diagnosis," *ORL*, vol. 55, no. 5, pp. 263–272, 1993.

[14] T. R. Kroeker and J. C. O'Brien, "Carotid resection and reconstruction associated with treatment of head and neck cancer," *Proceedings (Baylor University. Medical Center)*, vol. 24, no. 4, pp. 295–298, 2011.

[15] J. L. Roh, M. Ra Kim, S. H. Choi et al., "Can patients with head and neck cancers invading carotid artery gain survival benefit from surgery?" *Acta Oto-Laryngologica*, vol. 128, no. 12, pp. 1370–1374, 2008.

[16] C. H. Snyderman and F. D'Amico, "Outcome of carotid artery resection for neoplastic disease: a meta-analysis," *American Journal of Otolaryngology*, vol. 13, no. 6, pp. 373–380, 1992.

30

Oncoplastic Breast Reduction: Maximizing Aesthetics and Surgical Margins

Michelle Milee Chang,[1] Tara Huston,[2] Jeffrey Ascherman,[1] and Christine Rohde[1]

[1] *Division of Plastic Surgery, Columbia University Medical Center, New York-Presbyterian Hospital, New York, NY 10032, USA*
[2] *Plastic and Reconstructive Surgery Division, Stony Brook Medicine, Stony Brook, NY 11794, USA*

Correspondence should be addressed to Christine Rohde, chr2111@columbia.edu

Academic Editor: Joseph P. Crowe

Oncoplastic breast reduction combines oncologically sound concepts of cancer removal with aesthetically maximized approaches for breast reduction. Numerous incision patterns and types of pedicles can be used for purposes of oncoplastic reduction, each tailored for size and location of tumor. A team approach between reconstructive and breast surgeons produces positive long-term oncologic results as well as satisfactory cosmetic and functional outcomes, rendering oncoplastic breast reduction a favorable treatment option for certain patients with breast cancer.

1. Introduction

Surgeons who treat breast cancer strive to perform operations that are aesthetically pleasing without compromising oncologic outcome. Patients are more informed than ever and are encouraging their surgical teams to continue to evolve [1].

For treatment of their breast cancer, many women elect breast conservation therapy (BCT). BCT combines lumpectomy with postoperative radiation allowing a woman to preserve her breast. Factors leading to a greater use of BCT versus mastectomy include improved screening and earlier mammography which have resulted in an increased identification of small, early-stage breast cancers, an increased use of neoadjuvant chemotherapy which can shrink large tumors, and the patient's own preference to preserve her breast [2].

With breast preservation, cancer survival is affected by local control defined by appropriate clear margins. Despite a higher local recurrence rate, disease-free long-term survival is equivalent for patients undergoing total mastectomy and BCT. The premise of BCT involves both surgical excision and reconstruction, including an oncologically sound resection of the tumor, radiation of the resection bed, and preservation of the breast for enhanced aesthetic outcome [2].

To ensure clear margins of tumor resection in BCT, large volumes of breast tissue may need to be removed, leading to asymmetry, scarring, and deformity. Up to 30% of patients who have undergone BCT end up with a poor cosmetic outcome [3, 4]. Subsequent irradiation often then further compromises already suboptimal surgical results.

2. Oncoplastic Surgery

The initial reports of aesthetic techniques coupled with oncologic treatment were published in the 1990s [5]. The term "oncoplastic breast surgery" was coined in the mid-1990s [6]. Oncoplastic methods enable large tumor resections by marrying extirpative surgery with breast reduction surgery. Procedures are designed to anticipate and prevent unfavorable aesthetic outcomes, decreasing the rates to below 7% [7]. In addition, patients have the added benefit of a reduction mammaplasty, which may include a decrease in back, shoulder, and neck discomfort.

There are a number of oncologic advantages to oncoplastic breast reduction. A generous margin of tumor resection is feasible because a large volume of glandular tissue is removed [8, 9]. Furthermore, the resulting smaller breast size may improve the efficacy of radiation therapy. Lastly, reduction of the contralateral breast not only offers tissue sampling, but also theoretically reduces additional risk of breast cancer through removal of excess breast parenchyma [10]. The rate of occult breast cancers found in contralateral symmetrizing reduction specimens in patients undergoing breast reconstruction ranges from 4.6 to 11% [11–14].

Cosmesis in BCT (standard lumpectomy alone) is affected by breast size, with both very small- and very large-breasted women faring worst. Macromastia has been estimated in up to 40% of women treated with BCT [15]. In patients with macromastia, aesthetic outcome with lumpectomy alone might not be ideal. BCT in a large-breasted woman may leave an empty sac and can result in a ptotic breast, which can lead to a heterogeneous dose distribution. This is due to repeated positioning over an extended course of treatment [16]. Oncoplastic breast reduction has been found to circumvent these complications, relieving symptoms related to larger breasts, as well as treating the cancer itself [17].

Breast volume is important when considering oncoplastic surgery. Cochrane et al. has shown that as much as 10% of glandular breast volume can be removed without notable cosmetic deformities. In addition, the larger the breast is, the more tolerant it is to resection [18]. Delay and Clough demonstrated that up to 20% of breast volume can be excised, requiring local parenchymal rearrangement or skin excision for satisfactory results [19].

Communication between the breast and reconstructive surgeon is crucial. Preoperatively, this team approach is critical in defining areas of excision and in designing reduction techniques. The breast surgeon needs to be cognizant of breast aesthetics, volume, and symmetry, keeping in mind that referral to a plastic surgeon may be helpful. In turn, the reconstructive surgeon should understand oncologic surgical principles when creating a sound operative plan.

3. Patient Evaluation and Counseling

Numerous factors are considered in patient selection. The most important selection criteria include (1) a patient's desire for smaller breasts and (2) the degree of the cancer surgeon's concern about aesthetic irregularities while resecting adequate specimen size. An ideal candidate requires a large-volume resection and has symptoms of macromastia (chronic headaches, back pain, neck pain, shoulder grooving, or intertriginous rashes). However, any patients with moderate-to-large sized breasts are still possible candidates for selection [10]. The oncoplastic procedure is applicable to either patients who have had no prior surgical intervention or those who have attempted breast conservation with positive margins.

A detailed history is critical. Symptoms of macromastia should be documented as well as factors that can impact wound healing or breast tissue perfusion such as: steroid use, smoking, diabetes, prior breast surgery, connective tissue diseases, or irradiation to the thorax. The presence of any of these factors should prompt further counseling regarding increased risk of complications such as fat necrosis, nipple necrosis, or other wound healing complications. Also, because a history of smoking predisposes to increased nipple and flap necrosis, measures for smoking succession must be pursued if the patient is currently smoking. A focused physical exam is also important. Height, weight, and body mass index should be recorded. An emphasis on breast size, shape, prior scars, degree of ptosis, and position of lesion is important. In addition, measurements of breast width, sternal notch-to-nipple distance, nipple-to-inframammary-fold distance, and NAC width may be taken. Asymmetries should be documented and made evident to the patient. Photographs should be taken for the medical record.

Breast measurements are important as an indicator of breast size, ptosis, and volume. They help to point out preoperative asymmetries that may persist after surgery. There are no absolutes with breast measurements, but in general, patients with sternal notch-to-nipple (SN-N) distances of 35 or greater need to be counseled regarding the possibility of free nipple grafts. Greater SN-N distances risk poor perfusion to the nipple through the pedicle, leading to nipple/areola necrosis [20]. Patients for whom the SN-N distance will change by more than 10 cm are poorer candidates for vertical scar breast reductions because of the geometry of pedicle rotation within the skin reduction pattern.

After the decision for oncoplastic reduction has been made, the time course must then be considered. The immediate one-stage reconstruction approach is preferable, both for psychological and aesthetic reasons. Delayed reconstruction may be advisable for younger patients with extensive ductal carcinoma in situ (DCIS), as this group has a higher rate of positive margins. In such cases, preoperative counseling should be directed towards a two-stage procedure and reconstruction should be postponed until negative margins are confirmed [10].

Furthermore, both breasts should be integrated into the decision-making process and treatment plan. Immediate breast reconstruction on the contralateral breast is much more common, except in cases of patients with DCIS, as explained above. Symmetry is the most important factor for good cosmetic outcome. In order to spare additional surgery, surgeons will often reduce or symmetrize the contralateral breast in the first procedure. This, however, requires an educated approximation of the size and shape of the contralateral breast to the ipsilateral breast because it is impossible to know the final size of the ipsilateral breast following cancer ablation. Involution and edema of the breast following irradiation further exacerbates this situation. Following radiation, the treated breast will become firmer and often rise up on the chest wall. For this reason, some surgeons prefer to perform the contralateral symmetrizing reduction in a two-step delayed procedure. Fitoussi et al. showed a preferential shift from synchronous reconstruction to delayed contralateral symmetrizing reduction in 540 consecutive cases [21]. Despite these trends, studies show that immediate reconstruction is not only safe, but may also provide better aesthetic outcomes [22–24].

Patient counseling of possible complications, as well as the need for a total mastectomy (if margins are involved) is essential in the preoperative workup. After oncoplastic reduction, breast geometry is completely rearranged, potentially leaving margins unidentifiable. Patterns of recurrence can be significantly altered. Therefore, in our practice, if the margins are positive following this procedure, the necessary next step is usually a total mastectomy. In addition,

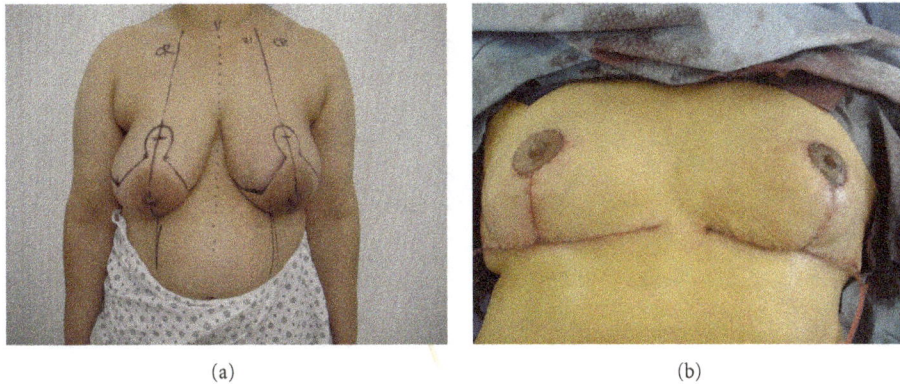

(a)   (b)

FIGURE 1: (a) Preoperative markings before Wise pattern superomedial pedicle oncoplastic breast reduction. The patient's breast cancer is located in the inferolateral breast. (b) Immediate on-table result after oncoplastic breast reduction showing location of scars.

decreased sensation, partial or total thickness skin loss, asymmetries, and wound-healing issues of the nipple are also complications that may arise from ablation, reduction, and subsequent radiation.

4. Planning

The two main surgical decisions that must be chosen when planning a breast reduction are the choice of incision and the type of pedicle on which the nipple areolar complex will be transposed. This is influenced by numerous elements. While tumor location is the most important factor, other considerations include previous scars/needle biopsy sites and whether these need to be excised, as well as the need for access to the axilla. While not always applicable, excision of skin overlying the tumor and its extent can also be included. The surgeon's comfort and preference for reduction mammaplastic techniques is an important factor as well. Lastly, thought must be given to the effect of radiation and the potential to change the eventual size of the breast. Radiation can lead to chronic edema and involution or shrinkage of the remaining breast tissue resulting in a smaller, firmer breast, which rides higher up on the chest wall.

5. Margin Evaluation

The most important goal of the oncoplastic approach is to resect the cancer with histologically negative margins. Oncoplastic breast reductions enable wider margins than standard lumpectomy alone. In our practice, to optimize positive margins, we try to remove the skin over the tumor whenever possible as well as the breast tissue and muscle fascia posterior to the tumor. Positive margins are associated with a significantly higher incidence of local recurrence [25, 26]. Intraoperative assessments of margins are advised, utilizing both pathologic specimen examination and radiologic imaging. Microcalcifications can be assessed via specimen mammogram with two 90-degree images. Intraoperative ultrasound use has shown a decrease in reexcision rate, especially in the cases with solid masses [27, 28].

Histologic evaluation is also useful. Currently, frozen sections with touch preparation are one of the most accepted methods of intraoperative histologic assessment of margins. Other recently developed technologies, such as the Spectroscopy or MarginProbe (Dune Medical Devices, Caesarea, Israel), are now being evaluated for real-time intraoperative margin assessment [28].

In our practice, we often mark the margins of resection with hemoclips. The clips serve as a guide to radiation oncologists for radiation therapy, especially in the delivery of an appropriate boost dose.

6. Skin Incision Types

Following a preoperative evaluation and determination of timing, the next major decision to be made is the location and size of the incision. There are numerous incisions to choose from, each with their advantages and disadvantages. The Wise pattern (or inverted "T") is the most commonly used incision for oncoplastic breast reductions because it offers the most opportunities for breast reshaping. This incision travels along the inframammary fold (IMF) and traverses up to the nipple (Figures 1(a) and 1(b)). The Wise pattern offers the surgeon much flexibility, with wide access to the breast parenchyma for use for a tumor in any location. This procedure also allows skin excision in both vertical and horizontal dimension and can be used with any pedicle. For lymph node sampling or clearance, a separate small incision may be needed in the axilla, depending on the pedicle and desire to avoid wide undermining.

The vertical scar mammaplasty, first introduced by Lassus and modified by Lejour, is the second most commonly used incision for oncoplastic breast reduction [29, 30]. This incision is made around the nipple-areola complex (NAC) and extended down to the IMF. The vertical scar technique also allows good access to the breast parenchyma; breast skin reduction is accessible in the horizontal axis, and vertical size reduction is possible through cinching closure of the skin. One drawback of this technique is that the axilla is not easily reached. The classic Lejour breast reduction includes

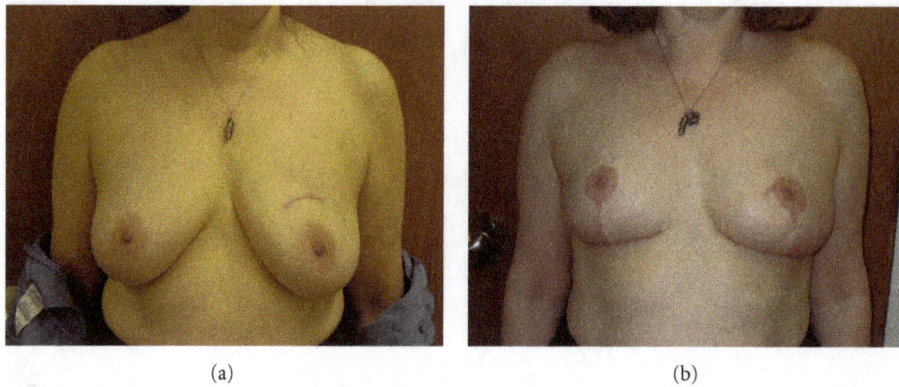

FIGURE 2: (a) Preoperative appearance of patient with left breast cancer. (b) Two-month postoperative appearance of patient after inferior pedicle Wise pattern breast reduction. Note incorporation of lumpectomy scar over superomedially located tumor into the incision for the areola.

a reduction in breast volume via liposuction. This step is not advisable in cancer operations because of the risk of seeding tumor cells.

The omegaplasty (or bat-wing incision) traverses above and alongside the nipple. While not cosmetically ideal, it does provide good access to superomedially located tumors [31]. Omegaplasty requires no undermining (which is better for radiation), but fails to decrease breast volume or address ptosis. This approach can also result in pseudoptosis if there is too much skin or parenchyma resected with an incision superior to the nipple.

The lateral mammaplasty incision runs from the nipple out laterally toward the anterior axillary line. It may also be extended superiorly to gain access to the axilla. Because most tumors are laterally located, this incision's lateral access makes it an important approach. One advantage of the lateral mammaplasty is the avoidance of thin, large surface area dermal flaps, creating thick flaps that are more tolerant to radiation. Medial mammaplasty incisions are the reverse of the lateral mammaplasty, traveling toward the sternum. This technique it the most useful for medially located tumors [32].

The periareolar approach is not as common because it does not permit a great deal of skin excision or volume reduction. The periareolar incision is solely around the nipple and does not extend out onto the breast. Still, this procedure has good access to the upper pole of the breast. Women with mild ptosis and for whom a mastopexy might be considered are good candidates for the periareolar technique.

7. Pedicle Options

After the location and size of incision has been determined, and the extent of tumor resection has been defined, a decision must be made for the origin of the dermoglandular pedicle on which the vascular and nervous supply to the nipple will be carried. The pedicle is important not only to achieve a satisfactory aesthetic outcome, but also to preserve the blood and nerve supply to the NAC. There is a myriad of pedicles, all of which have their cosmetic and sensory advantages or disadvantages. In oncoplastic breast reduction

surgery, the pedicle is chosen based on what remains after the ablation of the tumor. For example, a lower-pole tumor will require resection of glandular tissue in the lower half of the breast, leaving the reconstructive surgeon to choose between various superior pedicles. The pedicles most commonly used are superior, inferior, and medial.

The superior pedicle is preferred for being solid, reliable, and better able to preserve nipple sensation. Limitations of this pedicle arise from difficulty in moving the nipple long distances, especially in patients with significant hypertrophy of the breast. Use of this pedicle may be difficult with large reductions, where molding may result in only superior fullness. Superior pedicles are best for lower-quadrant tumors, particularly in moderate-sized breasts.

Inferior pedicles are reliable for tumors in any position. One caution to take is that it lacks parenchymal support and breasts may eventually sag or "bottom out," resulting in excess skin and tissue between the nipple and IMF. This technique is ideal for larger breasts with longer sternal notch-to-nipple distances as well as tumors located in the upper quadrants of the breast (Figures 2(a) and 2(b)).

The lateral pedicle is an option for medial tumors that extend into the upper or lower quadrants. This pedicle is not frequently used cosmetically because if the pedicle is too thick, the breast will be too full laterally. It is normally reserved for women with small-to-moderate-sized breasts and requires a mastopexy or a minor reduction.

Free-nipple grafting during reduction mammaplasty is most applicable for patients with gigantomastia. In such cases, preservation of blood supply and nerves to the nipple is limited by the length of the pedicle needed to carry the NAC into its new position and by the ability to reduce the breast with a large pedicle. The nipple-areola complex is removed as a skin graft, the breasts are reduced, and the NAC is then sutured in the appropriate position on the breasts. Nipple sensation is lost with this procedure, and hypopigmentation results, usually taking at least one year for pigmentation to return. In cases where oncologic margins require removal of the nipple-areola complex, it can be excised without negatively impacting breast shape, as long as adequate skin is

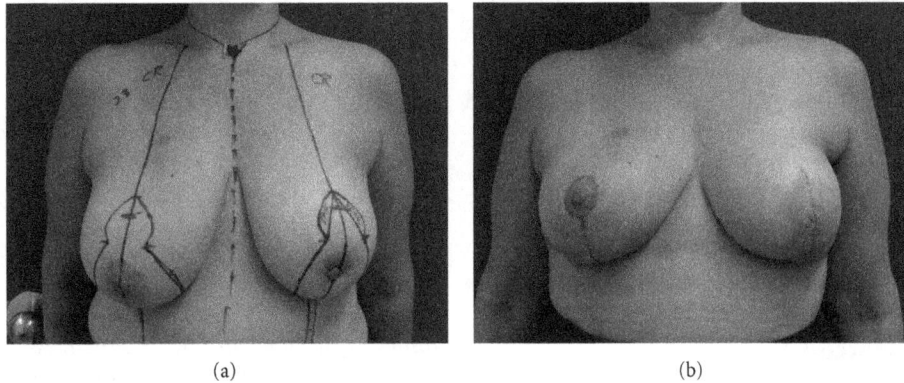

(a)   (b)

FIGURE 3: (a) Preoperative markings for Wise pattern oncoplastic breast reduction with planned excision of the left nipple areola complex. (b) Two-week postoperative result showing bilateral oncoplastic breast reductions with excision of left nipple-areola complex. Patient will then have nipple-areola reconstruction after completion of radiation.

preserved (Figures 3(a) and 3(b)). The nipple and areola can then be reconstructed after completion of radiation, using any standard method.

8. Postoperative Radiation

Radiation therapy is the second phase of BCT, starting 3 to 6 weeks after the reduction procedure once the incisions have healed. Therapy includes whole-breast irradiation, as well as a boost to the tumor bed to kill any residual microscopic deposit of cells that surgery may have missed. Cosmetically, radiation also tends to diminish scarring on the breast [33]. During surgery, surgeons should be mindful of imminent radiation by avoiding extensive skin-gland dissection and avoiding excessively long parenchymal pedicles that may be compromised and predisposed to fat necrosis. Patients should be informed that radiation therapy can result in chronic edema of the irradiated breast, or contraction and scarring, such that initial postoperative symmetry can be permanently affected.

9. Complications

In the literature, the complication rate for oncoplastic bilateral breast reduction ranges between 17% and 24% [7, 10, 34]. Common complications include skin necrosis, infection, partial or complete nipple areolar complex necrosis, and suture-line dehiscence. Like reduction mammaplasty patients without cancer, obese patients and regular smokers suffer from higher complication rates postoperatively.

If adjuvant chemotherapy is planned, it may begin once healing of the incisions has occurred and can be followed by radiation therapy. Complications that interfere with wound healing may delay the onset of chemotherapy or radiation therapy.

10. Oncologic Results

Fitoussi conducted the largest study to date, following 540 patients who underwent oncoplastic breast surgery for cancer, with a median followup of 49 months. Close

or positive margins occurred in 18.9%, with subsequent mastectomy being necessary in 9.4%. At five years, 90.3% reported a satisfactory aesthetic outcome. Five year overall and distant disease-free survival rates were 92.9% and 87.9% respectively, with local recurrence in 6.8% [21]. When compared to the standard BCT, comparable values have been found, demonstrating the equivalent oncologic safety between the two. Rietjens followed 148 women for a median 74 months to report a 3% rate of local recurrence [35]. Kayar recorded 116 patients over a period of 10 years, demonstrating overall survival rates at 100%, 89.1%, and 53.8% for stage I, stage II, and stage III, respectively [36].

Chakravorty et al. compared outcomes from 150 cases that had utilized the oncoplastic conservation techniques (77 of which were for oncoplastic reduction) with 440 cases, which used standard breast conserving surgery. At a 28-month followup and a subsequent projected 6-year local recurrence rate, oncoplastic breast conserving techniques were found to decrease reexcision rates, with oncological outcomes similar to that of standard breast conservation [37]. This finding of decreased reexcision rates is expected given the increased volume of tissue that can be removed with oncoplastic breast reduction and the need for mastectomy if there are positive margins.

11. Oncologic Surveillance

Less-experienced breast radiotherapists and radiologists may find the complex glandular reshaping from oncoplastic reduction techniques more challenging to examine on mammograms. Women with oncoplastic reductions are more likely to have a greater number of postoperative mammograms and ultrasounds as well as a greater rate of tissue sampling compared to women who have undergone partial breast reconstruction [38].

Oncoplastic breast reduction does not appear to affect cancer screening for recurrence. Although scar tissue, epidermal inclusion cysts, or fat necrosis may appear suspicious on physical exam, mammogram, ultrasound, or MRI, evaluation can be done with fine needle aspiration or core needle biopsy [39]. Typically, in postoperative healing, fat necrosis will present early on and slowly resolve with time, with complete or incomplete resorption. Because of such situations, each follow-up visit should be with the same oncologic surgeon. Mammographic findings from a study by Mendelsohn et al. found scarring and fibrosis in 50% of patients, fluid accumulations in 40% of patients, and dystrophic calcifications in 10% of patients [39]. Even though cancer screening is not compromised, patients who undergo oncoplastic reduction require more postoperative tissue sampling than those who receive traditional BCT [10].

12. Oncoplastic Outcomes

Currently, a widely accepted objective study for investigating cosmetic outcomes is not available. The BREAST-Q is a validated data set tool that may bring more insight into this matter. Through pre- and postoperative questionnaires, the BREAST-Q quantifies patient satisfaction and health-related quality of life experience in a psychometrically sound and clinically meaningful manner [40]. Patients report significantly improved body image, functional quality of life, and cosmesis when treated with BCT versus radical mastectomy [41]. More specifically for oncoplastic surgery, available publications indicate an overall satisfaction in treated patients. Chang et al. collected surveys from 20 patients with 70% rating the cosmetic outcome as excellent and 100% reported a high degree of satisfaction with cosmetic and functional results [42]. Goffman et al. established a panel, which included a surgical oncologist, an oncology nurse, a radiation oncologist, and a patient to evaluate cosmetic and functional results. Out of 55 patients, 72% evaluations gave excellent and very good marks [43]. Lastly, in a study conducted by Losken et al. 95% of women reported satisfactory aesthetic results after a six month followup [10].

13. Authors' Experience and Technique

All patients who the breast surgeons feel will have a significant deformity following lumpectomy are referred to a plastic surgeon. Small-breasted women generally decide to undergo mastectomy and reconstruction. For women with moderate-to-large sized breasts, there is an extensive discussion regarding relative advantages and disadvantages to an oncoplastic breast reduction versus mastectomy and reconstruction (as detailed in the rest of this paper).

Once the decision is made for oncoplastic breast reduction, a combined operation is scheduled. If wire localization is required, two wires are generally used at each tumor site to precisely localize the cancer within the breast. If the patient has had a prior lumpectomy, all efforts are made to incorporate the lumpectomy scar within the skin incision. Skin markings are made to include prior scars and biopsy sites whenever possible (Figure 2). This can sometimes mean adjusting markings more superiorly, laterally, or medially. Patients are counseled that the new position of the nipple-areola complex can be affected by these adjustments away from their ideal position at the breast meridian, inframammary fold, or near the midhumeral line. The choice of Wise pattern or vertical skin markings is made based on breast size, degree of ptosis, location of tumor, location of prior scars, and sternal notch-to-nipple distance. The Wise pattern incorporates a larger skin excision area. It is therefore more useful for incorporation of prior scars or skin over the tumors and is used more often in oncoplastic breast reductions.

The plastic surgeon and breast surgeon perform the lumpectomy together in order to maximize margins and aesthetics. The plastic surgeon starts the operation, making the incisions and creating the pedicle, with the guidance of the oncologic surgeon. When possible, the skin over the tumor is included in the specimen. As the wires or lumpectomy cavity are approached, the breast surgeon takes over to excise around the tumor. Posteriorly, the breast tissue is removed deep to the tumor, including muscle fascia, in order to maximize the posterior margin. The corresponding author prefers to use a superomedial pedicle whenever tumor location permits (personal preference), although the operation is similar with any pedicle. The reduction proceeds in a standard fashion [44]. The entire breast reduction specimen is removed as a single specimen incorporating the lumpectomy specimen, in order to avoid cutting across a margin. Once the specimen is removed, the breast surgeon reevaluates the remaining breast and removes any additional margins deemed necessary. Breast closure then proceeds in a standard fashion, with rotation of the superomedial pedicle into the keyhole and closure of the lateral and medial pillars. This technique enables the removal of multiple lumpectomy specimens, even the ones in completely different areas of the breast, since a wide area of skin and breast is removed. The plastic surgeon does not hesitate to remove more tissue than required by a standard breast reduction, in order to provide the needed oncologic margins.

To make up for the changes in geometry, additional tissue rearrangement within the breast may be necessary to provide the best shape and symmetry. Consequently, we advise all patients that a mastectomy would be needed if the margins return positive. Theoretically, a reexcision can be attempted depending on the original location of the tumor in relation to the reduction, and the location of the positive margin. Alternatively, the patient and oncologist may decide to give a radiation boost to the involved breast. However, we generally do not advise patients that a reexcision is likely possible, and we prepare them for the possibility of mastectomy if the margins are involved.

Over the last 4 years, we have performed over 30 oncoplastic breast reductions. There has been one positive margin at a nipple and the patient ended up with a mastectomy on that side. No other patients were reported with involved or close margins. Although we have performed a relatively smaller number of oncoplastic breast reductions compared with mastectomy reconstructions, our rate of 3.33% positive margins compares favorably with published rates of positive margins (11-12%) after lumpectomy [45, 46]. As discussed preoperatively, the patient presenting with positive margins ended up with a mastectomy. In retrospect, if there was high suspicion for involvement of the nipple with cancer, she could have had a breast reduction with central breast removal and later nipple reconstruction, as the patient in Figure 3 had. In an analysis of 540 cases, close or involved margins occurred in 18.9 percent, with mastectomy being necessary in 9.4 percent [17]. We postulate that our rate of positive and close margins is less than 18.9% because our techniques involve removing skin over the tumor site and/or fascia over the muscle, and we tend to use techniques that remove a large amount of surrounding tissue. Fittousi et al. described their experience with a variety of "aesthetic" and "combination" techniques for oncoplastic breast surgery, and it is not clear how many were specifically oncoplastic breast reductions [21]. The authors remark that one-half of the patients with involved margins were "satisfactorily managed oncologically with either repeated oncoplastic breast surgery or radiotherapy boost" [17]. The authors do not elaborate as to whether the patients who had repeat oncoplastic breast surgery initially had a reduction pattern surgery, or if they initially had a more limited tissue rearrangement that enabled repeat excision. In our practice, we counsel oncoplastic breast reduction patients that a mastectomy would likely be the next step if a margin is involved, but, of course, any case would be evaluated individually.

This issue of mastectomy if there is a positive margin would seem to argue against oncoplastic breast reductions, since patients usually have a chance at reexcision with lumpectomy alone. By agreeing to an oncoplastic breast reduction, they would seem to be agreeing to a single attempt at a lumpectomy only. However, for most patients in our practice choosing this procedure, the decision is not between a standard lumpectomy or oncoplastic breast reductions; it is a choice between oncoplastic breast reductions or mastectomy. Patients deemed candidates for oncoplastic breast reductions are those for whom standard lumpectomies would be too deforming (because of breast size, tumor size, multiple tumors, or tumor location) or those with symptomatic macromastia who desire breast reduction for the added symptom relief. Therefore, they are willing to try oncoplastic breast reductions as an alternative to mastectomy. Additionally, the rate of positive margins is much lower than that with standard lumpectomies, so it is rare that these patients do indeed go on to need a mastectomy.

14. Conclusions

In some parts of the United States, a potential lack of available reconstructive plastic surgeons limits combined treatment. Breast surgeons are then left with the choice of either referring their patients to larger centers or attempting to learn the reconstructive procedures themselves [47]. Despite these limitations, ideally, a combined approach with a breast surgeon and plastic surgeon provides the best results for the patient.

Management of patients with breast cancer is also changing. Surgeons are constantly looking for new, less invasive, and more cosmetically favorable techniques to help patients manage their disease and live with the results of their treatment.

References

[1] J. W. Canady, R. A. D'Amico, and M. F. McGuire, "Oncoplastic breast surgery: past, present, and future directions in the United States," *Plastic and Reconstructive Surgery*, vol. 124, no. 3, pp. 973–974, 2009.

[2] B. Fisher, S. Anderson, J. Bryant et al., "Twenty-year follow-up of a randomized trial comparing total mastectomy, lumpectomy, and lumpectomy plus irradiation for the treatment of invasive breast cancer," *New England Journal of Medicine*, vol. 347, no. 16, pp. 1233–1241, 2002.

[3] K. B. Clough, J. Cuminet, A. Fitoussi, C. Nos, and V. Mosseri, "Cosmetic sequelae after conservative treatment for breast cancer: classification and results of surgical correction," *Annals of Plastic Surgery*, vol. 41, no. 5, pp. 471–481, 1998.

[4] C. D'Aniello, L. Grimaldi, A. Barbato, B. Bosi, and A. Carli, "Cosmetic results in 242 patients treated by conservative surgery for breast cancer," *Scandinavian Journal of Plastic and Reconstructive Surgery and Hand Surgery*, vol. 33, no. 4, pp. 419–422, 1999.

[5] J. Y. Petit, M. Rietjens, C. Garusi, M. Greuze, and C. Perry, "Integration of plastic surgery in the course of breast-conserving surgery for cancer to improve cosmetic results and radicality of tumor excision," *Recent Results in Cancer Research*, vol. 152, pp. 202–211, 1998.

[6] W. Audretsch, M. Rezai, and C. Kolotas, "Tumor-specific immediate reconstruction in breast cancer patients," *Perspectives in Plastic Surgery*, vol. 11, no. 1, pp. 71–100, 1998.

[7] A. M. Munhoz, E. Montag, E. Arruda et al., "Assessment of immediate conservative breast surgery reconstruction: a classification system of defects revisited and an algorithm for selecting the appropriate technique," *Plastic and Reconstructive Surgery*, vol. 121, no. 3, pp. 716–727, 2008.

[8] P. L. Giacalone, P. Roger, O. Dubon et al., "Comparative study of the accuracy of breast resection in oncoplastic surgery and quadrantectomy in breast cancer," *Annals of Surgical Oncology*, vol. 14, no. 2, pp. 605–614, 2007.

[9] N. Kaur, J. Y. Petit, M. Rietjens et al., "Comparative study of surgical margins in oncoplastic surgery and quadrantectomy in breast cancer," *Annals of Surgical Oncology*, vol. 12, no. 7, pp. 539–545, 2005.

[10] A. Losken, T. M. Styblo, G. W. Carlson, G. E. Jones, and B. J. Amerson, "Management algorithm and outcome evaluation of partial mastectomy defects treated using reduction or mastopexy techniques," *Annals of Plastic Surgery*, vol. 59, no. 3, pp. 235–242, 2007.

[11] J. Y. Petit, M. Rietjens, G. Contesso, F. Bertin, and R. Gilles, "Contralateral mastoplasty for breast reconstruction: a good opportunity for glandular exploration and occult carcinomas diagnosis," *Annals of Surgical Oncology*, vol. 4, no. 6, pp. 511–515, 1997.

[12] B. L. Smith, M. Bertagnolli, B. B. Klein et al., "Evaluation of the contralateral breast: the role of biopsy at the time of treatment of primary breast cancer," *Annals of Surgery*, vol. 216, no. 1, pp. 17–21, 1992.

[13] J. A. Urban, D. Papachristou, and J. Taylor, "Bilateral breast cancer: biopsy of the opposite breast," *Cancer*, vol. 40, no. 4, pp. 1968–1973, 1977.

[14] H. J. Wanebo, G. M. Senofsky, and R. E. Fechner, "Bilateral Breast cancer. Risk reduction by contralateral biopsy," *Annals of Surgery*, vol. 201, no. 6, pp. 667–677, 1985.

[15] K. L. Dundas, J. Atyeo, and J. Cox, "What is a large breast? Measuring and categorizing breast size for tangential breast radiation therapy," *Australasian Radiology*, vol. 51, no. 6, pp. 589–593, 2007.

[16] M. E. Taylor, "Factors influencing cosmetic results after conservation therapy for breast cancer," *International Journal of Radiation Oncology Biology Physics*, vol. 31, no. 4, pp. 753–764, 1995.

[17] F. Hernanz, S. Regaño, A. Vega, and M. Gómez Fleitas, "Reduction mammaplasty: an advantageous option for breast conserving surgery in large-breasted patients," *Surgical Oncology*, vol. 19, no. 4, pp. e95–e102, 2010.

[18] R. A. Cochrane, P. Valasiadou, A. R. M. Wilson, S. K. Al-Ghazal, and R. D. Macmillan, "Cosmesis and satisfaction after breast-conserving surgery correlates with the percentage of breast volume excised," *British Journal of Surgery*, vol. 90, no. 12, pp. 1505–1509, 2003.

[19] E. Delay and K. B. Clough, "Oncoplastic breast surgery: conclusions and future perspectives," *Annales de Chirurgie Plastique et Esthetique*, vol. 53, no. 2, pp. 226–227, 2008.

[20] D. M. O'Dey, P. Baltes, A. Bozkurt, and N. Pallua, "Importance of the suprasternal notch to nipple distance (SSN:N) for vascular complications of the nipple areola complex (NAC) in the superior pedicle vertical mammaplasty: a retrospective analysis," *Journal of Plastic, Reconstructive and Aesthetic Surgery*, vol. 64, no. 10, pp. 1278–1283, 2011.

[21] A. D. Fitoussi, M. G. Berry, F. Famà et al., "Oncoplastic breast surgery for cancer: analysis of 540 consecutive cases," *Plastic and Reconstructive Surgery*, vol. 125, no. 2, pp. 454–462, 2010.

[22] K. B. Dough, S. S. Kroll, and W. Audretsch, "An approach to the repair of partial mastectomy defects," *Plastic and Reconstructive Surgery*, vol. 104, no. 2, pp. 409–420, 1999.

[23] S. J. Kronowitz, J. A. Feledy, K. K. Hunt et al., "Determining the optimal approach to breast reconstruction after partial mastectomy," *Plastic and Reconstructive Surgery*, vol. 117, no. 1, pp. 1–11, 2006.

[24] S. L. Spear, J. B. Burke, D. Forman, R. A. Zuurbier, and C. D. Berg, "Experience with reduction mammaplasty following breast conservation surgery and radiation therapy," *Plastic and Reconstructive Surgery*, vol. 102, no. 6, pp. 1913–1916, 1998.

[25] S. J. Schnitt, "Risk factors for local recurrence in patients with invasive breast cancer and negative surgical margins of excision: where are we and where are we going?" *American Journal of Clinical Pathology*, vol. 120, no. 4, pp. 485–488, 2003.

[26] S. E. Singletary, "Surgical margins in patients with early-stage breast cancer treated with breast conservation therapy," *American Journal of Surgery*, vol. 184, no. 5, pp. 383–393, 2002.

[27] A. Haid, M. Knauer, S. Dunzinger et al., "Intra-operative sonography: a valuable aid during breast-conserving surgery for occult breast cancer," *Annals of Surgical Oncology*, vol. 14, no. 11, pp. 3090–3101, 2007.

[28] F. D. Rahusen, A. J. A. Bremers, H. F. J. Fabry, A. H. M. Taets van Amerongen, R. P. A. Boom, and S. Meijer, "Ultrasound-guided lumpectomy of nonpalpable breast cancer versus wire-guided resection: a randomized clinical trial," *Annals of Surgical Oncology*, vol. 9, no. 10, pp. 994–998, 2002.

[29] C. Lassus, "Breast reduction: evolution of a technique—a single vertical scar," *Aesthetic Plastic Surgery*, vol. 11, no. 2, pp. 107–112, 1987.

[30] M. Lejour, "Vertical mammaplasty and liposuction of the breast," *Plastic and Reconstructive Surgery*, vol. 94, no. 1, pp. 100–114, 1994.

[31] B. O. Anderson, R. Masetti, and M. J. Silverstein, "Oncoplastic approaches to partial mastectomy: an overview of volume-displacement techniques," *Lancet Oncology*, vol. 6, no. 3, pp. 145–157, 2005.

[32] M. Ballester, M. G. Berry, B. Couturaud, F. Reyal, R. J. Salmon, and A. D. Fitoussi, "Lateral mammaplasty reconstruction after surgery for breast cancer," *British Journal of Surgery*, vol. 96, no. 10, pp. 1141–1146, 2009.

[33] K. B. Clough, C. Nos, R. J. Salmon, M. Soussaline, and J. C. Durand, "Conservative treatment of breast cancers by mammaplasty and irradiation: a new approach to lower quadrant tumors," *Plastic and Reconstructive Surgery*, vol. 96, no. 2, pp. 363–370, 1995.

[34] S. J. Kronowitz, K. K. Hunt, H. M. Kuerer et al., "Practical guidelines for repair of partial mastectomy defects using the breast reduction technique in patients undergoing breast conservation therapy," *Plastic and Reconstructive Surgery*, vol. 120, no. 7, pp. 1755–1768, 2007.

[35] M. Rietjens, C. A. Urban, P. C. Rey et al., "Long-term oncological results of breast conservative treatment with oncoplastic surgery," *Breast*, vol. 16, no. 4, pp. 387–395, 2007.

[36] R. Kayar, M. Cobanoglu, O. Güngor, H. Catal, and M. Emiroglu, "The value of breast reduction operations in breast conservation surgery, late results of 116 patients with breast cancer," *Meme Sağlığı Dergisi*, vol. 2, pp. 131–138, 2006.

[37] A. Chakravorty, A. K. Shrestha, N. Sanmugalingam et al., "How safe is oncoplastic breast conservation? Comparative analysis with standard breast conserving surgery," *European Journal of Surgical Oncology*, vol. 38, no. 5, pp. 395–398, 2012.

[38] A. Losken, T. G. Schaefer, M. Newell, and T. M. Styblo, "The impact of partial breast reconstruction using reduction techniques on postoperative cancer surveillance," *Plastic and Reconstructive Surgery*, vol. 124, no. 1, pp. 9–17, 2009.

[39] A. M. Mendelsohn, E. L. Bove, F. M. Lupinetti, D. C. Crowley, T. R. Lloyd, and R. H. Beekman, "Central pulmonary artery growth patterns after the bidirectional Glenn procedure," *Journal of Thoracic and Cardiovascular Surgery*, vol. 107, no. 5, pp. 1284–1290, 1994.

[40] A. L. Pusic, A. F. Klassen, and S. J. Cano, "Use of the BREAST-Q in clinical outcomes research," *Plastic and Reconstructive Surgery*, vol. 129, no. 1, pp. 166e–167e, 2012.

[41] D. Curran, J. P. Van Dongen, N. K. Aaronson et al., "Quality of life of early-stage breast cancer patients treated with radical mastectomy or breast-conserving procedures: results of EORTC trial 10801," *European Journal of Cancer*, vol. 34, no. 3, pp. 307–314, 1998.

[42] E. Chang, N. Johnson, B. Webber et al., "Bilateral reduction mammaplasty in combination with lumpectomy for treatment of breast cancer in patients with macromastia," *American Journal of Surgery*, vol. 187, no. 5, pp. 647–651, 2004.

[43] T. E. Goffman, H. Schneider, K. Hay, D. E. Elkins, R. A. Schnarrs, and C. Carman, "Cosmesis with bilateral mammoreduction for conservative breast cancer treatment," *Breast Journal*, vol. 11, no. 3, pp. 195–198, 2005.

[44] S. P. Davison, A. N. Mesbahi, I. Ducic, M. Sarcia, J. Dayan, and S. L. Spear, "The versatility of the superomedial pedicle with various skin reduction patterns," *Plastic and Reconstructive Surgery*, vol. 120, no. 6, pp. 1466–1476, 2007.

[45] A. B. Chagpar, R. C. G. Martin, L. J. Hagendoorn, C. Chao, and K. M. McMasters, "Lumpectomy margins are affected by tumor size and histologic subtype but not by biopsy technique," *American Journal of Surgery*, vol. 188, no. 4, pp. 399–402, 2004.

[46] H. Yang, W. Jia, K. Chen et al., "Cavity margins and lumpectomy margins for pathological assessment: which is superior in breast-conserving surgery?" *Journal of Surgical Research*, vol. 178, no. 2, pp. 751–757, 2012.

[47] A. Losken and M. Y. Nahabedian, "Oncoplastic breast surgery: past, present, and future directions in the United States," *Plastic and Reconstructive Surgery*, vol. 124, no. 3, pp. 969–972, 2009.

31

Neoadjuvant Chemotherapy in Locally Advanced and Borderline Resectable Nonsquamous Sinonasal Tumors (Esthesioneuroblastoma and Sinonasal Tumor with Neuroendocrine Differentiation)

Vijay M. Patil,[1] **Amit Joshi,**[1] **Vanita Noronha,**[1] **Vibhor Sharma,**[1] **Saurabh Zanwar,**[1] **Sachin Dhumal,**[1] **Shubhada Kane,**[2] **Prathamesh Pai,**[3] **Anil D'Cruz,**[3] **Pankaj Chaturvedi,**[3] **Atanu Bhattacharjee,**[4] **and Kumar Prabhash**[1]

[1]Department of Medical Oncology, Tata Memorial Hospital, Mumbai, India
[2]Department of Pathology, Tata Memorial Hospital, Mumbai, India
[3]Department of Surgical oncology, Tata Memorial Hospital, Mumbai, India
[4]Division of Clinical Research and Biostatistics, Malabar Cancer Centre, Kerala, India

Correspondence should be addressed to Kumar Prabhash; kumarprabhashtmh@gmail.com

Academic Editor: Kumar A. Pathak

Introduction. Sinonasal tumors are chemotherapy responsive which frequently present in advanced stages making NACT a promising option for improving resection and local control in borderline resectable and locally advanced tumours. Here we reviewed the results of 25 such cases treated with NACT. *Materials and Methods.* Sinonasal tumor patients treated with NACT were selected for this analysis. These patients received NACT with platinum and etoposide for 2 cycles. Patients who responded and were amenable for gross total resection underwent surgical resection and adjuvant CTRT. Those who responded but were not amenable for resection received radical CTRT. Patients who progressed on NACT received either radical CTRT or palliative radiotherapy. *Results.* The median age of the cohort was 42 years (IQR 37–47 years). Grades 3-4 toxicity with NACT were seen in 19 patients (76%). The response rate to NACT was 80%. Post-NACT surgery was done in 12 (48%) patients and radical chemoradiation in 9 (36%) patients. The 2-year progression free survival and overall survival were 75% and 78.5%, respectively. *Conclusion.* NACT in sinonasal tumours has a response rate of 80%. The protocol of NACT followed by local treatment is associated with improvement in outcomes as compared to our historical cohort.

1. Introduction

Sinonasal tumors are a rare entity [1, 2]. These tumors are usually not included in major head and neck cancer studies addressing questions regarding local management or systemic treatment [3–6]. Hence there is dearth of level 1 evidence in these tumors. Multiple small retrospective series have been published and certain facts are clear from these studies:

(1) The subclassification of sinonasal tumors into esthesioneuroblastoma, sinonasal tumor with neuroendocrine differentiation, and sinonasal tumor with poor differentiation helps as the outcome differs according to the exact subtype [7].

(2) In all these three subtypes surgical resection with or without adjuvant radiation remains the cornerstone of management [8, 9].

(3) The need for of systemic treatment is felt both with radiation when given in curative setting (only chemoradiation) and in adjuvant setting (chemoradiation postsurgical resection) in locally advanced tumors [10–12].

However the role of neoadjuvant chemotherapy (NACT) in locally advanced sinonasal malignancies is largely unaddressed. It is an interesting prospect considering anatomical proximity of sinonasal malignancies to vital structure and its locally aggressive behaviour both of which make gross total resection difficult. These tumors are responsive to chemotherapy in spite of the variable histologies seen at this site (esthesioneuroblastoma, sinonasal tumor of neuroendocrine differentiation, NUT midline tumors, and sinonasal tumor undifferentiated cancers).

Neoadjuvant chemotherapy before surgery may lead to regression of tumor and improvement in gross total resection rate in locally advanced tumors which in turn may improve the local control [7]. We routinely administer neoadjuvant chemotherapy in locally advanced resectable and borderline resectable sinonasal tumors with the aim of facilitating resection and improving local control. This audit was performed to study the efficacy (in terms of response rate), acute toxicity, and early outcomes with this strategy.

2. Methods

2.1. Selection of Cases. Sinonasal tumors are routinely discussed in a multidisciplinary clinic. Patients with the below mentioned criteria are referred for neoadjuvant chemotherapy before local treatment:

(1) Locally advanced sinonasal tumors with extension of tumor beyond nasal and paranasal sinus:

   (a) Resectable: but resection would been morbid requiring extensive surgery and would have chances of incomplete gross total resection.

   (b) Unresectable: frank involvement of any vital structure or surgically inaccessible site making upfront surgery not possible.

(2) ECOG PS 0–2.

(3) Without distant metastasis.

2.2. NACT Delivery. These patients were treated with neoadjuvant chemotherapy. NACT consisted of cisplatin and etoposide. Cisplatin dose of $33 \, \text{mg/m}^2$ D1 to D3 and etoposide dose of $100 \, \text{mg/m}^2$ D1 to D3 were administered intravenously. Cisplatin was replaced with carboplatin (AUC-5 or 6) if the calculated serum creatinine clearance was below 60 mL/min. The chemotherapy was administered with standard premedications and antiemetic prophylaxis. Patients were given 1 liter of 0.9% NaCl hydration with magnesium and potassium supplementation from D1 to D3. Secondary prophylaxis with G-CSF was administered for patients having febrile neutropenia in C1. Two cycles of NACT were administered.

2.3. Treatment Post NACT. Following 2 cycles of NACT, patients were assessed with axial radiological imaging (either CECT or PET-CT). These patients were then discussed in skull base multidisciplinary clinic. Patients who had adequate response, which would facilitate gross total resection

were offered surgical resection and adjuvant chemoradiation. Patients in whom, after 2 cycles, gross total resection was still not possible were offered radical chemoradiation. Patients who had progressed after NACT were considered for radical chemoradiation or palliative radiotherapy (RT) depending upon the patient's performance status and tumor volume. Palliative RT was delivered when tumor volumes were large and adequate tumoricidal RT doses could not be delivered without respecting the tolerance doses of nearby vital structures. These patients were followed up after treatment till death.

2.4. Data Collection. For this analysis, the data of these patients was acquired from a prospectively maintained head and neck cancer NACT database. Patients treated between August 2010 and August 2014 with sinonasal tumors and nonsquamous histology were selected. Data regarding baseline clinical details, staging, the indication of NACT, NACT details, response, adverse events, post-NACT local treatment details, pathological response, and outcome details were noted.

For this analysis, as NACT was given predominantly with the intention of having a gross total resection, the locoregional extent of tumor was charted. The charting was done with the following spaces being considered: involvement of cribriform plate, involvement of intracranial space with only extradural extension, involvement of intracranial space with intradural without involvement of brain, involvement of intracranial space with involvement of brain, involvement of orbit, and involvement of infratemporal fossa. This charting was done so that each of these space involvement would be analyzed as a factor predicting for achievement of resectability after NACT.

The response to NACT was noted in accordance with RECIST version 1.1. The adverse events during NACT were documented in accordance with CTCAE version 4.03. The pathological response rate was quantified as pathologic complete response (pCR) if no viable tumor was seen post-NACT and No-pCR if any viable tumor was seen post-NACT. The outcome data noted was progression free survival and overall survival. The progression free survival was calculated from date of start of NACT to date of progression (either locoregional or distant). Those patients who had not progressed were censored at their last follow-up. The overall survival was calculated from date of start of NACT to date of death. Those patients who had not died were censored at their last follow-up.

2.5. Statistical Analysis. Data was censored for analysis on September 30, 2015. Descriptive statistics was performed. Fisher's test was used to test whether there was a difference between response rate in the different histological subtypes considered. The analysis between achievement of resectability and different sites of involvement was also done by Fisher's test. The progression free survival and overall survival for each histology were computed by Kaplan Meier survival analysis. Log rank test was used for univariate analysis of PFS and OS. Cox regression analysis was used for multivariate analysis.

TABLE 1: Baseline details according to histological subtypes.

Variable	Esthesioneuroblastoma (n = 12 patients)	Sinonasal tumor with neuroendocrine differentiation (n = 13 patients)	Total (n = 25 patients)
Median age	40 years (IQR 36.5–42.75 years)	45 years (IQR 36.5–57.0 years)	42 years (IQR 37–47 years)
Gender			
Male	23	11	19
Female	04	02	06
ECOG PS			
PS 0-1	12	13	25
PS 2	00	00	00
Grade			
III-IV	10	13*	08

*All patients had high grade neuroendocrine tumors.

TABLE 2: Extent of locoregional spread.

Extent	Esthesioneuroblastoma (n = 12 patients)	SN-NEC (n = 13 patients)	Total (25 patients)
Involvement of cribriform plate	12 (100.0%)	13 (100.0%)	25 (100.0%)
Intracranial extension up to extradural region	06 (50.0%)	08 (61.5%)	14 (56%)
Intradural intracranial extension but brain parenchyma uninvolved	06 (50.0%)	04 (30.8%)	10 (40%)
Intradural extension with brain parenchyma involvement	02 (16.7%)	03 (23.1%)	05 (20%)
Involvement of orbit	06 (50.0%)	07 (53.8%)	13 (52%)
Involvement of infratemporal fossa	03 (25%)	03 (23.1%)	06 (24%)
Involvement of parapharyngeal space	01 (08.3%)	01 (7.7%)	02 (08%)
Involvement of regional lymph nodes	03 (25%)	05 (38.5%)	08 (32%)

3. Results

3.1. Baseline Details. Twenty-five patients of sinonasal cavity cancer were identified. The baseline details are shown in Table 1. The median age of the whole cohort was 42 years (IQR 37–47 years). The ECOG PS was 0-1 in all 25 patients. There were 12 esthesioneuroblastoma patients and 13 SNEC patients. The Hyams grading of esthesioneuroblastoma was grade 2 in 1 patient, grade 3 in 8 patients, grade 4 in 2 patients, and not available in 2 patients. In these 2 patients, one patient's tissue was inadequate for grading while in other slides and blocks was not available for review. Out of 25 patients, nine patients had some form of previous local resections. Previous radiation exposure was seen in one patient while one of the patients had prior chemotherapy exposure. This patient had received 2 cycles of cisplatin and etoposide previously. Out of these 25 patients who all had locally advanced disease, 11 patients (44%) were considered unresectable and 14 patients were considered resectable upfront (56%).

3.2. Extent of Locoregional Spread and Reason for NACT. The extent of locoregional spread is shown in Table 2. All patient had skull base invasion. Regional lymph node involvement

was seen in 08 patients (32%). Involvement of infratemporal fossa and parapharyngeal space was seen in 06 (24.0%) and 02 patients (08%), respectively.

The reason for NACT was dural involvement in 2 patients, brain parenchyma involvement in 4 patients, intracranial involvement in 5 patients, intracranial extension with orbital apex involvement in 2 patients, orbital involvement (extensive) in 1 patient, and infratemporal fossa involvement in 1 patient and extensive soft tissue disease in 10 patients.

3.3. NACT Compliance and Tolerability. Out of 25 patients 2 cycles of NACT were completed by all 25 patients. The median number of cycles delivered was 2 (IQR 2-3). Twelve patients (48%) received more than 2 cycles before locoregional treatment. The incidence of grade 3-4 toxicity in accordance with CTCAE version 4.03 was 76%. There was no grade 5 toxicity seen. The details of adverse events are shown in Table 3.

3.4. Response to NACT. The response was evaluable in all 25 patients after 2 cycles of NACT. The response was PR in 20 patients (80%, 95% CI 58.7%–92.4%), SD in 03 patients, and PD in 02 patients. The difference in response according to histological subtype is shown in Table 4. The response

TABLE 3: Adverse events in accordance with CTCAE version 4.03 observed during NACT. Numbers shown are actual patient numbers.

Toxicity	Grade 3	Grade 4
Anemia	02	00
Neutropenia	06	04
Thrombocytopenia	00	00
Febrile neutropenia	01	02
Nausea	00	00
Vomiting	00	00
Diarrhea	01	00
Increased serum creatinine	00	00
Transaminitis (raised SGOT/PT)	00	00
Hyponatremia	07	05
Hypokalemia	00	00
Hyperkalemia	00	00

rate in esthesioneuroblastoma and in SN-NEC was 66.7% and 92.3%, respectively (p value = 0.160). The response rate in upfront resectable patients was 85.7% (12 patients out of 14) while it was 72.7% (08 patients out of 11) in upfront unresectable patients (p value = 0.623).

3.5. Post-NACT Resectability.
Post-NACT 13 patients {n = 25, 52% (95% CI 33.5%–70.0%)} were resectable in the whole cohort of 25 patients. The achievement of resectability post-NACT with respect to the anatomical extent of the tumor is depicted in Table 5. Among the factors tested for achievement of resectability the resectability status before surgery had influence on achievement of resectability (Table 5). Resectability was achieved in 85.7% (12 out of 14) of patients who were considered resectable as opposed to 9.1% (1 out of 11) in patients who were considered unresectable (p = 0.136). Resectability was achieved in 60% (12 out of 20) of patients who responded to NACT as opposed to 20% (1 out of 5) in patients who did not respond to NACT (p = 0.136).

3.6. Post-NACT Treatment Details.
Post-NACT 13 patients were resectable but 1 patient opted for CTRT. Post-NACT treatment received was surgery followed by adjuvant treatment in 11 patients, surgery without adjuvant in 1 patient, radical chemoradiation in 9 patients, and palliative RT in 2 patients. Two patients did not take local treatment after NACT. One patient had progressive disease after NACT and was not suitable for any local treatment. The other patient had near complete response and he did not want any further treatment.

Surgery was performed in 12 patients. The type of surgery done was craniofacial resection in 06 patients, craniofacial resection with medial maxillectomy in 01 patient, medial maxillectomy in 03 patients, sinonasal resection in 01 patient, and radical maxillectomy with orbital exenteration in 01 patient. It was a gross complete resection in all 12 patients. The pathological response was pathological complete response in 03 patients. All 12 patients were offered adjuvant treatment consisting of chemoradiation. However one patient declined adjuvant treatment as there was risk of vision loss associated with RT. 11 patients received adjuvant chemoradiation. Out

of these 11 patients, 07 patients were treated with IMRT and 04 patients were treated with 3DCRT technique. The median dose to tumor bed (CTV) was 6000 cGy (IQR 6000-6000 cGy). All patients completed chemoradiation. The median number of weekly chemotherapy cycles (cisplatin 30 mg/m^2) received were 6 (IQR 6-6).

Radical chemoradiation was done in 09 patients. Out of these, 07 patients were treated with IMRT and 02 patients were treated with 3DCRT technique. The median dose to tumor bed (CTV) was 6000 cGy (IQR 6000–6600 cGy). All patients except one completed radical chemoradiation. This patient progressed after 10# of RT and hence his RT was stopped. The median number of chemotherapy (cisplatin 30 mg/m^2) cycles received were 5 (range 4–6).

Palliative RT was delivered by conventional method with the midline dose being 5500 cGy delivered in 22# in one patient and 5000 cGy in 25# in the other patient. Both patients had symptomatic relief postpalliative RT.

3.7. Outcomes.
The median follow-up was 1.7 years (IQR 1.0–2.2 years). There were 6 patients who had progression. The first site of progression was local in 2 patients, local with distant in 1 patient, regional in 1 patient, and distant in 2 patients. The sites of distant failures were bony metastasis in 2 patients and regional lymph nodes in 1 patient. Five patients had died at the time of analysis and all deaths were due to disease progression.

The 2-year progression free survival and overall survival were 75% and 78.5%, respectively. The influence of different factors on PFS and OS can be seen in Table 6. The 2-year progression free survival was 91.7% and 57.0% in patients with esthesioneuroblastoma and SNEC, respectively. The stage of disease and response to chemotherapy was not found significantly associated with median PFS. However patients who had sufficient response for the disease to be considered as resectable had a 2-year PFS of 92.3% as opposed to 50.0% in patients who did not have sufficient regression of disease to make it resectable (p = 0.015). Patients who had unresectable disease upfront had a 2-year PFS of 45.5% as opposed to 100% in patients who were considered resectable upfront (p = 0.002). Among patients who underwent local treatment with radical intent patients undergoing surgery had better 2-year PFS than patients who received radical chemoradiation. The 2-year PFS in surgery group was 100.0% as opposed to 64.8% in patients treated with radical chemoradiation (p = 0.348).

The 2-year OS (Figure 1) was 100% in patients who achieved resectability as opposed to 58.3% in patients who did not (p = 0.016). Similarly the 2-year OS was 100% in upfront resectable patients as opposed to 54.5% in unresectable patients (p = 0.008). Cox regression analysis failed to identify a single prognostic marker for PFS and OS. Both resectability achieved and upfront resectability status were considered for multivariate analysis.

4. Discussion

Sinonasal tumors have varied histology [1]. Squamous cell cancer histology seems to predominate [1]. We have

TABLE 4: Response rates according to histological type.

	Esthesioneuroblastoma (n = 12 patients)	SN-NEC (n = 13 patients)	Total (25 patients)
CR + PR	8 (66.7%)	12 (92.3%)	20 (80%)
SD + PD	4 (33.3%)	01 (07.7%)	05 (20%)

TABLE 5: Factors affecting achievement of resectability.

	Presence of factor	Resectability achieved	p value on Fisher's test (one sided)	p value on binary logistic regression analysis
Anatomical factors				
Intracranial extension up to extradural region	Yes: 14	8	0.430	Not included
	No: 11	05		
Intradural intracranial extension but brain parenchyma uninvolved	Yes: 10	06	0.404	Not included
	No: 15	07		
Intradural extension with brain parenchyma involvement	Yes: 05	03	0.541	Not included
	No: 20	10		
Involvement of orbit	Yes: 13	07	0.582	Not included
	No: 12	06		
Involvement of infratemporal fossa	Yes: 06	02	0.281	0.851
	No: 19	11		
Involvement of parapharyngeal space	Yes: 02	01	0.741	Not included
	No: 23	12		
Surgical pre-NACT status	Unresectable: 11	01	0.000	0.003
	Resectable: 14	12		
Biological factors				
Pathology	E: 12	08	0.157	Not included
	SNE: 13	05		
Response	CR + PR: 20	12	0.136	0.139
	SD + PD: 05	01		

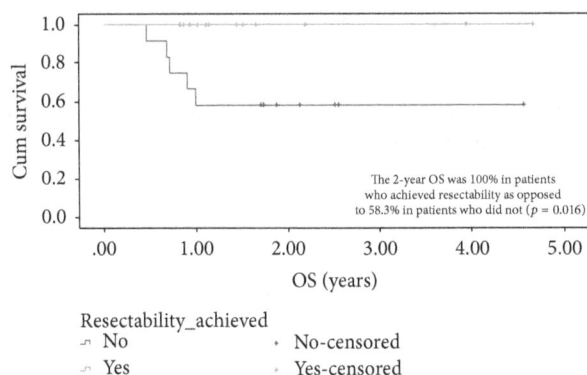

FIGURE 1: Two-year OS in accordance with achievement of resectability.

already reported our results of locally advanced maxillary squamous cell cancers who were treated with neoadjuvant chemotherapy followed by local treatment [13]. In this analysis we wanted to focus on nonsquamous sinonasal malignancies. Locally advanced sinonasal malignancies have varied prognosis according to histology and stage [7]. In our previous report of sinonasal malignancies we had very poor outcomes with nearly 75% of our patients having a recurrence within 2 years [14, 15]. Since then, emphasis has been placed on use of neoadjuvant chemotherapy in patients with locally advanced and borderline resectable tumors as a strategy to improve outcomes.

All of these patients had Kadish C or D stage disease. The extent of the local tumor is highlighted in Table 2, where it can be noted that all patients had skull base invasion, half had orbital involvement, and one-third had regional lymph nodes involvement. These features are independently associated with inferior outcomes [16]. Previous reports suggest that these patients, when treated only with upfront chemoradiation, experience suboptimal outcomes. In a report from Chao, it was seen that patients treated with chemoradiation had 5-year local control of 51.2% versus a local control of 87.4% for patients undergoing surgery and RT [8]. In another retrospective analysis reported from New York, it was seen that in esthesioneuroblastoma radiotherapy alone was associated with an inferior outcome compared to surgical treatment [17]. On a similar note Gruber et al.

TABLE 6: The influence of different factors on PFS and OS.

Factor	Division	Median PFS in years	2-year PFS	p value (log rank test)
Histological type (n = 25)	Esthesioneuroblastoma	NR	91.7%	0.094
	SNEC	NR	57.0%	
Stage (n = 25)	Kadish C	NR	60.0%	0.347
	Kadish D	NR	81.4%	
Response (n = 25)	CR + PR	NR	77.3%	0.266
	SD + PD	NR	60.0%	
Resectability achieved (n = 25)	Yes	NR	92.3%	0.015
	No	1.10	50.0%	
Upfront status (n = 25)	Resectable	NR	100%	0.002
	Unresectable	1.10	45.5%	

Factor	Division	Median OS in years	2-year OS	p value (log rank test)
Histological type (n = 25)	Esthesioneuroblastoma	NR	91.7%	0.169
	SNEC	NR	64.5%	
Stage (n = 25)	Kadish C	NR	79.6%	0.677
	Kadish D	NR	75.0%	
Response (n = 25)	CR + PR	NR	82.7%	0.185
	SD + PD	NR	60.0%	
Resectability achieved (n = 25)	Yes	NR	100.0%	0.016
	No	NR	58.3%	
Upfront status (n = 25)	Resectable	NR	100%	0.008
	Unresectable	NR	54.5%	

also have recommended in their publication that irradiation alone, even when doses were escalated to 7300 cGy, is not sufficient in esthesioneuroblastoma [16]. All these reports probably carried an unintentional bias in a sense that in many instances it was the unresectable tumors which were subjected to radical chemoradiation. However, in view of the poor outcomes seen in our series and others with radical chemoradiation alone in unresectable tumors, we routinely consider these locally advanced patients for neoadjuvant chemotherapy to improve rates of local control and gross total resectability.

The neoadjuvant chemotherapy used here was cisplatin and etoposide. This is a standard regimen for treatment of high-grade neuroendocrine carcinomas. This regimen either alone or in combination with radiation in accordance with stage is used. Different combinations of chemotherapy have been used in the literature with platinum backbone. Many of these combinations have infusional 5 FU [18–21]. However we have logistic issues in delivering infusional 5 FU; this regimen is mainly used for squamous cell carcinoma and hence the above regimen was selected. The response rates achieved with this regimen are comparable to those reported in other series. The heartening fact is that the regimen was well tolerated, there was no mortality associated with this regimen, and the response rates achieved with this regimen in such advanced tumors was 80%. There is a small chance of progression of disease with NACT; it is a matter of concern but it helps in biologically selecting patients for further treatment.

Esthesioneuroblastoma was associated with high response rates and better outcomes than SNEC. This finding is similar to that reported in other studies [7]. The 2-year PFS and OS are much better now in our locally advanced and/or technically unresectable sinonasal cancers than they were seen in our previous report. This may be due to contribution of neoadjuvant chemotherapy along with better surgical and radiation techniques. Such tailored approaches in locally advanced sinonasal tumors with neoadjuvant chemotherapy have been associated with improvement in survival [22]. The importance of multidisciplinary approach seems a necessity in these tumors.

Interestingly the factors which impacted both PFS and OS were the resectability status of the patients prior to both surgery and after surgery. All of these patients had extensive disease but these patients were classified in multidisciplinary clinic upfront into potentially resectable or unresectable. Unresectable patients were those whose tumors had frank invasion of vital structures making them not a candidate for surgery. However the involvement in these tumors in most occasions either were encasing vital structures (like optic nerve, orbital apex) or had frank invasion of brain making these tumors an unlikely candidate for surgery even if they showed excellent response to NACT. As opposed to these patients termed resectable implied that gross total resection may not have been possible and if attempted would have required an extensive mutilating surgery. This classification had an impact on PFS and OS very similar to that of post-NACT resectability status. Our data validates this upfront classification as only 1 out of 11 inoperable patients was considered resectable after NACT as opposed to 12 out of 14 resectable patients. This data emphasizes proper selection criteria for selecting patients for NACT when it is administered to make the tumor resectable. However we failed to provide objective assessment criteria for such classification upfront. Upfront invasion of none of the anatomical landmarks considered in the study could predict achievement of resectability after NACT.

This study though retrospective has its own strengths and limitations. This is one of the few studies reporting on nonsquamous locally advanced sinonasal tumors who have been selected with homogenous criteria (Kadish C and D) and have been treated with homogenous protocols. The treatment planning of these cases had been done in a multidisciplinary clinic and post-NACT treatment was also decided in the same clinic. The limitation of this study is its retrospective nature and short follow-up. It is known in sinonasal tumors, especially esthesioneuroblastoma, to have delayed recurrence, in some instances even 10 years after initial treatment [7].

5. Conclusion

Sinonasal tumors are a group chemosensitive tumors. NACT with cisplatin and etoposide can achieve response rate of 80% in nonsquamous sinonasal tumors and is well tolerated. The protocol of NACT followed by local treatment is associated with improvement in outcomes.

References

[1] J. H. Turner and D. D. Reh, "Incidence and survival in patients with sinonasal cancer: a historical analysis of population-based data," *Head and Neck*, vol. 34, no. 6, pp. 877–885, 2012.

[2] R. Goel, R. Karthikeyan, P. Ramani, and T. Chandrasekar, "Sino nasal undifferentiated carcinoma: a rare entity," *Journal of Natural Science, Biology and Medicine*, vol. 3, no. 1, pp. 101–104, 2012.

[3] J. B. Vermorken, E. Remenar, C. van Herpen et al., "Cisplatin, fluorouracil, and docetaxel in unresectable head and neck cancer," *The New England Journal of Medicine*, vol. 357, no. 17, pp. 1695–1704, 2007.

[4] M. R. Posner, D. M. Hershock, C. R. Blajman et al., "Cisplatin and fluorouracil alone or with docetaxel in head and neck cancer," *The New England Journal of Medicine*, vol. 357, no. 17, pp. 1705–1715, 2007.

[5] R. Haddad, S. Sonis, M. Posner et al., "Randomized phase 2 study of concomitant chemoradiotherapy using weekly carboplatin/paclitaxel with or without daily subcutaneous amifostine in patients with locally advanced head and neck cancer," *Cancer*, vol. 115, no. 19, pp. 4514–4523, 2009.

[6] R. Hitt, J. J. Grau, A. López-Pousa et al., "A randomized phase III trial comparing induction chemotherapy followed by chemoradiotherapy versus chemoradiotherapy alone as treatment of unresectable head and neck cancer," *Annals of Oncology*, vol. 25, no. 1, Article ID mdt461, pp. 216–225, 2014.

[7] S. Su, D. Bell, and E. Hanna, "Esthesioneuroblastoma, neuroendocrine carcinoma, and sinonasal undifferentiated carcinoma: differentiation in diagnosis and treatment," *International Archives of Otorhinolaryngology*, vol. 18, no. 2, pp. S149–S156, 2014.

[8] K. S. C. Chao, C. Kaplan, J. R. Simpson et al., "Esthesioneuroblastoma: the impact of treatment modality," *Head & Neck*, vol. 23, no. 9, pp. 749–757, 2001.

[9] D. A. Reiersen and M. E. Pahilan, "Meta-analysis of treatment outcomes for sinonasal undifferentiated carcinoma," *NOtolaryngology—Head and Neck Surgery*, 2012.

[10] B. S. Hoppe, C. J. Nelson, D. R. Gomez et al., "Unresectable carcinoma of the paranasal sinuses: outcomes and toxicities," *International Journal of Radiation Oncology, Biology, Physics*, vol. 72, no. 3, pp. 763–769, 2008.

[11] O. Guntinas-Lichius, M. P. Kreppel, H. Stuetzer, R. Semrau, H. E. Eckel, and R. P. Mueller, "Single modality and multimodality treatment of nasal and paranasal sinuses cancer: a single institution experience of 229 patients," *European Journal of Surgical Oncology*, vol. 33, no. 2, pp. 222–228, 2007.

[12] J. H. Kang, S. H. Cho, J. P. Kim et al., "Treatment outcomes between concurrent chemoradiotherapy and combination of surgery, radiotherapy, and/or chemotherapy in stage III and IV maxillary sinus cancer: multi-institutional retrospective analysis," *Journal of Oral and Maxillofacial Surgery*, vol. 70, no. 7, pp. 1717–1723, 2012.

[13] V. Noronha, V. M. Patil, A. Joshi et al., "Induction chemotherapy in technically unresectable locally advanced carcinoma of maxillary sinus," *Chemotherapy Research and Practice*, vol. 2014, Article ID 487872, 6 pages, 2014.

[14] S. Menon, P. Pai, M. Sengar, J. P. Aggarwal, and S. V. Kane, "Sinonasal malignancies with neuroendocrine differentiation: case series and review of literature," *Indian Journal of Pathology and Microbiology*, vol. 53, no. 1, pp. 28–34, 2010.

[15] T. Gupta, T. Wadasadawala, R. Phurailatpam et al., "Early clinical outcomes in midline sinonasal cancers treated with helical tomotherapy-based image-guided intensity-modulated radiation therapy," *International Journal of Head and Neck Surgery*, vol. 4, no. 1, pp. 6–12, 2013, http://www.jaypeejournals.com/eJournals/ShowText.aspx?ID=4232&Type=FREE&TYP=TOP&IN=~/eJournals/images/JPLOGO.gif&IID=332&isPDF=YES.

[16] G. Gruber, K. Laedrach, B. Baumert, M. Caversaccio, J. Raveh, and R. Greiner, "Esthesioneuroblastoma: irradiation alone and surgery alone are not enough," *International Journal of Radiation Oncology Biology Physics*, vol. 54, no. 2, pp. 486–491, 2002.

[17] D. Jethanamest, L. G. Morris, A. G. Sikora, and D. I. Kutler, "Esthesioneuroblastoma: a population-based analysis of survival and prognostic factors," *Archives of Otolaryngology—Head and Neck Surgery*, vol. 133, no. 3, pp. 276–280, 2007.

[18] P. LoRusso, E. Tapazoglou, J. A. Kish et al., "Chemotherapy for paranasal sinus carcinoma. A 10-year experience at Wayne State University," *Cancer*, vol. 62, no. 1, pp. 1–5, 1988.

[19] T. Bjork-Eriksson, C. Mercke, B. Petruson, and S. Ekholm, "Potential impact on tumor control and organ preservation with cisplatin and 5-fluorouracil for patients with advanced tumors of the paranasal sinuses and nasal fossa: a prospective pilot study," *Cancer*, vol. 70, no. 11, pp. 2615–2620, 1992.

[20] E. Y. Hanna, A. D. Cardenas, F. DeMonte et al., "Induction chemotherapy for advanced squamous cell carcinoma of the paranasal sinuses," *Archives of Otolaryngology—Head and Neck Surgery*, vol. 137, no. 1, pp. 78–81, 2011.

[21] L. Licitra, L. D. Locati, R. Cavina et al., "Primary chemotherapy followed by anterior craniofacial resection and radiotherapy for paranasal cancer," *Annals of Oncology*, vol. 14, no. 3, pp. 367–372, 2003.

[22] A. Al-Mamgani, P. van Rooij, R. Mehilal, L. Tans, and P. C. Levendag, "Combined-modality treatment improved outcome in sinonasal undifferentiated carcinoma: single-institutional experience of 21 patients and review of the literature," *European Archives of Oto-Rhino-Laryngology*, vol. 270, no. 1, pp. 293–299, 2013.

Permissions

The contributors of this book come from diverse backgrounds, making this book a truly international effort. This book will bring forth new frontiers with its revolutionizing research information and detailed analysis of the nascent developments around the world.

We would like to thank all the contributing authors for lending their expertise to make the book truly unique. They have played a crucial role in the development of this book. Without their invaluable contributions this book wouldn't have been possible. They have made vital efforts to compile up to date information on the varied aspects of this subject to make this book a valuable addition to the collection of many professionals and students.

This book was conceptualized with the vision of imparting up-to-date information and advanced data in this field. To ensure the same, a matchless editorial board was set up. Every individual on the board went through rigorous rounds of assessment to prove their worth. After which they invested a large part of their time researching and compiling the most relevant data for our readers.

The editorial board has been involved in producing this book since its inception. They have spent rigorous hours researching and exploring the diverse topics which have resulted in the successful publishing of this book. They have passed on their knowledge of decades through this book. To expedite this challenging task, the publisher supported the team at every step. A small team of assistant editors was also appointed to further simplify the editing procedure and attain best results for the readers.

Apart from the editorial board, the designing team has also invested a significant amount of their time in understanding the subject and creating the most relevant covers. They scrutinized every image to scout for the most suitable representation of the subject and create an appropriate cover for the book.

The publishing team has been an ardent support to the editorial, designing and production team. Their endless efforts to recruit the best for this project, has resulted in the accomplishment of this book. They are a veteran in the field of academics and their pool of knowledge is as vast as their experience in printing. Their expertise and guidance has proved useful at every step. Their uncompromising quality standards have made this book an exceptional effort. Their encouragement from time to time has been an inspiration for everyone.

The publisher and the editorial board hope that this book will prove to be a valuable piece of knowledge for researchers, students, practitioners and scholars across the globe.

List of Contributors

Olivier Nguyen, Lucas Sideris, Marie-Claude Gagnon, Guy Leblanc, Yves E. Leclerc and Pierre Dubé
Department of Surgery, Maisonneuve-Rosemont Hospital, Université de Montréal, 5415 boulevard de l'Assomption, Montr'eal, QC, Canada H1T 2M4

Pierre Drolet
Department of Anesthesiology, Maisonneuve-Rosemont Hospital, Université de Montréal, 5415 boulevard de l'Assomption, Montréal, QC, Canada H1T 2M4

Andrew Mitchell
Department of Pathology, Maisonneuve-Rosemont Hospital, Université de Montréal, 5415 boulevard de l'Assomption, Montréal, QC, Canada H1T 2M4

A. Mirza, S. Pritchard and I. Welch
Departments of Gastrointestinal Surgery and Histopathology, The University Hospital of South Manchester, Southmoor Road,Wythenshawe, Manchester M23 9LT, UK

Jennifer L. Agnew, Benjamin Abbadessa and I. Michael Leitman
Department of Surgery, Albert Einstein College of Medicine, Beth Israel Medical Center, 10 Union Square East, Suite 2M, New York, NY 10003, USA

A. Tsochrinis, D. T. Vassiliadou, E. Efstathiou and J. Spiliotis
1st Department of Surgical Oncology, Metaxa Cancer Hospital, 18537 Piraeus, Greece

E. Halkia
1st Department of Surgical Oncology, Metaxa Cancer Hospital, 18537 Piraeus, Greece
Peritoneal Surface Malignancy Unit, IASO General Hospital, 15562 Athens, Greece

A. Pavlakou
Department of Anesthesiology, Metaxa Cancer Hospital, 18537 Piraeus, Greece

A. Vaxevanidou
Department of Anesthesiology, Gennimatas General Hospital, 54635 Thessaloniki, Greece

A. Datsis
Department of Surgery, General Hospital of Messolonghi, 30200 Messolonghi, Greece

Mona P. Tan
Breast Surgical Oncology, MammoCare, 38 Irrawaddy No. 06-21, Singapore 329563

Nadya Y. Sitoh
MammoCare, 38 Irrawaddy No. 06-21, Singapore 329563

Yih Y. Sitoh
Medical Education, Mount Elizabeth Hospital, 3 Mount Elizabeth No. 17-16, Singapore 228510

Hassan Iqbal, Abu Bakar Hafeez Bhatti and Raza Hussain
Department of Surgical Oncology, Shaukat Khanum Memorial Cancer Hospital and Research Centre, 7A Block R-3,M.A. Johar Town, Lahore, Pakistan

Arif Jamshed
Department of Radiation Oncology, Shaukat Khanum Memorial Cancer Hospital and Research Centre, 7A Block R-3, M.A. Johar Town, Lahore, Pakistan

Mehrzad Namazi
Division of Surgical Oncology, Department of Surgery, Ottawa Hospital,Ottawa, ON, Canada

Angel Arnaout
Division of Surgical Oncology, Department of Surgery, Ottawa Hospital, Ottawa, ON, Canada
CancerTherapeutics Program, Ottawa Hospital Research Institute, Ottawa, ON, Canada

Christina L. Addison
Cancer Therapeutics Program, Ottawa Hospital Research Institute, Ottawa, ON, Canada

Mark Clemons
Cancer Therapeutics Program, Ottawa Hospital Research Institute, Ottawa, ON, Canada
Division of Medical Oncology, Department of Medicine, Ottawa Hospital and Ottawa Hospital Cancer Center, Ottawa, ON, Canada

Susan Robertson
Division of Anatomical Pathology, Ottawa Hospital, Ottawa, ON, Canada

Iryna Kuchuk and Demetrios Simos
Division of Medical Oncology, Department of Medicine, Ottawa Hospital and Ottawa Hospital Cancer Center, Ottawa, ON, Canada

Gregory R. Pond
Department of Oncology, McMaster University, Hamilton, ON, Canada

G. S. Simpson, R. Smith, A. Shekouh, C. McFaul, M. Johnson and D. Vimalachandran
Countess of Chester Hospital NHS Foundation Trust, Countess of Chester Health Park, Liverpool Road, Chester CH2 1UL, UK

P. Sutton
Countess of Chester Hospital NHS Foundation Trust, Countess of Chester Health Park, Liverpool Road, Chester CH2 1UL, UK
University of Liverpool, Liverpool, Merseyside L69 3BX, UK

Anthony Kodzo-Grey Venyo
North Manchester General Hospital, Department of Urology, Manchester, UK

Pier Federico Salvi, Laura Lorenzon, Salvatore Caterino, Laura Antolino, Maria Serena Antonelli and Genoveffa Balducci
Surgical and Medical Department of Translational Medicine, Sant'Andrea Hospital, Faculty of Medicine and Psychology, University of Rome La Sapienza, St. Andrea Hospital, Via di Grottarossa 1035-39, 00189 Rome, Italy

M. Re
Department of Otorhinolaryngology, Marche Polytechnic University, 60121 Ancona, Italy

A. Santarelli, M. Mascitti and F. Bambini
Department of Clinical Specialistic and Dental Sciences, Marche Polytechnic University, 60121 Ancona, Italy

L. Lo Muzio
Department of Sperimental and Clinical Medicine, University of Foggia, 71121 Foggia, Italy

A. Zizzi and C. Rubini
Department of Neurosciences, Marche Polytechnic University, 60121 Ancona, Italy

F. Corsi, L. Sorrentino, D. Bossi, A. Sartani and D. Foschi
Surgery Division, Department of Clinical Sciences, L. Sacco Hospital, University of Milan, Via G.B. Grassi 74, 20157 Milan, Italy

Preya Ananthakrishnan and Fatih Levent Balci
Breast Surgery Division, Department of Surgery, Columbia University College of Physicians and Surgeons, New York, NY 10032, USA

Joseph P. Crowe
Department of General Surgery, Cleveland Clinic Foundation, Cleveland, OH 44195, USA

J. R. Reddy, R. Saxena, R. K. Singh, B. Pottakkat, A. Prakash, A. Behari, A. K. Gupta and V. K. Kapoor
Department of Surgical Gastroenterology, Sanjay Gandhi Postgraduate Institute of Medical Sciences (SGPGIMS), Rae Bareily Road, Lucknow 226014, India

Mohammed Badruddoja
Department of Surgical Oncology, Rehabilitation Associates of Northern Illinois, Rockford, IL 61111, USA

S. Quadrelli, G. Lyons, D. Chimondeguy and A. Buero
Thoracic Oncology Centre, Buenos Aires British Hospital, Perdriel 74, C1280AEB Buenos Aires, Argentina

H. Colt
University of California, Irvine, CA 92697, USA

Melina Shoni
Department of Obstetrics and Gynecology, Division of Gynecologic Oncology, Brigham andWomen's Hospital, HarvardMedical School, Boston, MA 02115,USA

Taymaa May and Michael G. Muto
Division of Gynecologic Oncology, Dana-Farber Cancer Institute, Boston, MA 02115, USA

Allison F. Vitonis
Department of Obstetrics and Gynecology, Epidemiology Center, Brigham and Women's Hospital, Boston, MA 02115, USA

Charles M. Quick
Department of Pathology, University of Arkansas for Medical Sciences, Little Rock, AR 72205, USA

Whitfield B. Growdon
Department of Obstetrics and Gynecology, Division of Gynecologic Oncology, Massachusetts General Hospital, Harvard Medical School, Boston, MA 02214, USA

Dimitrios Zacharoulis
Department of Surgery, University Hospital of Larissa, Mezourlo, 41110 Larissa, Greece

Konstantinos Perivoliotis
Department of Surgery, University Hospital of Larissa, Mezourlo, 41110 Larissa, Greece

Postgraduate   Programme   (MSc):   Research
Methodology in Biomedicine, Biostatistics and Clinical
Bioinformatics, University of Thessaly, Larissa, Greece

Eleni Sioka
Postgraduate   Programme   (MSc):   Research
Methodology in Biomedicine, Biostatistics and Clinical
Bioinformatics, University of Thessaly, Larissa, Greece

Athina Tatsioni
Postgraduate   Programme   (MSc):   Research
Methodology in Biomedicine, Biostatistics and Clinical
Bioinformatics, University of Thessaly, Larissa, Greece
Research Unit for General Medicine and Primary
Health Care, Faculty of Medicine, School for Health
Sciences, University of Ioannina, Ioannina, Greece
Tufts University School of Medicine, Boston, MA, USA

Ioannis Stefanidis
Postgraduate   Programme   (MSc):   Research
Methodology in Biomedicine, Biostatistics and Clinical
Bioinformatics, University of Thessaly, Larissa, Greece
Department of Nephrology, Medical School, University
of Thessaly, Larissa, Greece

Elias Zintzaras
Postgraduate   Programme   (MSc):   Research
Methodology in Biomedicine, Biostatistics and Clinical
Bioinformatics, University of Thessaly, Larissa, Greece
Department of Biomathematics, University of Thessaly
School of Medicine, Larissa, Greece

Giulia Montori
General Surgery Department, Spedali Civili, Chirurgia
Generale 3, Piazzale Spedali Civili, 25121 Brescia, Italy

**Federico Coccolini, Marco Ceresoli, Nicola Colaianni,
Eugenio Poletti and Luca Ansaloni**
General Surgery Department, Papa Giovanni XXIII
Hospital, 42121 Bergamo, Italy

Fausto Catena
Emergency Surgery Department, Ospedale Maggiore,
43121 Parma, Italy

**Jia Lin Ng, Claramae Shulyn Chia, Grace Hwei Ching
Tan, Khee-Chee Soo and Melissa Ching Ching Teo**
Department of Surgical Oncology, National Cancer
Centre Singapore, 11 Hospital Drive, Singapore 169610

Whee Sze Ong
Division of Clinical Trials and Epidemiological Sciences,
National Cancer Centre Singapore, 11 Hospital Drive,
Singapore 169610

Anthony Kodzo-Grey Venyo
North Manchester General Hospital Department of
Urology, Delaunay's Road, Manchester, UK

L. Barr
Nightingale and Genesis Prevention Centre, University
Hospital   South   Manchester,   Southmoor   Road,
Manchester M23 9LT, UK

N. N. Basu
Nightingale and Genesis Prevention Centre, University
Hospital   South   Manchester,   Southmoor   Road,
Manchester M23 9LT, UK
Department of Breast Surgery, Queen Elizabeth
Hospital, Birmingham B15 2TH, UK

D. G. Evans
Nightingale and Genesis Prevention Centre, University
Hospital   South   Manchester,   Southmoor   Road,
Manchester M23 9LT, UK
University of Manchester Department of Genomic
Medicine, Institute of Human Development, St. Mary's
Hospital, Oxford Road, Manchester M13 9WL, UK

G. L. Ross
The Institute of Cancer Sciences, The University of
Manchester, Oxford Road, Manchester M13 9PL, UK

**Francesco Muratori, Leonardo Bettini, Filippo
Frenos, Nicola Mondanelli, Maurizio Scorianz and
Domenico Campanacci**
Divisione di Ortopedia Oncologica e Ricostruttiva
Ospedale, Azienda Universitaria Ospedaliera Careggi
Firenze, Firenze, Italy

Daniela Greto and Lorenzo Livi
Dipartimento di Radioterapia Azienda Ospedaliera
Universitaria Careggi, Firenze, Italy

Rodolfo Capanna and Alessandro Franchi
Dipartimento di Ricerca Traslazionale e delle Nuove
Tecnologie in Medicina e Chirurgia, Universit`a di
Pisa, Pisa, Italy

Giuliana Roselli
Divisione di Radiologia Ospedale, Azienda Universitaria
Ospedaliera Careggi Firenze, Firenze, Italy

**Evgeni Brotfain, Leonid Koyfman, Dmitry Frank,
Yoav Bichovsky and Moti Klein**
Department of Anesthesiology and Critical Care,
General   Intensive   CareUnit,   Soroka   Medical
Center,Ben-Gurion University of the Negev, Beer
Sheva, Israel

Gilbert Sebbag
Department of General Surgery B, Soroka Medical Center, Ben-Gurion University of the Negev, Beer Sheva, Israel

Michael Friger
Department of Public Health, Faculty of Health Sciences, Ben-Gurion University of the Negev, Beer Sheva, Israel

Boris Kirshtein
Department of General Surgery A, Soroka Medical Center, Ben-Gurion University of the Negev, Beer Sheva, Israel

Abraham Borer
Department of Infectious Disease, Soroka Medical Center, Ben-Gurion University of the Negev, Beer Sheva, Israel

Jochanan G. Peiser
Department of Medical Management, Soroka Medical Center, Ben-Gurion University of the Negev, Beer Sheva, Israel

Harsh Kanhere , Markus Trochsler and Guy Maddern
University of Adelaide Discipline of Surgery, The Queen Elizabeth Hospital,Woodville, Adelaide, SA, Australia

Raghav Goel and Ben Finlay
Division of Surgery, The Queen Elizabeth Hospital, Woodville, Adelaide, SA, Australia

Brian Shrager, Ghalib A. Jibara, Parissa Tabrizian and Sasan Roayaie
Division of Surgical Oncology, Department of Surgery, Mount Sinai School of Medicine, One Gustave Levy Place, New York, NY 10029, USA

Stephen C. Ward
Department of Pathology, Mount Sinai School of Medicine, 1468 Madison Avenue, Annenberg Building, 15th Floor, Room 92, New York, NY 10029, USA

Jianyi Li, Yang Zhang, Wenhai Zhang, Shi Jia, Rui Tian and Ye Kang
Department of Breast Surgery, Shengjing Hospital of China Medical University, Shenyang, Liaoning 110004, China

Yan Ma
Ultrasound Diagnosis Center, Shengjing Hospital of China Medical University, Shenyang, Liaoning 110004, China

Dan Li
Pathological Diagnosis Center, Shengjing Hospital of China Medical University, Shenyang, Liaoning 110004, China

Mariane Campagnari, Eduard R. Brechtbühl, Eduardo Bertolli and João P. Duprat Neto
Skin Cancer Department, AC Camargo Cancer Center, São Paulo, SP, Brazil

Andrea S. Jafelicci and Helio A. Carneiro
Surgical Oncology, AC Camargo Cancer Center, São Paulo, SP, Brazil

W. L. Lodder
Department of Head and Neck Oncology and Surgery, The Netherlands Cancer Institute-Antoni van Leeuwenhoek Hospital, Amsterdam, The Netherlands Department of Otorhinolaryngology/Head and Neck Surgery, The University Medical Center Groningen, University of Groningen, 9700 RB Groningen,The Netherlands

A. J. M. Balm
Department of Head and Neck Oncology and Surgery, The Netherlands Cancer Institute-Antoni van Leeuwenhoek Hospital, Amsterdam, The Netherlands Department of Otorhinolaryngology, Academic Medical Centre, University of Amsterdam, Amsterdam, The Netherlands

M. W. M. van den Brekel
Department of Head and Neck Oncology and Surgery, The Netherlands Cancer Institute-Antoni van Leeuwenhoek Hospital, Amsterdam, The Netherlands Department of Otorhinolaryngology, Academic Medical Centre, University of Amsterdam, Amsterdam, The Netherlands Institute of Phonetic Sciences, ACLC, University of Amsterdam, Amsterdam, The Netherlands

C. A. H. Lange and H. J. Teertstra
Department of Radiology, The Netherlands Cancer Institute-Antoni van Leeuwenhoek Hospital, Amsterdam, The Netherlands

F. A. Pameijer
Department of Radiology, University Medical Centre Utrecht, Utrecht, The Netherlands

Michelle Milee Chang, Jeffrey Ascherman and Christine Rohde
Division of Plastic Surgery, Columbia University Medical Center, New York-Presbyterian Hospital, New York, NY 10032, USA

Tara Huston
Plastic and Reconstructive Surgery Division, Stony Brook Medicine, Stony Brook, NY 11794, USA

Vijay M. Patil, Amit Joshi, Vanita Noronha, Vibhor Sharma, Saurabh Zanwar, Sachin Dhumal and Kumar Prabhash
Department of Medical Oncology, Tata Memorial Hospital, Mumbai, India

Shubhada Kane
Department of Pathology, Tata Memorial Hospital, Mumbai, India

Prathamesh Pai, Anil D'Cruz and Pankaj Chaturvedi
Department of Surgical oncology, Tata Memorial Hospital, Mumbai, India

Atanu Bhattacharjee
Division of Clinical Research and Biostatistics, Malabar Cancer Centre, Kerala, India

Index

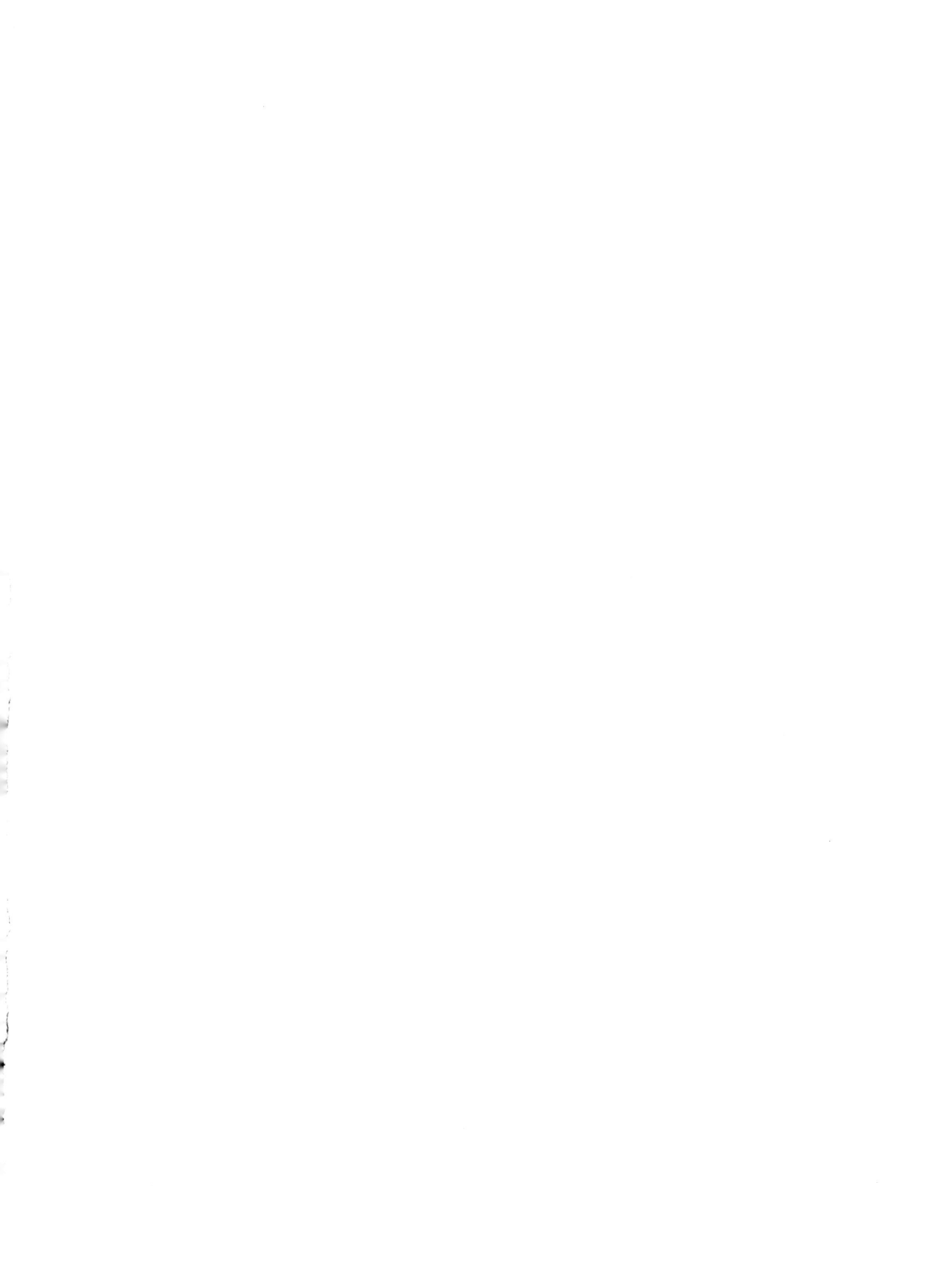